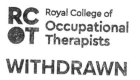

Rehabilitation of the Physically Disabled Adult

Rehabilitation of the Physically Disabled Adult

Edited by

C. JOHN GOODWILL

Consultant Rheumatologist and Consultant in Rehabilitation Medicine
Formerly at King's College Hospital, London, UK

M. ANNE CHAMBERLAIN

Professor of Rehabilitation Medicine, University of Leeds
Director of the Rehabilitation Unit of the Leeds Teaching Hospitals Trust, Leeds, UK

CHRIS EVANS

Formerly Consultant in Rehabilitation Medicine, Royal Cornwall Hospitals Trust, Cornwall, UK

Stanley Thornes (Publishers) Ltd

First edition published 1988 by Chapman and Hall
ISBN 0-412-49060-9

Second edition published 1997 by:
Stanley Thornes (Publishers) Ltd
Ellenborough House
Wellington Street
CHELTENHAM
GL50 1YW
United Kingdom

97 98 99 00 01 / 10 9 8 7 6 5 4 3 2 1

A catalogue record for this book is available from the British Library

ISBN 0-7487-3183-0

Typeset in 10/12pt Palatino by Acorn Bookwork, Salisbury
Printed and bound in Great Britain by Scotprint, Musselburgh

Contents

Part Two: Musculoskeletal Disability

Part Three: Energy-restricting Disability

Part Four: Sensory and Communication Disability

Part Five: Neurological Disability

Contributors

E.M. Badley
The Arthritis and Community Research
and Evaluation Unit
Wellesley Hospital Research Institute,
Wellesley Hospital, Toronto, Ontario, Canada

A.M.O. Bakheit
Senior lecturer and Consultant
Rehabilitation Research Unit
Southampton General Hospital
Southampton, UK

B. Bhakta
Senior Lecturer
Rheumatology and Rehabilitation Research
Unit
School of Medicine
University of Leeds
Leeds, UK

R. Birch
Orthopaedic Surgeon
Peripheral Nerve Injury Unit
Royal National Orthopaedic Hospital
Stanmore,
Middlesex, UK

E. Bower
Senior Research Fellow
Rehabilitation Research Unit
University of Southampton
Southampton, UK

A. Buller
Orthoptist
Ophthalmic Department
City Hospital
Truro, UK

E.G. Cantrell
Consultant and Senior Lecturer
Rehabilitation Research Unit
Southampton General Hospital
Southampton, UK

S. Casley
Practice Development Unit Leader
Department of Medicine
Seacroft Hospital
Leeds, UK

M. Anne Chamberlain
Charterhouse Professor of Rehabilitation
Rheumatology and Rehabilitation Research
Unit
School of Medicine
University of Leeds
Leeds, UK

R.L. Coakes
Consultant Ophthalmic Surgeon
Kings College Hospital
London, UK

A.K. Coughlan
Consultant Clinical Psychologist
St James' University Hospital
Leeds, UK

J.A. Cozens
Consultant in Rehabilitation Medicine
Grampian Healthcare Trust
Woodend Hospital
Aberdeen, UK

P. Crawford
Consultant Neurologist
Department of Neurosciences
York District Hospital
York, UK

P. Eames
Consultant Neuropsychiatrist
Grafton Manor Brain Injury Rehabilitation
Unit
Grafton Regis
Northamptonshire, UK

P. Enderby
Professor of Community Rehabilitation
Community Sciences Centre
University of Sheffield
Sheffield, UK

C.D. Evans
Former Consultant in Rehabilitation Medicine
Royal Cornwall Hospitals Trust
Cornwall, UK

E. Evans
Social Worker
Cornwall Stroke and Rehabilitation Unit
City Hospital
Truro
Cornwall, UK

J. Fisher
Senior Physiotherapist
Rehabilitation Unit
Chapel Allerton Hospital
Leeds, UK

J. Gaylor
Proof-reader
Penzance
Cornwall, UK

L. Gerber
Chief, Rehabilitation Medicine Department
National Institutes of Health
Bethesda
Maryland, USA

J. Goodwill
Consultant in Rheumatology and
Rehabilitation
Sloane Hospital
Beckenham
Kent, UK

C. Green
Assistant Clinical Neuropsychologist
Cornwall Stroke and Rehabilitation Unit
Truro
Cornwall, UK

A.R. Harvey
Consultant Rheumatologist
Pontefract General Infirmary
Pontefract, UK

P. Helliwell
Senior Lecturer in Rheumatology
Rheumatology and Rehabilitation Research
Unit
School of Medicine
University of Leeds
Leeds, UK

H. Henderson
Consultant in Plastic Surgery
The Leicester Royal Infirmary
Leicester, UK

R. Langton Hewer
Professor of Neurology
Department of Social Medicine
University of Bristol
Bristol, UK

P.N. Hirschmann
Consultant Dental Surgeon
Leeds Dental Institute
Leeds, UK

J. Hunter
Consultant in Rehabilitation Medicine
Rehabilitation Medicine Unit
Astley Ainslie Hospital
Edinburgh, UK

G. Jackson
Consultant Cardiologist
Guys Hospital
London, UK

M. Jackson
15 Highwood Grove
Leeds 17
(Formerly Superintendent Physiotherapist,
The General Infirmary at Leeds)

P. Jay
Occupational Therapist
London, UK

S. Kahtan
Rehabilitation Compensation Advisor
London, UK

M. Lord
Senior Lecturer
Department of Medical Engineering and
Physics
King's College
London, UK

R. Luff
Consultant in Rehabilitation Medicine
Disablement Services Centre
King's College Hospital
London, UK

J. Malone-Lee
Professor of Geriatric Medicine
University College London Medical School
St Pancras Hospital
London, UK

L. Marks
Consultant in Rehabilitation Medicine
Royal National Orthopaedic Hospital
Stanmore
Middlesex, UK

W. El Masry
Consultant in Spinal Injuries and Senior
Lecturer, Keele University; Director
Midlands Centre for Spinal Injuries
Oswestry
Shropshire, UK

J. McCarthy
Vice President
St Loye's College Foundation
Exeter
Devon, UK

E. McClemont
Consultant in Rehabilitation Medicine
Ashby Rehabilitation Centre
Lincoln, UK

L. McLellan
Europe Professor of Rehabilitation
Rehabilitation Research Unit
University of Southampton
Southampton, UK

J. McMullan
General Practitioner
Amersham
Buckinghamshire, UK

S. Middleton LLB
Solicitor
Truro
Cornwall, UK

G.A. Morgan
Consultant Anaesthetist
Royal Cornwall Hospitals Trust
Treliske Hospital
Truro, Cornwall

T. Morley
Consultant in Orthopaedic Surgery
Royal National Orthopaedic Hospital
Stanmore
Middlesex, UK

J. Moxham
Professor of Respiratory Medicine
Department of Respiratory Medicine
King's College Hospital
London, UK

C. Murray-Leslie
Consultant in Rehabilitation Medicine
Derbyshire Royal Infirmary
Derby, UK

S. Peters
Occupational Therapist
Hampshire County Council
Southampton, UK

J. Phillips
District Advisor in Tissue Viability
Lincoln District Healthcare Trust
Lincoln, UK

F.T. Ponton
Senior Orthotist
Nuffield Orthotics and Rehabilitation
Engineering
Nuffield Orthopaedic Centre NHS Trust
Oxford, UK

R. Potter
Head of Clinical Engineering
Department of Medical Physics and
Engineering
Community Rehabilitation Centre
Lincoln, UK

M.J. Powers QC
One Paper Buildings
Temple
London, UK

M. Roberts
Consultant in Rehabilitation Medicine
City General Hospital
Carlisle, UK

M. Sansom
Team Leader
Marie Therese House
St Michael's Hospital
Cornwall, UK

J. Shindler
General Practitioner
Thornton Heath
Surrey, UK

P.E.M. Smith
Consultant Neurologist
University Hospital of Wales
Cardiff, UK

L.H. De Souza
Professor of Physiotherapy
Dept of Health Studies
Brunel University College
Middlesex, UK

S.D.G. Stephens
Consultant in Audiological Medicine
Welsh Hearing Institute
University Hospital of Wales
Cardiff, UK

A.M. Stewart
Neurology Counsellor
Dept of Neurosciences
York District Hospital
York, UK

F. Struthers
Orthoptist
Ophthalmic Department
City Hospital
Truro
Cornwall, UK

C. Tarling
Patient Handling Adviser and Care Manager
(Occupational Therapist)
Social Services Department
Durham County Council
Durham, UK

A. Tennant
Charterhouse Principal Research Fellow
Rheumatology and Rehabilitation Research
Unit
School of Medicine
University of Leeds
Leeds, UK

C. Turton
Regional Director
Habinteg Housing Association Ltd
London, UK

A. Tyerman
Consultant Clinical Psychologist
Community Head Injury Services
Aylesbury,
Buckinghamshire, UK

D.T. Wade
Consultant in Neurological Disability
Rivermead Rehabilitation Centre
Oxford, UK

A.E. Ward
Consultant/Senior Lecturer in Rehabilitation
Medicine
North Staffordshire Rehabilitation Centre
Stoke-on-Trent, UK

A. Wasti
Senior Registrar
Rheumatology and Rehabilitation Research
Unit
School of Medicine
University of Leeds
Leeds, UK

M. Winchcombe
Senior Project Officer
The Disabled Living Centres Council
London, UK

C. Wisdom
Formerly Art Therapist
Cornwall Stroke and Rehabilitation Unit
City Hospital
Truro

Preface to the second edition

The first edition of this book was produced in the hope that it would help professionals in many fields through the complexities of bringing good care and rehabilitation to those who sought their help. The evidence is that it has done so and become an important source of information.

There have been many changes since 1988. There is better recognition of the potential of those with disability, information about services is more easily available, and expectations are higher. Care in the Community has been introduced, and there has been anti-discrimination legislation on both sides of the Atlantic designed to help those with disability. At the same time as there is pressure to spend less within Health and Social Services, new technologies are providing exciting possibilities for people with disabilities to achieve greater independence. Distance learning, working from home, using the Internet for communication and exchanging information will soon become routine. The opposing forces of the need for economy and the wealth of new possibilities, make it imperative we can give the best advice to encourage and support independence.

This edition of the book will reflect these trends, and offers a wide range of techniques for rehabilitation and a great deal of factual information about services, and how they may be found.

John Goodwill
Anne Chamberlain
Chris Evans

Acknowledgements

Our grateful thanks are expressed to all who have written so ably for us, some at very short notice, to those who have commented on contributions and to those who have helped in many other ways.

In Leeds we particularly wish to thank Mrs J. Packter who, together with Mrs B. Glossop, word-processed large amounts of text. Thanks also go the Senior Registrars in Rehabilitation Medicine, who not only wrote, but also bore some of the service commitments of MAC when the pressures of the book were particularly heavy. MAC dedicates this, the second edition, to David, whose love has made so much possible.

In London our particular thanks go to Mrs B. O'Sullivan and Dr Steve Novak, Senior Registrar in Rehabilitation Medicine, who kindly helped and advised, also at short notice.

Down in Truro, Michelle and Helen dealt with great enthusiasm and good humour with the information which arrived by letter, fax, e-mail and disks in an amazing quantity. The outpourings of the many different word processors were eventually translated into a common language! Thanks also to Pam Kitch, the librarian at the Post Graduate Medical Centre in Treliske Hospital for her support and hard work on the references. Dr Liz Winterton very kindly checked the telephone numbers in Chapter 55.

The authors of the first edition would like to record their appreciation of the Truro Team and of Chris Evans' expertise with the computer, which has produced a single text out of the massive amount of contributions.

We are grateful to Mr J. Rowley for his original design for the cover of our book. We also thank Bill Thornton who let us use his picture. When it was taken he had just covered 1000 miles from Paris to Compostela in a fund-raising bid.

Finally, we would like to thank our long-suffering families who have tolerated the intrusion into our homes of the writing and editing of this textbook. Their hospitality, catering skills and encouragement have been essential in the production of the book.

Note

Addresses and telephone numbers in Chapter 55 and elsewhere were checked for accuracy at the time of going to press. We apologize for any inconvenience caused if they subsequently change.

PART ONE

REHABILITATION: SETTING THE SCENE

1 Introduction: the aims of rehabilitation

M.A. Chamberlain

Disability limits choice: rehabilitation restores choice to the individual. Medicine has not always concerned itself with dramatic cures: it is not so long ago that physicians were unable to intervene in conditions such as lobar pneumonia that now seem routine. They had to watch and hope that the patient weathered the crisis. Not until the 1930s and 1940s could such situations be averted with any regularity. Modern medicine continues to change rapidly. Health services in the last quarter of the twentieth century are concerned with diseases and operations that differ greatly from those prevalent at their inception. Then there was much infectious disease, including tuberculosis, high maternal and child mortality and the management of arthritis had barely begun. There was no provision for younger patients who were chronically ill; dependency from osteoarthritis of the hip could not be relieved by arthroplasty, nor angina by coronary artery bypass. Rheumatic heart disease caused much morbidity; polio was feared for its ability to kill and maim the young.

A different picture has now emerged: tuberculosis is largely curable (though pockets of it are re-emerging, often associated with social deprivation) and many older infectious diseases are curable or less virulent. AIDS presents us with sad and dramatic new fears. The management of arthritis is much improved, and even since the first edition of this book, there have been changes. The problems associated with severe spina bifida are rarely seen in those below their mid-twenties, and phocomelia is mostly confined to a cohort chronologically just ahead of this. Most small-for-date babies survive with a good prognosis but, unfortunately, some have severe disabilities that will persist when they are adults. Cerebral palsy (CP) is not becoming rarer worldwide and most of those with it do not have access to sophisticated surgery, either in childhood or young adulthood. The high usage of roads and technical abilities of intensive care mean that, worldwide, people survive road accidents but have a reduced quality of life; their demands on services are high. Although lifespan is increasing, evidence shows that so is the length of time a person can expect to be disabled. There is much to be done.

The caring tradition is old. The first evidence that early humans exhibited compassion is some 600 000 years old, and comes from Northern Iraq. There, the bones of an old man with severe arthritic changes and a congenital abnormality that would have rendered his right arm useless, lie beside those of another with recent injury. Both these and five other skeletons are surrounded by

Rehabilitation of the Physically Disabled Adult. Edited by C. John Goodwill, M. Anne Chamberlain and Chris Evans. Published in 1997 by Stanley Thornes (Publishers) Ltd, Cheltenham. ISBN 0-7487-3183-0.

pollen, showing that floral tributes had been paid to the dead (Passmore, 1979). Sometimes admirable traditions become insidiously inappropriate. The wheelchair and limb fitting centres of the UK were designed for young fit veterans of the First World War, not for elderly arteriopaths who mostly use them now. The McColl Report (McColl, 1986) suggested that changes were required. These are now in place.

Rehabilitation is about more than caring. It is interventionist, aiming to maximize the person's abilities in all spheres, physical, intellectual and social. The World Health Organization definition, which is widely accepted, includes '. . . all means aimed at reducing the impact of disabling and handicapping conditions and at enabling disabled people to achieve optimal social integration'. There is an alternative definition: 'freedom to make decisions regarding the way of life best suited to an individual disabled person's circumstances' (Prince of Wales Advisory Group on Disabilities, 1985). It will be increasingly appropriate to remember this definition as people with disabilities press for their civil rights.

These definitions are important: they encourage us to use all means, medical, social and technological, to give patients a better lifestyle. Most wish to be as independent as possible, exercise control over their own lives and to be involved in decisions about their lives and those of their families. In the future patients may hold copies of their notes. Rehabilitation should help the acquisition and preservation of peoples' roles within society. It should also reduce the burden of dependency on patient, carer, social services and health services.

How may this be done? When the first edition of this book was being prepared, rehabilitation in the UK was just emerging as a defined specialty. Its academic base was very small. Over the next decade there were considerable changes: the specialty is now recognized, its function is clearly defined and

Table 1.1 Facilities required in a comprehensive rehabilitation service

Communication aids
Continence care
Disabled living centre
Driving assessment
Environmental controls
Equipment loan centre
Head injury services
Hearing impairment services
Housing and housing modification
Orthotics
Prosthetics
Rehabilitation engineering
Services for young adults with physical disabilities (transition services and full range for 16–64 years)
Sexual counselling
Stoma care
Tissue viability
Visual impairment services
Vocational assessment
Wheelchairs and seating

its academic base has been enlarged. The framework for comprehensive provision has been laid out in the Royal College of Physicians Report *Physical Disability in 1986 and Beyond* (Royal College of Physicians, 1988). This points to the need for a range of services, some local, and some at regional level which will provide the professional help and technology needed. Table 1.1 represents an up-to-date version of the recommendations.

Effective organization of services is essential. People with complex cognitive and physical disabilities will require this range of services at various times, and need clear access points to them. Some conditions, like traumatic brain injury, start from a catastrophic event and will require various responses from clinical teams, which may be delivered in different places as the patient progresses from acute hospital to the community. Not all patients will need all the services in Table 1.2, but the services need to be accessible when they are needed.

Table 1.2 Head injury services – a model for services for disability which is complex and has catastrophic onset

Phase 1	Acute (hospital) care
Phase 2	Intensive, inpatient rehabilitation focused and multidisciplinary
Phase 3	Community rehabilitation Specialist community team Community resources (often with LA or voluntary organization) Training/education and work introduction
Phase 4	Care, respite Access to intermittent assessment, rehabilitation

Also primary and secondary prevention, reduction of risk

Those who have fluctuating or declining conditions will depend on rehabilitation services to maintain function and independence as long as possible. This is a most important part of rehabilitation, which is too often forgotten with consequent unnecessary dependency and much misery.

Profound changes are taking place in the organization of health services in many parts of the world. Within an increasingly knowledge-based culture, those who pay for services will ask what evidence exists about the value of rehabilitation. We have yet to provide all the answers (the specialty is not alone in this). Some answers have been found, some await better definition of outcome measures; others will be more difficult if it is not recognized that outcome includes patient's wishes and expectations. Questions have to be asked about the value patients and families place on our services. Cost-effectiveness studies are needed, and in the equation the long-term benefits of rehabilitation, which are substantial, must be included. Many benefits will be outside the field of health, in housing, employment and social integration.

The necessity for rehabilitation in the presence of new or deteriorating complex physical disabilities is now undisputed, but the size of the problem is only beginning to be recognized. Rehabilitation has the potential for helping many people, of all ages, both in the developing and industrialized parts of the world.

Populations are ageing, and where censuses have been done it has been shown that the prevalence of disability increases sharply with age. The UK figure of one in eight having some disability (Martin and White, 1988) may not be very different in other countries at different stages of development. However, the causes of disability and desired outcomes of rehabilitation will be different, partly because rehabilitation is a culture-based specialty.

Hospitals are far from user-friendly to people with disabilities. However, the Royal College of Physicians of London with the Prince of Wales Advisory Group on Disability (1992) have published a charter and checklist to encourage audit of suitable facilities.

The best available technology should be used, as should the resources of the local community. Family members can be taught much and will be keen to help. In richer countries the trend to professionalization should be resisted if it leads to an unwillingness to teach families and share skills, as the professionals treating the patient can never be available on a one-to-one basis. There will always be a greater need for practical help than can be provided by the health and social services. We should regard ourselves as teachers, researchers and advisers and, to be effective, the best teaching methods available need to be used (Figure 1.1).

The move towards community rehabilitation is welcome. This does not mean that the patient's home should be invaded by an army of uncoordinated workers, nor that community teams should not have a base. The acute hospital or rehabilitation unit will often provide intensive coordinated rehabilitation programmes for short periods after trauma or

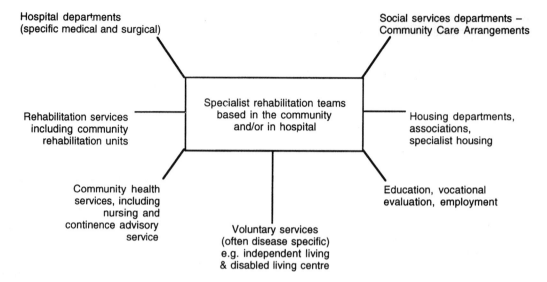

Figure 1.1 Relationship between specialist community outreach teams and other services.

acute illness. It should be viewed as a resource of expertise, teaching and research. Often, expensive and developing technologies will have to be concentrated there to be effective. There, as in the community, new methods and treatments have to be tried.

It is hoped that this book will not only give a clear picture of standard treatments, but also present new ways of thinking about old problems. Also, it is anticipated that the book will continue to be of use to a wide variety of people in health, social services and voluntary organizations. Readers' comments are welcomed.

REFERENCES

McColl, I. (1986) *Review of Artificial Limb and Appliance Service Centres*, DHSS, London.

Martin, J. & White, A. (1988) *The Prevalence of Disability among Adults*. OPCS Surveys of Disability Report 1, OPCS Social Survey Division, HMSO, London.

Passmore, R. (1979) The declaration of Alma-Ata and the future of primary care. *Lancet*, ii, 1005–8.

Prince of Wales Advisory Group on Disability (1985) *Living Options: guidelines for those planning services for people with severe physical disabilities*, Prince of Wales Advisory Group on Disability, London.

Royal College of Physicians (1986) Physical disability in 1986 and beyond. *Journal of the Royal College of Physicians*, **20**, 3–37.

Royal College of Physicians of London and Prince of Wales Advisory Group on Disability (1992) *A Charter for Disabled People Using Hospitals*. Royal College of Physicians, London.

2 Epidemiology

E.M. Badley and A. Tennant

INTRODUCTION

Epidemiology is the study of the patterns of disease occurrence in the population and the factors that influence these patterns (Lilienfeld and Lilienfeld, 1980). An epidemiological perspective on disablement can help clinicians in various ways. Disablement describes the consequences of a disease, disorder or injury on three planes, impairment, disability and handicap, following the World Health Organization's (WHO) *International Classification of Impairments, Disabilities, and Handicaps* (ICIDH) (WHO, 1980). Information on the frequency and characteristics of conditions which give rise to disablement provides the background for diagnostic assessment. Knowledge of the natural history and outcome enlightens management and guides development of prognosis. Clinicians are also concerned to secure the resources needed to assist individuals with disabilities, a group that has generally not fared well in obtaining an equitable share of medical services and technology, or of social welfare provisions. This moves into the field of policy and planning. Different types of information are needed for these various purposes. This chapter will try to cover these different aspects, so far as available data allow.

A series of questions need to be considered:

1. *Why is an appraisal being undertaken?* If the emphasis is to be placed on understanding the origins of disablement, then the clinical picture has to be completed by information on the occurrence of mild as well as severe disablement. On the other hand, if the concern is with the outcomes or consequences of illness and their amelioration, i.e. with the service needs of disabled individuals, only those with degrees of severity requiring special services have to be taken into account.

2. *Who is disabled?* This question may be answered by documenting the characteristics of affected individuals in terms such as age, sex and ethnicity. If only particular subgroups of the population are affected, this may shed light on the origins of the problem, and such findings will also indicate vulnerable subgroups on whom attention may be preferentially focused (such as by screening).

3. *How are people affected?* This calls for measurement of the extent of the severity of the problem, of the needs that ensue and of associated phenomena – including the consequences of various actions by physicians and other health professionals and the responses by people with disabilities to their own circumstances.

4. *Where are the affected people?* Identifying the situations in which disablement is encountered might reveal geographical variations, for example, which in turn could draw attention to influences on

Rehabilitation of the Physically Disabled Adult. Edited by C. John Goodwill, M. Anne Chamberlain and Chris Evans.
Published in 1997 by Stanley Thornes (Publishers) Ltd, Cheltenham. ISBN 0-7487-3183-0.

expression of the problem, while more localized variations may indicate the role of the environment in determining handicap.

5. *When does the problem get recognized?* This calls for review of trends in variation of disability-related phenomena, as well as considering the sensitivity of their detection at various levels of health or social services organization.

6. *What is the impact of disablement?* In other words, quantification of the size of the problem, which establishes its scale and is helpful when trying to resolve conflicts in priorities.

INFORMATION ON DISABLEMENT IN THE POPULATION

The prevalence of disablement and its impact upon the population needs to be established. This has been done for some countries, mostly by national population surveys. This chapter will refer mainly to data from two surveys, the 1986 Office of Population Censuses and Surveys (OPCS) surveys of disability in Great Britain (Martin, Meltzer and Elliot, 1988) and the 1986 Canadian Health and Activity Limitation Survey (HALS) (Statistics Canada, 1989).

The UK data are drawn from two surveys addressing disability in adults living in private households and in institutions. For those living in private households 100 000 addresses were selected and a screening questionnaire was sent by post to 80% of these (Martin, Meltzer and Elliot, 1988). In the remaining 20%, who were mostly in inner urban areas, screening questions were completed by interview. This led to approximately 18 000 adults being approached for interview, together with a further 3533 adults living in institutions. The survey identified 13 types of disability based on the ICIDH scheme. Severity of disability was determined by a complex model of comparative judgements made by teams of professionals, dis-

abled people and their carers (Martin, Meltzer and Elliot, 1988). A weighting system was designed to provide an overall severity grade, ranging from 1 (least severe) to 10 (most severe).

The Canadian HALS used a similar methodology. The target population was all persons with physical or psychological disabilities aged 15 years and older who were living in private households in Canada at the time of the 1986 Canadian Census (Statistics Canada, 1989). An additional segment of the survey covered individuals living in health-related institutions. The first stage comprised a question in the 1986 census to identify individuals with any activity limitation. In the second stage a sample of individuals was seen for a detailed face-to-face interview. In all, 132 337 people aged 16 years and older were covered by the survey. Those with disability include those responding affirmatively to: (a) a non-specific activity limitation question referring to restriction in the kind or amount of activity lasting, or expected to last, 6 months or more, and (b) any of 18 activity-specific questions (based on OECD disability indicators) (McWinney, 1982). Severity of disability is a variable derived by Statistics Canada which is an overall weighted score of activity restriction and disability in specific activities.

PREVALENCE OF DISABLEMENT IN THE POPULATION

THE 1986 UK national survey found that the prevalence of disability among adults was 135 per 1000 population aged 16 years and over and 142 per 1000 including those living in institutions (Martin, Meltzer and Elliot, 1988). These estimates are very similar to the 132 per 1000 (including those living in institutions) in the population aged 15 years and over found in the 1986 HALS (Statistics Canada, 1990).

Age-specific estimates for 13 different types of disability in the UK survey are given in Table 2.1. The prevalence increases with age

Table 2.1 Estimates of prevalence of disability in Great Britain by type of disability and age for the total population, including those in establishments: expressed as rates per 1000 population (physical disability types are in bold). (Source: Martin, Meltzer and Elliott, 1988)

Type of disability[a]	Age group			
	16–59	*60–74*	*75+*	*All adults*
Locomotion	31	198	496	99
Hearing	17	110	328	59
Personal care	18	99	313	57
Dexterity	13	78	199	40
Seeing	9	56	262	38
Intellectual function	20	40	109	34
Behaviour	19	40	152	31
Reaching and stretch	9	54	149	28
Communication	12	42	140	27
Continence	9	42	147	26
Disfigurement	5	18	27	9
Eating, drink and digesting	2	12	30	6
Consciousness	5	10	9	5

[a]Types of disability as specified by the ICIDH (the OPCS types are slightly different).
Behaviour, which includes aspects such as self-awareness, personal safety or family role.
Communication, which includes understanding of, and lack of ability in speaking, listening and seeing.
Personal care, including incontinence, and many of the traditional areas of Activities of Daily Living (ADL), such as bathing, dressing and feeding.
Locomotor including ambulation and transfer.
Body disposition, which includes domestic tasks such as shopping or laundry, picking up objects and maintaining posture.
Dexterity, including opening and closing doors, lighting fires and handling money.
Situational, which includes need for a special diet, difficulty in sustaining positions, as well as intolerance to heat or light.
Particular skill, which is primarily concerned with occupation-related disabilities, and was not fully developed in the original classification.
Other activity restrictions, which is designed to pick up any disabilities not classified in the above.

for each disability. Physical disability is the most relevant in the context of this book, and comprises locomotion, personal care, dexterity, reaching and stretching and disfigurement disabilities. Over three-quarters (77%) of disabled people were found to have one or more of these physical disabilities, implying a prevalence rate of 104.1 per 1000 aged 16 years and over living in the community, or 109 per 1000 including those in institutions.

Locomotion disabilities are the most common with a prevalence in the total adult population (including those in institutions) of 99 per 1000 people, with the highest prevalence for all age groups, and is reported by

half of all people aged 75 years and older. Personal care disabilities are reported by 57 per 1000 of all adults, and by almost a third of those aged 75 years and older. The prevalence of dexterity disability is shown to be 40 per 1000 adults, including nearly 1 in 5 of those aged 75 years and over. Disfigurement disabilities are rare, affecting only 9 per 1000 adults.

Physical disability is also likely to occur in combination with other types of disability, especially sensory disabilities. An estimated 44.6 per 1000 adults have physical disability only (Table 2.2). A further 20.3 per 1000 have physical and hearing disabilities. However, it

Table 2.2 Estimated prevalence of physical disability and other concurrent disabilities in the adult population living in private households. (Source: Martin, White and Meltzer, 1989)

Type of disability	Rate per 1000
Physical (only)	44.6
+ Hearing	20.3
+ Seeing + hearing	9.5
+ Seeing	8.1
+ Mental	8.1
+ Mental + hearing	5.4
+ Mental + seeing + hearing	5.4
+ Mental + seeing	2.7
Total (all physical disability)	104.1

Columns and subtotals are subject to rounding error.

is the combination of physical and mental disabilities (affecting 21.6 per 1000) that appears to be most disabling (Table 2.3).

For example, while 39% of those with severity category 1–2 have physical disability only, this falls to 18% for those at severity categories 9–10. In contrast, while only 2% of those at severity category 1–2 have physical + mental disabilities ($\pm$ sensory disability), this rises to 56% of those most severely disabled.

The major causes of disability found in the UK are shown in Table 2.4, overall, and for the types of disability related to physical disability. Musculoskeletal disorders were the most frequently reported cause, followed by disability due to disorders of the ear and eye. However, a large proportion of these sensory disabilities occur in conjunction with physical disabilities, and the resulting communication problems may have implications for rehabilitation. On the other hand, musculoskeletal disorders have their principal impact upon physical disabilities, with two-thirds of dexterity disabilities due to this cause. Circula-

Table 2.3 Types of disability by severity category expressed as a percentage within each severity group: adult population living in private households. (Source: Martin, White and Meltzer, 1989)

Type of disability	Severity (%)[a]					
	1–2	3–4	5–6	7–8	9–10	Total
Other disability (not physical)	38	26	17	5	0	23
Physical	39	35	31	25	18	33
Physical + sensory	21	31	30	36	28	28
Physical + mental ($\pm$ sensory)	2	8	24	34	56	18
Total (all types)	100	100	100	100	100	100

Columns and subtotals are subject to rounding error.
[a]Examples of Severity Scores (Martin and White, 1988):
Severity category 2: Woman aged 71 with angina and eye problem. Cannot walk 200 yards (182 m) without stopping or severe discomfort. Cannot see well enough to recognize a friend across the road.
Severity category 6: Man aged 65 years. Arthritis in spine and legs. Stroke affecting right side and heart condition. Always needs to hold on to something to keep balance. Cannot bend down and pick something up off the floor and straighten up again. Can only walk up and down a flight of 12 stairs if holds on and takes a rest. Cannot walk 200 yards (182 m) without stopping or severe discomfort. Has difficulty holding either arm in front to shake hands with someone. Has difficulty picking up and pouring from a full kettle or serving food from a pan using a spoon or ladle. Has difficulty unscrewing the lid of a coffee jar or using a pen and pencil. Can pick up a small object such as a safety pin with one hand but not the other.
Severity category 9: Man aged 79. Arthritis of the spine and deafness. Cannot get in and out of bed without help. Finds it impossible to understand people who know him well. Has difficulty hearing someone talking in a loud voice in a quiet room. Cannot follow TV programme with volume turned up. Cannot use the telephone. Loses control of bladder at least once every 24 hours. Has difficulty serving food from a pan using a spoon or ladle. Has difficulty unscrewing the lid of a coffee jar. Cannot bend far enough down to touch knees and straighten up again. Can only walk up and down a flight of 12 stairs if holds on and takes a rest. Has difficulty seeing to read ordinary newspaper print.

Table 2.4 Frequency of complaints (in disease groups) causing physical disabilities[a] and all disability, for adults in private households: expressed as the percentage with complaints within each disability group. (Source: Martin, White and Meltzer, 1989)

Disease (ICD) group	Type of disability				
	All types	Locomotor	Research and stretch	Dexterity	Disfigurement
Musculoskeletal	46	56	64	67	61
Ear	38	1	0	0	1
Eye	22	2	0	1	2
Circulatory	20	23	10	7	5
Mental	13	3	2	3	1
Nervous system	13	12	21	22	12
Respiratory	13	14	3	2	1
Digestive	6	2	2	1	5
Other/vague	6	5	3	4	1
Genitourinary	3	1	1	0	2
Neoplasms	2	1	3	2	4
Endocrine	2	2	1	1	1
Infections	1	1	1	1	3
Blood	1	0	0	0	0
Skin	1	1	0	0	4
Congenital	0	0	0	0	3

[a]Data on complaints associated with personal care disabilities have not been published.

tory disorders and nervous system disorders also contribute to physical disability. Whilst the impact of the former probably arises from deficits in energy and endurance, nervous system disorders (which include stroke) have a more global impact with disabilities in reaching and stretching, and dexterity.

Many complex disabilities arise from multiple pathology. Guralnik and colleagues, working on analysis of the National Health Interview Survey in the USA, showed that the proportion of the population aged 60 years and over with two or more conditions increased by age, and was higher for women than for men (Guralnik *et al.*, 1989). Arthritis and hypertension, the two conditions with the highest prevalence, coexisted in almost one-quarter (24.1%) of those aged over 60. Work by Verbrugge and colleagues shows that as the number of chronic conditions experienced by older people rises, the prevalence of disability rises almost exponentially (Ver-

brugge *et al.*, 1989). Rehabilitation of people with physical disabilities is therefore likely to be complicated by comorbidity and the presence of other types of disability, particularly in older adults.

VARIATIONS IN PREVALENCE OF DISABLEMENT

The variation by age has already been noted. Variations by sex also occur. Overall there are more women with disabilities than men, although this varies by underlying cause of disability. In the UK study the prevalence of disability amongst males (including those in institutions) was 121 per 1000, and 161 per 1000 females (Martin, Meltzer and Elliot, 1988). Rates also varied by ethnic grouping with a prevalence of 151 per 1000 for West Indian (age standardized), living in private households, compared to 126 per 1000 for Asian groups, although these differences

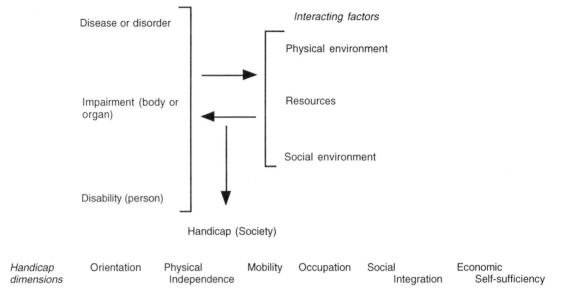

A model for the consequences of disease,
disorders, or injuries

Disease or disorder

Interacting factors

Physical environment

Impairment (body or organ)

Resources

Social environment

Disability (person)

Handicap (Society)

| Handicap dimensions | Orientation | Physical Independence | Mobility | Occupation | Social Integration | Economic Self-sufficiency |

Figure 2.1 A model of the consequences of disease.

failed to reach statistical significance. The UK study also found that the overall prevalence of disability for all ages varied by region; age-standardized rates for the Northern region at 162 per 1000 were 36% higher than the London (GLC) area, with a prevalence of 119 per 1000. Furthermore, the onset of most of the common causes of disability is after the completion of formal education. Thus the low socioeconomic status (SES) of many people with disabilities is a pre-existing circumstance of their lives and not a result of their disability. In the UK survey disabled people were more likely to be in manual occupations. While almost two-thirds (63%) of men with disability had manual jobs, this compares to just over a half (54%) of men generally (Martin, White and Meltzer, 1989). These differences in prevalence of disability as reflected by occupation, low educational attainment and low income are well known and found throughout the western world

(Black *et al.*, 1982; La Vecchia *et al.*, 1987; Pincus, Callahan and Burkhauser, 1987; House *et al.*, 1990; Leigh and Fries, 1991). Low SES is a risk factor for disability (Badley and Ibañez, 1994) and indeed more generally for chronic disease (La Vecchia *et al.*, 1987; Pincus, Gallahan and Buckhauser, 1987; Leigh and Fries, 1991). The lesson for rehabilitation is that the population of people with disabilities is skewed towards those who have the least resources (Department of Health and Social Security, 1971; Statistics Canada, 1994).

THE NATURE OF DISABLEMENT

The challenge is to describe disablement in such a way as to illuminate possible strategies for reducing the impact, at both individual and societal levels. The ICIDH provides such a framework (Figure 2.1) (Badley, 1995).

Impairment is concerned with abnormalities in the structure or functioning of the body or parts of the body. It is characterized by the existence or an occurrence of an anomaly, defect or loss of a limb, organ, tissue or other structure of the body (WHO, 1980). For example, limited range of motion in the arm, grip strength, pain and fatigue are all impairments.

Disability is concerned with the performance of activities, with tasks, skills and behaviours, and the way the performance of activities departs from the norm, as a result of an impairment or disorder. Disability is the process by which impairment expresses itself as a reality in everyday life. Disabilities include the whole range of activities of daily living, as well as instrumental activities of daily living such as shopping, housework and so on.

Handicap is used to describe the disadvantage experienced by the individual as a result of impairment and disabilities, and represents the more social consequences to the individual. Handicap has been described as 'the circumstances in which people with disabilities are likely to find themselves, circumstances that can be expected to place such individuals at a disadvantage in relation to their peers when viewed from the norms of society' (WHO, 19809; Badley, 1995). This description reinforces the social and contingent nature of handicap, and the fact that handicap is an interaction between the individual with impairments and disabilities and the social and cultural setting.

Handicap can be experienced in several dimensions. For people with physical disabilities, there may be a loss of **physical independence**, with the need to rely on the help of other people. **Mobility**, the ability to move around effectively in the environment, may be reduced. **Occupation** including work, leisure and obligations in the home, may be affected, as may **social integration**. There may be reduced **economic self-sufficiency**, not only through reduced earning power, but also as a result of the extra expenses incurred. Finally, **orientation handicap** may be present.

Handicap is not an inevitable and direct consequence of impairment and disability (Badley, 1995) (Figure 2.1), as it arises from an interaction of impairment and disability with other external factors. The physical environment, such as steps or stairs, architectural barriers and housing, is one such factor. Here, the impact of disabilities in climbing stairs will be less for someone who lives in a single-storey house with no external or internal steps or stairs. Other interacting factors include the availability of resources such as assistive devices, personal help, education, personal attributes, money and possessions. The social environment can also affect the development of handicap, and includes the attitudes of others, both within the family and the more general population, and is influenced by cultural background and values, and expectations. The impact of physical disability on the life of an individual is therefore neither just a function of the severity of the disease, nor the number of disabilities. Many people severely affected by physical disabilities lead full and rich lives, whereas others with minimal disabilities may be utterly devastated. There is indeed a school of thought which would view handicap as society's failure to design and accommodate to the range of human ability, which leads to many of its members being disadvantaged.

IMPACT ON INDIVIDUALS IN THE POPULATION: INDICATORS OF DISADVANTAGE

The ICIDH conceptual model can be used to illustrate the impact of physical disability on the lives of those affected. Unfortunately, few data exist which directly address handicap, but some data are available to enable assignment to certain points on the handicap scales. Other indicators of likely handicap can be gleaned by looking at the implications of certain types of disability. These various 'indicators' are listed in Table 2.5 and are grouped into domains reflecting the dimen-

Table 2.5 Indicators of disability: expressed as percentage of disabled adults in private households. (Source: Martin, White and Meltzer, 1989, Statistics Canada, 1990)

Handicap	OPCS	HALS
Mobility		
Restricted to dwelling without help	22	19
Disability in climbing a full flight of stairs	34[a,b]	58[c]
Cannot walk more than 400 yards (364 m)	69[b]	60
Physical independence		
Needs at least occasional help	18	17[d]
Social integration		
Live alone	30	19
Receive visitors once a month or less	15	13[e]
Goes out < once a week	15	
Occupation		
Employed	31[f]	25[f]
Full-time education	1	
Homemaking	11	
Unable to work	34	35
Economic self-sufficiency		
Out-of-pocket expenses because of disability	60	35[g]
Base prevalence/1000	135	132[h]

[a]Without stopping or severe discomfort.
[b]As a result of locomotor disability.
[c]Occasional dependence because of a health problem (excludes other reasons for dependence): heavy household chores; looking after personal finances (e.g. banking, paying bills).
[d]Weekly or more frequent dependence because of a health problem (excludes other reasons for dependence): shopping for groceries or other necessities; everyday housework; personal care (e.g. washing, grooming, dressing, feeding); moving about within own residence; preparing meals.
[e]Never visits relatives or friends.
[f]Under pension age.
[g]Out-of-pocket expenses: includes for medication, special aids or supplies, health and medical services not covered by insurance, modifications to residence, transportation, personal services (e,g, attendant, housekeeping services, etc.).
[h]Age 15 years and over, including those in institution.

sions of handicap. The selected data on handicap indicators presented show the proportion of those with disablement who have specific problems, using data from both UK and Canadian surveys.

Many of the categories are not strictly comparable, as indicated in the footnotes, but when the categories are similar, so too are the levels of handicap. For example, the proportion of disabled people who are housebound without assistance; who need at least occasional help; and who are permanently unable to work. Where differences are observed, for example in employment, part of this will be a reflection of the different contexts of the two surveys, but part could well be a reflection of international differences in the circumstances of people with disabilities.

Mobility

Mobility handicap reflects individuals' ability to move about effectively in their surroundings. It is concerned not so much with the practicalities of ambulation, as individuals' ability to move in the environment. Just over one in five (22%) of disabled adults in the UK survey were restricted to their dwelling without help (Table 2.5); this includes 8% of all disabled adults who were housebound, even when help was at hand. The Canadian experience is of the same order of magnitude, with almost a fifth (19%) of disabled people unable to leave their residence without help.

Physical independence

Physical independence handicap reflects the individual's ability to sustain a customarily independent existence, particularly in day-to-day activities of daily living (ADL). Disabilities in ADL can mean that help may be needed, or the person may be unable to do certain tasks at all. Help may also be needed if the person can only do the activity so slowly, or with such expenditure of energy, that it impinges on other areas of life. For example, someone who can dress themselves, but would be so tired out that they could do nothing else, is likely to seek help for the task. Rather than look at individual items, the WHO Handicap Classification (WHO, 1980) attempts to get a global picture by looking at the frequency and urgency with which help would be likely to be required.

In the OPCS survey physical independence handicap was ascertained by direct questioning with regards to the amount of help the disabled person required. Table 2.5 shows that 18% of disabled adults needed help at least occasionally. This comprises 1% who needed help all day and night, 4% who needed help day or night, and a further 4% who needed regular help throughout the day, but could be left alone for an hour or so. A further 9% need at least occasional help. In the HALS, 17% were dependent on help weekly or more often. As might be expected, there was an association with severity, so that three-quarters of those with severe disability were dependent. In another study, it was found that the proportion of people reporting that they were not responsible for carrying out household and kitchen activities increased with increasing levels of disability. This suggests that there may be some reallocation

of tasks within households of people with disability which minimizes perceived dependence (Badley and Tennant, 1991).

Social integration

Social integration is the individuals' ability to participate in and maintain social relationships. It is difficult to obtain information on this dimension as it is not well covered in surveys, and is dependent on many factors other than disability, such as finance and personality. However, some indication of social integration can be obtained by looking at the converse, social isolation, and one can assume that living alone implies some measure of isolation (even though this varies with culture). In the UK survey 3 in 10 of disabled people, and almost a fifth (19%) of those with disability in the HALS survey, lived alone, the latter compared with only 8.5% in the Canadian non-disabled population. Many people with disability are older and may be living alone because of the loss of a spouse. The lower overall rate in Canada may reflect the lower proportion of the population that are aged 65 years and older (Badley and Crotty, 1995). The fact that such a sizeable proportion live alone is of relevance in view of the level of dependence described above.

The UK study also highlighted the paucity of contacts for some disabled people. Fifteen per cent of disabled adults received visitors only once a month or less often, and 15% reported that they, themselves, went out less than once a week (Martin, White and Meltzer, 1989). Thirteen per cent of disabled people in Canada never visited family or friends.

Occupation

Occupation concerns the individual's ability to occupy his/her time in the manner consistent with age, sex and culture. It includes recreation, paid employment, as well as domestic tasks. In the UK study, just under a third (31%) of disabled adults under pension age were working. 1 in a 100 were in full-time education and 11% (virtually all female) were engaged in homemaking (Martin, White and Meltzer, 1989). That is, approximately 43% of disabled adults could be construed as being fully 'occupied' in ICIDH terms. Just over one in three disabled people reported that they were permanently unable to work. Similarly, in the HALS, of those aged less than 65 years, over a third were not in the labour force specifically because their health problem prevented them from working in a job or business. The proportion increased with increasing severity of disability, to almost 70% of those with severe disability.

Almost two-thirds of the Canadians never attended sporting events, concerts, plays or films at cinemas. Likewise two-fifths never participated in arts, crafts, gardening or other hobbies, and 18% never engaged in social activities. This could only partly be related to the older age of those with disability, as there was a gradient with severity of disability. In the UK half reported that they had not taken a holiday or had being given respite care during the previous year (Martin, White and Meltzer, 1989).

Economic self-sufficiency

Economic self-sufficiency handicap is defined as the individual's ability to sustain customary socioeconomic activity and independence. People with disability had lower incomes than the non-disabled population. In the HALS survey almost a half had an income in 1986 of less than $20 000 compared to only 24% of the non-disabled population. The UK survey found that incomes of disabled pensioners were only slightly lower than those of pensioners in the general population, but those of working age had income levels reduced to 72% of that of the general population (Martin and White, 1988). The proportion of income gained from

employment by all disabled adults of working age decreased as severity of disability increased. Whilst over half (56%) of income for disabled adults in severity categories 1–2 came from employment, just 18% was derived from this source for those in severity categories 9–10. Reliance on state benefits increased by level of severity, rising from 30% of income in severity categories 1–2, to 73% of income for the highest categories. Pensioner family units derive most of their income from benefits, irrespective of their level of severity.

A considerable proportion of people with disability reported incurring extra expenses because of disability; 60% in the UK and over a third of people in the Canadian survey. The UK survey found that the poorest families were paying out the largest proportion of their income on disability-related expenditure (Martin and White, 1988). In both Canada and the UK all basic medical services, including all physician charges and some rehabilitation services, are covered by the health service. However, the increased expenses because of the disability point to disadvantage for those who may be already financially less well endowed than their non-disabled peers. In countries, such as the USA, without universal health services, the proportion with disability-derived expenses is likely to be very much higher than in countries with a national health service, and often causes great poverty and distress.

THE GLOBAL BURDEN

The analysis so far has been confined to the western world, using the UK and Canada as examples. A number of factors will affect the prevalence of disablement. The first is patterns of mortality and morbidity. The experience in less developed countries is dominated by the consequences of infectious disease, malnutrition and trauma (including war). In contrast, in western countries the community burden is dominated by chronic and generally

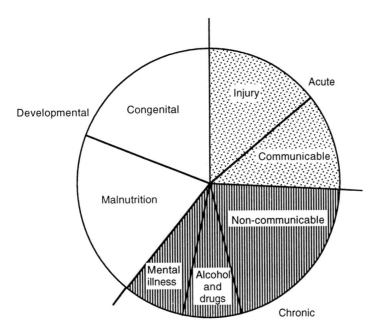

Figure 2.2 Classes of disorder giving rise to disability in the world (from Wood, 1983). (WHO estimate of population affected: 450–500 million.)

non-fatal illness, with their bigger and more persistent toll of disability. The second influence is demographic. The prevalence of disability is related to the proportion of the population who are elderly (over 65 years). The world's population is ageing (Verbrugge, 1989; US Bureau of Census, 1991), so a growing burden of disablement is scarcely surprising.

As far as numbers are concerned, WHO has estimated that about 1 in 10 of the world's population are disabled. The precision of this estimate is understandably open to some question. It is probably more appropriate to recognize that about a third of the world's population is impaired in some way, a third of those with impairment are disabled to some degree (which is close to the 1 in 10 estimate) and a third of the latter experience sufficiently severe restrictions in activity as to suggest handicap.

An approximation to the situation in the world is offered in Figure 2.2, which shows

the underlying causes of disability. The marked difference from the situation in the UK is due to the predominant distribution of the world's population in less developed countries. In fact, one-third of those affected are children, and four-fifths of people with disabilities live in developing countries. It can be seen that the total burden is subdivided into three groups of roughly similar size – developmental, acute and chronic conditions, with the two former groups accounting for 64% of the total. A large part of the developmental and acute conditions could be prevented by application of conventional public health insights, and particularly by immunization and improved nutrition. By far the biggest challenge, therefore, is to learn more about why what is possible is not put into effect, a conclusion that probably applies with almost as much force to controlling chronic disorders and their consequences in the UK and Canada as it does to other conditions elsewhere in the world.

Table 2.6 Selected examples from a strategy for the control of disablement (from Wood, 1983)

Primary control (to prevent) – largely a function of social policy, particularly through such means as development of appropriate services
  (i) **Health promotion**, which may be:
    (a) handicap-oriented (enablement), through urban design (re. isolation), educational and employment opportunities, transport policies, social attitudes, etc.
    (b) disease-oriented, through family planning, antenatal care, breast feeding, immunization, adequate diet, prophylactic replacement (e.g. salt for workers under thermal stress), and physical activity
  (ii) **Protection** (hazard containment), which may be:
    (a) collective, by repression (e.g. clean water), reduction (speed limits), restriction (sanitation), regulation (alcohol), evasion (pedestrianization), separation (surgeon's gloves), modification (product design, such as cot slats) and awareness (e.g. domestic illumination – fuller examples are given in Wood (1983)
    (b) individual, by limiting access (such as to domestic fires) and by genetic counselling, contact tracing, avoiding ototoxic drugs, prophylaxis (e.g. penicillin for rheumatic fever) and identification of risk factors

Secondary control (to arrest)
  (i) **Reaction** – identifying damage, which is largely a function of social policy
    (a) prompt response, such as automobile seatbelts and emergency (rescue) services
    (b) screening, for early detection and treatment
  (ii) **Stabilization** – countering damage, related to the availability of health services
    (a) cure – many conventional medical initiatives (e.g. hormone replacement)
    (b) amelioration – (avoiding impairment and disability by arrest of disease progression (part of WHO's first level 'disability prevention')
Tertiary control (to repair) – control of disablement
  (i) **Restoration** – control of disability (WHO's second level 'disability prevention'), a function of the availability of health and remedial care
    (a) reconstruction (e.g. total hip replacement)
    (b) rehabilitation (e.g. remedial services, provision of aids)
  (ii) **Maintenance** – control of handicap (WHO's third level 'disability prevention'), largely a function of social policy
    (a) continuing care (e.g. monitoring for deterioration)
    (b) enablement (e.g. extension of opportunities, vocational resettlement)
    (c) support (e.g. welfare provision, assistance, aid to family)

CHALLENGES FOR POLICY

A comprehensive strategy for the control of disablement is outlined in Table 2.6. If the overall goal is to reduce handicap, a number of possibilities are revealed. Health may be promoted in non-specific ways by measures that benefit those without illness as much as the sick. Policies that minimize social disadvantage include broad areas such as urban design, educational and employment opportunities, transport policies and initiatives directed at public attitudes. In a more conventional vein, opportunities for control of disablement arise from control of the underlying disorders. This highlights the importance of prevention of disease and trauma, and where this is not possible, appropriate medical and rehabilitation care.

If the impact of a disorder is viewed solely in terms of impairment and disability, the options for interventions for people with disability are narrow. Interventions to control the extent of impairment and disability are part of conventional medical and rehabilitation services. By intervening at the level of handicap and considering the interaction of the social and environmental setting with the impairment and/or disability of the individual, the options are greatly expanded. Some of the other factors that might influence outcome are indicated in Figure 2.1. These include modifications to the physical environment, and the provision of resources including assistive devices and education. Facilitation of education regarding the experience of disability in the wider social setting of the community may also be important, by minimizing the degree of handicap in individuals.

In summary, this analysis draws attention to some major policy issues to reduce the impact of disablement. Using the ICIDH framework it is apparent that one can reduce resultant handicap at many levels, ranging from the individual to society as a whole, and that there is room not only to react to what has occurred, but also for preventive strategies at all these levels.

REFERENCES

Badley, E.M. (1995) The genesis of handicap: definition, models of disablement, and role of external factors. *Disability and Rehabilitation*, **17**, 53–62.

Badley, E.M. and Crotty, M. (1995) An international comparison of the estimated impact of the ageing population on the major causes of disablement, musculoskeletal disorders. *Journal of Rheumatology*, **22**, 1934–40.

Badley, E.M. and Ibañez, I. (1994) Socio-economic risk factors and musculoskeletal disability. *Journal of Rheumatology*, **21**, 515–22.

Badley, E.M. and Tennant, A. (1991) A survey of disablement in a British population using an action-orientated measure, physical independence handicap: problems with activities of daily living and level of support. *International Disability Studies*, **13**, 91–8.

Black, D., Morris, J.N., Smith, C. and Townsend, P. (1982) *The Black Report*. Penguin, London.

Department of Health and Social Security (1971) *Health Management Circular HM45/71*, DHSS, London.

Guralnik, J.M., LaCroix, A.Z. and Everett, D.F. (1989) Comorbidity of chronic conditions and disability among older persons – United States, 1984. *Morbidity and Mortality Weekly Report*, **38** 788–91.

House, J.S., Kessler, R.C., Herzog, A.R. *et al.* (1990) Age, socio-economic status, and health. *The Milbank Quarterly*, **68**, 383–411.

La Vecchia, C., Negri, E., Pagano, R. and Decarli, A. (1987) Education, prevalence of disease, and frequency of health care utilisation. The 1983 Italian National Health Survey. *Journal of Epidemiology and Community Health*, **41** 161–5.

Leigh, J.P. and Fries, J.F. (1991) Occupation, income, and education as independent covariates of arthritis in four national probability samples. *Arthritis and Rheumatism*, **34**, 984–95.

Lilienfeld, A.M. and Lilienfeld, D.E. (1980) *Foundations of Epidemiology*, 2nd edn, Oxford University Press, New York.

Martin, J., Meltzer, H. and Elliot, D. (1988) *The Prevalence of Disability Among Adults. OPCS surveys of disability in Great Britain Report 1*. OPCS Social Survey Division, HMSO, London.

Martin, J. and White, A. (1988) *The Financial Circumstances of Disabled Adults Living in Private Households. Report 2*. OPCS Social Survey Division, HMSO, London.

Martin, J., White, A. and Meltzer,, H. (1989) *Disabled Adults: services, transport and employment. OPCS surveys of disability in Great Britain Report 4*. OPCS Social Survey Decision, HMSO, London.

McWinney, J.R. (1982) *Measuring Disability. The OECD social indicator development programme. Special studies no. 5*, Organisation for Economic Co-Operation and Development, Paris.

Pincus, T., Callahan, L.F. and Burkhauser, R.V. (1987) Most chronic diseases are reported by individuals with fewer than 12 years of formal education in the age 18–64 United States population. *Journal of Chronic Diseases*, **40**, 865–74.

Statistics Canada (1989) *Health and Activity Limitation Survey Microdata User's Guide Adults in Household*. Statistics Canada, Ottawa, Ontario.

Statistics Canada (1990) *Health and Activity Limitation Survey. Highlights: disabled persons in Canada*. Catalogue 82-602. Canadian Government Publishing Centre, Ottawa, Ontario.

Statistics Canada (1994) *Selected Characteristics of Persons with Disabilities Residing Households: 1991 Health and Activity Limitation Survey.* Catalogue No. 82-555. Statistics Canada, Ottawa, Ontario.

US Bureau of Census (1991) *Global Ageing: Comparative indicators and future trends.* US Department of Commerce, Economics and Statistics Division, Washington.

Verbrugge, L.M. (1989) Recent, present and future health of American adults. *Annual Review of Public Health,* **10,** 333–61.

Verbrugge, L.M., Lepkowski, J.M. and Imanaka, Y. (1989) Comorbidity and its impact on disability. *The Milbank Quarterly,* **67,** 450–84.

WHO (1980) *The International Classification of Impairments, Disabilities and Handicaps.* WHO, Geneva.

3 Social factors

E. Evans

INTRODUCTION

The social factors affecting disability considered in this chapter are primarily about attitudes and the environment. It draws attention to the need for change and examines the difficulty in producing it. Disabled people seek change and the professions should help and support them in this. If the able-bodied world is to become less hostile to those with disabilities, changes are needed. This chapter aims to draw out some relevant issues which society as a whole has to address.

In 1990 George Bush, then President of the USA, signed the 'Americans with Disabilities Act'. It gave those with disabilities in America comprehensive civil rights and a legal right to challenge discrimination. It followed extensive political lobbying. Currently in the UK people with disabilities are seeking antidiscriminatory legislation. If successful, it would at least, in theory, give disabled people equal rights and opportunities. Yet there is political reluctance to respond and apathy (happily decreasing) among the general population. In other areas of the world, often where there are pressing issues of resources, especially poor medical care, disabled people may find little or no interest in their abilities or rights.

DEFINITIONS

Until about the 1970s there was little awareness of disability issues in the UK. Indeed many, both professionals and lay people, failed to make a distinction between chronic disease and disability. Early in the 1980s the World Health Organization (WHO, 1980) produced the International Classification of Impairments, Disabilities and Handicaps (ICIDH). This has enabled distinctions to be drawn between **impairment** (defined as disturbance of the normal structure and function of the body), **disability** (inability to carry out tasks) and **handicap** (where the role of the person is disadvantaged). This has cleared thinking on the subject greatly, especially about assessment and treatment.

However, the classification has been criticized (or at least the handicap dimension has) by some people with disabilities. They maintain that the problem lies not with the disadvantaged individual but with society. Thus someone is not disabled because they are paraplegic and cannot walk, the disability is because the environment is not wheelchair accessible. They suggest that if physical barriers were removed many more disabled people could have freedom of movement and equal opportunities to use their abilities. The Disabled People's International suggests that 'disability has too long been viewed as a problem of the individual and not the relationship between an individual and his/her environment'. They state handicap is more related to physical and social barriers.

Rehabilitation of the Physically Disabled Adult. Edited by C. John Goodwill, M. Anne Chamberlain and Chris Evans. Published in 1997 by Stanley Thornes (Publishers) Ltd, Cheltenham. ISBN 0-7487-3183-0.

The Union of the Physically Impaired Against Segregation (UPIAS) defines disability as 'the disadvantage or restriction caused by a contemporary social organisation which takes no or little account of people who have physical impairments and thus excludes them from participation in the mainstream activities. Physical disability is therefore a particular form of social oppression.' The Prince of Wales Advisory Group on Disabilities (1985) suggests it is important to remember the need for 'freedom to make decisions regarding the way of life best suited to an individual disabled person's circumstances'.

Such ideas are challenging and need to be acknowledged. However, they may be less relevant when working with people who have, for example, a lack of insight, inattention problems or memory difficulties. Nevertheless, a poor environment affects the lives of all and its improvement will enhance life for others who are not physically disabled (such as mothers with prams using public transport). Similarly, an awareness of disability, a tolerance of those who are different and a recognition that all have an equal right to opportunities should be features of a humane society.

Advances in medical technology, particularly neonatal care and intensive care of adults, present us with new situations and often new ethical dilemmas. There are issues around prenatal screening and the treatment of small-for-date babies, some of whom will be severely disabled and require considerable support throughout life. Increasingly we have the power to keep people alive by interventions that include tracheotomy and percutaneous endoscopic feeding. Many who survive after such treatments are severely disabled and the length of their survival with disability (and morbidity) has risen. The presence of significant numbers of young adults in persistent vegetative states (or states little removed from this) is creating much debate and generating discussion about Living Wills.

ATTITUDES

Historical influences

Several strands are present in the history of how people with disabilities were viewed by society. One response to those who are different has been to isolate them. Sometimes fear, particularly of infection, invokes this response. Lepers were forced to live in communities away from the general population. In Truro the Leper's Arch (which still exists) marked the boundary through which they were not allowed to pass (Figure 3.1). There is an echo of this segregation in the reaction to AIDS today. Another response was that of providing care. This was traditionally associated with the major religions. Part of their ethos was to call their members to provide such services. It often led to a paternalistic approach, placing those in need of care in a submissive role.

Although it is not entirely clear what happened in the Middle Ages, the numbers of disabled people remained relatively small because of high infant mortality and little medical expertise. Individuals were looked after by their families and by institutions such as monasteries. The Industrial Revolution led to a break up of the extended family. Economic changes and increased mobility of the population meant less support was available and emphasized the division between disabled and able-bodied people. The problems caused by the death of a carer or the loss of work because of disability resulted in the growing need for residential care. Many people found themselves living in workhouses, sometimes the forerunner of local hospitals and geriatric units.

Residential homes for disabled people were, like the Leper's Gate, often placed on the boundaries of the main community and hidden behind high walls. It was presumed disabled people were unable to look after themselves and this became reinforced by the prevailing philosophy of care. Although this was well meaning, it would now be seen as

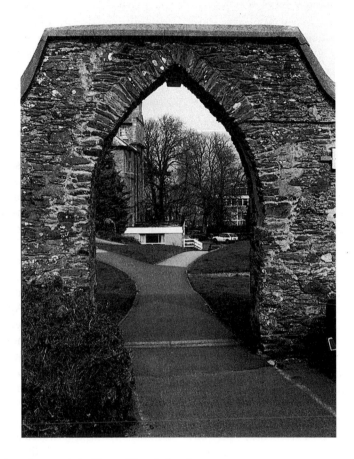

Figure 3.1 Lepers' Arch, as it is in Truro Hospital today.

oppressive. Upon admission, the disabled person was expected to hand over control of all aspects of his life, with able-bodied people assuming professional roles of providing care and management of the institution. The removal of disabled people from normal society led to a lack of understanding, patronizing attitudes and prejudice, some of which can still be detected today. It is easy to look back and be critical of such ideas and establishments, but at the time those men and women who pioneered homes to care for disabled people were responding to the need in the only way they knew.

During the 1970s a survey was undertaken by Miller and Gwynne, two social researchers from the Tavistock Institute, to look at how homes were run (Miller and Gwynne, 1972). They defined two models of care: the 'warehousing' and the 'horticulture'. They condemned the former because the person had no say over their lifestyle (what they ate and wore, how they occupied their time and when they had to go to bed). The body was well cared for but the soul was starved; it was social death and commonly found. The horticultural model was preferred. It allowed the person more choice and involvement and catered for their social needs. Many residential institutions began to change to the 'horticultural' model.

However, articulate people with disabilities felt the survey had failed to realize that disabled people were capable of independence and that other options should be considered. Wherever possible everyone should live within the community and be supported there as needed. The provision of services in Sweden (the Fokus scheme) showed acceptable ways of living within the community. Since then disabled people have continued to press for better provisions and greater awareness of their problems. They want recognition of their worth and are challenging the views that disabled people are unable to control their lives or earn a living.

Current influences

The provision of services in the UK is undergoing profound changes. This is shown by the Care in the Community policies and the move towards antidiscriminatory legislation. Resources are often scarce and support insufficient, so people continue to struggle. There is, however, an acceptance, in policy and in practice, that this is the way to progress.

Disability issues are complex. The paternalistic attitudes described earlier are still held by many, often subconsciously. In modern industrialized society, advertisements relentlessly promote the perfection of the body beautiful; success is measured too often by financial and work status. Those who are disabled, unemployed or poor (or all three) are at a major disadvantage. The abilities of people with disabilities vary widely but it is still the case that many people associate any physical problem with diminished under-standing. Political and legislative changes may help improve our awareness of those with disability, but changes in attitude will be hastened by a greater understanding of disability issues.

Staff attitudes

There is a need for training in disability awareness. This applies even, or perhaps especially, to those who work in hospitals or social services. Studies suggest that attitudes to disability are no better in the health services than in the general population. There is also a suggestion (Kahtan *et al.*, 1994) that unless medical students are specifically taught about disability, their attitudes will worsen, not improve, over the time of their training (Horden, 1994). Emotions such as pity, disgust, rejection and even fear are sometimes displayed by professionals, and it is necessary to be aware of these primary responses. Disability awareness training can help to produce a better response.

Our own experience of meeting or working with disabled people will modify and develop our perception of attitudes and needs. While many accept that a person with visual impairment may use Braille or be accompanied by a guide dog, fewer are tolerant of, or willing to adapt to, those with hearing difficulties, speech defects or who have to use a communication aid. In part, this may be due to associated factors; it requires great time and effort to communicate with a profoundly dysarthric patient and eye contact may be lost when using a communication aid. The cues coming back from a disabled person may be distorted, few or absent. Pentland *et al.* (1987) found that physiotherapists unconsciously smiled less and gave less time to patients with Parkinson's and thought this was probably due to the immobile face and lack of response.

The relationship between the professional worker and the patient should ideally be a partnership in which the worker provides information and options and the disabled person agrees the goals and plan of action for treatment. If the professional is constantly seeking to control and direct the individual, it suggests that the views of the disabled person are not being heeded. There may be occasions where the professional may have to take the initiative. This may occur when the effects of trauma or illness may be so severe that the person is unable to understand or actively participate or communication is impossible. There will be occasions when the aspirations of people will be seen as unrealistic or containing too many risk elements (such as the wish of a person with severe memory impairment and poor insight to live alone). However, it is to be accepted that the disabled person should be able to take risks, as in normal life, but the risk to carers and professionals should not be unmanageable.

Differences in attitudes and reactions by disabled people

Within the disabled population there will be those who passively accept their limitations, those who refuse to acknowledge the difficulties and those who feel the limitations are caused by 'society'. The following – punishment, grief, a challenge – are just a few examples of how disabled people perceive disability.

Is it a punishment

Some newly disabled people, and parents of disabled babies, often express a concern that disability is a form of punishment for some imagined wrong doing. One lady who had suffered a stroke felt it was her punishment for not having afforded and placed a headstone on her husband's grave. While counselling may be available to help work through such negative feelings, this idea of disability needs to be challenged.

Grief

Grief is a common reaction to disability. Many disabled people talk of adjusting to life with a disability rather then accepting it. It is important that professionals and carers can acknowledge the grief and allow time for the person to work through their feelings. This is a continual process, reflecting the changes in a person's situation. Such changes may be caused by a deteriorating condition with increased loss of function or by the gradual realization of loss. This may well be happening during the process of rehabilitation and returning home.

Case history

This is illustrated in the case of a divorced 48-year-old man living on his own who had sustained a left CVA. At the end of his rehabilitation this man still had a right-sided weakness, dysphasis, dyspraxia, a hemianopia and severe mobility problems. He wanted to go back to his own bungalow. He achieved this goal using the supporting services that were set up by the multidisciplinary team. His dysphasia and dyspraxia meant he lived with some risk and was unable to resume former hobbies of bridge and chess. Joining new clubs proved difficult for the same reasons. Rambling, another former interest, could not be resumed because of hemiparesis. His hemianopia and right-sided neglect meant he could not drive. Despite the relative success of enabling him to return home, this man constantly grieved for what he had lost and at one point attempted suicide. He felt the loss of language and communication most keenly. His discharge was an excellent example of risk management.

A challenge

There are many disabled people who respond in a positive manner. They can reintegrate back into their former lifestyle, return to work, drive and continue with former relationships and activities. Modifications may be required, physically and emotionally, but active participation in their former environment is maintained.

Some disabled people wish to develop their own distinct culture based on their disability. They resist negative statements about the experience of disability, there is not the same wish for integration and it can be difficult for society to sympathize with this approach.

Attitudes expressed by carers

Family members and other unpaid carers are relied upon heavily to support disabled people in the community. Financial benefits may be paid to carers, but these are often not comparable with the lost salary or the hours of caring involved.

Some disabling conditions may cause changes in the person and in turn affect their relationships. This may include personality changes or problems such as incontinence or memory impairment. Carers can feel trapped looking after someone who is no longer the same and may not be as likeable. The dependency of the disabled person and the associated responsibility of caring may be irksome to the individual and the carer. There are also some carers who enjoy their role and prevent the disabled person from achieving their potential.

The growth in carers' support groups and the introduction of legislation is to ensure that needs of carers are specifically addressed gives recognition to the needs and concerns of those involved in the care of a disabled person. Some may argue that the growth in concern about carers emphasizes the negative aspects about disability and maintains the divide between disabled and able-bodied people.

ENVIRONMENTAL ISSUES

General

Do environmental barriers create disability? This question has caused some disabled

groups to suggest that an apartheid structure exists and is maintained by society creating physical barriers. It is more likely that such environments existed long before the use of wheelchairs and that there has been a lack of appreciation of the needs of such users rather than a designed malevolence to exclude them. Some of the main environmental problems are to do with access, communication systems, housing and transport facilities.

It is increasingly felt by disabled people that it is not sufficient for able-bodied people to plan services which will affect them; too often practical mistakes are made which would have been avoided if they were consulted throughout (such as in the building of a new hospital). However, many reasons are still found to resist their involvement.

Access

Many buildings were built before the emergence of equipment for mobility and even in recent times many designers fail to allow for the needs of those with young children, the elderly or people who have disabilities. It follows that if wheelchair users or those who have difficulties managing steps cannot enter shops, toilets or public buildings, they will not have the same opportunities to participate as others. Even if problems of access can be overcome at an alternative entrance, many people would see this as second rate and segregating.

Once access is gained, users have to feel confident of receiving a normal quality of service. This will so often depend on the attitudes of service providers and other service users. The environment may be physically suitable but the interplay of attitudes may still pose problems; for example, eating in restaurants.

Communication

Individual systems such as Braille, loop systems, Minitel, signing, communication aids and environmental controls are all dis-cussed elsewhere in this book. Systems are sometimes found in churches and public places of entertainment, but they need to be more routinely available. One might pause to ask how the deaf person with a relative in hospital is to enquire about their progress. Routine use and familiarity with the different types of communication aids should help to dispel embarrassment and increase under-standing and acceptance.

Domestic housing

With the emphasis on community care comes a need for adapted and individually tailored housing in both public and private schemes. A range of living options needs to be available to meet the various needs of people (Chapter 54). It is important that the different forms of accommodation and the external environment near the disabled person's home are also barrier free.

Transport

The ability to get to work, to shops, to visit friends and so forth is essential and often taken for granted. For those with mobility problems the means and availability of trans-port become crucial. Many feel that private transport provides the best solution, tailored to the individual's needs. However, it is also important to recognize that users of public transport include those on low income, the old, disabled or mothers with young children. Simple design features, such as lowered steps, adequate rails, better shock absorption, would be helpful. There are some practical issues, like simply allowing the person to walk to their seat before the bus starts, which would help many people. Some taxis are wheelchair accessible. Some cities have Access buses and schemes such as Shopmobility where powered chairs are available for hire to facilitate shopping.

Accessible transport benefits all and wheel-chair-accessible transport should also be routinely available.

PROBLEMS IN PRODUCING CHANGE

Legislation

There have been various attempts to try and promote change through legislation. However, in the field of employment it has proved to be piecemeal and ineffective. The Disabled Persons (Employment) Act 1944 was the only legislation specifically aimed at protecting disabled workers. It established a register of disabled workers and imposed a system whereby if companies employed more than 20 staff at least 3% should be disabled. Exemption required a permit from the Employment Department. The Act was also designed to prohibit the dismissal of registered disabled workers if it meant the 3% quota was not maintained. Under the Act disabled people were only allowed to complain to the Employ-ment Department and only the Secretary of State could prosecute employers. This Act had little impact on the employment of disabled people. There were very few prosecutions and the quota system was not strictly enforced. At this time unemployment was very low, about 300 000, and there were also many unskilled and semi-skilled jobs available. These factors worked to the advantage of people with disabilities wishing to work.

Part of the problem relates to attitudes held by potential employers about disabled workers. Assumptions are sometimes made that disabled workers are less productive, have more sick leave or require expensive work modifications. These are described in an information pack entitled 'Disability and Discrimination in Employment' (available from RADAR). A study of the Americans with Disability Act by Veronica Scott shows how the USA has adopted a more positive approach to employing people with disabil-ities and legislation to enforce it (Scott, 1994). Chapter 52 will discuss employment in greater detail.

Legislation with the power to enforce, together with a positive shift in attitudes, is required to promote change.

Financial costs

In the introduction to this chapter it was stated that in many parts of the world there are problems in resourcing even basic medical care, let alone funding for the social and physical needs of those with disabilities. Even where there are seemingly plentiful resources, the cost of making changes in existing systems can be huge. For example, it is cheaper and easier to legislate that all future buildings are wheelchair accessible rather than to include and enforce access alterations to all existing buildings. Financial restrictions will inevitably limit the range of services available. This is true of many service provisions, whether for the disabled or for other sectors of the population.

Perceived needs of people with disabilities

It is difficult when a minority group has diverse needs. Attitudes held by different groups of non-disabled people may be at variance, as may be their goals. This is paralleled by disabled people. For example, a person with paraplegia may seek the removal of any physical barriers so as to gain freedom within their environment. They may seek control of the management and funding of practical care services. This is beginning to happen in some areas and enables people to direct their own lives. Those who have head injuries, with resulting cognitive problems and physical limitations, would require a similar care service but might be unable to manage and supervise it. Indeed part of the care package should include safeguards to prevent exploitation by others. This suggests that those who are vulnerable because of cognitive deficits will require the support of others, which to some extent weakens the argument of those who wish

disability to be seen as being caused by the environment. It is however possible to identify common needs and to have agreement about areas requiring change and goals to be achieved.

CONCLUSION

This chapter has addressed some of the social and political issues surrounding disability. It has discussed the many negative features that still exist in our society. This has included the inadequate and poorly monitored legislation, the lack of housing and transport options. It has also looked at the various attitudes about disability issues and how these influence change.

However, there are positive features. Portrayals in the media of personalities such as Stephen Hawking, the Professor of Mathematics who uses computers to communicate, and the abilities of many disabled people are helping their ability to become better recognized by society. Although there is anxiety about the cost of antidiscriminatory legislation, there is a recognition that this cannot be delayed for too long and that it will be demanded by people with disabilities as a right. The climate of opinion is very different from that when Gwynne and Miller were writing. There needs to be a continuing partnership working towards full integration.

REFERENCES

Horden, L. (1994) Attitudes of medical students to disability. *British Journal of Rheumatology*, **33**, 203–4.

Kahtan, S., Inman, C., Haines, A. and Holland, P. (1994) Teaching disability and rehabilitation to medical students. *Medical Education*, **28**, 386–93.

Miller, E.J. and Gwynne, G.V. (1972) *A Life Apart*, Tavistock Publications, London.

Pentland, B., Pitcairn, T.K., Ray, T.M. and Riddle, W.J.R. (1987) First Impressions of Parkinson's Disease Patients, Paper presented at the meeting of the Society for Research into Rehabilitation.

Prince of Wales Advisory Group on Disabilities (1985) *Living Options. Guidelines for those planning services for people with severe physical disabilities.* Prince of Wales Advisory Group on Disabilities, London.

Scott, V. (1994) *Lessons from America*, RADAR, London.

WHO (1980) *World Health Organisation International Classification of Impairments, Disabilities and Handicaps*, WHO, Geneva.

FURTHER READING

Oliver, M. (1991) *Social Work – Disabled people and disabling environments*, Jessica Kingsley, London.

USEFUL ADDRESSES

*RADAR (Royal Association for Disability and Rehabilitation)*12 City Forum, 250 City Road, London EC1V 8AF, UK.

4 Psychological factors

A.K. Coughlan

INTRODUCTION

This chapter has been written mainly with physical disability in mind, but its contents are also generally applicable to sensory and cognitive disabilities.

The way in which people react to acquiring a disability and the extent to which they adjust to it varies enormously from person to person. This chapter attempts to outline the major factors that influence their reactions and abilities to adjust. These will be considered under the following headings:

Nature of the disability:
    type;
    severity;
    mode of onset, knowledge of condition and expectations;
    progression.
Psychological factors:
    personality and coping style;
    self-image and self-esteem.
Brain damage (if applicable)
    personality change;
    cognitive impairments;
    lack of insight;
    neglect.
Reaction of others.
Supportive network.
Financial security.
Quality of professional care.

NATURE OF THE DISABILITY

The nature of the disability comprises four components:

- type, e.g. blindness, paraplegia, ataxia, memory loss;
- severity;
- mode of onset – acute or gradual;
- progression – improvement, static, intermittent decline or steady decline.

Each component will have an effect on how the person reacts and copes. Different conditions involve these components to varying degrees, so this chapter aims to give a broad account of their effects.

Type

Each type of disability brings its own hindrances and frustrations to everyday life with the consequent likelihood of outbursts of temper or tearfulness. Over time, as the person learns new ways of carrying out old tasks or adopts routines that avoid some of the difficulties, these reactions subside, though some particular difficulties may always remain irksome and a cause of irritation. Some disabilities will also preclude certain occupational or recreational activities, leading possibly to isolation, loss of self-esteem and feelings of lack of fulfilment. For some people there may also be a strong

Rehabilitation of the Physically Disabled Adult. Edited by C. John Goodwill, M. Anne Chamberlain and Chris Evans. Published in 1997 by Stanley Thornes (Publishers) Ltd, Cheltenham. ISBN 0-7487-3183-0.

interaction between the type of disability and their self-esteem. Some disabilities are intensely threatening to a person's view of their own worth. In such instances problems in adjustment are likely to occur. This is discussed further below in the section on psychological factors.

Severity

As a general rule, the more severe the disability the more frustration it will cause and the greater is the likelihood that occupational or recreational activities will be affected. Enforced dependence on others for activities of daily living may give rise to a variety of emotions, particularly those of anger, sorrow and lowered self-esteem. Nonetheless, after an initial period of shock and despair, many people bear severe disablement with great fortitude and dignity. Others, however, are devastated by relatively trivial handicaps and become preoccupied by them. These differences arise predominantly from the interaction of the type and severity of the condition with the robustness of the person's personality and with his/her self-image.

Mode of onset, knowledge of condition and expectations

Acute onset confronts the sufferer with a sudden alteration in circumstances. This can produce a variety of reactions – most commonly shock, bewilderment and disbelief – and may result in a state of mental numbness akin to that experienced by people who lose a loved one through sudden bereavement. This phase is likely to be followed by a period of anxiety and uncertainty when a multitude of thoughts and worries about the future will occur: 'will I get better', 'how will I cope with my job?', 'what will others think of me?', 'am I going to be in a wheelchair for life?', 'how will my family cope?', 'will I ever find a partner now?', 'will my husband/wife stick by me?', 'will I need an operation?'. The

extent to which these anxieties can be dispelled will vary from condition to condition and with the individual's circumstances. In the early stages the prognosis may be unclear and uncertainty becomes unavoidable.

When the onset is gradual much will depend on the type and severity of the condition and the person's understanding of it. In some cases diagnosis is delayed due to investigations. During this time optimism that a cure will be available may be felt or anxiety that something dire will be revealed. If a cure is not available the effect of this information may well produce feelings of shock similar to those in the acute conditions, although some uncertainty will be relieved. If the condition is progressive (e.g. multiple sclerosis or motor neurone disease) the reaction will also be influenced both by the information given and the way it is done. If a diagnosis is given the person's knowledge about the condition will be important. Many people harbour notions about the way a condition might progress that may be quite unrealistic. In some instances an unrealistically rosy view may serve as a defence against anxiety and the costs and benefits of introducing realism have to be carefully considered. In other cases there will be fears about unpleasant developments that are unlikely or impossible and these will give rise to much unnecessary anxiety. It is important to be on the look out and probe for such fears as they are not always volunteered, especially in busy clinics.

Progression

If improvement occurs the person may be left with little or no disability. In such cases the anxieties and the uncertainties following the onset will usually disappear and a return to the normal emotional state will take place. However, for some people the event may have a prolonged emotional impact. This may take the form of a specific anxiety about a recurrence (even though this may be highly unlikely) or a more general neurotic disturbance, possibly arising from feelings of reduced control over one's fate and a heightened sense of vulnerability.

If permanent disability ensues the person is faced with having to adapt to the altered circumstances. There may be difficulties at the practical, the social (see 'Reactions of Others' below) and the psychological levels. The weeks or months following onset may be likened to the period of mourning that follows a bereavement; the person in this instance mourning the loss of part of his/her identity and having to adjust to continuing life without it. The duration of this phase will vary enormously from person to person but, as in bereavement, it can sometimes be made more bearable by counselling. Some people may develop a clear depressive illness during this period and treatment with antidepressant medication may be warranted. Motivation will be variable during the mourning phase but improve as it is passed through. Eventually a more accepting state should be reached in which the person acknowledges his/her limitations but is able to adopt a more positive approach to learning any necessary new skills and to preparing for an altered lifestyle. However, some people will never come to terms with their disability despite the passage of time and the continued efforts of family, friends and professionals. Instead they may become locked in protracted unhappiness, self-pity, withdrawal or difficult (usually demanding or irritable) behaviour. In such cases it is likely that self-esteem is strongly linked to a rigid self-image and that deviation from this image is intolerable. Disability which is the result of someone else's carelessness or negligence may prove particularly difficult to adjust to.

For those who are faced with a progressive condition reaction will be influenced by the person's expectations concerning the condition (whether true or false), the stage (or severity) that the condition has reached, the rate of decline and whether it is steady or intermittent. Many of the progressive disabling conditions are neurological and involve some cerebral deterioration in their later stages, so that reaction will also depend on organic changes in personality, emotional reactivity and degree of insight. It is therefore difficult to make more than vague general statements about the course of the reaction to progressive conditions. However, bouts of demoralization or anxiety are likely to occur throughout the course of the condition, particularly in response to any sudden deterioration, and feelings of frustration and resentment are also likely to increase in line with increasing limitations.

PSYCHOLOGICAL FACTORS

Personality and coping style

People will generally cope with acquired disability in accordance with their personalities and with their usual methods of dealing with stressful situations. For example, the person who bears adversity with fortitude is less likely to lapse into depression or self-pity than one who is less robust or who tends to feel dissatisfied with life, though exceptions do occur. The person who prides him/herself on being independent may prefer to struggle laboriously to do tasks rather than ask for help or may fail to take medication, for example analgesics, that might offer relief. The perfectionist may seek to impose the standards he/she can no longer maintain for him/herself on family or carers, usually to their annoyance. The influence of such characteristics is related to issues of self-image and self-esteem, which are discussed later.

Faced with a progressive condition, some people will be optimistic that the course will, for them, be slow and mild. Others will be pessimistic and may feel that life is already over, well in advance of any substantial disability. Some will believe, rightly or wrongly, that their actions will influence its outcome and so may engage in particular regimes of behaviour, for example of exercise or diet, and may seek new forms of treatment. Others will adopt a more passive attitude, assuming that 'what will be will be'. Some will contemplate and discuss constructively how they will cope as the condition progresses, some will wait to see what happens and others will merely worry. Some will feel unwilling to accept substantial disability and seriously consider suicide. For some, the prospect of suicide as a way out may be sufficient to allow them to cope. Plans for suicide at a certain stage in the condition may be revised once that stage is reached and deferred to the next stage, and so on. For a minority, suicide will have been regarded as the only sensible option.

Self-image and self-esteem

The extent to which disability disrupts a person's self-image, and thereby self-esteem, is probably the most important factor in determining how the person copes with disability. Each person has a view of him/herself, with perceptions of his/her physical and cognitive attributes, character, achievements and relationships with others. By self-image is meant the person's evaluation of him/herself, based on these perceptions, on a multitude of dimensions. These dimensions can be considered as descriptive bipolar scales, such as 'good–bad', 'strong–weak', 'lucky–unlucky'. By self-esteem is meant that part of his/her evaluation that is based on the dimensions that he/she considers particularly important, i.e. on those dimensions that relate to a sense of intrinsic worth. Which dimensions a person considers to be important will vary from individual to individual, being a reflection of the many influences and experiences that over the years have helped shape the person's personality. However, common ones are 'attractive–unattractive', 'strong–weak', 'clever–stupid', 'masculine–feminine', 'competent–incompetent', 'interesting–dull', 'sexually desirable–sexually undesirable',

'independent–dependent', 'important–insignificant' and 'successful–unsuccessful'. The set of dimensions that contributes most to the person's self-esteem will be referred to as 'core' dimensions. It is essential to realize that how a person relates particular physical and cognitive attributes, particular aspects of character, and particular achievements and relationships to points on any dimension is an idiosyncratic matter. Thus physical strength and financial success may be associated with being highly sexually desirable, competent and clever for one person but not for another. It is also the case that a person's rating of him/herself on a particular dimension may bear little relationship to any objective assessment or how other people would evaluate him/her. Thus two people may obtain equal examination results or be equally attractive to a third person, but may well evaluate themselves very differently on the 'clever–stupid' and 'attractive–unattractive' dimensions.

Whilst being aware of some aspects of themselves they might wish to change, most people have a generally positive self-esteem, i.e. they have a sense of intrinsic worth as humans, although the intensity and robustness of this positive self-image will vary from person to person. If particular physical or cognitive attributes, aspects of character, achievements or relationships with others are associated with strong positive evaluations on core dimensions, then loss or impairment of these will probably be associated with strong negative evaluations. Such losses or impairments will then give rise to a devalued self-esteem, i.e. a devaluation of one's sense of intrinsic worth. If substantial devaluation occurs then a negative self-esteem, i.e. a loss of one's sense of intrinsic worth, will result and emotional disturbance is likely to arise. This will often take the form of depression, but may take other forms such as anger, irritability or generally difficult and erratic behaviour.

Disability can disrupt a person's self-esteem

if the person holds stereotyped views about disabled people or people with particular disabilities, so that such people are generally viewed by the person as rating poorly on his/her core dimensions. Stereotypes get built up over the years and will contain the person's knowledge, fears and fantasies about different disabilities as derived from experience, education, gossip, media coverage and society's and peer-group values. These stereotypes may differ from disability to disability, or all be rather similar, coming under an umbrella stereotype of 'disabled' with little differentiation between conditions. Many of these stereotypes may well have considerable negative connotations and so be viewed with unease or distaste by the person. If the person then acquires a disability that he/she has endowed with strong negative connotations, it will be difficult for him/her to maintain a positive self-esteem.

Self-esteem is nonetheless still vulnerable to disability in persons who have no strong stereotyped notions about disabled people. Self-image will probably be altered by the disability, but whether self-esteem is affected depends on whether the disability involves those cognitive attributes that the person values most, i.e. those that are related to strong positive evaluations on his/her core dimensions. (The difference between this and holding a stereotype is that the person may not regard other disabled people with the same disability in a negative way, but nonetheless has negative views of him/herself because of his disability). As noted earlier, it is an idiosyncratic matter as to which physical and cognitive attributes contribute most to a person's sense of worth, so the effect of any particular disability on an individual's self-image and self-esteem will vary. An important corollary of this is that a mild disability in one sphere may be more devastating to a person's self-esteem than a severe disability in another. For example, if a person places high value on verbal skills because they imply for him/her cleverness, competence and strength,

then a mild dysphasia, causing hesitancy in speech and occasional muddling of words, will give rise to feelings of stupidity, incompetence and weakness, and may cause more distress than loss of use of a hand. Of course, the loss of a hand is unlikely to be received lightly, but the person will come to terms with this loss more quickly, and while periodic frustration might be suffered because of the limitations the loss imposes, it will not devalue his/her sense of worth or prevent him/her from feeling he/she can lead a fulfilling life to the same extent as the dysphasia will. For another person the reverse may apply; a substantial dysphasia will be reasonably well tolerated but partial functioning of the hand will be viewed as a major catastrophe.

The effect of disability on self-esteem may be direct or indirect. Some physical or cognitive attributes may be valued for their own sake, for example a person may associate physical mobility with independence and arithmetical ability with competence, so that loss or impairment of these attributes leads directly to a devaluation in self-esteem. Indirect effects arise when the disability interrupts some other aspect of life that contributes strongly to self-esteem. For example, the person may set great store on success in business or an athletic prowess, so any disablement that prevents these achievements will lead to a devaluation in self-esteem. Of course, prevention of these achievements may have other implications, such as future financial problems or loss of social contacts, which in themselves will be a cause for concern. However, it is important not to overlook self-esteem; it may be this component which underlies some problems in long-term adjustment.

The extent to which self-esteem can remain preserved following onset of disability will depend on how many other things contribute to the person's self-esteem which remain intact, for example aspects of character, achievements, relationships and other physical and cognitive attributes. The more that remain, the less devastating the particular loss or impairment will be. Counselling may assist the person to modify his/her self-image and to be flexible to those aspects that constitute self-esteem. This may help the person to regain some fulfilment in life. However, some people will maintain a very rigid and narrow view of what attributes make them worthwhile, and be impervious to counselling, possibly resenting any attempt to encourage them to examine their view.

Disablement may also cause disruption to a person's self-esteem by preventing the person from realizing fantasies or ambitions. These may be dispensable for many people, in that fantasies may be accepted as unattainable dreams and ambitions which, although desired, do not have the status of personal necessities, that is if they fail to be realized they would probably not greatly detract from self-esteem. For some people, however, fantasies or ambitions may act as a defence against a weak or negative self-esteem – 'there may not be much to me at the moment, but one day...' self-esteem would be greatly enhanced by their realization. If loss or impairment of a physical or cognitive attribute necessary to the realization of such a fantasy or ambition occurs then, whether the fantasy or ambition had any chance of success or not, the person's defence against his/her negative self-esteem will be reduced and problems in adjustment may follow.

BRAIN DAMAGE

In many conditions brain damage is either the cause of disabilities, as in stroke, or a contributor to the overall picture, as may occur in multiple sclerosis. However, as well as giving rise to disabilities, brain damage may influence how the person reacts to and copes with them. The main influences are described below.

Personality change

Personality change resulting from brain damage can be regarded as a disability in its own right (in that the change is usually in an adverse direction) and it may also colour the reaction to other disabilities.

Among the common changes are reduced tolerance to frustration and thus a greater tendency to be angry or tearful when the disability causes inconvenience; an increased tendency to worry or to become absorbed in one's own problems so that the person becomes preoccupied with the difficulties caused by the disability; an increased disposition to depression so that in the case of progressive disability deterioration will be harder to bear; rigidity of thought, such that the person becomes less flexible in approaching problems caused by the disability and less amenable to practical advice or counselling.

In some cases, however, most noticeably those involving frontal-lobe damage, the change may give rise to emotional blunting or euphoria so that the person, although aware of the disability and the limitations caused by it, seems to lack appropriate concern. This could perhaps be confused with a good adjustment to the disability if it were not for the fact that the lack of concern will extend to many other problems that might confront the person, and there will be a lack of motivation to deal with them. In addition, other aspects of the 'frontal-lobe syndrome' may well be present, such as contented apathy, impulsiveness or disinhibition. In cases of very severe disability lack of concern may be regarded as a blessing, but it will also mean that in instances where remedial therapy could potentially make a useful impact there will be a lack of motivation to engage. This type of personality change is often seen with head injuries. It may also occur in progressive conditions, for example in the later stages of multiple sclerosis where it sometimes supersedes an earlier depressive change.

Cognitive impairments

As with personality change, cognitive impairments can themselves be regarded as disabilities but they may sometimes also affect how people adjust to other disabilities. For example, severe dysphasia may make it difficult or impossible for the person to comprehend relevant information as regards prognosis or decisions about treatment and so give rise to anxiety or lack of cooperation. Severe dysphasia may also prevent detailed discussion of feelings and circumstances and so hinder counselling or render it impossible. Similarly, memory problems may limit the use of counselling because of the person's difficulty in retaining information from session to session.

Two specific forms of cognitive impairment which have considerable bearing on adjustment to disability, i.e. lack of insight and neglect, are discussed in the following sections.

Lack of insight

Brain damage can result in lack of insight into the various other problems caused by the brain damage. Partial lack of insight will result in the person failing to appreciate the full extent of the disability and its implications. Complete lack of insight will result in denial of disability. In such cases the person may claim that his/her personality is unchanged despite friends and relatives describing him/her as 'completely different', claim that his/her memory is normal despite being blatantly amnesic or claim that he/she can walk despite being paralysed. Confrontation may elicit some fleeting acknowledgement of the problem, but little interest in it, and it may be rationalized as reasonable, 'I wouldn't expect to remember that', or temporary, 'the leg seems a bit stiff today'. As with lack of concern, lack of insight can seem a blessing if disability is very severe but it can also reduce motivation to engage in therapy.

Neglect

Substantial cerebral lesions that involve the parietal lobes can produce neglect of the contralateral side of the body or of the contralateral visual field. Severe neglect may, for example, result in failure to groom the contralateral side of the body, failure to move the contralateral limbs and failure to respond to any stimuli in the contralateral hemispace, such that objects placed there are ignored and food on that side of the plate is left uneaten. Thus, the person behaves as if he has a hemiparesis or hemianopia of which he is unaware. Actual hemiparesis or hemianopia are not essential for the phenomenon of neglect to be present but they often coexist with it. When mild, neglect will be more sporadic or be manifest as 'inattention', i.e. be discernible only when the person is required to devote attention to the ipsilateral side of the body or hemispace simultaneously. Neglect or inattention are most commonly seen following stroke, and particularly following stroke within the right hemisphere. Severe neglect usually declines over the course of weeks or months but may leave a persistent residual inattention. Whilst it is possible that neglect or inattention may occasionally have a psychodynamic origin, they are generally considered to reflect dysfunction of cognitive attentional or representational processes.

REACTIONS OF OTHERS

The reaction of family, friends and other acquaintances, for example work colleagues, will have an important bearing on how the person copes. Generally, the closer the relationship the more important the reaction of the other person will be. If the person is accepted by others despite his/her disability, then this will help to maintain self-esteem, although sometimes even the most sincere and committed efforts by those with the closest relationship are insufficient to overcome a severe loss of self-esteem. However, if the person meets with rejection then self-esteem is, not surprisingly, liable to be devalued. Rejection at a sexual level may be particularly dispiriting (and frustrating). Some people find disablement in others renders them sexually unattractive, so although they may wish to continue living and caring for their disabled partner, they feel unable or unwilling to indulge in a sexual relationship.

Those with close relationships to the disabled person, i.e. spouses, parents or children, are likely to be the carers if the disablement necessitates this. Mostly this care is carried out with understanding and good grace, but sometimes the carer feels over-burdened or unjustly burdened. If such feelings are communicated to the disabled person, he/she in turn is likely to feel guilty, insecure or rejected. Sometimes the disabled person feels rejected despite no such communication from the carers. This can arise because the person had a low self-esteem or was prone to anxiety before the onset of disablement or has developed these features since.

Those who care for the disabled sometimes react by over-protection or over-caring. This may arise through pity, a desire not to see the disabled person suffer any more, concern that the person might become more disabled or die (e.g. if the person has suffered a heart attack or stroke) or it may be an attempt to assuage feelings of guilt that one's actions or negligence might have caused or contributed to the disability. Unless the disabled person enjoys a dependent and fussed-over existence, over-protection will tend to foster anger and irritation.

Often non-disabled people feel uncomfortable when talking to disabled people because they find the disability repulsive or because they feel great pity and therefore do not know what to say. They may be afraid they will say something upsetting, such as talking about activities that the disabled person is unable to enjoy. Some able-bodied people will deal with their feelings by avoiding disabled people, looking away from them, ignoring them in conversation or talking to them in a patronizing manner. These actions are likely to give rise to feelings of rejection and anger in the disabled person. As time goes on the able-bodied person may overcome his/her discomfort and interaction will be less painful for both. However, further awkward encounters may become a long-term hazard for disabled people as they encounter new people. For some it may always rankle, whilst others will rightly interpret it as a problem of the non-disabled person and either ignore it or actively seek to put the non-disabled person at ease.

SUPPORTIVE NETWORK

The more severe the disability the more likely the person will have to give up occupation or leisure activities. This may considerably reduce opportunities for social interaction and may therefore lead to social isolation. If mobility is substantially impaired then opportunities for socializing will be further reduced. Visits to relatives and friends and outings will become difficult or impossible, and the person will become reliant on others for social contact. A supportive network of family and close friends may be vital. Visits from work colleagues and friends made through specific leisure pursuits are liable to tail off over the course of a year while relatives and long-standing friends, assuming they live reasonably close at hand, tend to be more regular visitors.

People vary in how much they value social contact, but for those to whom it is important but lack nearby close friends and relatives, feelings of loneliness, boredom and even worthlessness may result. Many will deal with these problems by attendance at day centres, but for some this will be an unacceptable solution as mixing with other disabled people will be seen as distasteful or second best, and may be more threatening to self-esteem than the loneliness.

Depending on the nature and the severity of disablement there may be partial or total dependence on others for the needs of everyday living such as shopping, cooking, cleaning and self-care. Those with a supportive network are likely to be more able to remain living at home, either with their family or by themselves. Therefore, despite the dependence, there will be opportunity to retain as much home comfort, community contact and independence as possible which will help to preserve a sense of well-being. For those without family or friends to help out there may be no alternative but to give up their home and accept residential or nursing-home care, a move which may be strongly resented and resisted.

Reactions to dependence are likely to be mixed. Dependence may be resented because it devalues the self-esteem or because it makes the person feel a burden to others (whether or not others communicate such a message). This resentment may be expressed in various ways, such as demoralization, guilt, and hostility to the carers. On the other hand the person may feel grateful to his/her carers and, because of his/her dependence, also concerned not to upset them in case of rejection by them. This may cause anxiety and the need for reassurance that the carers want him/her, and may produce a state of passive compliance with the carer's wishes, with the person feeling unable to complain or express negative feelings. Not uncommonly both types of feelings will be present, i.e. resentment and concern not to upset, and this may give rise to forms of 'passive' aggression, by which is meant difficult behaviour for which the person cannot seemingly be blamed. An unexplicable worsening of physical symptoms, such as incontinence, might be an example. However, it must be emphasized that such an interpretation should not be made lightly, and should have supporting evidence from enquiry into the person's feelings.

FINANCIAL SECURITY

Despite the persisting truth of the cliché that money does not buy happiness, the material comforts money can buy may help to give freedom from some of the demoralizing effects of deprivation. Disability may result in loss of employment. Spouses or parents may find themselves giving up work in order to care for the disabled person. Disability may therefore give rise to indefinite financial hardship for the disabled person and his family. This can exacerbate frustration and social isolation and lead to additional strain on self-esteem and on relationships. Most disabled people and their families are forced to rely on state benefits and allowances but these are usually insufficient to allow more than a basic level of subsistence. Although local authorities provide various forms of support in order to allow people to continue to live at home, there are often shortages and waiting lists and, increasingly, the individual is being expected to contribute to the cost of care. Thus, being financially well off can allow the person to remedy the inadequacies of state provisions and to have more control over his/her life. It can also help give freedom from guilt and worry over how dependents are to be supported and thereby help to retain self-esteem.

QUALITY OF PROFESSIONAL CARE

From the onset of the condition the disabled person will come into contact with a variety of professional carers. The person's physical and material well-being will be influenced by their competence, but unless substantial negligence occurs it is the manner in which they give their care that will have the greatest impact on the disabled person's well-being.

The person's level of anxiety is most likely to be influenced by the behaviour of professionals. This is particularly important in the days or weeks following the onset of disability. At that time the person will have been faced with a sudden change in circumstances or will perhaps be undergoing a series of seemingly mysterious investigations. He/she is likely to feel frightened and have many questions about the future, and will hope that the professionals will have at least some of the answers. The willingness of the professional staff to sit and listen to worries, to accept and understand them without censure and, if possible, to proffer information and advice, will go a long way in helping to reduce anxiety. Conversely, if professional staff appear abrupt, remote, too busy to listen, or uninterested or even dismissive of the person's worries (so that he/she is made to feel stupid or inadequate), then anxiety is likely to be raised and motivation or morale may decline. There may, of course, be many instances in which the professionals are unable to provide the information or give the reassurances that the person seeks. In such instances some professionals will prefer to be remote in order to not appear useless or to avoid unpleasant feelings of helplessness. This remoteness is unlikely to help. It may be better to sit and discuss the limitations on providing what the patient seeks in a sympathetic and unhurried manner.

Most people will readily talk about their worries if given a secure (i.e. sympathetic and unhurried) atmosphere. Some, however, will still hold back because they fear their anxieties will make them seem stupid. It is, therefore, important to enquire about the person's apprehensions in a manner that actively and sincerely reassures him/her that they are natural. It is also important to explore and acknowledge the anxieties that anyone who will be caring for the disabled person may have and, providing there is no conflict with confidentiality, to proffer advice and information. Any reduction in the carer's anxiety will be beneficial to the person being cared for. Even if there are questions that cannot be answered, or problems that cannot be solved, the fact that the professional is prepared to listen and shows understanding can give comfort to both the disabled person and the carer.

FURTHER READING

Robertson, S.E. and Brown, R.L. (eds) (1992) *Rehabilitation Counselling: approaches in the field of disability*, Chapman & Hall, London.
Stewart, W. (1985) *Counselling in Rehabilitation*, Croom Helm, London.

5 Rehabilitation in primary care

J. McMullan and S. Kahtan

WORKING AND LEARNING TOGETHER

This chapter considers the way in which those in primary care work with one another; with disabled people and their families and associates; and with relevant agencies in hospital and community. It goes on to explore how these working relationships may be used to further undergraduate, vocational and continuing education.

When the NHS began in 1948 most general practitioners had surgeries in their own homes and many had access to cottage hospitals. There have been substantial developments since (Hasler, 1994). In the 1960s some Medical Officers of Health (who then employed district nurses) began to attach nurses to practices, one of the earliest attachment schemes being in Winchester (Swift and McDougall, 1965). The 1966 contract helped to modernize and enlarge premises and paid 70% of general practitioners' staff salaries.

Hasler identified a core team composed of general practitioners, nurses and practice managers, and a support team. He includes in the support team, amongst others, occupational therapists, physiotherapists, psychologists and speech therapists. A report published after wide consultation by the Royal College of General Practitioners (Stott, 1996) adopts this concept but is less specific about the support team. Practice nurses are firmly established, an increasing role for nurses is likely, and future developments must allow for the professional aspirations of nurse practitioners now in training.

Attachment of district nurses helped to overcome some of the problems, especially those of communication, described by Hockey (1966). District nurses remain the most important source of help in primary care for disabled people. It is they who ensure adequate aftercare for patients discharged from hospital and work in liaison schemes with hospitals. These have improved greatly in recent years. These nurses are the best point of contact for the rehabilitation team and should be invited to team meetings.

The role of the general practitioner

Basic competence in diagnosis and treatment is essential, but management of problems needs personal support, not just pure science:

1. Early treatment of disease which can also prevent or limit disability.
2. Help with practical problems.
3. Obtaining specialist advice.
4. Supervision of continuing treatment.
5. Coordination of help in the community.
6. Personal support for patients and helpers.

This can be illustrated by arthritis. When help is first sought for painful joints, clarifying the effects on daily life and responding to under-

Rehabilitation of the Physically Disabled Adult. Edited by C. John Goodwill, M. Anne Chamberlain and Chris Evans. Published in 1997 by Stanley Thornes (Publishers) Ltd, Cheltenham. ISBN 0-7487-3183-0.

lying concerns are as fundamental as the diagnosis. Discussion, a treatment plan and the way a prescription is given are at least as important as the drug chosen. At this stage help is needed to allay anxieties, to foster healthy attitudes and to continue normal life. If the arthritis does not settle down the general practitioner must judge the time for referral, preferably before the patient asks for a second opinion, and well before avoidable damage has occurred.

In established severe rheumatoid arthritis, the general practitioner will have sought specialist advice and, as well as medication, there will often have been splinting, counselling, aids to daily living and social work arranged at the hospital. The general practitioner must know what has been done to support the patient's efforts to remain independent and fill in any gaps. Attention to the details of problems of daily living, reinforcing the advice of the nurse and community occupational therapist, is needed. Interest in the wider aspects of patients' lives, such as work, family, sport, hobbies and clubs, is rewarding. This may often be part of any consultation but can be of particular importance and help to a severely disabled person.

EXPERIENCE TEACHES

There are many aspects of severe disability which were not covered in the undergraduate training of many general practitioners now established in practice. Awareness, understanding, knowledge and teamwork are linked and overlapping. They are important in all general practice but especially in helping disabled people. They may come with experience but must be fostered in training. Disabled people seek normal human rights such as access, choice, involvement in decision making and autonomy. Understanding this makes it easier to help appropriately and to evaluate barriers to acceptance of help. Concern about apparent trivialities may hide undisclosed anxieties. Many people tend to play down their disability and this is healthy. This must be taken into account whilst bolstering abilities and attitudes.

AUTONOMY

Disability is not the same as illness. When a stable situation is reached, disabled people may not seek medical advice very often. They may save up their problems, large and small, for one consultation. It may suit the disabled person to be visited at home, although the general practice building should be accessible. Sufficient time can then be given and home surroundings appreciated so that a warm and mutually supportive relationship develops over the years.

A disabled person usually become expert in managing their disability and this needs to be recognized by professionals. Anyone admitted to hospital loses some autonomy and this may affect disabled people disproportionately if hospital staff do not understand (Prince of Wales Advisory Group on Disability, 1992).

LISTENING AND COMMUNICATION

Sensitive listening and observation are basic (Fletcher and Freeling, 1988). It is necessary to listen carefully to what is said, the choice of words, the inflexion and the context. An apparently offhand remark may be full of meaning. It is important to note any specific problems or requests, whether from patients, relatively or colleagues.

Telling the diagnosis

Good communication is important, especially in telling the diagnosis. This involves both giving information and being sensitive to the response of the patient. Eye contact is needed. Whenever possible, the partner or closest relative should be present. Often bad news has to be broken. Useful advice on doing this has been published (Brewin, 1991).

The Romford Neurocare Plan (Findley and Oxtoby, 1990) has developed a coordinated process to explain to patients the implications of their diagnosis and a 20-minute video is available. This shows the team telling a man with early Parkinsonism and his wife the suggested management, so that the manner and timing of advice will help them to accept things they do not want to hear. Above all, they must be involved in a full assessment of all the relevant factors.

INFORMATION

To know how to obtain help is more important than having detailed factual knowledge (which fast becomes outdated). It is necessary to know of the existence of aids to daily living, home adaptations, orthotics, special footwear, wheelchairs, speech aids, environmental controls and other equipment for disability. The details of how these are obtained are set out by Mandelstam (1991), and information is available from rehabilitation medicine departments and therapy staff and from Disabled Living Centres, whose work includes advice on equipment (Part Eight). Knowledge about special centres, for example for driving assessment, head or spinal injury, epilepsy or respiratory failure, may be needed. Sources of respite care must be established.

Housing, clubs, day care, holidays, recreation, sheltered work and financial matters such as benefits are best dealt with by social workers (Chapter 53).

ASSESSMENT

Full assessment may require consideration of a range of factors, listed below.

Social background

- Family, neighbours, friends
- Housing: suitability and security of tenure

- Occupation, income, allowances
- Church, clubs, social activities, holidays

Current state

- Diagnosis, medication
- Mobility, hearing, vision
- Activities of daily living
- Hobbies, interests
- Mood, orientation, mental state
- Personal relationships, sex

Services

- Nurse, bath helper, home carer, daily help, night attendant
- Physiotherapist, occupational therapist, speech therapist
- Meals on wheels, day centre, day hospital
- Volunteers, societies, charities

Aids and adaptations

- Walking aids
- Hearing aids, telephone adaptations, low visual aids
- Stair rail, bath or toilet facilities
- Door opener, emergency call system, environmental controls

The general practitioner will not assess all these factors personally, but needs to be aware of them. The assessment will be a team effort by doctor, nurse, therapists and social worker with the disabled person and the principal carer. A record of the facts and an initial list of problems with possible solutions is agreed. Some items can be dealt with immediately, others must await discussion by the team as a whole.

TEAMWORK

For teams to work well the composition of the team must be known, the various members should understand one another's roles and have sufficient time together to establish common objectives and working methods. The disabled person and any carers are part of the team and their interests are central. Working in interdisciplinary teams is considered more fully in Chapter 6.

Nurses, physiotherapists, occupational therapists and speech therapists all have practical skills; they also have much to offer by way of advice and support. Therapists spend longer with patients and get to know their problems, physical and psychological, more intimately. Doctors who listen to them will learn much about their patients and sometimes about themselves. This can happen in teamwork and is essential for the team if it is to function effectively. Some medical students now learn about working in teams, but most general practitioners and those passing through general practitioner vocational training need to know more. Clinical psychologists and social workers are less well known to doctors and yet have much to offer. Meetings of the team are the best way to find out how they work.

MEETINGS

Full team meetings are very time consuming but may be the most efficient method of organizing help for severely disabled people when they first join the practice or after a major change in the level of disability. If possible, the disabled person and principal carer should be present at these meetings. Meetings should be structured, kept to an agreed time, be properly led and decisions recorded.

Whilst the general practitioner's first assessment will cover the usual clinical features and must include nutrition, continence and pressure areas, three other aspects may be considered.

1. How does the patient spend the day? What help is needed at various times? If alone what fills the time? How are the nights?
2. What sort of life was led before the disability? How close were family, friends and work colleagues? What hobbies, interests or social activities existed? How have these changed?
3. What are the needs and aspirations of the disabled person? Are they realistic?

A keyworker may be chosen to aid implementation and as a reference point for future action. After the first meeting of the full team, the keyworker keeps in touch with the disabled person and arranges any further help needed. This obviates a confusing series of calls by various members of the team. Further full meetings may not be essential, but it may be useful if the team meets at predetermined intervals (Ward, Crates and Skeates, 1993).

When a stable situation is reached the general practitioner should not withdraw entirely. Visits at long intervals, perhaps at an anniversary, are welcomed and good practice. Willis (1986) describes a simple computer listing to help this. It is also important to visit promptly for key episodes such as skin problems, urinary or respiratory infections.

Clear and accessible records of disabled people are necessary to monitor care. Any member of the practice team should be able to add a name to the list if the disability is causing problems significant to the patient and they agree. Usually only the first three points below need to be considered initially:

- identification: name, date of birth, etc.;
- nature and severity of disability, e.g. mobility, ADL, sensory deprivation;
- causative disease or impairment;
- family and social background, including carer;
- services required or used;
- aids, adaptations, etc.;
- unmet needs.

The patient should never be the passive recipient of services, but must be actively involved, with the relatives, in the process of assessment, the setting of goals and the development of a plan. They should, whenever possible, help map out the future, and this will help them to adjust their aspirations and fears to reality. The problems of each patient must be worked out with them and, although many situations may be similar, there is no place for rigidly set regimes.

TOWARDS A COMPREHENSIVE SERVICE

For the majority of adults with physical disability hospital care is a short episode, albeit of considerable importance. Rehabilitation however may be a lengthy phase in the life of a disabled person. It may have variable outcomes: some will be fully restored to their previous state, but more often the person will have to adapt to residual disability and build on their various remaining abilities. Some will have to contend with progressive disability, and effective rehabilitation will be most important to them. This means that plans for rehabilitation have to be comprehensive and use general practice skills and those of community and hospital rehabilitation. All are required, and the primary care team is central to providing the advice and services that the patient needs.

The general practitioner will work closely with the community nurse, and other members of the team will be the physiotherapist who will particularly work with problems of mobility, the occupational therapist particularly involved in activities of daily living, aids, appliances, wheelchairs and home adaptations. A speech therapist is needed for those with speech and/or swallowing problems, a social worker for housing, benefits and social needs, and a counselling and/or clinical psychology service will also be of value where it is available. The consultant in rehabilitation medicine will be

needed if the disability is complex and persisting.

Voluntary organizations are invaluable in helping those with chronic disability. Meetings are essential in order to agree the problems to be solved and the possible solutions to be offered to the patient so that goals may be agreed by all those involved. If there is inconsistency in the approach and advice from different professionals there will be major problems for the patients.

MEDICAL EDUCATION

The General Medical Council has for many years advocated a reduction in the amount of factual data to be memorized and urged self-education, critical thought and the evaluation of evidence. The Council says (General Medical Council, 1992) that general clinical training should enable pre-registration house officers to 'investigate patients' problems and plan and carry out treatment, including the requirement for rehabilitation when appropriate. They should learn how to involve patients in decisions about themselves. They must also learn to communicate effectively with patients' families and with medical and other colleagues involved in patient care.' Similar and more detailed recommendations about communication skills, teamwork and problem solving are made for undergraduate education and the training of specialists.

'I have learned much from my teachers, and from my colleagues more than my teachers, and from my students more than from all' (Haggadah, 4th Century). If the word 'patients' is substituted for 'students' this makes a good text for the rehabilitation team. Unfortunately, the principle of learning from one another has not been prominent in the education of the medical and allied professions. Certainly we all learn much from patients, but learning from one another has tended to be limited by traditional divisions. The rehabilitation team is an ideal setting for remedying these defects. The UK

Centre for the Advancement of Inter Professional Education (CAIPE) was founded in 1987 and became a registered charity in 1991. Its purpose is to 'promote and support high quality developments in the practice and research of interprofessional education and training in health and social care in order to improve user and carer focused collaborative care' (CAIPE, 1995).

The following sections discuss, with special reference to primary care, the situation in undergraduate, vocational and continuing education and suggest ways forward.

Undergraduate education

The undergraduate years are among the most intensive learning experience in medical, nursing and therapy education. They are formative years, when students observe their elders and absorb philosophies as well as bald facts. Unfortunately many of their teachers and examiners will have scant interest in rehabilitation medicine. This prevailing attitude needs to be countered strongly with charismatic and effective teaching on disability medicine and rehabilitation.

The end result of a good, all-round education should be a graduate who looks at every patient and immediately asks:

1. How does this patient's condition affect lifestyle?
2. Are there likely to be long-term consequences of this condition, and how will those affect lifestyle?
3. What can the team do to reduce the effect on lifestyle?

Rehabilitation should be as much a part of patient management as the more historical components such as drug or surgical treatment.

Much has been written about the aims of education on disability and rehabilitation (McCrory and Marrone, 1984; Inman and Kahtan, 1994; General Medical Council, 1980). Many papers have also documented the remarkably limited rehabilitation information conveyed during an average undergraduate medical education (Marshall, Haines and Chamberlain, 1991; British Society of Rehabilitation Medicine, 1992). More recently, there have been a large number of experiments in the best approach to achieving educational goals in this area.

A study of current practice in undergraduate medical education on disability and rehabilitation (Inman and Kahtan, 1994) showed a tendency to focus excessively on disabling conditions which produce gross locomotor disability. Medical students are most likely to meet rehabilitation teams and consider the rehabilitation needs when they study conditions such as spinal injury and stroke. Nursing students seem to fare better, with increasing emphasis on completing ADL (Activities of Daily Living) assessments of **every** patient they 'clerk', while therapist training encourages a broad view of the patient's problems. It may be partly for this reason that some of the more successful developments in this field have involved multidisciplinary education (Inman and Kahtan, 1994).

Nurses are directly involved in helping those with difficulties in ADL, and tasks such as feeding and washing are far more likely to fall to a student nurse than to a medical student. Medical students can benefit from the increased awareness of nursing students who have had such experiences. Conversely, nursing students will benefit from a more analytical approach to the causes and consequences of disabling diseases. Education offers an ideal opportunity for medical, nursing and therapy students to begin learning together as much as possible.

The outcome of combined education is refreshing, as witnessed in a series of medical students who were shown a 'short case' patient with cerebellar ataxia. The examiner's question was 'What strikes you about this patient?' after they had seen him walk across the room and attempt to shake the examiner by the hand. The medical students responded variously, according to their different aptitudes and levels of preparation, with remarks about the nature of the gait disturbance, the intention tremor and the possible underlying causes. One student proved an exception; her immediate response was 'Excuse me, but would you like me to pass you your stick?' These floors are a bit slippery, aren't they?' Her comment was directed at the patient, not the examiner. In a split second, this student had grasped the essential facts, that the patient was wobbly on his legs and unsupported; she had looked around, spotted the patient's walking stick next to his coat, and suggested this as a solution to prevent the fall she anticipated. It transpired that this student was a former nurse who had subsequently decided to study medicine. Such pragmatism, combined with a knowledge of other aspects of medicine, would produce an ideal member of the primary care team.

Assuming that medical, nursing and therapy establishments are prepared to organize combined educational sessions, which core issues should be addressed? To some extent the factual content is of less importance than conveying the right attitude towards the subject.

KEY AREAS IN TEACHING ABOUT REHABILITATION OF THE DISABLED ADULT

- Epidemiology
- Disability awareness and communication skills
- Assessment of function (including ADL)
- Prevention of further disability
- Aids and adaptations for ADL, finance, employment, driving and outdoor mobility
- Bladder and Bowel continence and sexual function
- Seminars with disablement facilitators/disability simulation exercises

This needs some amplification:

Epidemiology

Students can usefully discuss the prevalence of common conditions which lead to physical disability among adults, including heart disease, chronic obstructive airways disease, obesity, sensory impairment, arthritis, as well as neurological disorders such as stroke, epilepsy, multiple sclerosis and motor neurone disease. Students should discuss the relative prevalence of these disorders so that they are less prone to focus on the obvious disabilities and can learn to understand physical disabilities which may be invisible. They can be asked to consider whether the disability is mild or severe, static, fluctuating or progressive.

Disability awareness and communication skills

Students need to grasp that every patient, and indeed every person, has abilities and disabilities. These may be physical, intellectual, psychological or social, major (e.g. total blindness) or minor (mild presbyopia). Students may then be asked to consider their own abilities and disabilities. Depending on the group rapport and size, these analyses may be shared among the group. The end result should be to dissolve the false dichotomy between patients seen as disabled and those people seen as able-bodied. This has two advantages. For the obviously disabled patient, it will result in less obtrusively 'special' treatment. For the apparently able-bodied patient, it will result in a more creative approach to the impact of disease on their lifestyle and addressing their minor disabilities.

Assessment of function (including ADL)

It is fortunately undeniable that after the undergraduate years, increasing pressure on time will prevent all members of a primary care team from going through this assessment with all patients. Nevertheless, if they all understand what is involved in assessments, and have experience of making such assessments, they will be better able to interpret their colleagues' findings. Primary care is becoming more multidisciplinary than ever before and it is necessary for all to have a basic understanding of the skills and contributions made by other members of the rehabilitation team. All need to realize that there are problems such as incontinence which the patient may not mention unless asked.

When considering the physically disabled adult, screening systems such as the GALS locomotor screening system are useful (Doherty *et al.*, 1992). This enables any health care professional to make a rapid assessment of a patient's locomotor abilities and impairments, and to record them briefly and comprehensively.

Prevention of further disability

It is suggested that only moderate emphasis is placed on aspects such as preventing heart disease and obesity, which will be covered in other sectors of the curriculum. Instead, the emphasis should be placed on preventing deterioration in adults who have a physical disability: for example, for patients with respiratory disease, prophylaxis may include vaccination against influenza; for patients who are bedbound or chairbound, teaching may concentrate on preventing pressure sores and managing incontinence.

For all those with major disability, psychological prophylaxis is of critical importance. All health professionals should be encouraged to think about the impact of disability, the concepts of secondary gain, the patient's support systems and how these can be supplemented. Staff should understand the vicious cycle of disability, depression, lack of motivation, increasing disability and increasing isolation.

Aids and adaptations, ADL, finance, employment, driving and outdoor mobility

It is the underlying attitude to these topics which must be taught, rather than the details. The intended result is that every student should look at every patient and consider them. If the patient is experiencing difficulties in any of these areas, are there ways in which they could be helped to overcome these difficulties?

If aids and adaptations could help, does the patient want them? A Disabled Living Centre can help by showing alternatives. It is useless to prescribe orthoses which will not be worn, and hearing aids which will not be used. All aids and adaptations have attendant costs, both for the original provision and for repair, maintenance and replacement. Many disabled people have poor financial resources, yet fail to claim needed allowances, and health staff do not usually understand the details of the various benefits but should know where to refer for help. One needs to know when disability is threatening a person's employment or when isolation is due to lack of transport, finance or support.

The aim of teaching is not to produce a graduate who knows everything about the subject, but a graduate who knows where to refer the patient for specialist advice.

Bladder and bowel continence and sexual function

The causes of these problems may range from complex neurological lesions to simple housing difficulties, such as a toilet being accessible to a patient with a prostate problem and osteoarthritis. Primary care personnel are well situated to study the situation within which continence poses difficulties. They can assess the relative contributions of the patient's environment and the underlying condition. Undergraduate attachments to general practice can help the student to understand such interactions and the difficulties that those with continence problems have when they try to go outside the home to work, to shop or for social activities.

Most importantly, students should be taught to probe a little, particularly about matters of continence and sexual function. This approach will benefit a wide range of people without any ostensible physical disability. Post-menopausal women, for instance, may feel unable to consult their general practitioner about vaginal dryness; they may feel that the problem is trivial or that it would be too embarrassing to broach the subject. Much suffering could be relieved if more doctors and nurses could offer a matter-of-fact but sympathetic approach to these areas.

Seminars with disablement facilitators/ disability simulation exercises

These two exercises are offered as alternatives since each has its supporters and its detractors. The aim of this session should be integrative, rounding off the student's appreciation of the impact of physical disability and the value of rehabilitation. Talking with users of services is one method of achieving this. Small group seminars, of six to ten students, meet with a disablement facilitator who needs to be carefully chosen. It is important to avoid a facilitator who merely outlines dreadful treatment by doctors and nurses in the past. The session should focus on what transforms medical, nursing and therapy contact into a positive experience. Students should feel unintimidated and able to ask questions, rather than being on the receiving end of a tirade or a monologue.

This method has advantages, but it has significant disadvantages. Recruitment of suitable facilitators is difficult but is central to the success or failure of the seminars. Interviewing and selecting potential facilitators, and training them in the necessary techniques, is time-consuming and outside the realm of accustomed practice. Some of the difficulties

can be surmounted by consulting organizations of disabled people which offer a rich source of highly motivated and confident people with disabilities. Students will remember what a competent person with disability tells or shows them. Even so, the small group seminar is not an easy option. When it is good, it is very very good, but when it is bad, it is truly horrid.

Disability simulation exercises are much easier to organize. Many medical schools have introduced such schemes (Inman and Kahtan, 1994) in which students spend a day in a wheelchair or move round a shopping precinct with opaque glasses. Again, there are positive and negative aspects. Many students do learn something of the frustrations and limitations of physical disability. Others find the experience traumatic; they feel fraudulent and uncomfortable that their activities may cause offence to people who are really confined to wheelchairs or who genuinely have a major visual handicap. Furthermore, the experience is necessarily short lived, so it teaches nothing of the long-term issues. It can also be argued that students would do better to achieve their understanding of patients' limitations and frustrations by listening to patients, rather than trying to extrapolate from their own brief experience of being 'diabetic for a day' with marbles in their shoes and three pairs of rubber gloves on their hands.

When these exercises are performed, they should be sensitively organized. No student should be made miserable by being compelled to adopt a role in which they feel uncomfortable. As a rough guide, the tutor or facilitator should not ask the students to do anything which they would not do themselves. If the students spend the day in a wheelchair, so should their tutor or facilitator. Such exercises are probably best kept within the medical or nursing school premises, and they should be optional.

A combination of both techniques may be most effective, but is also difficult to organize.

If there is nobody available who has the necessary time, motivation and charisma, it may be better not to attempt either. Badly organized sessions may have a net negative effect. On the other hand, well-organized sessions may have a lasting impact on the way a student thinks about disability (Inman and Kahtan, 1994). Sessions such as these can be extremely powerful and are useful in overcoming the inertia of established thought patterns, particularly in postgraduate education.

VOCATIONAL TRAINING FOR GENERAL PRACTICE

The Leeuwenhorst Group appointed by the second European Conference on the Teaching of General Practice (1975) produced 21 educational aims for general practitioner training. At least one-third of these are relevant to physical disability and many are similar to the General Medical Council recommendations relating health to personal, family and social circumstances, with diagnoses taking account of physical, psychological and social factors. They emphasize cooperation, understanding and problem solving.

To become a principle in general practice in the UK, 3 years training in approved posts must be completed satisfactorily and at least one of these years must be spent as a registrar in general practice. General practitioner trainers are themselves trained in educational methods and they and their practice premises and organization must be approved. Registrars have one tutorial with their trainer and one-day or half-day for group study a week. General practitioner course organizers supervise the whole programme and advise trainers and registrars. Study sessions may amount to only 60 or less half-day sessions in the year, and the many topics to be covered are decided jointly, but with considerable regard to the suggestions of the learners. Clearly physical disability offers important practical and educational opportunities, but

course organizers and trainers who have had little or no education themselves in physical disability may not realize this. Nor will the topic be suggested by registrars who have had little undergraduate experience. This may alter with improved undergraduate education.

General practitioner trainers

The Royal College of General Practitioners in the UK has a register of special interests declared by college members. In 1992, 54 trainers with an interest in physical disability were asked by postal questionnaire to give three points they considered important for doctors entering general practice (McMullan, 1993). The replies suggested that tutorials should cover the following areas:

1. The patient as a person, family background, aspirations and goals.
2. Assessment of the personal and home surroundings, linking this to help with practical psychological and sexual problems.
3. Equipment, occupational and recreational opportunities, holidays, respite care, allowances and many other practical issues. Helping the team to provide the appropriate help and monitoring long-term care.

Practical experience is also needed. When registrars first join their practices they may spend a day visiting patients with the attached community nurse. This will usually include visits to disabled people and give an opportunity to see and discuss problems with them in their homes. This early experience may not mean a lot to doctors fresh from hospital medicine, and the trainer should, after a few weeks, introduce the topic. Most can be learned direct from the disabled person and the problems of one or two such patients can form the basis for a tutorial. The registrar will need to be directed towards suitable patients and to spend about an hour in their home. They will pick up more information if they have a list of important points to discover (McMullen, 1993).

The young doctor will learn much about good discharge planning by following a person disabled by a condition such as stroke from the hospital into their home in the community. If the registrar is informed when the patient is admitted to hospital, it should be possible to visit and to be involved in at least one of the hospital team meetings before discharge, to see the various members of the team working together, and later, in conjunction with the patient, carers, community nurse and others concerned, how well the patient's needs have been met. A good account of stroke management for general practice gives, in less than 100 small pages, what must be considered, and sets out concisely general principles for helping where disability is due to other causes (Wade, 1988). Such an exercise can be instructive and encouraging to the patient.

Some disabled people become very independent; much can be learned from these patients, and visiting them allows insight into their ways of maintaining their independence.

Day-release courses

Only one report of vocational training has been found (Heyes, 1992). Dr Janet Heyes continued as a general practitioner trainer, practising from a wheelchair, after a sudden paraplegia. She says 'hospital training in undergraduate medical teaching may perpetuate the belief that if some degree of cure is not possible then there is "nothing to be done". This sense of futility is very unpleasant and almost always wrong but, because it is unpleasant, it leads to unease, avoidance and less than optimum care.' The aim of this special addition to a Liverpool vocational training course was 'to change the medical model from diagnosis and care to improvement in qualify of life and function'.

There are many possible approaches to learning about physical disability. The one suggested here (McMullen, 1993) seeks active involvement to discover the essentials. There are three main elements:

1. **Catching the attention**. This may be done by a short video of one or two disabled patients, by asking them to present their problems in person (see undergraduate education, above, for difficulties), or a nurse, therapist or doctor may give the essentials of the subject.

2. The small **body of knowledge** about aids and equipment, home adaptations, wheelchairs, speech aids, environmental controls and other equipment can then be covered. Ideally an occupational therapist will do this describing their schemes of assessment. A nurse or social worker may give their special insights and deal briefly with housing, occupation, clubs, recreation, day or respite care, finance and allowances. Emphasis will be on where to find information, not learning details.

3. The third element is a **sharing of the experience** gained by each registrar personally. It is helpful if some disabled people in their practices have been visited before the first session. Within the next few weeks one or two other visits can be made. A second session, about 2 months after the first, will allow the registrars to share what they have learned. It is best if at least one of the resource speakers from the first session is present. The registrars run the session themselves, but will need guidance.

Learning objectives should be agreed at the first session and reviewed at the second. Topics such as awareness of the needs of people with disabilities, finding resources to respond to these needs and monitoring outcome can be covered. More specific aims will evolve and should include:

1. The home surroundings and emotional climate.
2. The main clinical features with their bearing on the disability. An hour by hour account of events from dawn to dawn is informative.
3. The steps by which the various members of the team have assessed the situation and worked out the management with the patient and carer.
4. Residual problems, with suggestions for improvement.
5. A summary of what has been learned.

Sometimes visits are made to facilities such as a Disabled Living Centre, a young disabled unit or a hospital rehabilitation service, but there is no substitute for active learning from patients and the local team. For learning to take place, aims and objectives should be agreed before the visit and discussed before the visit ends. If time can be found, it is probably more effective to accompany one disabled person than to participate in a group visit.

Therapists have specific knowledge, skills and attitudes to impart and nurses are even closer to patients; they and the disabled people are the best teachers. Consultants in rehabilitation medicine will provide valuable advice for those with more complex disabilities, and this will be part of a team and community approach. This contact will help to increase the local cooperation that is so important in maintaining the independence of the disabled person at home.

Continuing education

In many areas of medicine, continuing education is using new technology. For instance, distance learning courses may be based on interactive computer programs and CD-ROM publications. Disability and rehabilitation are less suited to this approach than many other topics, because the key to success in this area is in the underlying philosophy. Nevertheless, new teaching methods can be used creatively and can include video films of the progress of patients undergoing innovative procedures such as implantation of anterior sacral root stimulators, or an artificial cochlea, as well as patients describing more routine but equally important treatments. Discussion on the value of technological advances will raise many issues about their ability to reduce disability and handicap.

May there never develop in me the notion that my education is complete but give me strength and leisure and zeal continually to enlarge my knowledge.

(Moses Maimonides, 1135–1204).

REFERENCES

Brewin, T.B. (1991) Three ways of giving bad news. *Lancet*, **337**, 1207–9.

British Society of Rehabilitation Medicine (1992) *The Teaching of Rehabilitation of Medicine to Medical Students*, British Society of Rehabilitation Medicine, Royal College of Physicians, London.

CAIPE (1994) *Annual Report September 1995*, CAIPE, London.

Doherty, M., Dacre, J., Dieppe, P. and Snaith, M. (1992) The 'GALS' screen. *Annals of Rheumatic Diseases*, **51**, 1165–9.

European Conference on the Teaching of General Practice (1975) *The General Practitioner in Europe*. A statement by the working party appointed by the Second European Conference on the Teaching of General Practice, Leeuwenhorst Group, Netherlands.

Findley, L.J. and Oxtoby, M. (1990) Community care and patients with progressive conditions. *British Medical Journal*, **301**, 1329.

Fletcher, C.M. and Freeling, P. (1988) *Talking and Listening to Patients*, Nuffield Provincial Hospitals Trust, London.

General Medical Council (1980) *Recommendations on Basic Medical Education*, General Medical Council, London.

General Medical Council (1992) *Recommendation on General Clinical Training*, General Medical Council, London.

Haggadah (4th Century) *Palestinian Talmud*.

Hasler, J.C. (1994) *The Primary Health Care Team*, John Fry Trust Fellowship, Royal Society of Medicine Press, London.

Heyes, J. (1992) Teaching trainees to deal with handicap and impairment. (*Postgraduate*) *Education for General Practice*, **3** 125–32.

Hockey, L. (1966) *Feeling the Pulse*, Queens Institute of District Nursing, London.

Inman, C. and Kahtan, S. (1994) *Medical Education on Disability*. A Report from the University College London Medical School and the Prince of Wales Advisory Group on Disability, POWAG, London.

McCrory, D.J. and Marrone, J.A. (1984) The physician and the disabled patient: a challenge to medical education. *Journal of Medical Education*, **59** 429–31.

McMullan, J.J. (1993) *Physical Disability: an approach for general practice*. A report to the Nuffield Provincial Hospitals Trust. (Unpublished, but available from the Royal Society of Medicine Library, 1 Wimpole Street, London, W1M 8AE.)

Mandelstam, M. (1991) *Equipment for Disability. A guide to provision*, Nuffield Provincial Hospitals Trust, Disabled Living Foundation, London.

Marshall, J., Haines, A.P. and Chamberlain, A. (1991) Undergraduate medical education on disability and rehabilitation in the UK. *Clinical Rehabilitation*, **5**, 251–4.

Prince of Wales Advisory Group on Disability (1992) *A Charter for Disabled People using hospitals*, Royal College of Physicians, London.

Stott, N. (Chairman). (1996) *The Nature of General Medical Practice: working party report from general medical practice 27*, Royal College of General Practitioners, London.

Swift, G. and McDougall, I.A. (1965) The family doctor and the family nurse. *British Medical Journal*, **1**, 697.

Wade, D.T. (1988) *Stroke. Practical guides for general practice 4*, Oxford University Press, Oxford.

Ward, C.D., Crates, P. and Skeates, S. (1993) Development of a disability team in general practice. *Clinical Rehabilitation*, **7** 157–62.

Wills, J. (1986) Bringing the visiting diary up to date. *British Medical Journal*, **292** 1715–16.

USEFUL ADDRESS

The UK Centre for the Advancement of InterProfessional Education (CAIPE)
344 Gray's Inn Road, London, WC1 8BP, UK.

6 Working in teams

A.R. Harvey

Interdisciplinary working is central to rehabilitation. It is often assumed that the ability to fit into a team and work closely alongside other professional colleagues comes automatically with a health professional qualification. This is not the case because the mutual trust and interdependence essential for effective teamwork cannot be learned in the classroom. The more experienced therapists, nurses or doctors may find it particularly difficult to adapt from individual to team-working patterns. Working as a team appears to take time from patient contact, so some may decry it as inefficient. Do benefits outweigh the risks and penalties? What are the aspects of rehabilitation for which team work is essential? How do we ensure that team working is efficient in use of time without losing the many potential benefits?

It is not surprising that many developing teams struggle to work effectively together. There is very little teaching or discussion about the benefits and risks of team working at undergraduate level in the health professions, and little training in team work is generally available to qualified rehabilitation staff. This chapter aims to fill this gap. It is in three sections.

- The reasons for working in teams, especially in rehabilitation.
- Theories and research outcomes about team working and team development. Much of this derives from manufacturing industry rather than service delivery, but the key issues of clear goals, good communication, interpersonal interaction and leadership/management styles are common to all areas of team work.
- The application of the general principles to rehabilitation, both for inpatients and in community-based team work.

WHY TEAM WORK?

It can be very satisfying and motivating, can acknowledge and make good use of an individual's skills in new ways, and can promote the introduction of new ideas more effectively than when individuals work independently. Team working is particularly relevant in rehabilitation because of the needs of the patient requiring complex therapy, and the mechanisms of service delivery.

Patients' needs

A patient with new or established disability may experience difficulties in many aspects of his or her life (e.g. physical mobility, continence, work, personal relationships), each of which merits careful and expert assessment and all of which may require specialist input. Although the alternatives to team work (discrete assessments by separate specialists

Rehabilitation of the Physically Disabled Adult. Edited by C. John Goodwill, M. Anne Chamberlain and Chris Evans. Published in 1997 by Stanley Thornes (Publishers) Ltd, Cheltenham. ISBN 0-7487-3183-0.

without integration, or one individual such as the general practitioner taking on all roles) may work to an extent, successful *team working* gives greater potential for patient satisfaction and effective problem solving.

Service mechanisms

The process of rehabilitation work also argues strongly for the coordination of different professions into close working teams. Some specific benefits are:

1. **Information** from the assessment by one discipline may help the work of another.
   Example: Improved posture and tone following physiotherapy assessment may enhance swallowing, and care of personal hygiene; clarification of cognitive deficit by a psychologist may lead to improved communication and cooperation with other staff and relatives.

2. **Information** from assessment by one discipline may determine the agenda for another.
   Example: An occupational therapy home visit indicating that the ability to walk a short distance will be essential for living at home; medical assessment indicating that cardiac reserve is not sufficient to allow certain activities or goals.

3. One discipline is able to observe, apply and reinforce the successful outcome from another discipline's work.
   Example: Utilizing recovering hand function in daily living activities.

Costs versus benefits

These potential benefits come at a cost. It is important to recognize the potential drawbacks of team working, so that they can be minimized or avoided. The costs of team working may include:

- The time spent in interdisciplinary *communication* rather than patient treatment.
- Marginalization of the influence of patient and *carer* on the rehabilitation process; this may be helped by using a key worker.
- Using everybody's time to resolve limited issues.

Team working brings with it risks to personal and professional confidence which may require careful monitoring and sensitive resolution. These include:

- Conflicting assessments from different professionals.
- Overlap of therapeutic skills with another team member, with the need to decide 'who does what'.
- Allocation of responsibility for day-to-day details (someone has to do it).

Team work is particularly relevant in the following situations:

- When working with a patient with complex disabilities, where more than two activity areas (e.g. communication, mobility, continence, dexterity, cognition) need expert assessment and management.
- When a patient's clinical status is unstable and disability may change, with the requirement for rapid communication.
- When the patient's social or psychological status is under stress (e.g. being discharged from hospital with recently acquired severe disability, or when communication problems are severe, or when there has been bereavement).

Rehabilitation, of all health care areas, demands interdisciplinary working. The risks are an integral part of the process of interdisciplinary working and cannot be avoided by the staff any more than patients can avoid risk taking during the process of rehabilitation. Managing risks and minimizing penalties are important aspects of effective team work. **Training** in these aspects of health care should be developed within all undergraduate courses as well as during specialist postgraduate experience. The Centre For Advancement of Interprofessional Education in Primary Health and Community Care (CAIPE 344–354, Gray's Inn Road, London, United Kingdom. WC1X 8BP) provides a lead in the UK.

The following section aims to present some of the knowledge and experience available to help understand the processes operating in a team at work and the stages through which a new team must develop in order to be successful. It also describes the characteristics and attributes that team members may bring in order for them to get the best out of their work in the team, and for the team's work to benefit most from their input.

WHAT DOES TEAM WORK REQUIRE FROM ME; WHAT CAN I EXPECT FROM IT?

What is a team?

Sport is often used to illustrate the purpose of working as a team, because the complementary contributions of players with different physical skills can be easily recognized. This metaphor translates easily to a manufacturing situation. It prompts the comment 'a team … ultimately ·has one objective – to score more than the opposition. So it is in the work situation even though the line may not be so clearly defined' (Margerison and McCann, 1984). In service industry it is less easy to apply. Timeliness, value for money, quality and client satisfaction are all measurable outcomes against which performance of a restaurant could be measured, but timeliness is the only goal that can be objectively measured and agreed. In health care provision current service evaluation has focused on timeliness (according to the Patients' Charter) but such measures will not report anything about the appropriateness or value of team working. *Building a Better Team. A handbook for managers and facilitators* offers a different

starting point for discussing team work in the health service (Moxon, 1993). It is a valuable introduction to the theory of team working and is a practical manual for team development. Moxon's definition of a team is provided below.

A *team* is distinct from a group when it has the following attributes:

- a common purpose;
- recognition by each individual as belonging to the same unit (i.e., team identity);
- interdependence functions;
- agreed norms or values which regulate behaviour (…a common code of practice about communication, decision making, handling conflict, etc.).

This definition looks within the team at the identities and interactions of the team members, concentrating on getting it right locally, rather than on the external goal and its competitive connotations. It indicates the need for individuals to adapt in order to work with others in the group.

Many teams are established in order to develop a new, or different style of, service. This brings with it stresses and reactions resulting from the introduction of change to traditional systems of care. **Innovation** is an important characteristic of new team work but introduction of new practice in itself may be the easy part; managing the reaction, facilitating others in their adaptation and rebuilding links and networks take time and emotion. It has been said that for change to be successfully managed, the rate of learning has to be greater than the rate of change. The process requires careful management based on knowledge, previous experience of team development, and anticipation of pitfalls as well as rewards.

WHAT DO TEAMS DO TOGETHER?

There are certain behaviours that characterize effective and innovative team work. In a study of innovation among hospital management teams, other health care teams and a commercial management team, West and Anderson (1994) found that the following characteristics predicted effective innovation:

- Active individual participation in decision making (including decisions about the team as well as about the clients).
- Information sharing.
- Consensus decision making based on constructive controversy and critical self-appraisal.
- Verbal and practical support for innovation.

In addition, clear objectives and a clear commitment to excellence in performance were features of the successful teams. These characteristics highlight the importance of enabling the individual team member to contribute, valuing his or her skills and knowledge and providing constructive feedback on performance, including encouragement for good work. Success in any joint venture depends on enabling individuals to achieve what is important for them.

INDIVIDUAL PERFORMANCE VERSUS TEAM COLLABORATION

We enjoy our work more and perform better when we meet our own standards and aspirations, and when we get encouragement from people with whom we work (colleagues and clients). We all wish our contribution to be seen in its best light, but the process of working in a team inevitably requires compromise and may initially necessitate altering our own standards, suppressing our own aspirations and foregoing some of the individual positive feedback that we had previously enjoyed.

One key issue in developing team work is to achieve a balanced group of individuals whose skills are complementary and whose aspirations are not mutually exclusive. A number of universal work-related activities or characteristics can be identified. A parti-

cular team will require some or possibly all of these for effective functioning. Margerison and McCann (1984) developed a system for analysing team structure as an aid to team management. They propose four key work-related personality traits:

- relating;
- gathering and using information;
- making decisions;
- organizing selves and others.

Their work suggests that these four characteristics may each distribute somewhere between two poles. Each of us will fall somewhere on the spectrum between introversion and extroversion in how we relate to others, between practical and creative in how we gather and use information, between analytical and belief dependent in how we make decisions, and between highly structured and flexible in how we prefer to organize ourselves and others. This allows us to reflect on how we may as individuals interact with others and contribute to the work of the team.

Margerison and McCann identified five key areas of activity that a team must demonstrate if it is to be successful as a unit. These five activities, advising, exploring, organizing, controlling and linking, can be further divided into more specific team roles as illustrated in the team management wheel (Figure 6.1). Any individual may feel strong in three or four of these roles and may feel weak in one or two. Expression of these strengths at an early stage in team development will help in producing an overall balance in the team's work, and acknowledgement of weakness will avoid the risk of taking on unsatisfying roles resulting in poor performance. Each individual member may take on two or three of the 'team' roles so the model can be applied to small as well as large teams.

These roles may seem mainly relevant to industrial or commercial organizations, but they are also relevant to health care teams. A rehabilitation team may have to organize case

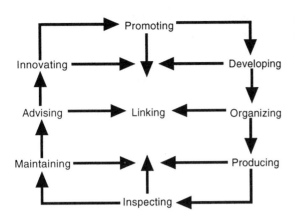

Figure 6.1 The team management wheel. Interdependent roles in an innovating team.

conferences, record and pass on information, undertake audit, give training, and learn about and apply new techniques. They will do research and be aware of the need for public relations. These tasks can be mapped onto the team management wheel. Others, such as counselling or synthesizing a multi-disciplinary management plan, do not fit easily into this analysis. These 'team' roles are separate from an individual's professional role; there is no inherent link between any particular team role on this model and any health care profession's duties.

TEAM RELATIONSHIPS: DEVELOPING TRUST AND COLLABORATION

Many of the personal characteristics and behaviours relevant to team working (e.g. openness to feedback, self-disclosure, willingness to take risks) are those that we ask of our patients during the rehabilitation process. They contrast with the characteristics that we often associate with individual success. This is because the team must become, to an extent, a single organism and its strength and effectiveness is determined by the interdependence of its members and the development

of its own integrity. Only then can it become greater than the sum of its parts. This enhancement can be seen in simple practical terms by the abolition of the duplication of effort, and the development of good communication and clear targets.

THE NATURAL HISTORY OF TEAM DEVELOPMENT

Peter Moxon, in his book *Building A Better Team* (Moxon, 1993), amplifies work by B.W. Tuckman and describes the following stages of team development:

- Forming (initial awareness of each other and agreement about the team's purpose).
- Storming (sorting out jobs and strategies and bidding for control and power).
- Norming (self-organization with transition from competition to collaboration).
- Performing (maturing and mutual acceptance).

New teams must recognize that this process takes time. An understanding of the stages of team evolution, recognition of the risks involved and the barriers to progress at each stage, and acknowledgement of the tasks and behavioural changes needed to progress may smooth the process of team development and prevent the occasional disaster of team failure and disbanding. The following is a summary of his description of these stages and recommendations for proactive team development.

Forming

This stage represents the initial establishment of a team but may also need to be renegotiated when new members join. For each individual member the main question at this stage is 'will I be accepted?' and behaviour will be characterized by avoidance of controversy and confrontation and preservation of one's own identity while getting to know the others. Ideas are kept simple, serious topics are avoided. Self-disclosure and the giving of feedback is tightly controlled. Personal needs and wishes may be suppressed. Cliques may develop but are not usually a threat to the developing team at this stage. This period is characterized by dependence on the team leader since group identity has not developed and each individual's uncertainties and anxieties push them to seek reassurance and direction. Leadership and a clear goal (even temporary or short term) are critical to the success of this stage of development, and their absence will prolong or threaten it.

Storming

This stage is characterized by competition and conflict as the mechanisms for decision making and control are determined. Aspirations, suppressed during the forming stage in order to allow mutual acceptance without conflict, may now be asserted in order to preserve or restore individuality and to satisfy the need for respect from others. Behaviour will often appear negative or defensive with challenging views expressed strongly by some, withdrawal by others, emotional expression and poor listening and collaboration. Leadership may be challenged. Cliques established by this stage may interfere with and threaten the progress of team development. Group identity is still poor and the concept of team work as an effective way of achieving the proposed goal may itself be rejected. The team's work is achieved through compromise and the outcome may be seen by many as poor quality. Creative or innovative suggestions may be suppressed as bids for control or leadership.

Norming

This stage is heralded and characterized by a shift in attitude and interaction from competition to collaboration. The team (as opposed to the individuals within the group) begins to build and strengthen its own identity. The leadership role may be shared and may change, as the team finds its own direction, to facilitator and guide. Members participate more actively, listen to each other's ideas and start to view disagreements as subjects for joint problem solving. Willingness to self-disclose (see 'Openness and mutual trust as the basis for effective team work' below) will develop gradually as trust between members increases and each individual's unique abilities are recognized and accepted. Roles become more fluid, a willingness to shift preconceived ideas leads to greater creativity and the quality and speed of decision making increases. The benefits of team working may only begin to emerge clearly at this stage.

Performing

Striking changes in interaction and relationships between team members will be apparent when compared with the forming and storming stages. The team is much less dependent on formal structure, individual contribution is more flexible, difference of view and other expressions of individuality become accepted again because, within the context of trusting relationships, they no longer represent a potential threat. A strong sense of loyalty develops which may carry the risk that, to outsiders, the team appears closed and unapproachable.

Progression from stage to stage can be recognized and developed and barriers may be anticipated and pre-empted. This process cannot be forced. As Moxon says: '.... each member must be prepared to give up something at each step in order to move forward'. Moving from stage one (forming) to stage two (storming) involve team members becoming aware of each other and of the differences between them. Sharing feelings may seem particularly risky at this stage. Moving from stage two to stage three (norming) requires that an individual no longer feels the need to fiercely defend his or her own view and recognizes that other ideas may work better in some situations. Progress may be blocked by one subgroup or clique seeking to dominate the agenda, or by the leader or other team members avoiding conflict and burying issues that need to be resolved. Progress from stage three to stage four (performing) depends on the development of mutual trust.

Openness and mutual trust as the basis for effective team work

These are not just nice ideas that allow people to feel good. They are necessary for practical day-to-day effectiveness. They '.... provide a ... climate in which conflicts and differences can be dealt with quickly ensuring all the team's energies can be focused on the task' and they '... allow individuals to work effectively on their own or in subgroups on issues that directly affect the whole team' (Moxon, 1993). The development of trust among team members can be encouraged, but the details of team building are outside the scope of this chapter.

A useful model of interpersonal interaction is the Johari Window (Figure 6.2). The aim throughout the team development process is for an individual to increase the arena (the area of their interactive personality known to themselves and to others) by reducing the facade (the area they do not disclose) and the blind spot (the area that others see but they do not recognize) through self-disclosure and acceptance of feedback. 'In a working relationship within a team the more each person understands the needs, preferences and perspectives of others the more effectively they can all work together. They do not have to agree with each other but they do need to understand why each will behave in a particular way.'

Moxon suggests that in the different stages of team development members may present a changing 'front'. Based on the Johari Window model, during the forming stage individuals present a large unknown, during the storming phase an excessive blind spot may be evident,

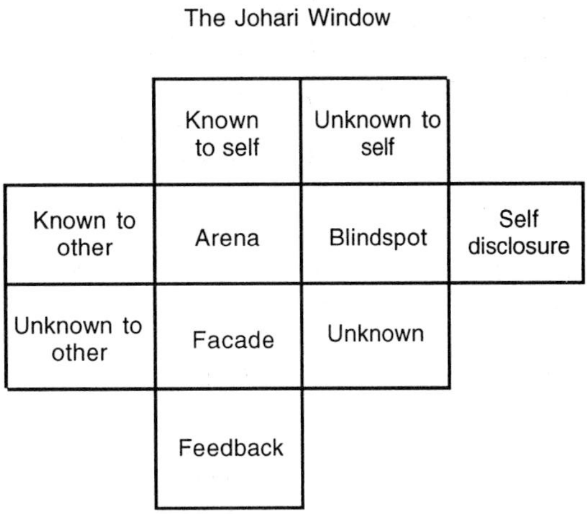

The Johari Window

Figure 6.2 The Johari window illustrates the interpersonal space within which human interaction takes place. One aim of team building and development is to increase the arena (and decrease other arenas) by facilitating self-disclosure and the giving and receiving of constructive feedback. (Source: Luft, 1961.)

during the norming phase the facade is still considerable and finally by the performing stage the arena is the main area within which individual work and team interrelationships take place (Table 6.1). There are personal as well as professional rewards resulting from this process of developing self-knowledge and confidence in personal interaction.

Problems arising in team development

These have been categorized into four areas by Irwin, Plovnik and Fry (1974):

1. **Goals.** The main issues with goals are clarity and whether they encourage collaborative working as opposed to individual direction and effort.

2. **Roles.** When goals are clear, roles can usually be agreed but issues around overlap and autonomy needs to be discussed and clarified early and reviewed as the team develops.

Table 6.1 Characteristic behaviours: changing Johari profiles during team development. (Source: Moxon, 1993)

Forming	
Large unknown	Avoiding conflict
	Politeness
	Low risk taking
	Views and feelings withheld
	Reserved behaviour
Storming	
Large blindspot	Defending, withdrawal
	Win–lose confrontations
	Distrust and suspicion of others
	Poor listening/minimal seeking of feedback
	Asserting own views
Norming	
Large facade	Desire to help others
	Aversion to conflict
	High interpersonal support
	Receptive to others' needs
	Seeking feedback
Performing	
Large arena	Openness – two-way
	High trust
	Good listening
	Sharing of feelings
	Risk taking

3. **Process**. Problems with processes can be sorted into those relating to decision making (with issues such as rights to consultation, rights of veto, the need for consensus and what is a quorum), to communicating and meeting (including balancing lack of information with information overload, and organization of, and attendance at, team meetings) and to leadership style.
4. Moxon states 'for the team to develop and for a climate of openness and trust to exist the leader must be prepared to seek and accept feedback both on his or her style and on the impact it is having on the group'.

Relationships

Failure to give and receive feedback and for self-disclosure will hinder team development (see Figure 6.2 and Table 6.1).

APPLICATION OF THE PRINCIPALS OF TEAM WORKING TO REHABILITATION PRACTICE

The skills required by a rehabilitation team will vary depending on the case mix of the target population and on the location of the work. Skills common to all teams will include assessment and management of impaired physical mobility, dexterity, communication, eating and swallowing, cognition, continence, tissue viability and emotional well-being, including the skills of counselling. Medical knowledge of diagnosis, prognosis and drug treatment and its complications must be readily accessible. These professional skills must be supplemented by other team-related skills. These include good information recording, communication, public relations, teaching, evaluation and monitoring of outcomes, and research and development. Skills of mediation, performance review, career counselling and leadership must also be available.

Developing a team profile

Rehabilitation is a complex activity. It is helpful when establishing a team to develop a profile of the skills and roles (patient directed and team directed) needed. The nine roles in the team management wheel of Margerison and McCann (Figure 6.1) may help in translating health needs into team roles required.

Once the profile is developed the recruitment process must seek to meet the team profile, not just to select on individuals' characteristics. A team may be established from a group of staff currently employed in a different setting or structure (e.g. deploying staff from a ward closure into a day hospital or community-based team). Skills may be identified within the profile (e.g. psychological assessment and counselling, technical occupational therapy support) which are not present within the starting establishment. With a flexible approach and expert advice this situation can often be redeemed. A nurse may be willing to undergo training in counselling and to develop this as a specialized nursing role; a health care assistant may welcome the change in work offered by the occupational therapy technician role and could be offered in-service training to develop appropriate skills. Nursing staff may feel that their numbers are being unjustifiably depleted, but this is effectively a redistribution of work. Specialist needs will be met by individuals with specialist training rather than, as previously, handled within the workload of the generic staff. Blurring the demarcation between professional roles is a characteristic of all good team work. The establishment of a key worker system, through which any patient relates primarily to one particular member of the team, will be appreciated by patients and carers. It will also streamline communication and will help maintain the central influence of the patient and carer in the rehabilitation process.

Getting the process organized

West and Anderson (1994) have defined the characteristics of effective health care teams. Their recommendations are:

1. Clarify the 'common purpose' or goal and make it explicit to all team members through discussion and consensus agreement.
2. Establish the mechanisms for team collaboration through face-to-face information sharing and decision making.
3. Provide opportunities for feedback to members and leaders. Encourage some informal social contact to facilitate the process of self-disclosure.

4. Involve team members in decision making about the team and its direction as well as about patient management. This is particularly important if changes are taking place in the parent organization. Encourage individual members to identify clearly with the team.
5. Include a mechanism for individual and team self-appraisal to ensure progress and innovation.
6. Provide encouragement and resources for reasonable innovation, particularly research-based development.

TEAM LEADERSHIP: TEAM MANAGEMENT: TEAM BUILDING AND DEVELOPMENT

Rehabilitation is not only complex but also emotionally charged. The team's support system is very important. The distinct roles of manager and leader are both important. They may both be carried out by the same individual but experience suggests that separating the roles works better.

Leadership

The leader's role is critical early in the development of the team (the 'forming and storming' stages in Moxon's definitions). It includes maintaining a clear vision of the goal and presenting this to old and new team members; ensuring the day-to-day processes are working smoothly (personally or by delegation); and ensuring team-related issues are identified, aired and resolved as far as possible even if this necessitates some initial conflict. The linking role in the Team Management Wheel model is part of the leader's job. As the team develops its identity and direction the leadership role will become more a facilitatory role and is often shared or rotated among members. Leadership should always be from within the team. This does not have to be a doctor, and the doctor does not have to be the leader. The key requirements are **time** to give to the task, interpersonal listening and communication skills, and the authority and wisdom to make appropriate delegation.

Management

The manager's role is mainly to do with resources and maintaining links with the parent organization and with other related services or agencies. A good manager is a great asset, often working behind the scenes on behalf of the team but willing to stand up and speak for them in the central planning committees of the organization, and keeping them informed of opportunities for additional funding for research, development and training which may be available. Occasionally, there is uncertainty about loyalties for team members derived from different agencies and organizations when their line manager may have no personal involvement with, or other financial interests in, the team's work. In this situation a good line manager will make herself or himself aware of the team, its purpose and its leadership mechanisms and on the basis of that knowledge agree to relinquish some control over the areas of the team members' work to the team's leadership. She or he will request feedback through the member of the team.

Team building and development

Team working is a constantly evolving process as changes take place in patients' needs and expectations, forms of treatment, styles of clinical management and structures of the parent organization and related agencies. Team building and development should be seen as a continuing process, not a once-only start-up requirement. In general, team interventions may include components of the following four approaches based on different models of team working, each focusing on a different aspects. The **goal setting** model is based on the identification of barriers to achieving set objectives and using this to develop an action plan. This is allied to the

problem-solving approach, which seeks to assign and develop tasks such as identifying and analysing problems, developing options for solving them and choosing and implementing action plans. The **interpersonal** model emphasizes development of openness, trust and high-quality communication, aiming to promote team strength through integration. The **role model** emphasizes the team as a set of interdependent roles and seeks to make them explicit, and to improve mutual understanding of them through role definition and role negotiation.

Moxon suggests that 2 or 3 days should be given to initial team development, then a day or month for several months (as the team is going through the storming and norming phases), then 1 day every 6 months. This should be supplemented by about 1 hour each month in regular team meetings reviewing the team's working, and identifying issues for the team development day.

Interaction with other service providers

One danger in becoming successful as a team is that other people with whom the team should be working closely may feel excluded and unconfident about approaching the team. It is the team's responsibility to ensure that this does not happen. One strategy is to offer teaching sessions based on the expertise and experience that the team has developed. Other strategies may be to seek joint training opportunities including shared case discussions, to establish joint working opportunities for care planning with shared patients, and to provide positive feedback to the other agency for successful work. This should be offered to relevant voluntary and independent providers, as well as groups from other statutory agencies and health care services.

RECORD KEEPING

Another important area of interaction with other service providers is the recording and circulation of clinical notes through the patient case record.

The purposes for note keeping are to record initial assessment, to record goals, to detail the management plan, and to record progress through outcome measures and new goals and management plans as abilities change. Current problems with notes include difficulty in getting notes when needed (leading to every unit keeping their own notes), duplication of recording in different agencies and by different staff in the team (which is irritating for the patient), the use of different outcome measures, many of which are non-standardized, and the different cultures of confidentiality existing in different organizations, leading to reluctance to share information without the patient's written consent.

Having common notes across all agencies is a worthy goal and the key issues for achievement of this are:

1. Identifying a core set of clinical and social data, appropriate to all agencies, and a common 'language' or structure for recording it.
2. Having a system flexible enough to incorporate some additional specialist information, necessary for each discipline to have continuity from visit to visit.
3. Agreement of simple and relevant progress and outcome measures, which can be recorded reliably by members of different disciplines.
4. Reliable transfer of notes for visits to different locations.
5. Agreement of confidentiality issues, including stipulation of the types of information which may need to be kept out of common notes.

The use of patient-held records has a number of potential advantages. The location of the notes is always known and transfer from unit to unit should be reliable (although this may be erratic initially, until it becomes second nature to all involved). Confidentiality becomes less of a problem, in that the patient can be asked before recording, that she/he is happy for the information to be shared and he/she would have access to it. This would bring the additional advantage of involving the patient more closely in the process of goal setting and the recording of achievement of progress.

One potential disadvantage of this system is that statutory records (e.g. hospital case notes, housing agency files) may not receive information about the rehabilitation process at all and deliberate efforts will be required to ensure that users of these notes have summaries of progress or key management decisions available to them.

Evaluating team effectiveness

Health care teams are more complex than many other work groups because individuals have different training backgrounds, and join the team from hierarchical work systems with different professional expectations and prejudices. They may also have different criteria for judging effectiveness. Outcomes should measure performance and viability, the latter relating to success at the team working process. They should include measures of goal clarity, satisfaction of team members and quality of communication and decision making. Research under way at the MRC/ESRC Social and Applied Psychology Unit, University of Sheffield, has identified four domains of measurable outcomes:

1. Issues related to patients and carers (e.g. timeliness, access, information and continuity).
2. Quality of care (standard setting, multi-disciplinary audit, protocols).
3. Staff development and team viability (skills profile, training, equal opportunities).
4. Organization and planning of care (health needs assessment, innovation in practice, achieving Department of Health targets, interagency collaboration).

A questionnaire to evaluate these areas has been developed for the primary health care team (Poulton and West, 1994) which could be adapted for rehabilitation teams. The research in Sheffield continues, and may provide a broader model for health care team evaluation.

Community rehabilitation: team working without a team

Some community rehabilitation teams are constituted as a single unit, often following joint funding agreements and with a specific target patient group in mind (e.g. patients with traumatic brain injury or young adults with severe disability). More commonly, the need is to develop the process of team working among staff already 'on the ground' in a particular locality. The greatest challenge in rehabilitation service development is making community-based management of people with progressive disabilities proactive, introducing health promotion, and coordinating the contributions of disciplines from different backgrounds employed in different agencies. It has been practised successfully in the UK and elsewhere.

The principles are the same as for formally constituted teams working within a hospital setting and can be summarized:

1. Agree and clarify the purpose and goals of the collaborative work and make it explicit. This agreement will require a consensus from a number of senior staff and/or managers from different agencies who have identified the need for such a service development.
2. Develop the skills profile, including an emphasis on networking, linking and other team-work skills.
3. Develop a profile of the agencies (including voluntary agencies) from which staff will be involved, and which may be stake holders in the team members' work.

4. Form the team. The membership will be determined by who is already involved in the locality but 'recruitment' should endeavour to include representatives from all the main agencies, in particular from social services (in the UK this agency has financial responsibility for community care). The project must be supported by field staff, middle managers and senior management in all agencies if it is to be successful. The current political climate around health and social care provision supports this approach, at least in the UK. Any funding requirements, for example, training, secretarial support, must be agreed at this stage. Preparing an information leaflet listing the team members and the agencies they represent will symbolize the achievement of this stage as well as being an important mechanism for advertising.
5. The team members and supporting managers must now work through the process issues. First, the team development needs must be agreed and a programme instituted. Second, initial leadership of the team should be clarified; it will often be shared between two or three individuals representing the main agencies involved. Third, the location and format for team meetings must be agreed.
6. Systems for monitoring the work of a community team must be developed even though the task will be difficult. Principles being developed for primary health care team monitoring may be applicable (Poulton and West, 1994).

Professional versus unqualified team members: skill mix and the generic health care worker

Skill mix in rehabilitation teams will vary depending on the work style and location. The main differences between community-based and working in a hospital-based team are the larger numbers of patients, the greater difficulty in getting to them, and the differences in assessing patients in their own home compared to a hospital assessment facility. The first two points argue for the introduction of generic rehabilitation staff, who are not highly trained, to work on behalf of, and under the direction of, professional team members in order to 'cover the ground'. The third point reminds us that skilled clinical assessment must always be the basis on which a management plan is based. Getting this mix right will be critically important for the continued development of community-based rehabilitation. A number of models have already been developed and research to evaluate the benefits and drawbacks of each is urgently needed.

SUMMARY

Rehabilitation is a particularly complex area of health care delivery, as it is essentially interdisciplinary, protracted and often carried out across diverse locations. Team working should be the aim in organizing and delivering services. Good team working is usually satisfying. The early stages of team evolution and development may be difficult for several reasons. Individuals taking part should understand about interactions within teams and appreciate the importance of open com-munication and self-disclosure. They should be able to give and accept criticism. The development of a team specification of skills and roles must precede its establishment. Ideally, recruitment should aim to identify the important team roles as well as relevant professional skills. Team building and development is a continuing process.

REFERENCES

Irwin, I.M. Plovnik, M.S. and Fry, R.C. (1974) *Task-orientated Team Development*, McGraw Hill, New York.

Luft, J. (1961) The Johari Window, in *Human Relations Training News, 5–7, Of Human Interaction*, National Press Books, Palo Alto, CA.

Margerison, C. and McCann, D. (1984) *The Team Management Index*, MCP University Press, Bradford.

Moxon, P. (1993) *Building a Better Team. A handbook for managers and facilitators*, Gower Publishing, Aldershot, Hants, UK.

Poulton, B.C. and West, M.A. (1994) Primary health care team effectiveness; developing a constituency approach. *Health and Social Care*, 2: 77–84.

West, M. and Anderson, N. (1994) Measures of invention. *Health Services Journal*, 20 October, 26–7.

USEFUL ADDRESS

The Centre for Advancement of Interprofessional Education in Primary Health and Community Care (CAIPE) 344–354 Gray's Inn Road, London WC1X 8BP, UK.

7 Clinical assessment

J. Shindler and J. Goodwill

The clinical consultation is the most important source of information for effective diagnosis of medical conditions as well as for management of disabilities. It may be based on one of a number of models, from the strict anatomical/biomedical description of the systems that do not work to the whole-of-life description of the current emotional and physical state of the patient in the context of their entire life. The functional model describes problems and needs in the context of specific losses relative to the previous lifestyle. In practice, time is the biggest constraint, and a compromise is forced.

THE BIOMEDICAL MODEL

The conventional medical history begins with the presenting symptoms and continues with direct questioning, examination and investigations. This will establish the diagnosis of an illness, for example an arthritis causing pain, stiffness and swelling in a particular group of joints over a particular time course. The description may be sufficiently characteristic of a particular disease and should be adequate to indicate possible further investigations and interventions.

However, this model does not always consider the impact of disease on the patient's lifestyle, so if the patient and the doctor confine their discussion within this framework the mismatch of the patient with his/ her environment is left unexplored. Thus the young mother with arthritis in her wrists may not disclose her fears that she may drop the baby, or someone with multiple sclerosis may not admit that the lack of accessible public lavatories precludes going shopping or visiting normally. The limitations of the biomedical model of assessment is that it fails to account for the patient's perceptions or the doctor's understanding of those perceptions of their disease process and its effect on their patient's lifestyle.

THE FUNCTIONAL MODEL

The functional model allows a description of the patient's current state of overall ability in the context of their life, and includes that of their immediate family and their environment. Loss of function is the result of a disease process on a person's body. The features that are necessary to describe disability are not necessarily the same as those required to describe a disease. If we consider the patient with multiple sclerosis, diagnosis traditionally requires that lesions are separated chronologically and anatomically in the nervous system (though modern diagnostic methods may make it possible to make a positive diagnosis after one episode). The patient's life can remain undisturbed even after the several minor episodes that establish the diagnosis (events such as transient paraesthe-

Rehabilitation of the Physically Disabled Adult. Edited by C. John Goodwill, M. Anne Chamberlain and Chris Evans. Published in 1997 by Stanley Thornes (Publishers) Ltd, Cheltenham. ISBN 0-7487-3183-0.

siae or numbness). The onset of paraplegia, urgency/frequency or severe ataxia may, however, mean that the patient loses job, independence and the ability to mix in society and attention has to be focused on the resulting handicap. Despite accurate diagnosis and specific medical or surgical treatment, very many patients remain disabled.

A medical condition may cause temporary or permanent disability, the disabilities may be static, fluctuant or progressive. The main groups of physical impairment are:

- cardiac, e.g. myocardial ischaemia;
- respiratory, e.g. chronic obstructive airways disease;
- sensory deprivation, e.g. reduction of vision or hearing;
- communication and speech disorders, e.g. stroke;
- locomotor disability, e.g. arthritis, amputation;
- neurological, e.g. stroke, multiple sclerosis, cerebral palsy, spina bifida, paraplegia;
- multiple disabilities.

Many diseases cause a mixture of locomotor, sensory, intellectual or other problems. These disabilities require assessment, without which advice and management may be inadequate. It requires time and patience to assess all the problems of the disabled person, medical and social, arising from the illness or injury. Once the problems and their priority order have been found, the solutions may become clearer.

Consideration of prognosis for mortality and morbidity is required when planning advice and intervention. A knowledge of risk factors, such as smoking and hypertension, which may cause disease deterioration is needed, as they may interfere with rehabilitation.

The assessment process should include the functional implications of each symptom. The assessment of disability is a very different procedure from the process required to establish a medical diagnosis. A complete assessment will describe the patient in terms of impairment (diagnosis), disability (specific objective deficits of function, e.g. weak arms), and handicap (which defines the social disadvantage). To complete the assessment, the emotional state of the patient and an understanding of the effect of the disabilities in the context of the patient's normal environment are needed. While the diagnosis and initial assessment will often be done by a doctor, either general practitioner or specialist, other health and social service professionals will be involved in assessing the patient later.

WHAT DOES THE PATIENT WANT AND EXPECT?

It is vital to find out how the patient views the problems in everyday life arising from the condition. Prompting of patients is required because often they will suppress many of the real problems, believing that the doctor will not be interested or will not be able to help or that the matter is insoluble. The medical assessment may gradually disclose other problems which patients had not mentioned or of which they have been unaware. Problems may be clinical or social; they should be listed together logically with the setting of realistic goals and methods of achieving these goals.

Patient's expectations are important

Patients have been known to come to a clinic merely for a repeat prescription for special shoes, but have found themselves examined from head to toe by an enthusiastic doctor who, finding a wealth of abnormalities for investigation, quite irrelevant to the patient's immediate problem, has then forgotten to order the shoes.

Several expectations lie buried in a consultation and those of the patient may differ from those of the carers (markedly so in head injury) and again these may be at variance with those of the referring general practitioner, the hospital doctor and other involved professionals. Questions such as the following can yield helpful, and at times, strange and sad replies. 'What can I do for you?', 'What have you come for?' (appropriately said!) and 'What have they said about your coming to this clinic?'

It is helpful if a patient does not come alone to a rehabilitation clinic, for disability rarely involves only the patient. The whole family will be involved and it is important to have some indication of their characters, strengths, weaknesses and roles. It helps to have them present with the patient when an attempt is made to explain the disease and its consequences. It helps if all agree on the aims of treatment and the priorities.

Many patients with disabilities are best assessed in their home environment. It is helpful if their general practitioner can be present who can provide background information on the health and social situation of the family. This can then lead on to assessment under the Community Care Act (1990), in which the responsibility is given to the Social Service Department for assessment of the person's needs and the provision of appropriate aids and a Community Care Plan.

PERSONALITY AND INTELLECTUAL FUNCTION

Knowledge of the previous education, work experience and recreations will help to understand the impact of the condition on the individual patient. Prior to the disability some patients may have been very active and independent. Others may have been content to sit at home doing relatively little with modest ambitions. The latter may appear to do less well with rehabilitation management; however, they may be more easily satisfied than the former, who may well set unrealistic goals and be disappointed if they cannot achieve them. In the absence of brain damage personality does not change with the occur-

rence of disability, but behaviour may be altered. Patients may be less able to repress the undesirable features of themselves, although sometimes hidden strengths are revealed to understand and cope with the disability.

At the end of the interview one should be in a position to make some assessment of the patient's intellect, orientation in time and space, cognitive function, short- and long-term memory, ability to concentrate, to synthesize information, to structure it, to sort and sequence it, to communicate and to follow advice. Affect should be noted: is the patient depressed (and if so, is this appropriate), anxious, lacking in confidence, unrealistic, apathetic, or unmotivated. What is the perception of self? Of the problems listed, which are of most concern to the person and/ or to the family? Critical to the understanding of this perception is a knowledge of the person's response to the onset of the disability, their 'sense of loss' (Worden, 1991).

Assessing comprehension and emotional response

The emotional responses of individuals and their carers to disability have been compared to the stages of mourning (Parkes, 1970; Bowlby, 1980). A critical feature of assessment is to establish the current emotional state and the extent to which an adjustment to the new circumstances has been made. There are successive stages of grieving. In the context of disability they may be described as follows:

- A feeling of numbness and denial of the reality of the illness.
- Working through the pain of grief at reduction of future life possibilities.
- Accepting the reality of the disability (loss of function).
- Adjusting to a new environment with the disability, the actual physical environment and/or the changes in work and social possibilities.

- Emotional adjustment and moving on with life, looking to the residual possibilities in the future. The planning and success of the rehabilitation process is dependent on these adjustments being achieved.

A patient in shock and emotional turmoil may appear to be more disabled than the observer would think justified and an angry denying patient may play down some features or completely deny the existence of disability. The examination of the mental state may reveal evidence of major depression which would colour response to the assessment and which should then be appropriately treated with antidepressants.

If there is evidence of maladjustment to the disabling process, then it may be appropriate to plan early therapy in conjunction with counselling and to delay a definitive assessment to such time as the patient has reached a stable emotional state with respect to the disability. One must aim for an active acceptance of disability coupled with a desire to use remaining abilities.

The cognitive competence of the patient is important. Organic brain damage due to stroke, head injury or multiple sclerosis will affect the patient's reactions to the disability. This may vary from aggression to emotional lability. Reduction of memory and learning ability due to brain damage also cause misunderstandings. Any of these may make it difficult for the patient to realistically understand how and what can be achieved. Perhaps in some severe disabilities denial is the only psychological response that makes life possible and occasionally this must be accepted by those treating the patient. Honesty and a full explanation of the treatment goals are essential to success.

Understanding of the condition is an important determinant of the response to disability. It is important to establish that the patient has a realistic understanding of the illness or injury, the specific treatment for the condition, and the management of the handicap and disability arising from it. There will be occasions after brain injury, however caused, when the patient is not sufficiently aware to be able to make sound decisions. This is a medicolegal minefield (Chapter 10).

THE REACTION OF THE RELATIVES AND FRIENDS

This may be as important as that of the patient. Usually acceptance of reality is easier if there is a clear cause -and -effect, paraplegia due to trauma being easier for people to understand than that due to a virus causing transverse myelitis. Where there is no apparent cause for the condition, relatives or the patient may construct a framework which may include their guilt or others' failure. Where the patient or a relative is not entirely satisfied with the explanation of the cause of the illness, anger, frustration and even complaints may persist. Many angry complaints about management are manifestations of a grief response.

The patient and family may listen attentively, but not be able to remember all the information given. Furthermore, memory can be selective and sometimes only things that are welcome are remembered. Honest discussion is vital. This may take several appointments, with ample time for discussion and questions on what can and what cannot be achieved. Accurate information is important, but may need to be imparted gradually. Untruths must be avoided or the trust which is essential will not be built up. It is important to concentrate on maximizing the function that remains and what can be achieved with rehabilitation. It is important that the patient, family and staff aim for the same goals.

Counselling may be very valuable for family and friends as well as the patient. If the psychological reaction of the patient or family appears unusual, assessment and advice from a clinical psychologist may be of value. Sometimes a tape or video given to the patient after interview or treatment acts as a useful reminder or it can be kept and given with a later tape to show improvement.

THE AIM OF ASSESSMENT

1. To establish the diagnosis and to record disabilities, their nature and their character (static, fluctuant, deteriorating) in the context of the person's previous lifestyle, past life and future expectations.
2. To produce a problem list.
3. To draw up treatment plans for the disease and the resulting disabilities.

The topics detailed below should be explored at assessment.

Mobility

Limitation may be due to a number of different problems in any one disease. The amount of difficulty due to each must be assessed to allow treatment of these specific problems. In rheumatoid arthritis it may be pain requiring systemic drug treatment, limitation of joint movement requiring splintage and physiotherapy, or so much pain or instability of one or more joints that surgery or an orthosis is required. Alternatively weakness may be due to neurological complications of neuropathy or myelopathy, the latter requiring evaluation of the cervical spine. With neurological conditions such as stroke or multiple sclerosis there may be muscle weakness requiring exercise, spasticity or contracture requiring physiotherapy, drugs or even surgery, or it may be that incoordination or sensory loss pose far greater problems, and are relatively more resistant to treatment. Frequently there is a combination of problems, so that treatment needs to be directed at each, depending upon their relative importance. For instance, sensory loss or astereognosis, often with body-image problems on the same side, cause much greater difficulty in everyday life than a moderate degree of muscle weakness.

When assessing mobility, the following questions should be asked:

Mobility on foot
How far does the patient walk?
Is a helper required?
Are mobility aids needed?
Are there any other problems?
Check problems of access to and from the home, work/school and leisure pursuits.

Wheelchair mobility
Which wheelchair(s) does the patient have?
Do these satisfy the needs? If not, what might?
Are they in good repair?

Private transport
What transport is used?
Is the patient passenger or driver?
What are the problems?
What aids or help are necessary to get in/out of the vehicle; what modifications are needed?

Public transport
Is public transport available?
Is it accessible?

Vision

Visual acuity can be judged by the patient's behaviour in the consulting room, the ability to read a paper or by formal testing with test charts. Visual fields can be tested by confrontation, but small defects or scotomata will be missed. Where there is doubt, especially about brain damage or perceptual problems, formal testing is needed.

Hearing

Bilateral loss of hearing is usually obvious, but it is quite possible to miss a complete unilateral loss, for example after head injury. This may need formal checking (Chapter 19).

Communication

In everyday life communication is through speech, hearing and vision. If one or other channel of information is reduced, the patient may have to communicate in different ways. Both the patient and those around him/her will probably use non-verbal communication.

The distinction should be drawn between dysphasia and dysarthria. In the former there is a loss of language which may be expressive or receptive; it will not matter whether the patient tries to speak or write. If the patient is dysarthric, then writing, reading and understanding are unimpaired and he or she can understand and formulate correct words though articulation is flawed. Detailed speech assessment will be done by the speech and language therapist.

The patient may understand more by visual than aural communication, so gesture, body language and other non-verbal communication will be important. If the patient does not speak English, an independent translator is essential. A member of staff may be more helpful than the patient's family who will often not ask the questions as given or will give their own reply rather than that of the patient, which can be very misleading. The translator should not modify question or answer.

Breathlessness and fatigue

These may coexist due to cardiac and/or respiratory disease, which is relatively easily assessed, but fatigue occurring with neurological conditions such as multiple sclerosis, stroke or rheumatoid arthritis may be an underestimated problem. Fatigue is a subjective phenomenon and it is not easy to quantify. Severe fatigue may make treatment more difficult. It may be worsened by depression; but treatment may help.

Activities of daily living (ADL)

ADL may be formally tested by the occupational therapist (OT) who can arrange for supply of technical aids or appliances. It is important that the doctor asks key questions to indicate whether there is a need for an OT assessment. Personal care, i.e. dressing, washing, bath and toilet needs, as well as cooking, eating and drinking, will be considered by the OT, together with other activities around the home that we all take for granted. If necessary, with the aid of a home visit, the OT will be able to advise on modifications and will assess the ability to operate the telephone, front door, radio, television, lights and heating.

Home aids and modifications are provided by the Social Services Department, but Environmental Control Equipment is supplied by the Health Service (Chapter 49).

Bowels and micturition

Patients with urinary problems require careful assessment to identify the cause. The patient may be asked to keep a daily micturition chart to determine when and how often it occurs and further investigation, including urodynamics, may be required.

Some patients, particularly the elderly, may consider that some of their problems are due to their age and nothing can be done about them. The professionals treating that patient must not make the same mistake. Even if specific treatment cannot be given to improve control, improvement in mobility or the provision of easily accessible toilet facilities may solve the functional problem (Chapter 35). More help may be provided by a builder than a urologist!

Dental problems

Hirschmann (Chapter 42) gives six good reasons for checking dental problems. In addition to preventing pain, improving appearance and making eating easier, he suggests it can help speech, oral hygiene and maybe maintaining teeth as an accessory limb.

Tissue viability

Sensory loss, immobility or incontinence will predispose to skin breakdown and pressure sores. Areas at risk need to be examined (Chapter 36).

Sexual problems

It is important that this issue is not ignored. However, an outpatient clinic may not be the ideal venue. Causes of sexual problems may be physical, due to spasticity, muscle weakness, sensory loss, pain or joint limitation, or psychological. They may be caused by anxiety or depression or they may be due to prescribed drugs, notably hypotensives. Lack of understanding of the underlying condition with its consequent disability will compound the problem; concentration on residual abilities will help. Some patients have a poor self-image, seeing themselves as incomplete and damaged, which impairs their psychological and sexual function as well as every other aspect of their life.

The possibility of abuse in childhood needs to be borne in mind as a cause for unexplained symptoms: it happens, and may trigger a roundabout request for help. Disabled children may be abused, this happens too, it is important to be aware of the possibility, and to know where there are specialist counsellors accessible. There are now books available to help professionals and patients (see 'Further reading').

Work and finance

Work will involve consideration of return to the previous employment, possibly modified, placement in an alternative occupation or training for a new job (Chapter 52).

Finance is a major problem for people with disability as this often results in additional costs for transport, clothing, food and heating, and a reduced income. For advice on allowances or other benefits available, the patient may be directed to the Welfare Rights Adviser at the Citizens' Advice Bureau or to the social worker who can offer up-to-date advice as benefits change frequently. While money does not solve disability, lack of it certainly compounds the problem. Frequently patients do not claim all the benefits to which they are entitled.

Family and social relationships

Once management of the most severe problems is under way, other problems can be considered. It is important to help the patient to take part in social activities (in work, sports and leisure). However, considerable help and encouragement may be needed. A disabled person affects the whole family to some degree. Explanation to the family jointly with the patient about the remaining abilities and the treatment programme is vital from the beginning. The family will obviously consider the needs of the disabled person, but these must not be so dominant that the other members of the family are neglected.

CONCLUSION

Caring for a patient with a disability involves a network of professional carers. Each have different roles and responsibilities and needs to make their own role-orientated assessment. The assessment and management of disability is an area in which team work is essential (Chapter 6).

Rehabilitation is an enabling process which allows the disabled person to gain maximum independence and enjoyment of life. The disabled person may frequently underestimate residual ability and acceptance by others, which will lead to social isolation and a rapid worsening of medical and social functioning.

Adequate medical and social assessment of the disabilities arising due to the illness or injury will lead to better management. Even if problems remain, the patient will benefit from knowing that someone cares enough to spend time and trouble finding out what the problems really are and explaining to the patient and family which problems can be overcome and which are insoluble. We should aim for acceptance of the true situation and restoration of choice in life as far as possible.

REFERENCES

Bowlby, J. (1980) *Attachment and Loss: loss, sadness and depression*, vol. 3, Basic Books, New York.

Parkes, C.M. (1970) The first year of bereavement: a longitudinal study of the reaction of London widows to death of husbands. *Psychiatry*, **33**, 444–67.

Worden, J.W. (1991) *Grief Counselling and Grief Therapy*, 2nd edn, Routledge, London.

FURTHER READING

Bass, E. and Davis, A. (1988) *The Courage to Heal*, Mandarin Paperbacks, London.

Doyle, C. (1994) *Child Sexual Abuse*, Chapman & Hall, London.

Wakley, G. (1991) *Sexual Abuse and the Primary Care Doctor*, Chapman & Hall, London.

8   Locomotion: analysis of gait

J. Goodwill and M. Lord

INTRODUCTION

Walking is an activity which we all take for granted. Yet its performance requires complex coordination of the neuro-skeletomotor system, adequate to maintain an inherently unstable structure in an upright position, and to do this during an activity involving no less than lifting one of the two supporting struts off the ground. During walking, the body is not in a quasi-static balance, but rather proceeds with a series of controlled falls from one limb to the other.

Disruption of any part of the system, from damage to the basic mechanical structures of bone and joint, through loss of muscle power or altered sensory feedback, up to pathology of the integrating centres of the CNS, will all be reflected in some form of gait abnormality. This might be demonstrated by:

- unusual timing or variation of the normal sequence of walking;
- abnormal ranges of motion at joints;
- asymmetry of gait;
- slowness, jerkiness;
- erratic repetition of the gait cycle and loss of rhythmicity;
- difficulty with compensation for disturbances such as irregular ground;
- tripping or falling.

Clinical gait analysis is used to describe and quantify these abnormalities as a basis for patient assessment and the planning, monitoring and evaluation of treatment (Whittle, 1991).

THE GAIT CYCLE

The swing and stance phases

For each leg walking is a cyclic repetition of two phases of gait. The **stance phase** is that part of the cycle when the foot is in contact with the ground, and the **swing phase** is when it is lifted clear and propelled forward. Since the stance phase typically lasts for 60% of the walking cycle, there is an overlapping **double-support** period when both feet are on the ground (Figure 8.1)

Sagittal plane motion

The most easily described gait events occur in the sagittal plane. In normal gait, the stance phase commences at heel contact. The knee is close to full extension and the ankle dorsiflexed with the foot partially supinated, so the lateral border of the heel touches the ground first. The foot comes smoothly flat to the ground during the first 15% of the stance phase under a controlled co-contraction of the ankle dorsi-and plantar-flexor muscles. In this early stance phase, the forward velocity of the body drops slightly and hence this is also referred to as the deceleration state.

Rehabilitation of the Physically Disabled Adult. Edited by C. John Goodwill, M. Anne Chamberlain and Chris Evans. Published in 1997 by Stanley Thornes (Publishers) Ltd, Cheltenham. ISBN 0-7487-3183-0.

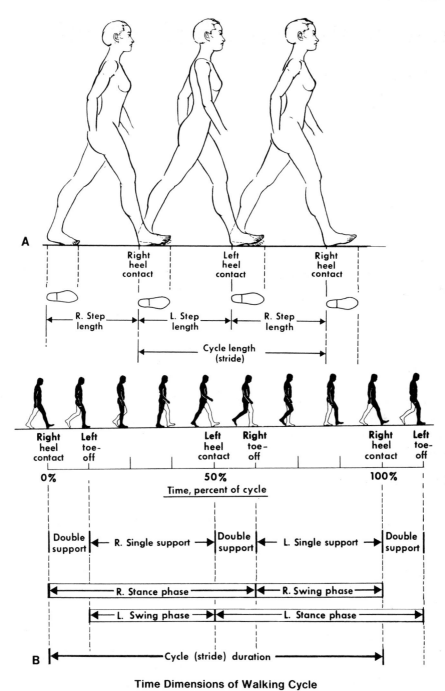

Figure 8.1 Distance and time dimensions of walking cycle. A, distance (length); B, time.

As the body progresses forward over the foot the knee of the supporting leg is flexed to 12–15° (Figure 8.2). This helps to maintain a smooth forward progression of the pelvis by reducing rapid 'vaulting' over the limb. By mid-stance both knee and hip are approaching their neutral position; the hip then starts to extend. At about 70% of stance phase the knee begins to flex again allowing the heel to lift off the floor and the foot pronates. The body is accelerated forward: hence the term **push-off** is sometimes used for this stage. **Toe-off** normally occurs from the medial border under the great toe with the knee flexion at 40–50°. Once the foot leaves the ground it enters the swing phase. The thigh is rapidly accelerated forward by flexion of the hip. The foot initially trails behind with knee flexion increased up to 60° at mid-swing. This knee flexion, in combination with dorsi-flexion at the ankle and abduction at the hip, ensures that the foot remains clear of the ground during swing through (Chao *et al.*,1983). Maximum hip flexion of 25° is reached by mid-swing and maintained while the knee extends to bring the foot forward to its full extent before the next heel contact ends the cycle.

Coronal plane motion

The body also moves from side to side during each step. The distance between successive steps, measured between the centre-heel of the left and right foot perpendicular to the direction of progression, is a measure of the **stride width**. Stride width may be subconsciously increased if the stability of gait is threatened as, for example, when walking on a rocking boat or when walking with a limb prosthesis. As a consequence of the mediolateral motion, acceleration of the body in late stance phase is directed not only forward but also towards the contralateral limb. Similarly deceleration in early stance phase is directed posteriorly

and medially. **Stride length** is the distance between successive heel contacts.

Transverse plane motion

Rotations of the femur and tibia result partially from sideways body motion while the foot is weightbearing and stationary with respect to the ground; partially from the effect of the oblique angle of the subtalar joint in the hindfoot complex, this leading to conversion of inversion/eversion of the hindfoot into external/internal rotation respectively of the tibia. Hence, after heel contract, the tibia rotates internally as the foot pronates to the foot flat position (Inman, Ralston and Todd, 1981; Moseley *et al*, 1995): in the last 25% of the stance phase the tibia rotates externally 8–9° as the hindfoot inverts at heel-off. In the course of stance phase rotation at the hip immediately passes from near neutral to 6° external, reversing back to 4–5° internally (Smidt, 1990) to facilitate the anteromedial direction of push-off. In swing phase the hip moves in a sequence of external then internal rotation back to the neutral position before heel contact.

Opposing trunk and pelvic rotations are observed in normal gait. As the left leg swings forward, the accompanying clockwise rotation of the pelvis is balanced by an anticlockwise rotation of the trunk of approximately 7°. Right arm swing accompanies the trunk rotation, with flexion at the shoulder and elbow of approximately 30°. The counter-rotation of the pelvis and trunk, and the counterbalancing of leg and arm swing, are both essential elements of an efficient gait. Without these upper-body compensatory motions, a net twisting moment would be generated on the body which demands extra muscular effort to counter. Jackson, Joseph and Wyard (1983) found that walking was difficult if the ipsilateral arm moved forward with the leg or if the arms were strapped to the trunk.

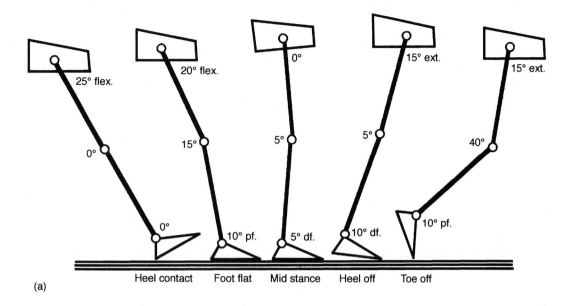

(a)

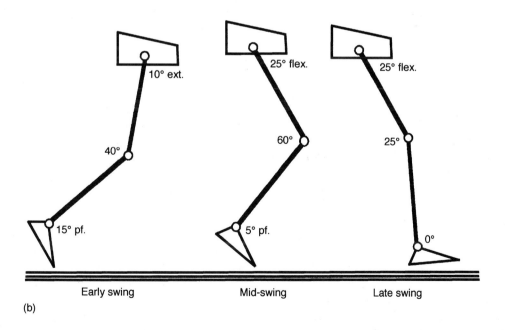

(b)

Figure 8.2 Position of leg joints. (a), In stance phase; (b), in swing phase. Showing angle of hip flexion or extension, knee flexion, and ankle plantarflexion (pf) or dorsiflexion (df).

RANGES OF MOTION

For normal gait, adequate ranges of motion are required at the hip, knee and ankle. In summary these are :

- Hip: 15° extension in late-stance, up to 25° flexion in late swing/early-stance phase
- Knee: a few degrees flexion at early-stance, up to 60° flexion in mid-swing
- Ankle: up to 15° plantar flexion at heel-off, up to 20° dorsiflexion at toe-off and early swing phase.

FORCES AND ENERGY

The ground reaction force (GRF) acting between foot and floor opposes both the vertical pull of gravity and the inertial forces generated in acceleration of the body. The GRF is greatest in the vertical direction, but horizontal components in the anteroposterior and mediolateral directions are not negligible at about 15% bodyweight.

After heel contact, the vertical component of force under the heel shows a sharp transient rise due to the shock of impact; it then rises more gradually to a first peak at foot-flat as the limb takes the weight of the body. The vertical force falls off slightly in mid-stance, then reverses back to a second peak at the commencement of push-off before dropping again to zero at toe-off. **This produces a characteristic double-humped shape in the plot of vertical force versus time.** Both of the peaks are slightly greater than body weight in normal gait. The patterns are often a sensitive indicator of gait abnormalities such as asymmetry between left and right, or loss of push-off acceleration due to hip problems. In the horizontal direction, the force is consistent with the deceleration at early-stance phase and acceleration at push-off in the fore-aft direction, and is predominantly directed medially towards the contralateral limb.

If the GRF is shown as a vector, its line of action is instructive about the moments which are sustained about the major joints of the body (Figure 8.3). For example, in spastic gait

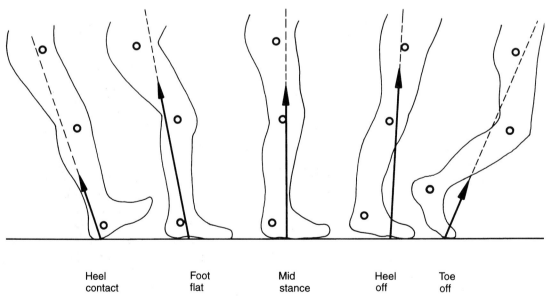

| Heel | Foot | Mid | Heel | Toe |
| contact | flat | stance | off | off |

Figure 8.3 Ground reaction force vectors relative to joint positions during stance phase: the vector represents the magnitude and line of action of the force.

the GRF vector may be seen to fall well ahead of the knee joint in early-stance phase: this results in the knee characteristically snapping and locking into hyperextension throughout early- and mid-stance phases. In this case, an ankle-foot orthosis may be appropriate to prevent excessive ankle flexion and bring the GRF into the more normal line close to the knee.

Walking speed and energy consumption

Most people adopt the gait pattern which is most energy efficient, unless pain or loss of joint stability are dominant. This includes a preferred speed from which deviations, either faster or slower, result in a higher metabolic cost per unit of distance travelled (Ralston, 1958, Margaria 1976). On average, walking is most efficient at about 80 m min^{-1} requiring about 0.8 cal/m per kg of body mass. A disabled person may walk more slowly to maintain a level of oxygen consumption which does not cause breathlessness (Fisher and Gullickson, 1978)

Faster forward progress cannot be achieved by maintaining the same cadence (steps min^{-1}) and increasing the stride length only, because energy consumption is then unduly increased; the cadence as well as the stride length must be increased (Saunders *et al.*, 1953). As cadence increases there is a reduction in both stance phase and double support phase time as a percentage of the gait cycle. Conversely double support may be much longer in slow or hesitant gait (Kirtley, Whittle and Jefferson, 1985)

The centre of gravity of the body undulates, moving upwards during stance phase and falling again during swing phase by approximately 20–50 mm (Inman, Ralston and Todd, 1981). The resultant oscillations in potential energy of the body are partially offset by the antiphase fluctuations in kinetic energy as forward velocity changes. By this means an efficient gait is maintained. Abnormalities of gait which prevent this regular exchange, as with those which require excessive and irregular movements, will reduce efficiency.

MUSCLES USED IN WALKING

Anterior tibial muscles are used throughout swing phase to dorsiflex the ankle and in early-stance until foot-flat. **Calf muscles** act mainly in mid-stance to provide heel-off.

The **quadriceps** contract in early stance to stabilize the knee, and in late-stance and early-swing to bring the flexed knee forward to gain step length, whilst the **hamstring** muscles are used particularly in late-swing and early-stance to help stabilize the knee. **Hip abductors and extensors** contract mainly in early-stance to support the body weight; **hip flexors** in swing phase to bring the leg forward, while the **hip adductors** contract mainly in the late-stance phase.

Walking up or down steps requires a greater range of movement and muscle strength than walking on a level surface. When going up the calf muscles have to lift the body weight on to the next step, and the ankle of the supporting foot plantarflexes more than the 15° required in level walking; conversely when descending, the ankle of the supporting foot dorsiflexes more than the usual 20°. The hips and knees flex less on going downstairs than when walking on level ground, but when going upstairs may have to flex up to 80° or 90°, or even more for a high step. On stairs the quadriceps and hip muscles need to contract more strongly than when walking on flat ground, so as to lift the body weight up, or to support the stance leg while the other leg is lowered on to the next step. The latter is often the bigger problem, and may cause more pain in the arthritic knee or hip than going upstairs. In the same way weakness of hip or knee muscles from neurological or other diseases can make it more difficult to go downstairs than upstairs; moreover, when going up the body is leaning forwards and the patient is less likely to fall.

The neurological control of gait is complex and only partly understood. It is coordinated by interneurones and fixed at an early stage in infant development. There are rhythm-generating centres in the spinal cord, one for each limb, leg flexion occurring mainly in swing phase and extension in the stance phase of gait, with inhibition of the opposite muscle groups. These centres are controlled by descending pathways from the brainstem and cerebral hemispheres. Sensory input from joint muscle and skin receptors and vestibular apparatus is needed for normal gait and visual input is important, particularly if either of these are damaged. The cerebellum influences timing and coordination of gait, and the basal ganglia influence posture so that disease of the latter causes immobility (Martin, 1967). The neurological control of gait was well reviewed by Joseph (1985)

CLINICAL GAIT ANALYSIS

Simple observation of gait by a skilled clinician can be highly informative in a single patient assessment. More quantifiable measures are desirable for planning and monitoring of complex treatment. Protocols and methodology for gait analysis are arguably still in their infancy as regards standard practice and verification; although these have been used in research laboratories for many years, there are few examples of routine clinical use. Of these, planning of tendon transfer operations and alignment of lower-limb orthoses can be cited.

The well-equipped gait laboratory will be equipped with a walkway, a motion analysis system to record kinematics and a force plate to record the ground reaction force. It may have facilities for EMG or foot-pressure studies. Technically all this equipment is undergoing rapid development and a multi-media approach is now producing exciting clinical possibilities. The 'visual vectorgram' concept which originated at Moss Rehabilita-

tion Hospital in Philadelphia (Cook, 1978) makes the information given in Figure 8.3 a simple procedure to capture; the modern version of this incorporates the output of the force plate with a video recording of the patient's gait or even a 'stickman' produced from the motion analysis system.

ABNORMAL GAIT

Arthritis

A leg that is short by 3–5 cm or more causes obvious dipping of the pelvis towards that side during stance phase, the patient leaning towards that side, while excessive flexion of the opposite knee and hip is used to clear the ground with the contralateral foot.

Pain in the hip or knee will be worse in stance than swing phase, the proportion of the former being decreased causing asymmetry of gait. In walking, joint movement and step length are reduced (Tesio, Civuschi and Tessari 1995).

Also, during stance on the painful side, the hip may not be able to support the body weight adequately, giving rise to excess dipping of the pelvis towards the opposite leg, i.e. waddling.

Pain in the ankle or tarsal joints is felt mainly during the early-stance phase as the force of the body weight is taken on the hindfoot; the pain may ease as the heel leaves the ground. It is at this time, later in stance phase, that the metatarsophalangeal joints are passively dorsiflexed as the body weight moves forward over them. Because of this movement and the extra force through the forefoot, pain at these joints is worse late in the stance phase, although it can be reduced by a rocker sole on the shoe (Chapter 47)

Limitation of joint movement

Fixed flexion at the hip will require increased lumbar lordosis to maintain an erect posture when the knee is straight and weightbearing. If the hip is so much flexed that the knee cannot be fully extended normally in the first part of the stance phase, the flexed knee can only be stabilized by stronger contraction of the quadriceps or by the patient leaning forward on a stick, resulting in reduced step length on the normal side.

Fixed hip adduction causes an inability to abduct the hip during the swing phase, the patient tilting the pelvis to the opposite side to compensate.

Fixed flexion or adduction of the hip causes apparent shortening of the leg. In the stance phase, severe flexed adduction may make the patient unstable; falling to the affected side is prevented by use of a stick on that side.

Limitation of hip flexion is not a problem for walking because the joint only needs to flex 25–30°, and by the time this severity of limitation occurs the associated hip pain is usually the bigger problem. However, going up steps or sitting down requires up to 90° of hip flexion, and will be difficult for many patients.

Fixed flexion of the knee over 25° causes the ground reaction force to lie behind the knee axis during the stance phase, requiring stronger quadriceps contraction to support the body weight and the patient to lean forward. In addition, the heel stays clear of the ground so that the stance phase starts with the toe hitting the ground rather than with the normal heel contact. In the swing phase the leg cannot reach out as far as normal to gain a normal step length.

Limited flexion of the knee, or pain on flexion, limits the normal joint movement in late-stance and early swing phase of gait, causing a reduction in step length on both sides and an inefficient gait pattern. With a fixed straight knee the ipsilateral pelvis has to rise excessively in the swing phase and gait may improve with a heel raise on the opposite side. It is easier with a knee fixed in 15° flexion; however, there is still greater movement of the centre of gravity than is normal.

Ankle joint limitation on its own causes little problem until the movement is reduced to 10° up or down, when the foot tends to be put down and taken up in one piece, with loss of the normal heel-toe gait. There is a small increase in knee and hip flexion to compensate (Saunders *et al*, 1953). However, there is often limitation of tarsal joint movement as well, which limits the normal pronation-supination of the foot.

FLACCID MUSCLE WEAKNESS

Flaccid foot-drop as in common peroneal nerve paralysis, poliomyelitis or muscular dystrophy, requires excessive lifting of the leg during the swing phase in order to clear the ground; this is done by lifting the pelvis on the ipsilateral side with excessive flexion of the hip and knee. Stance may start with toe rather than heel contact, unless there is only moderate dorsiflexion weakness, when the whole foot may reach the ground at one time, causing a slapping sound.

Calf muscle weakness limits the force available to lift the body weight up during attempted heel-off. Heel-off on the weak side is delayed until heel contact occurs on the opposite side, and the ground reaction force passing through the foot is kept further back for longer than is usual. There is an increased flexor moment about the knee, requiring increased quadriceps contraction to counteract it. Excessive ankle dorsiflexion may result, which can be controlled by an ankle-foot orthosis limiting dorsiflexion (Lehmann *et al*, 1985)

Quadriceps weakness: the knee axis passes through the femoral condyles 2–4 cm above the joint line, being forward in extension and moving back as the knee flexes. Knee stability during the stance phase is normally maintained by quadriceps power, although weakness may be partly or wholly compensated by strong hip extensor muscles. During the stance phase this moves the knee joint axis back behind the line of body weight as the centre of gravity moves forward rapidly. This will then prevent knee flexion while the cruciate ligaments prevent excessive extension. During the late swing phase normal knee extension is helped by the inertia of the forward-moving leg; strong hip extensors decelerate the thigh. allowing the lower leg to swing forward to heel contact.

Weakness of hip and knee flexor muscles: this causes reduced hip flexion in the swing phase and reduced knee control in the swing and early-stance phases, resulting in excessive lifting and forward rotation of the ipsilateral pelvis with a forward 'flip' of the leg, including some circumduction.

Hip girdle muscle weakness causes a waddling gait because the hip is not supported normally in the stance phase, allowing excessive dipping of the opposite side of the pelvis. This is seen in muscular dystrophies and in other myopathies such as osteomalacia and hypothyrodism. Often the quadriceps muscles are also weak, causing additional problems with knee stability. When standing still, any attempt to stand on one leg causes dropping down of the contralateral unsupported side of the pelvis, because the hip on the stance side is not supported normally by the hip abductors and extensors. (Trendelenburg sign).

PARAPLEGIA

If the patient has complete leg weakness he/she may walk using elbow or Canadian crutches and knee–ankle–foot orthoses with the knees locked in extension; the ankles are supported to prevent plantarflexion. This stiff-legged gait works because the pelvis is lifted for each step by the latissimus dorsi, and the remaining abdominal and spinal muscles, the point of fixation being the shoulders which are supported by strong downward thrust on the arms through straight elbows to the crutches. The higher the lesion, the more

energy is required for walking, and above T11–12 it usually becomes a wasteful activity for most adults, although there are a few exceptions (Chapter 47). Even normal subjects use twice the normal amount of energy when walking with either under-arm or elbow crutches; no difference was found between these two types of crutches (Fisher and Patterson 1981). However, Dounis, Steventon and Wilson (1980) found that in five normal subjects the Canadian crutch (with a rigid complete circular top) was more energy efficient than the elbow crutch; the distance walked per litre of oxygen used was on average 61.3 m compared with 53.3 m. Children can walk efficiently with higher lesions than adults, as is seen in many children with spina bifida who walk when young but stop doing so when they reach their teens. These children may use plastic or metal above-knee orthoses (KAFO), a hip guidance orthosis or a swivel walker (Rose, 1986)

Cauda equina lesions produce a wide variety of patterns of leg weakness; although they have flaccid paralysis, contractures can be a major problem if these are not prevented. If the quadriceps are spared, ankle–foot orthoses will provide foot and ankle support, and the normal knee control will allow a near-normal gait pattern using a walking aid. If quadriceps are weak, then KAFO are needed, and the patient will walk with a stiff-legged gait as described above.

SPASTIC MUSCLE WEAKNESS

Spastic drop foot causes the foot to catch during the swing phase, and the spasticity of the calf muscles produces an inversion moment about the subtalar joint causing the foot to go into equinovarus. At the start of the stance phase, the toe rather than the heel reaches the ground first, and the outer border of the foot may reach the ground before the inner border; if the spasticity is mild, the foot may then be forced flat by the body weight. If there is severe varus, the body weight pushes the foot into more inversion and the patient may bear all or most of his/her weight on the outer border of the foot throughout the stance phase. The axis of the subtalar joint passes about 45° downwards and 12° outwards from the navicular, backwards, out and down to the outer posterior aspect of the calcaneum, so that the tendo Achilles has a medial (inversion) movement about this axis (Hall, 1959). Although the vertical distance from the line of pull of the tendo Achilles to the joint axis is small, the strength of the muscles is so much greater than that of the other invertors, that this vector of force provides the main mechanical force inverting the subtalar joint (Lapidus, 1955), at the same time as it plantarflexes the foot at the ankle joint (Alexander *et al*, 1982)

Most commonly spastic equinus is part of hemiplegia due to stroke, in which there is not only spastic weakness of the arm and leg but often also impairment of skin sensation, muscle and joint position sense and often of body image, all of which affect gait. The stance phase is shortened on the affected side but the duration of single-leg support does not correlate with the degree of motor recovery. If there is some remaining power in the quadriceps and hip muscles, the patient may learn to keep the knee locked in extension to help weight to be taken through the affected leg; however, this makes it impossible to walk with anything approaching a normal pattern. Measurement of the ground reaction force reflects accurately the degree of recovery and is useful in evaluating gait in these patients (Morita, Yamamoto and Furuya, 1985). The ipsilateral side of the pelvis is also rotated backwards which aggravates the problem (Wall and Ashburn, 1979; Brandstater *et al*, 1983). Slow movement of the paretic leg during the swing phase prolongs stance on the opposite leg; the latter is also prolonged due to the slower than normal weight transferance from the weak to the good leg during the period of double support (Eke-Okoro and Larsson, 1984). Step

length on the weak side is shortened to 67–92% of normal (Tesio, Civaschi and Tessari, 1985). There are thus many abnormalities of gait with which patient and therapist have to contend, and clearly the ability to maintain single leg support while the good leg swings through is the main determinant of gait (Perry, 1969; Turnbull and Wall, 1985).

The combination of stroke and leg amputation is not uncommon (Varghese *et al*, 1978) and presents a considerable challenge to rehabilitation, Nevertheless, in that series of 30 patients, 10 achieved useful walking in their home, although only three were able to walk outside the house, all of the latter having the hemiplegia and the amputation on the same side.

EFFECTS OF CONTRACTURE

Fixed plantarflexion due to contracture of the calf muscles, as may occur with prolonged spasticity due to stroke or head injury, causes the tibia to be angled back if the foot is flat on the ground. This helps to lock the knee in extension in early-stance and weight-bearing, but later in the stance phase it precipitates early heel-off and impedes knee flexion. This either effectively increases leg length and increases rise and fall of the centre of gravity or greatly limits step length in the other leg.

Fixed flexion of the knee and/or hip can occur even with good physiotherapy, more often due to head injury than stroke; more than 25° fixed flexion of either will cause gait problems. The knee is bent in the stance phase in either case, and even if fixed equinus is absent the heel is off the ground in order to keep the line of body weight over the supporting foot. Step length is shortened because the knee cannot extend in the latter part of the swing phase, and walking aids are often needed to maintain stability.

PARKINSON'S DISEASE

Bradykinesia and the rigidity results in difficulty in initiating movement and a slow shuffling flat-footed gait. Knuttson (1972) found the reduced walking speed and prolonged gait cycle were due to diminished stride length, with an increased period of double support and reduction of associated trunk and arm movement. In normal gait right and left steps are equal, but he found only 4 of 21 subjects with Parkinson's disease has a symmetrical gait pattern. Ankle plantar-flexion was reduced at the end of the stance phase, causing difficulty in initiating swing, and there was also a reduction in hip flexion and knee flexion and extension. These combine to reduce the speed and amplitude of leg movement, and the gait problems are aggravated by the variability of the disease.

CEREBELLAR ATAXIA

This condition presents considerable problems. The patient walks on a wide base, the incoordination affecting all parts of the gait cycle and encouraging a prolonged stance phase to prevent falling. If a stick is used, the support base can be kept wide while the feet are brought into a more normal position. The gait problem is largely unresponsive to physiotherapy, even using biofeedback with the patient viewing his/her gait pattern in a mirror placed in front of him/her. The difficulties may be aggravated by ataxia of the arms and/or trunk, or by muscle weakness or position sense loss, all of which often occur in the diseases that cause cerebellar ataxia.

AGEING

With an ageing population, gait in the elderly has come under closer scrutiny, particularly with respect to the lift-threatening phenomena of falls. The basic changes in gait were noted by Murray, Kory and Clarkson, (1969); Murray, Kory and Sepic, (1970) in studies of men up to age 87 and women up to 70. On average the preferred walking speed decreases from middle age, but this must be viewed against normal variability in gait parameters (Dobbs *et al*, 1993). The gait characteristics are not noticeably different in healthy elderly subjects from those at the same speed of walking in a younger person (Finley, Cody and Finizie, 1969). If asked to walk faster, this is achieved by increasing cadence rather than stride length. Stride width also increases in elderly subjects (Payne and Blanke, 1985)

Physiological changes which obviously affect gait in the elderly include a loss of flexibility and shock absorption properties of the connective tissue, loss of muscle bulk and strength, and deterioration in coordination. Nevertheless, the changes in normal gait parameters of the elderly are not particularly striking until well into the 80s, provided that there is no underlying pathological condition. Why then are the elderly apparently more prone to falls? This is more readily understood from the viewpoint of Overstall (1978) who describes a fall simply as an uncorrected displacement. If gait is regarded as a series of controlled falls, then it is the loss of control that is crucial. When the centre of gravity has moved outside the stable base, rapid corrective action is needed (Winter, 1984). It is not yet established whether the deficit is in the voluntary or involuntary reactions, in the sensing and coordination of a response, or the production of a rapid muscle contraction.

In any event, the critical time for falls during walking is as the foot either reaches or leaves the floor. At heel contact the danger is one of the shoe sliding, at toe-off of catching; polished vinyl floors and deep carpets are equally hazardous. Twenty-five per cent of all falls have been reported to occur on the stairs (Nickens, 1985), where corrections for deviations in position are naturally occurring against a background of very high force levels in the muscles (Freedman, Wannstedt and Herman, 1976). For this reason, it is important that steps be as even in height and contours as possible to minimize the disturbances, with the height kept low to reduce the demands on muscles.

SUMMARY

Detailed descriptions of human locomotion available at this time can be used to illuminate abnormalities due to pathological conditions. Studies in gait laboratories have augmented experienced clinical observation to provide a deeper understanding of the skeletomotor action, neuromuscular integration and biomechanical factors in the maintenance of posture and walking. Recognition of clinical conditions and correct attribution of abnormalities to causative factors is a vital part in the treatment or management of the resulting disability.

REFERENCES

Alexander, M.C., Battye, C.K., Goodwill, C.J. and Walshe, J.B. (1982) The ankle and subtalar joints. In measurement of joint movement. *Clinics in Rheumatic Diseases*, **8**, 3.

Brandstater, M.E., de Bruin, H., Gowland, C. and Clark, B.M. (1983) Hemiplegic gait: analysis of temporal variables. *Archives of Physical Medicine and Rehabilitation*, **64**, 583–7.

Chao, E.Y., Laughman, R.K., Schneider, E. and Stauffer, R.N. (1983) Normative data of knee joint motion and ground reaction forces in adult level walking. *Journal of Biomechanics*, **16**, 219–33.

Cook, T.M. (1978) Force visualisation as a method of gait analysis, in *Disability* (Eds. R.M. Kenedi, J.P. Paul and J. Hughes), Macmillan, Basingstoke, pp. 124–30.

Dobbs, R.J., Charlett, A., Bowers, S.G., O'Neill, C.J.A., Weller, C., Hughes, J. and Dobbs, S.M. (1993) Is this walk normal? *Age and Ageing*, **22**, 27–30.

Dounis, E., Steventon, R.D. and Wilson, R.S.E. (1980) The use of a portable oxygen consumption meter (Oxylog) for assessing the efficiency of crutch walking. *Journal of Medical Engineering and Technology*, **4**, 296–8.

Ede-Okoro, S.T. and Larsson, L.E. (1984) A comparison of the gaits of paretic patients with the gaits of control subjects carrying a load. *Scandinavian Journal of Rehabilitation Medicine*, **16**, 151–8.

Finley, F.R., Cody, K.A. and Finizie, R.V. (1969) Locomotion patterns in elderly women. *Archives of Physical Medicine and Rehabilitation*, **50**, 140–46.

Fisher, S.V. and Gullickson, G. (1978) Energy cost of ambulation in health and disability, a literature review. *Archives of Physical Medicine and Rehabilitation*, **59**, 124–33.

Fisher, S.V. and Patterson, R.P. (1981) Energy cost of ambulation. *Archives of Physical Medicine and Rehabilitation*, **62**, 250–6.

Freedman, W., Wannstedt, G. and Herman, R. (1976) EMG patterns and forces developed during step down. *American Journal of Physical Medicine*, **55**, 275–90.

Hall, M.C. (1959) The normal movement at the subtalar joint *Canadian Journal of Surgery*, **2**, 287–90.

Inman, V.T., Ralston, H.J. and Todd, F. (1981) *Human Walking*, Williams & Wilkins, Baltimore.

Jackson, K.M., Joseph, J. and Wyard, S.J. (1983) The upper limbs during human walking. Part 2: Functional. *Electroencephalography and Clinical Neurophysiology*, **23**, 435–46.

Joseph, J. (1985) Neurological control of locomotion. *Developmental Medicine and Child Neurology*, **27**, 822–9.

Kirtley, C., Whittle, M.W. and Jefferson, R.J. (1985) Influence of walking speed on gait parameters. *Journal Biomedical Engineering*, **7**, 282–8.

Knuttson, E. (1972) An analysis of Parkinsonian gait. *Brain*, **95**, 475–86.

Lapidus, T.W. (1955) Subtalar joint, its anatomy and mechanics. *Bulletin for the Hospital for Joint Disease* **16**, 179–95.

Lehmann, J.F., Condon, S.M., de Lateur, B.J. and Smith, J.C. (1985) Gait abnormalities in tibial nerve paralysis: a biomechanical study. *Archives of Physical Medicine and Rehabilitation*, **66**, 80–5.

Margaria, R. (1976) *Biomechanics and Energetics of Muscular Exercise*, Clarendon Press, Oxford.

Martin, J.P. (1967) *The Basal Ganglia and Posture*, Pitman, London.

Morita, S., Yamamoto, H. and Furuya, K. (1995) Gait analysis of hemiplegic patients by measurement of ground reaction force. *Scandinavian Journal of Rehabilitation Medicine*, **27**, 37–42.

Moseley, L., Smith, R., Hunt, A. and Gant, R. (1995) Three dimensional kinematics of the rearfoot during the stance phase of walking in normal young adult males. *Clinical Biomechanics*, **11**, 39–45.

Murray, M.P., Kory, R. and Clarkson, B. (1969) Walking patterns in healthy old men. *Journal of Gerontology*, **24**, 169–78.

Murray, M.P., Kory, R.C. and Sepic, S.B. (1970) Walking patterns of normal women. *Archives of Physical Medicine and Rehabilitation*, **51**, 637–50.

Nickens, H. (1985) Instrinsic factors in falling among the elderly. *Archives of Internal Medicine,* **145**, 1089–93.

Overstall, P.W. (1978) Falls in the elderly–Epidemiology, aetiology and management, in *Recent Advances in Geriatric Medicine* (ed. Isaacs, B.), Churchill Livingstone, Edinburgh, p. 61.

Payne, P. and Blanke, D. (1985) Comparison of gait parameters of young and elderly women *Physical Therapy,* **65**, 686. (abstr).

Perry, J. (1969) Mechanics of walking in hemiplegia. *Clinical Orthopaedics,* **63**, 23–31.

Ralston, H.J. (1958) Energy–speed relation and optimal speed during level walking. *Zeirschmt für Angewandte Bäder and Klimaheilkunde,* **17**, 277–83.

Rose, G.K. (1986) *Orthotics: principles and practice,* Heinemann, London.

Saunders, J.B. deC., Saunders, M., Inman V.T. and Eberhart, H.D. (1953) The major determinants in normal and pathological gait. *Journal Bone and Joint Surgery,* **35A**, 543–58.

Smidt, G.L. (ed) (1990) *Gait in Rehabilitation,* Churchill Livingstone, Edinburgh.

Tesio, L., Civaschi, P. and Tessari, L. (1985) Motion of the centre of gravity of the body in clinical evaluation of gait. *American Journal of Physical Medicine,* **64**, 57–70.

Turnbull, G.I. and Wall, J.C. (1985) The development of a system for the clinical assessment of gait following a stroke. *Physiotherapy,* **71**, 294–8.

Varghese, G., Hinterbuchner, C., Mondall, P. and Sakuma, J. (1978) Rehabilitation outcome of patients with dual disability of hemiplegia and amputation. *Archives of Physical and Medical Rehabilitation,* **59**, 121–3.

Wall, J.C. and Ashburn A. (1979) Assessment of gait disability in hemiplegics. *Scandinavian Journal Rehabilitation Medicine,* **11**, 95–103.

Whittle, M. (1991) *Gait Analysis: An Introduction,* Butterworth Heinemann, Oxford.

Winter, D.A. (1984) Kinematics and kinetic patterns in human gait: variability and compensating effects. *Human Movement Science,* **3**, 51–76.

FURTHER READING

Antonsson, E.K. and Mann, R.W. (1985) The frequency content of gait. *Journal of Biochemistry,* **18**, 39–47.

Inman, V.T. (1967) Conservation of energy in ambulation. *Archives of Physical Medicine and Rehabilitation,* **48**, 484–8.

Murray, M.P., Drought, A.B. and Kory, R.C. (1964) Walking patterns of normal men *Journal of Bone and Joint Surgery,* **46A**, 335–60.

Winter, D.A. (1987) *The Biomechanics and Motor Control of Human Gait.* University of Waterloo Press, Canada.

9 Outcome, indices and measurements

J. Hunter

INTRODUCTION

Research in rehabilitation lags about 25 years behind most organ-specific specialities and 50 years behind laboratory-based clinical investigations. This is largely due to the relatively primitive state of development of appropriate tools to measure many aspects of the consequences of disease. Within the last 20 years, however, a large number of instruments have been developed and validated and it is now possible to measure most of the physical and psychological consequences of disease. Our ability to measure social performance, however, remains very limited. Progress in the field has been complicated by the variety of terms used to describe similar consequences of disease, for example functional ability, functional status, health status, quality of life, etc. Although in many instances the variation in use of terms may reflect genuine differences of concept, for example in the individual and societal definitions of disability, commonly, as in the use of the term **outcome measures**, it may hide a lack of clarity of thought.

However, improvement is occurring, some being traceable to the development in the 1960s and 1970s of psychometric and statistical techniques which have established a framework for developing many of the measures used today. The delineation of the concepts of impairment, disability and handicap by the World Health Organization (WHO) in 1980 has also provided a rational framework for many of the more recent developments. Whilst it is useful to be clear whether various outcome measures are measuring impairment, disability or handicap, many measures, particularly older ones, measure attributes in more than one of the ICIDH classifications.

MEASUREMENT

The phrase outcome measures has been used in two separate ways, first to describe the instruments by which a particular function may be measured, and second as a shorthand way of describing the results of these assessments. For the purpose of this chapter the term **tools of measurement** will be used to describe the techniques used, and **outcome** to refer to the results obtained using these instruments. It is also worth defining **measurement** – the use of a standard to quantify an observation. The **quantitative** approach was a major factor leading to the rapid advances made in physics and chemistry, and more recently in biological and biomedical sciences. 'When you can measure what you are speaking about, and express it in numbers, then you know something about it, and when you cannot measure it, and you cannot express it in numbers, then your

Rehabilitation of the Physically Disabled Adult. Edited by C. John Goodwill, M. Anne Chamberlain and Chris Evans. Published in 1997 by Stanley Thornes (Publishers) Ltd, Cheltenham. ISBN 0-7487-3183-0.

knowledge is of a meagre and unsatisfactory kind' (Lord Kelvin).

The rest of this chapter will be devoted to outlining some of the more useful quantitative tools in use today in rehabilitation but it is worth reflecting beforehand on the relevance, and importance of qualitative research in this field. **Qualitative research** is essentially a descriptive process which focuses on the interaction of complex factors, from which some general inferences can be drawn. Proponents of this approach eschew the pre-eminence of numbers in determining conclusions – 'the curse of Kelvin'. In placing reliance solely on the quantitative approach, we may be guilty of the sin of Procrustes. (He was an innkeeper in Greek mythology who only had one bed to let. It was therefore only of one size, and if the guest was too tall he chopped off his feet and/or his head in order to make him fit into it.) Advocates of the quantitative approach counter with criticisms of the softness and subjectivity of qualitative data. The qualitative approach is neither better nor worse than the quantitative one, merely a different way of looking at problems, the two are complementary. Qualitative research can provide a strong skeletal framework of knowledge, while the quantitative approach provides details and nuances which colour the interpretation of the data. Indeed, it may be a necessary precursor to the production of an outcome measure, to collect qualitative data systematically from patients, using focus groups, for instance. In this way the outcome measure derives from patient experience of the effects of disease or disability and not from what professionals believe is happening. Having said this, it should be emphasized that it is now rarely necessary to devise new measures and much better to use established validated ones.

TYPES OF QUANTITATIVE MEASURE

There are four categories of measurement levels – nominal, ordinal, interval and ratio.

The choice of level of measurement depends on the questions which one is attempting to answer and the way in which the results will be applied and interpreted.

In a **nominal** scale the numbers are used simply to classify a characteristic. They have no meaning except within the context in which they are being used. The code used in the International Classifications of Disease is an example of the application of numbers to the task of categorization. Nominal scales may be used when the frequencies or proportions of a particular characteristic within a sample are being studied (e.g. number of patients discharged to their own home, to residential care, to long-term care, transferred to another unit or who died while undergoing treatment). If statistical analysis is required non-parametric techniques such as chi square should be used.

An **ordinal** scale ranks the order so that adjacent scores signify that the parameter being measured is either better or worse than the other. A simple example is:

1	None
2	Mild
3	Moderate
4	Marked
5	Severe

The intervals between the numbers on the scale are not necessarily uniform. Thus, an increase in the number of points at one end of the scale may not be the same improvement as a similar change in score at a different part of the overall scale. Once again, non-parametric techniques are required for data analysis. If groups are being compared, tests such as the Willcoxon or Mann–Whitney U test are appropriate, while correlation coefficients based on the rank order of results, for example Spearman or Kendall rank correlations, are used when hypotheses are being examined. It is also more appropriate to compare the median values of scores, rather than their mean, since this reflects the number of recordings above and below, rather than their mathematical weight.

Many scales for measuring disability are of this type. They may assess a particular hierarchy of activity, e.g. the level of assistance required in order to carry out a particular activity. More often the tools are produced by summating scores awarded to capabilities in the items which comprise the scale. The Barthel Index and Functional Independence Measure are good examples. Ordinal scales have substantial limitations, but they are nevertheless, an improvement on clinical assessments based solely on impressions. It is perfectly valid to use them provided their limitations are understood, not only in relation to their measurement characteristics but also to their content. Statistical techniques are available to measure and compensate for the non-linearity of these scales (Rasch, 1980) but are beyond the scope of this chapter.

An **interval** scale is truly quantitative. An interval scale has a common and constant unit of measurement and the intervals between the points on the scale are uniform. The zero point is however arbitrary, as are the units of measurement. The Fahrenheit and Celsius scales of temperature are good examples of true interval scales. The freezing point of water is 0° on the centigrade scale and 32° on the Fahrenheit scale, while its boiling points are 100° and 212° respectively. The common parametric statistics such as mean, standard deviation, Pearson correlation coefficients, etc. can be used with interval scales as well as statistical tests of significance such as *t* test, etc. provided the data are normally distributed. Some of the scales used in rehabilitation attempted to convert from ordinal to interval scales by weighting the value attached to a particular score, for example the OPCS Disability Scale or the Symptom Impact Profile.

A **ratio** scale is an interval scale with a true zero at its origin, for example weight. The ratio of any two points on two interval scales is independent of the unit of measurement. In clinical practice speed (distance over time) is a very useful ratio scale, while many of the measures used in health economics, such as cost per case, are also of this type. Parametric tests are again appropriate for analysis.

In summary, these different levels of scales may be used in the following ways: a nominal scale is sufficient to measure the proportion of a population achieving a particular outcome; an ordinal scale can describe how x compares with y; an interval scale defines how x differs from y; while a ratio scale tells us how proportionally different x is from y.

DESIRABLE CHARACTERISTICS OF SCALES

The primal attributes of a good scale are:

- sensitivity
- specificity
- reliability
- appropriateness
- acceptability
- robustness.

Sensitivity is the ability of a method to identify those who have the condition, while **specificity** is the ability of the scale to identify correctly those who do **not** have the condition in question. Sensitivity thus gives the true-positive and the specificity the true-negative rate. In the field of disability research, false-positive and false-negative findings are common. Changing the cutting point in an analysis can increase the sensitivity and reduce the specificity, or vice versa. Thus if the true-positive rate (sensitivity) is plotted against the false-positive rate (1 – specificity) at different cutting points, a curve is produced which illustrates the trade-off between sensitivity and specificity. These are aspects of the more general concept of validity.

Validity is concerned with whether the scale measures the attribute under study or not – does it measure what it is supposed to? It therefore requires a standard criterion against which the attribute may be assessed.

In most areas of disability research there is no such gold standard. Validity can be subcategorized into a number of components – face, content, criterion, concurrent, predictive, construct and convergent/discriminant validity are all terms which may be encountered in the research literature.

An instrument used in rehabilitation research should measure a specific and defined aspect of the consequences of disease based on the satisfactory concept or theoretical foundation. The theoretical basis of the scale determines its **construct** validity. It may be inferred by correlating the scale which is being assessed with related scales and variables with which the items under test should not correlate, which is called **discriminant validity.** More recently Rasch methodology has become available, allowing construct validity to be proved by fit to the model.

The practical direct assessment of validity involves the assessment of content and criterion validity. **Content validity** assesses whether the components of the scale cover all aspects of the factor being studied. The simplest level of content validity is whether or not the meaning and relevance of the scale is reasonably self-evident to all who would use it. This is called **face validity.** The acceptability to the subject plays an important role in determining compliance with the test and satisfactory completion of the study. In general, people prefer simple tests which do not take too long to complete. In the course of its development, a scale is usually examined critically by experts in the field. When the experts agree that it is complete and has been written clearly, it is then tested for the next level of content validity, called **criterion validity.** Criterion validity is a measure of the accuracy of the scale and it is usually assessed by the correlation of the scale with some well-established measure of the same factor. Concurrent and predictive validity are subsections of criterion validity. **Concurrent validity** involves correlating a new scale with

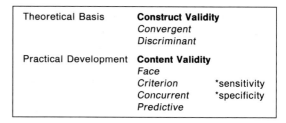

Figure 9.1 Elements of 'validity'.

a criterion measure, both being administered to the same subject simultaneously. **Predictive validity,** on the other hand, assesses whether the measure predicts future differences. By definition this can only be assessed retrospectively when a particular end point of the study or experiment has been reached. Sensitivity and specificity are other important elements of content validity. The elements of the concept of validity are shown in Figure 9.1.

Reliability is the degree to which the scores obtained using a measure can be replicated. There are two main types of inconsistency which need to be assessed – inter-rater reliability and test-retest reliability. **Inter-rater reliability** is assessed by correlating the judgments of different raters studying a sample of subjects using the instrument. In rehabilitation, inter-rater reliability is of particular importance as those measuring (e.g. therapists and doctors) have had different training, and possess different skills and attitudes (usefully so), to the same problems. **Test-retest reliability** (also known as repeatability or reproducibility) is studied by one observer by measuring the same subjects (selected because their condition or situation is considered to be stable) on two occasions, the interval between the test being judged in relation to the problem being studied. In laboratory tests very high correlations for both these forms of reliability would be required. Using rating scales on humans, however, some degree of inconsistency is unavoidable and lower levels of reliability are acceptable. The internal consistency of the items of the test should also be examined (e.g. using Cronbach's coefficient alpha after uni-dimensionality has been proven) when a scale is being developed – how far do the questions it contains measure the same theme? The more specific the topic under test, the higher should be the internal consistency; conversely, more global instruments are likely to have lower measured levels of internal consistency. It is important to be consistent about the method of administering a test: if it has been validated using a **trained** observer to question and record data face to face, it cannot be assumed that the test will give consistent results administered (for instance) by tele-phone, or by asking patients to fill in forms themselves. Furthermore, there are also important questions of language. Informal translations, even in the same language, of tests may destroy reliability. A formal process of translation must be undertaken when the test is to be used in another language. Usually the **culture** of the people using the translation will also be different and modifications, particularly of the Activities of Daily Living (ADL) tests (e.g. use of toilet), may present major obstacles which have to be recognized and formally dealt with.

The appropriateness of the instrument selected depends on the nature of the study to be undertaken. This has to be considered when designing the research. The accept-ability to the subjects plays an important part in determining compliance. In general people prefer short, simple tests. They also appreciate being able to comment on their problem and on the test. Such qualitative information is worth recording.

The **robustness** of measures is also worth commenting on. Some simple measures are found to be consistently useful. Thus speed of walking can be quickly determined and relates closely to the usefulness the person derives from getting around on foot (e.g. to shops, to visit neighbours). Another measure, return to work, is easy to determine but is less

useful in times of high unemployment – indeed results will vary widely over time for this external reason rather than reflecting a change in the severity of disease or disability or the effectiveness of management. Robust measures are usually considered to be those which continue to be used in the clinical situation over many years: there are usually good reasons for such clinical preference.

SELECTING SCALES FOR SPECIFIC PURPOSES

A very large number of instruments and techniques have been used to measure almost every aspect of rehabilitation but a relatively small number have passed the requisite tests of validation and reliability described above. Nevertheless, it is almost always better to use an available established instrument than to try to develop one *de novo*, although the development of new measures should not cease. On the contrary, much effort needs to be put into this field of research, but it is a time-consuming and painstaking exercise which has to be done systematically.

In selecting a scale for a specific study a balance has to be struck between various competing tensions, for example brevity versus completeness or a disease-specific measure versus a generic one. It is important to consider what the scale is actually mea-suring, that is its construct and content validity.

In fact any test should be 'checked out' to determine in what circumstances it has been used, and more particularly tested. For instance, was it designed for research or for clinical use, for inpatients or outpatients or, indeed, for any particular diagnostic group or disability level? Is it a test which one expects to be incorporated into routine clinical mea-surements in the proposed study? If so, how long will it take to do and is this feasible given the proposed number of subjects. Or will a researcher be using the test? Is it to be administered by a professional or by the patient, or by the carer? Will there then be problems because of comprehensive deficiencies? Will the test be sent by post (if so, is the language comprehensible to most of the population?) or administered by telephone or by interview?

Within a tool of measurement there may be subscales. Debate often occurs about the usefulness of adding together scores from subscales. The Symptom Impact Profile, for instance, contains subsections which assess specific functions and results with a subscale which can point to areas of difficulty the subjects are experiencing which then become the focus of treatment, the success of which can be monitored by repeat estimations. Such information can be lost if one is merely presented with a global score.

It is not possible to describe or discuss all of the scales which may be applied to the measurement of human function. However a number of tools of measurement have gained widespread acceptability in the last few years, and are used across a spectrum of diseases and disabilities. Recommendations about scales which may be used in specific diseases or particular clinical or other situations are made in other chapters of this book. The reader is referred to specialist texts and compendia for advice on specific topics (McDowell and Newell, 1987, Bowling, 1991, 1995; Wade, 1992).

The United Kingdom Clearing House for Information in the Assessment of Health Outcomes is an excellent resource which can give informed advice on particular scales and areas of research activity.

A number of different terms have been used to describe particular consequences of disease, for example health status, functional ability, quality of life, etc. There is much uncertainty and ambiguity in the literature about the meaning of many of these terms. In this chapter, therefore, selected areas will be considered. Unfortunately many tests, including the majority used in psychological and psychometric assessments, are covered by copyright restrictions and have to be bought from the firms which publish them.

Measures of impairment

This may be measured by objective studies, often timed, in which the disabled person is observed carrying out a particular task. More commonly it is recorded in simple scales, some of which form part of more wide-ranging measures of impairment.

Upper limb/hand function

In many conditions such as injury, arthritis or post surgery the power of grip is reduced. Its response to therapy needs to be determined.

Grip strength (more accurately power grip) can be measured using a simple Douglas bag attached to a sphygmomanometer. This is useful but not very reliable and certainly for research purposes should be replaced by a dynamometer of known accuracy (Izquierdo-Avino *et al.*, 1995). MIE has the advantage of also giving a printed record of fall-off in power over time which can be informative. Of course, these tests give no information about the impairment in the various involved joints or muscle groups, nor can they predict the ability of an individual patient to perform particular tasks. This may depend on a wide variety of influences such as motivation, apraxia and specific nerve damage.

The nine-hole peg test reflects the ability to perform fine movements and coordination, rather than grasp. The patient is asked to place nine wooden pegs, each 9 mm in diameter, into the corresponding number of holes, each of which are 10 mm in diameter, and are spaced 15 mm apart in three rows of three. The time taken to complete the test is recorded (in seconds); if the test has not been completed in 50 seconds it is terminated. It is widely accepted in neurological rehabilitation (Wade, 1992) but could equally well be used as a test of hand function in arthritis and other causes of disability.

The **arm section of the Motricity index** (Demeurisse *et al.*, 1980; Collin and Wade, 1990), which is now widely used in clinical practice to record recovery after stroke, is an example of a measure of arm and hand impairment. Other scales may include substantial sections on hand and upper limb function, such as the 'reaching and stretching' and 'dexterity' sections of the OPCS Disability Scale.

Spasticity is usually tested in the arm (Ashworth, 1969). This is not easy to do and the reliability of even the **modified Ashworth test** is not high (Bohannon and Smith, 1987). Nevertheless as yet there is no satisfactory replacement. Muscle power in the leg muscles can be conveniently if crudely measured without instrumentation using MRC gradings. This is often sufficient to assess patients such as those recovering from Guillain–Barré disease, though quite insufficient when dealing with athletes.

Lower limb walking

Accurate measurement of maximum power in various muscle groups can be made using standard commercial dynamometers. However, **speed of walking** is probably of more use in many rehabilitation situations, particularly where endurance is more important than maximum power. It is probably the single best measure of locomotor disability. This may be assessed in a number of ways, the two principal approaches being to measure walking speed over short distances or to ask the patient to walk for 2, 6 or 12 minutes. Speed of walking over 10, 15 and 20 m (10 m forward, turn, then 10 m back) are all valid and reliable measures. A variation on this theme is the **timed get up and go** test (Podsiadlo and Richardson, 1991), which includes the time taken to rise from a chair and start walking, as well as the speed when walking actually starts. The longer walking tests as originally devised were measures of endurance. The person was asked to walk at

their own speed but, if they stopped, the stopwatch was also arrested and re-started when they started to walk again, until the predetermined time (2, 6 or 12 minutes) had elapsed; the distance walked in the fixed time was then recorded (McGavin *et al.*, 1978). An alternative approach which better reflects a disabled person's abilities (and ensures their cooperation in future tests) is to ask him/her to walk at his/her own place until limited by pain, dyspnoea or distress. The distance recorded is that covered before stopping (or after 12 minutes if still going), and the time taken is recorded (Hunter, 1986), from which the speed can be calculated.

The **lower limb section of the Motricity index** is a useful measure of lower limb impairment. Although there are many detailed scales of walking and lower limb disability, those contained within the FIM (which are sensitive to small improvements in function among severely disabled people) and the OPCS Disability Scale – a broad ranging measure of locomotion – suffice for many studies.

Effort

The measurement of **oxygen consumption** under standardized conditions (VO_2) is the gold standard for the measurement of exertion. However it is valid and reliable only after the subject has been walking for at least 2 minutes at a steady speed. Its measurement involves the use of breathing masks and either Douglas bags or specialized equipment in a laboratory and it is often considered too cumbersome for routine clinical use. **Heart rate changes** at steady state correlate very well with VO_2 but many of the studies in rehabilitation research involve people who can only walk for short distances or times and never reach a steady state. Assessments of change in pulse rate may be used for studies on individuals but are not reliable for studies on groups of patients. A semiquantitative measure – the **Physiological Cost Index (PCI)**

– was developed by McGregor (1979), and has proved useful in disability research.

$$PCI = \frac{\text{pulse rate (beats per metre) during activity–pulse rate (at rest)}}{\text{speed}}$$

The lowest PCI is found when the subject is walking at his preferred speed. More effort is required (with a corresponding increase in pulse rate and PCI) not only at faster, but also at slower, walking speeds. It is now widely used in studies on prosthetics and orthotic devices (Butler *et al.*, 1984); a variation on the theme – The Physiological Cost of Wheelchair Propulsion – has also been shown to be useful in studies on wheelchair users (Mattison, Spence and Hunter, 1989).

Subjective estimates of the effort expended are also useful in practice. **The Borg Scale of Perceived Exertion** (Borg, 1970) is widely used and is acceptable to staff and subjects. It is shown in Figure 9.2.

Psychological measures

Measure of organic brain function, mood and

6	
7	*Very very light*
8	
9	*Very light*
10	
11	*Fairly light*
12	
13	*Somewhat hard*
14	
15	*Hard*
16	
17	*Very hard*
18	
19	*Very very hard*
20	

Please circle the number which corresponds best to how hard you found the activity.

Figure 9.2 The Borg Scale of Perceived Exertion.

subjective feelings may all be considered under this heading.

The **mini-mental** state examination is widely used as a screening measure of cognitive impairment in clinical practice in rehabilitation units. It includes many elements of higher cortical function such as memory, attention, language etc. and is a useful basic tool for inclusion in any battery of tests of cognitive function (Wade, 1992). Other clinically useful tests, such as **Hodkinson Mental Test** (Hodkinson, 1972) and **Digit Span** (a test of attention which is part of the Wechsler Adult Intelligence Scale), are relatively blunt for research studies. The great majority of neuropsychological tests have to be purchased and have to be administered by a trained observer. They are considered in Chapter 29. Similar considerations apply to tests of speech and language, although the **Frenchay Aphasia Screening Test** (FAST) (Enderby *et al.*, 1986) is simple to use, particularly for untrained doctors.

Anxiety and depression are common and important consequences of physical disability, as well as being presenting symptoms in their own right. There is a large number of tests but the two which have proved to be most useful in disability research are the Hospital Anxiety and Depression Scale (Zigmund and Snaith 1983) and the General Health Questionnaire (Goldberg, 1978). The Beck Inventory is also frequently used (Beck *et al.*, 1961).

The Hospital Anxiety and Depression Scale (HAD) is proving useful in the field of rehabilitation research since it has only one question which may be answered inappropriately because of physical disability. It has been validated for stroke but not in many other physical conditions. It is not known how well it performs in adolescence. A score of 7 or below for anxiety or depression (scored separately) is normal, while scores of 11 and above are abnormal.

The General Health Questionnaire (GHQ) is a widely used, well-validated, reliable, simple and quick measure to apply. The 28-

question version which has four subscales and an overall cut-off at 4/5 has now all but replaced the original 60-item version. Full details may be obtained from NFER Nelson of Windsor. There are cut-off points for 'caseness' but scores within the 'abnormal but not a case' range are very common, not only in disabled people but also in their carers.

Responses to illness, disability or some other stress in life, such as change in employment status, are many. 'Life satisfaction' encompasses this wider area of the individual affective response to everyday experience. It is an important component of the concept of 'quality of life'. A number of scales have been developed to measure the degree to which a person reports being satisfied with the salient feature of his/her everyday life and personal environment. The **Affect Balance Scale** developed by Bradburn (1969) is based on the concept that psychological well-being depends not only on the absence of negative feelings such as worry, loneliness or unhappiness, but also on the presence of positive affects such as excitement, interest and elation. This test has been validated extensively.

The **Philadelphia Geriatric Centre Morale Scale** (Lawton, 1979) has been recommended for use in geriatric rehabilitation centres by a joint working party of the British Geriatric Society and the Royal College of Physicians in London. People's beliefs about illness and how far they are in control of their own lives are major determinants of outcome. **Locus of control** has been measured in a number of ways (Wallston, Walston and De Vellis, 1978; Rotter, 1986; Partridge and Johnston, 1989) and studies have established this is an important area for research, particularly on the interaction between psychological and social factors in determining outcome.

Personality inventories, such as the **Minnesota Multiphasic Personality Inventory** (Hathaway and McKinlay, 1990) and the somewhat shorter **Eysenck Personality Questionnaire** (Eysenck and Eysenck, 1985), have

been used extensively as a way of measuring how personality characteristics may vary in response to symptoms or health problems, particularly chronic pain. Other emotional reactions such as fear as a determinant of behaviour are likely to be studied more extensively in the future.

Most of the psychological measures discussed above are mainly measures of impairment. Following this, measures which are mainly of ability and disability and are task orientated are considered.

DISABILITY MEASURES

Measurement of 'restriction or lack of ability to perform an activity in a way or within the range considered normal' may be undertaken in various ways. Three main approaches are based on the assessment of:

1. Activities of daily living (ADL).
2. Activities undertaken in a period of time such as the preceding week.
3. Function in other areas of bodily activity.

The selection of a tool of measurement depends on the nature of the question which is being addressed in the study, and the level of ability under assessment.

Personal ADL measures

There are numerous ADL indices, some appropriate for general use, while others have been developed for specific diseases or disabilities. The most widely used measure is the **Barthel Index** (Mahoney and Barthel, 1965; Wade and Collin, 1988). It measures dependence or the extent of reliance on help from others and is a simple and reliable instrument to use.

There is, however, a ceiling effect when the patient is independent in self-care and basic mobility but may still be quite disabled, perhaps in other areas such as communication skills which are not included within the

Index, or when no further improvement, even in the areas such as mobility can be registered. Not withstanding these limitations it is used successfully in hospital and community and is one of the range of measures recommended for use in geriatric medicine units. There are different versions such as the Extended Barthel (Shah, Vanclay and Cooper, 1989) which may be more sensitive. A telephone version has been validated (Korner Bitenslay and Wood Dauphinee, 1995).

Dissatisfaction with the limitations of the Barthel Index led to the development of the **Functional Independence Measure** (FIM) (Grainger *et al.*, 1986). This is now the most widely used measure in rehabilitation units in America. It records the burden of care required in the following areas of activity – self-care, sphincter control, mobility/transfer, locomotion, communication and social cognition, each subscale having seven levels of function.

The FIM was developed to be sensitive to small improvements in dependency during treatment of severely disabled people. A comprehensive manual has been developed to aid categorization of performance in the areas studied. Users must receive training from a person approved by the developers of the system (Uniform Data Set for Medical Rehabilitation, New York). It is based on direct observation of the disabled person's performance in the range of tasks specified. For this reason its applicability in the community is less certain, although a telephone version and one developed for paediatric use (wee FIM) are available. The subscales recording physical function have been accepted widely but some doubts remain over the psychosocial components. An expansion of the psychosocial items has been proposed (Functional Activities Measure) but the resulting FIM + FAM is very time consuming and cannot be recommended.

The Barthel Index and FIM are both ordinal scales.

Instrumental ADL measures

Instrumental ADL measures go beyond activities associated with personal care, and include domestic and household management activities. The **Extended Activities of Daily Living Scale** (EADL) is one example of this approach, developed originally for use with stroke patients in the community (Nouri and Lincoln, 1987) and validated in this group of patients (Gompertz, Pound and Ebrahim, 1994), but it can be applied to other groups of patients. The specified areas of study are mobility, kitchen, domestic and leisure pursuits. Its appropriateness for use with hospitalized patients is questionable. An alternative activity measure is the Frenchay Activity Index (Wade, Leesmith and Langton Hewer, 1985), also developed for use with stroke patients but somewhat gender dependent.

The **OPCS Disability Scale** differs from those already described in a number of ways. In the first place it is based on a theoretical model of disability (as defined by ICIDH; WHO, 1988). It does however include a mix of impairments and disabilities. The scale was developed by the Office of Population Censuses and Surveys (OPCS) in the UK, who operationalized the 'D' categories of the ICIDH and applied it in a major community study of disability in 1987 (Martin, Meltzer and Elliot, 1988). The underlying concept is loss of function, it includes an assessment of difficulty in performing an activity, as well as the level of dependence of the disabled person. A weighting was applied to the severity of dysfunction in the following areas – locomotion, reaching and stretching, dexterity, personal care, continence, seeing, hearing, communication, behaviour, intellectual functioning, consciousness, eating, drinking and digestion, disfigurement. This generated a profile of severity scores in these different areas. An overall severity score is calculated by selecting the three highest non-zero scores and applying the following formula:

Overall severity score = highest score + 0.4 (second highest score) + 0.3 (third highest score)

Because of the weighting which has been allocated to the various scores in each dimension it has been analysed as an interval scale. It can be applied successfully in hospital (McPherson *et al.*, 1993) as well as community settings after a period of familiarization with the scale. Those who are used to thinking in terms of activities of daily living find it difficult to use initially but will appreciate its importance once they overcome the conceptual difficulties. There is, for example, no single measure of difficulty in propelling a wheelchair. On the other hand, the disability of a tetraplegic person can be compared with that of a paraplegic person. Both are likely to be unable to walk and be incontinent. They would therefore be awarded the highest possible scores in the subscales of locomotion and continence. The person who is paraplegic will however score well on tests of reaching and stretching, dexterity, and relatively well in personal care, and therefore be able to use a wheelchair efficiently, while a tetraplegic patient will score poorly in these latter areas, the details depending on the level of the spinal cord lesion and recovery, and have difficulty propelling a chair.

Measurement of handicap

The dimensions named in the ICIDH (WHO, 1980) are:

- orientation;
- physical independence;
- mobility;
- occupation;
- social integration;
- economic self-sufficiency.

The rules of assignment to the different categories within these nominal scales were specified in detail in the ICIDH and summarized in Wade (1992).

Several scales are derived from them. The **London Handicap Scale** (Harwood *et al.*, 1994), which is quickly completed by the patient, is validated and of promise for community studies. The **Leeds Assessment Scale for Handicap** (J.M.L. Geddes, 1994) (using four dimensions only) is useful for inpatients with neurological disorders and in stroke may prove to have prognostic significance (J.M.L. Geddes, 1996, personal communication). Roy, *et al.*, (1992) have also shown that the ICIDH handicap profile itself improves in the course of a hospital-based rehabilitation programme. The **Edinburgh Rehabilitation Status Scale** (Affleck *et al.*, 1988) has been based on the same theoretical concept of handicap. A validated potentially useful alternative approach to the measurement of handicap is described by Harwood, Gompertz and Ebrahim (1994).

The social integration component of the ICIDH measures integration dependent on behaviour. Patients without affective or personality disorders may yet lead impoverished social lives so that a measure of **social function** is required. These may include the use made of social networks and support. The **Frenchay Activities Index** is such a measure, but many more have been described.

Many measures, particularly older ones, do not lie neatly within one ICIDH domain but straddle impairment, disease and handicap. Nevertheless, tests such as the **Arthritis Impact Measurement Scale** (AIMS) (Meenan, Gertman and Mason, 1990; Meenan and Mason, 1991) are widely used. The reader should consult full texts such as those of McDowell and Newell (1987), Bowling (1991, 1995) and Wade (1992).

Self-report measures of health status

Health is not merely the absence of disease and WHO has reminded us that the ultimate aim of rehabilitation is full social integration of the disabled person.

There is unfortunately no accepted definition of **positive health** and the literature is bedevilled in this area, as in so many others, by the use of related multifaceted concepts such as social well-being, social health, quality of life, etc. However, the importance of assessing people's views on areas that are important to them is accepted fully and explored in a large number of studies. The Sickness Impact Profile (Bergner *et al.*, 1981), and its anglicized equivalent of the Functional Limitations Profile (Patrick and Peach, 1989), are benchmark indices. An alternative but similar approach by the RAND Corporation led to the development of a number of batteries of tests (Donald and Ware, 1984). Over the years these have been distilled into a relatively simple questionnaire, the **SF36** (Ware and Sherbourne, 1992). This was recommended in 1993 by the UK Clearing House as the preferred global index of health status, but it is not necessarily of use in all situations: for instance, it does not work well in community studies of stroke survivors. It examines a number of areas of human experience but should be seen as complementary to, for example, disability indices rather than as being the only tool of measurement which should be applied irrespective of the patient population or problem being studied. Details of the test and scoring may be obtained from the Medical Outcomes Trust.

In the UK the *Nottingham Health Profile* (NHP) was developed to measure perceived health problems and the extent to which they affect normal activities (Hunt *et al.*, 1980). It has been used in a variety of studies on many patient groups. The responses to Part 1 of the questionnaire are allocated weightings in the scoring system, details of which may be obtained from Dr Stephen McKenna of Galen Research. In addition to this well-used generic quality of life measure, disease-specific variants based upon the developmental methodology of the NHP are now available. Hopefully these will more accurately reflect improvements after medical and other interventions.

The conceptual continuum dependent on the ICIDH is a useful framework for considering measures one proposes to use in a study.

Tests and measurements of themselves have little value. The context in which they are used is of great importance. Proposing a study the researcher has to be clear: is this audit or research? Is it in the clinical arena or epidemiological? Is it to be done in hospital or at home? Is it done by testing function or using face-to-face interviews (will these be written and self-completed?) or perhaps by telephone?

Study design is of great importance: good studies require much preparation and are not easy to do well. The reader is referred to Hicks (1988). Similarly, the message resulting from the hard work involved in any study will not be heard unless the material is presented well either audiovisually or in written form (Andrews, 1993).

The choice of study design is large: the study may be qualitative, and descriptive, or quantitative. Within the latter category there are variants such as single case design, case-controlled studies, cohort studies, and single and double blind studies. All have use in advancing knowledge on the value and effectiveness of rehabilitation interventions.

REFERENCES

Affleck, J.W., Aitken, R.C.B., Hunter, J.A.A., McGuire, R.J. and Roy, C.W. (1988) Rehabilitation status: a measure of medico-social dysfunction. *Lancet*, **i**, 230–3.

Andrews, K. (1993) Writing for medical journals. *Clinical Rehabilitation*, **7**, 91–8.

Ashworth, B. (1994) Preliminary trial of carisoprodol in multiple sclerosis. *Practitioner*, **192**, 540–42.

Beck, A.T., Ward, C.H., Mendelson, M. *et al.*, (1961) *An inventory for measuring depression. Archives of General Psychiatry*, **4**, 561–71.

Bergner, M., Bobbit, R.A., Carter, W.B. and Gibson, B.S. (1981) *The Sickness Impact Profile: development and final version of a health status measure. Medical Care*, **19**, 787–805.

Bohannon, R.W. and Smith, M.B. (1987) Inter-rater reliability of a modified Ashworth Scale of Muscle Spasticity. *Physical Therapy,* **67**, 206–7.

Borg, G. (1970) Perceived Effort as a measure of somatic stress. *Scandinavian Journal of Rehabilitation Medicine,* **2**, 92.

Bowling, A. (1991) *Measuring Health: A Review of Quality of Life Measurement Scales,* Open University Press, Milton Keynes.

Bowling, A. (1995) *Measuring Disease,* Open University Press, Milton Keynes.

Bradburn, N.M. (1969) *The Structure of Psychological Wellbeing,* Aldine Publishing, Chicago.

Butler, P.B., Englebrecht, M., Major, R.E., Tait, J.H., Stallard, J. and Patrick, J.H. (1984) Physiological cost index of walking for normal children and its use as an indicator of physical handicap. *Development Medicine and Child Neurology,* **26**, 607–12.

Collin, C. and Wade, D. (1990) Assessing motor impairment after stroke: a pilot reliability study, *Journal of Neurology, Neurosurgery and Psychiatry,* **53**, 576–9.

Demeurisse, G., Demol, O. and Robaye, E. (1980) Motor evaluation in vascular hemiplegia. *Europoean Neurology,* **19**, 382–9.

Donald, C.A. and Ware, J.E. (1984) The measurement of social support. *Research in Community Mental Health,* **4**, 325–70.

Enderby, P.M., Wood, V.A., Wade, D.T. and Langton Hewer, R. (1988) *The Frenchay Aphasia Screening Test: a short simple test for aphasia appropriate for non specialist. International Rehabilitation Medicine,* **8**, 166–70.

Eysenck, H.J. and Eysenck, S.B.G. (1985) *Manual for the Eysenck Personality Questionnaire,* Hodder and Stoughton, London.

Geddes, J.M.L. and Chamberlain, M.A. (1994) Proceedings of Society for Research in Rehabilitation *in* Clinical Rehabilitation 1995; **9**, 177–178 'Categorisation of patients in a neurorehabilitation unit according to the Handicap Classification of the ICIDH.

Goldberg, D.P. (1978) *Manual of the General Health Questionnaire,* NFER-Nelson, Windsor.

Gompertz, P., Pound, P. and Ebrahim, S. (1994) Validity of the extended activities of daily living scale. *Clinical Rehabilitation,* **8**, 275–80.

Grainger, C.V., Hamilton, B.B., Keith, R.A., Zielezney, M. and Sherwin, F.S. (1986) Advances in functional assessment for medical rehabilitation. *Topics in Geriatric Rehabilitation,* **1**, 59–74.

Harwood, R.H., Gompertz, P. and Ebrahim, S. (1994) Handicap one year after stroke: validity of a new scale. *Journal of Neurology, Neurosurgery and Psychiatry,* **57**, 825–59.

Harwood, R.H., Rogers, A., Dickinson, E. and Ebrahim, S. (1994) Measuring handicap: The London Handicap Scale, a new outcome measure for chronic disease. *Quality in Health Care,* **3**, 11–16.

Hathaway, S.R. and McKinley, J.C. (1990) *Minnesota Multiphasic Personality Inventory,* 2nd edn.

Hodkinson, H.M. (1972) *Evaluation of a mental test score for assessment of mental impairment in the elderly. Age and Ageing* **1**, 233–8.

Hunt, S.M., McKenna, S.P., McEwen, J., Backet, E.M., Williams, J. and Papp, E. (1980) A quantitative approach to perceived health status: a validation study. *Journal of Epidemiology and Community Health,* **34**, 281–6.

Hunter, J. (1986) *What does 'virtually unable to walk' mean? British Medical Journal,* **292**, 172–3.

Izquierdo-Avino, Spencer Jones, R., Jensen, B. and Schwemm, E. (1995) Hand grip analysis: a comparison of two methods. *Journal of Orthopaedic Rheumatism,* **8**, 203–6.

Korner-Bitensky, N. and Wood Dauphinee, S. (1995) Barthel Index Information elicited over the telephone. Is it reliable? *American Journal of Physical Medicine and Rehabilitation,* **74**, 9–18.

Lawton, M.P. (1979) The Philadelphia Geriatric Centre Morale Scale: a revision. *Journal of Gerontology,* **30**, 85–9.

Mahoney, F.I. and Barthel, D.W. (1965) Functional evaluation: The Barthel Index. *Maryland State Medical Journal,* **14**, 61–5.

Martin, J., Meltzer, H. and Elliot, D. (1988) *The Prevalence of Disability Among Adults,* Office of Population Censuses and Surveys, HMSO, London.

Mattison, P., Spence, S. and Hunter, J. (1989) Development of a realistic method of assessing the effort of wheelchair propulsion. *International Journal of Rehabilitation Research,* **12**, 137–45.

Meenan, R.F., Gertman, P.M. and Mason, J.H. (1980) Measuring health status in arthritis: The Arthritis Impact Measurement Scales. *Arthritis and Rheumatism,* **23**, 146–52.

Meenan, R.F. and Mason, J.H. (1990) *AIMS 2 Users Guide,* Boston University School of Medicine, Department of Public Health, Boston, M.A.

McDowell, I. and Newell, C. (1987) *Measuring Health: a guide to rating scales and questionnaires,* Oxford University Press, Oxford.

McGavin, C.R., Artvinli, M., Naoe, H. and McHardie, J.G.R. (1978) Dyspnoea, disability and distance walked: comparison of estimate of exercise performance in respiratory disease. *British Medical Journal,* **2**, 241–3.

McGregor, J. (1979) The Objective Measurement of Physical Performance with Long Term Ambulatory Physiological Surveillance Equipment, in *Proceedings of 3rd International Symposium on Ambulatory Monitoring* (eds F.D. Stott, E.B. Rattery and L. Goulding), Academic, London, pp. 29–39.

McPherson, K., Sloan, R.L., Hunter, J. and Dowell, C.M. (1993) Validation Studies of the OPCS Scale: more useful than the Barthel Index? *Clinical Rehabilitation*, **7**, 105–12.

Nouri, F.M. and Lincoln, N.B. (1987) An Extended Activities of Daily Living Scale for stroke patients. *Clinical Rehabilitation*, **1**, 301–5.

Partridge, C. and Johnston, M. (1989) Perceived control of recovery from physical disability: measurement and prediction. *British Journal of Clinical Psychology*, **28**, 53–9.

Patrick, D.L. and Peach, H. (eds) (1989) *Disablement in the Community*, Oxford University Press, Oxford, appendices I and II.

Podsiadlo, D. and Richardson, S. (1991) The Timed Get up and Go: a test of basic functional mobility for frail elderly persons. *Journal of the American Geriatrics Society*, **39**, 142–8.

Rasch, G. (1980) *Probabilistic Models for some Intelligence and Attainment Tests*, University of Chicago Press, Chicago.

Rotter, J.B. (1986) Generalised expectancies for internal versus external control of reinforcement. *Psychological Monographs*, **80**, 1–23.

Roy, C.W., Hunter, J., Arthurs, Y. and Prescott, R. (1992) Is handicap affected by a hospital based rehabilitation programme? *Scandinavian Journal of Rehabilitation Medicine*, **24**, 105–12.

Shah, S., Vanclay, F. and Cooper, B. (1989) Improving the sensitivity of the Barthel Index. *Journal of Clinical Epidemiology*, **42**, 703–9.

Wade, D.T. (1992) *Measurement in Neurological Rehabilitation*, Oxford University Press, Oxford.

Wade, D.T. and Collin, C. (1958) The Barthel ADL Index: a standard measure of physical disability? *International Disability Studies*, **10**, 64–7.

Wade, D.T., Leesmith, J. and Langton Hewer, R. (1985) Social activities after stroke: measurement and natural history using the Frenchay Activities Index. *International Rehabilitation Medicine*, **7**, 176–81.

Wallston, K.A., Walston, B.S. and De Vellis, R. (1978) Development of the Multi-Dimensional Health Locus of Control (MHLC) Scales. *Health Education Monographs*, **6**, 160–71.

Ware, J.E. and Sherbourne, C.D. (1992) *The MOS 36 Item Short Form Health Survey (SF 36) – one conceptual framework and item selection. Medical Care*, **30**, 473–83.

WHO (1988) *International Classifications of Impairments, Disabilities and Handicaps*, World Health Organization, Geneva.

Zigmund, A.S. and Snaith, R.P. (1983) The Hospital Anxiety and Depression Scale. *Acta Psychiatrica Scandinavica*, **67**, 361–70.

FURTHER READING

Grainger, C.V., Hamilton, B.B. and Sherwin, F.S. (1986) *Guide for the Use of the Uniform Data Set for Medical Rehabilitation*, Uniform Data System for Medical Rehabilitation Project Office, Buffalo General Hospital, New York.

Jebsen, R.H., Taylor, N., Trieschmann, R.B., Trotter, M.J. and Howard, L.A. (1969) An objective and standardised test of hand function. *Archives of Physical Medicine and Rehabilitation*, **50**, 311–19.

Mays, N. and Pope, C. (1995) *Qualitative Research in Healthcare*, BMJ Publishing Group, London.

Ottenbacher, K. (1986) *Evaluating Clinical Change*, Williams & Wilkins, London.

Roy, C.W., Arthurs, Y., Hunter, J., Parker, S. and McLaren, A. (1988) The work of a rehabilitation medicine service. *British Medical Journal*, **297**, 601–4.

USEFUL ADDRESS

Galen Research
Southern Hey, 137 Barlowmoor Road, West Didsbury, Manchester M20 8PW, UK.
Medical Outcomes Trust
PO Box 1917, Boston, MA 02205, USA.
NFER Nelson
Darvil House, 2 Oxford Road East, Windsor, SL4 1DF, UK.
Uniform Data Set for Medical Rehabilitation
Department of Rehabilitative Medicine, State University of New York, Buffalo General Hospital, New York, NY 14203, USA.
The United Kingdom Clearing House for Information in the Assessment of Health Outcomes
Nuffield Institute for Health, University of Leeds, Fairburn House, 71–75 Clarendon Road, Leeds LS2 9P, UK.

10 Legal problems

S. Middleton

INTRODUCTION

The purpose of this chapter is to look at the mechanics of decision making for those with some form of mental incapacity whether from mental or physical causes and the legal and medical difficulties that can arise. It is important at the outset to distinguish between those people who are capable of making a decision but need some assistance to ensure that there is control in the decision that is made and those people who are unable to make legally effective decisions. This chapter deals with the latter, with reference to the law in England and Wales.

In an era increasingly reliant on care in the community it is worth stressing that supervised discharge schemes figure in the category of decision making with assistance. Indeed, The Law Commission Report on Mental Incapacity states categorically that 'Neither the existing guardianship scheme nor the proposed supervised discharge scheme revolve around the concept of legal incapacity'. In other words, guardianship and supervised care in the community are not to be seen as forums for substitute decision making but simply to assist in the making of the decision.

Two frequent types of decision are about financial and medical matters. This chapter looks at possible ways of dealing with these decisions by those who are gradually pro-gressing to incapacity rather than those who make an immediate transition by virtue of sudden trauma. Also, it will look at what the future may hold and try to give some guidance in this area. In the space of this chapter only some aspects of decision making will be examined.

Before moving to those areas of decision making it is necessary to define what is meant by mental incapacity. The starting point is the Mental Health Act 1983. Section 1 (2) defines 'mental disorder' for the purposes of the statutory provisions for care and treatment of the so-called disorders, the management of patient's property and affairs and related matters. Mental disorder is defined as 'Mental illness, arrested or incomplete development of mind, psychopathic disorder and any other disorder or disability of mind'. Sadly, though, the terms 'mental illness', 'arrested or incomplete development of mind' and 'any other disorder or disability of mind' are not further defined in the statute. It is plain that the statute is not to be applied to those whose disorder is caused solely by either sexual deviancy or dependence on alcohol or drugs.

Interestingly, despite the above comments, the same definition is used in the Mental Health (Patients in the Community) Act 1995 (Law Com No 231 1995), which came into force on 1 April 1996 and deals with supervised discharge.

Rehabilitation of the Physically Disabled Adult. Edited by C. John Goodwill, M. Anne Chamberlain and Chris Evans. Published in 1997 by Stanley Thornes (Publishers) Ltd, Cheltenham. ISBN 0-7487-3183-0.

In essence therefore the Mental Health Act definition does not greatly assist the question of deciding who has mental incapacity. Until one can define those whose decisions need to be made for them, one cannot begin to address how to make the decisions themselves. Therefore this chapter looks at separate areas of decision making. It is only by looking at specific areas that one can identify those upon whose behalf decisions need to be made, the specific areas in which the decision can be made, and then how to make those decisions.

WAYS OF DEALING WITH SPECIAL DECISIONS

Financial decisions

There are various types of financial decisions that may need to be made on behalf of those with incapacity and various mechanisms by which those decisions may be made. These may be considered under the following headings:

● Court of Protection
● Wills
● State Benefits
● The Court

The Court of Protection

The Court of Protection is probably the most widely known forum for decision making for those with incapacity but there is much misconception about its function. It is a Court within the auspices of the Supreme Court but it is only empowered to deal with the property and affairs of those with mental incapacity. The case of *Re F*[2] [1990] (mental patient; sterilization), which will be looked at in detail later, confirms beyond doubt that in this context the definition includes only business matters, legal transactions and other dealings of a similar kind. In other words not welfare and health care decisions. Similarly the jurisdiction of the Court of Protection can only be invoked when the

Court is satisfied, on medical evidence, that a person is already incapable by reason of mental disorder (including brain damage) of managing and administering his or her property and affairs. The test requires not only mental disorder but that the inability to manage and administer property and affairs arises from that disorder. It is of course not inconceivable that those with mental disorders can manage their affairs. Certainly everyday one sees proof that those with no mental disorder are incapable of managing their own affairs! Ultimately determination on incapacity is decided upon by the Court in each individual case, although based on examination of the medical questionnaire submitted.

It is important to note that the test of whether someone has incapacity is an all or nothing test. If the Court of Protection decides that someone is incapable then that person will become a patient of the Court of Protection. If though a patient does not meet the standard of that test then that person retains all decision-making power over property and affairs. Where does one draw the line? What of those who only narrowly miss satisfying the incapacity test of the Court of Protection? It would appear that they remain free to make any decisions whatsoever in respect of their property and affairs unless and until their condition deteriorates. The Court of Protection has no power to intervene in some decisions only and not others. It must intervene in full or not at all.

This creates problems not only for those with partial incapacity but perhaps with more difficulty for those who have lucid intervals. Once the Court has determined someone is incapable the Court will exercise its powers for all purposes with no provision for a person during a lucid interval to make his or her own decision.

Once the Court of Protection has determined that someone is incapable then under the powers given to it under the Mental Health Act, section 95 it can deal with all such things as appear necessary or expedient for the maintenance or other benefit of the patient, for the maintenance rather than benefit of members of the patient's family, for making provision for other persons or purposes for whom or which the patient might be expected to provide if he or she were not mentally disordered or otherwise for administering the patient's affairs. In essence one looks primarily at the interest, benefit and requirements of each patient.

It is customary that a Receiver is appointed to act on behalf of a patient. However there are occasions when the Court of Protection will fill this role or if a person's estate is simple and straightforward a procedure without the need for a Receiver may be adopted. Where a Receiver is appointed quite frequently that Receiver is a close relative of the patient. Again the Receiver has to be appointed with Court approval and has only limited powers to make decisions without needing to seek Court of Protection approval to safe-guard the patient.

To obtain a discharge from the Court a patient, save on death, is subject to the Court determining on state of capacity. The test is simply reversed; the Court has to consider whether the patient is now capable of managing and administering his/her property and affairs. Again this is an all-or-nothing test.

It is not the place of this chapter to look in detail at the functions which the Court of Protection can carry out nor the mechanisms for carrying them out. Halsbury's Laws of England 30 carries detailed insight into this for those wishing to explore further. However on the whole the incapacity test is taken at the outset and there is then little medical involvement thereafter save to query return to capacity.

Wills

One of the functions that the Court of Protection can exercise is the creation of statutory wills. Application is made satisfying the Court of Protection incapacity test and also showing that as a result the applicant is incapable of making a valid will for him or herself. The Court will require evidence not only of incapability to manage affairs but also incapacity to make a valid will. These tests are separate and the fact that a person is already a patient of the Court of Protection does not necessarily mean that that person also lacks testamentary capacity.

It is therefore necessary to look at what constitutes testamentary capacity, particularly as quite often a member of the medical profession will be asked by solicitors to witness a will where there is any doubt as to testamentary capacity.

The primary criteria for testamentary capacity were laid down in *Banks* v. *Goodfellow* (1870). The Lord Chief Justice defined such capacity in the following terms:

> It is essential that a testator shall understand the nature of the act and its effects; shall understand the extent of the property of which he is disposing; shall be able to comprehend and appreciate the claims to which he ought to give effect; and, with a view to the latter object, that no disorder of mind shall poison his affections, pervert his sense of right, or prevent the exercise of his natural faculties – that no insane delusion shall influence his will in disposing of his property and bring about a disposal of it which, if the mind has been sound, would not have been made.

It is worth stressing that even the so-called rational may make unwise and unexpected dispositions. it is therefore essential when looking at the capacity to make a decision to remember not to look at the decision itself and reverse the test by deciding whether the decision reached evidences a failure of testamentary capacity.

Solicitors are often instructed at short notice where there is an imminent possibility of deterioration in condition. This can result in instructions being taken when there clearly is capacity but by the time the will is prepared for execution the testator's capacity has become questionable. The case of *Parker v. Felgate* (1883) confirms that in such a situation, provided that the testator satisfies one of the following three criteria, a will will be valid even if there was only an understanding that previous instructions were given and that the will accords with those. The three criteria are:

1. When the will was executed that the testator remembers and understands the instructions given to the Solicitor.
2. If it had been thought advisable to stimulate the testator that the testator could have understood each clause of the will when it was explained.
3. That the testator was capable of understanding, and did understand, that the testator was executing a will for which that testator has previously given instructions to the Solicitors.

Testamentary capacity also becomes relevant in the context of revocation of a will. **A will can be revoked in three ways**, by marriage, by preparing another will or simply by destruction of the existing will. In each case capacity of some form is required either to consent to marriage, to have testamentary capacity to make a fresh will or to have the capacity to understand the act of destruction of the will. It would seem that the degree of capacity required to revoke a will by destruction is no lower than that required to obtain testamentary capacity.

No examination of will-making procedure would be complete without looking at statutory wills to which there has been brief allusion. In essence **when creating a statutory will** a Court of Protection must adopt the following principles.

1. It is to be assumed that the patient is having a brief lucid interval at the time when the will is made.

2. It is to be assumed that during the lucid interval the patient has a full knowledge of the past and a full realization that, as soon as the will is executed, he or she will relapse into the actual mental state that previously existed, with the prognosis as it actually is.
3. It is the actual patient who has to be considered and not a hypothetical patient.
4. During the hypothetical lucid interval the patient is to be envisaged as being advised by competent solicitors.
5. In all normal cases the patient is to be envisaged as taking a broad brush to the claims on his or her bounty rather than an accountant's pen.

State Benefits

Inevitably a large number of those suffering from incapacity are entitled to state benefit. It is recognized that it is difficult for such people to make application to the Department of Social Security for their entitlement and to deal with their entitlement. Accordingly, under the Social Security (Claims and Payments) Regulations 1987, the Secretary of State for Social Security may appoint another person to act on behalf of that person who is in receipt of or entitled to benefit provided that the recipient is unable to act. Again this appears to be a wholly discretionary test with no definition in the regulation. It is also interesting to note that it is a test that does not adopt in any form the wording used in the Mental Health Act. Internal guidance in the Department of Social Security suggests that people may be unable to act if 'they do not have the mental ability to understand and control their own affairs, for example, because of senility or mental illness'. It would appear, somewhat inexplicably, that there is no set requirement for the production of medical evidence to show that a person is unable to act. There is certainly no standard form of certificate such as the one required to be completed by the Court of Protection.

The Court

Whilst the Court of Protection forms part of the Supreme Court it is not the only Court dealing with those with mental incapacity. Both County Court and High Court do have certain mechanisms to assist in the management of financial affairs to ensure that any litigation conducted on behalf of a person with incapacity is dealt with properly. Initially this involves the appointment of a next friend to pursue any claim or a guardian *ad litem* to defend any claim. This means that there is somebody available to make decisions in the conduct of any litigation on behalf of the incapacitated party. Clearly though where such a party is also a patient of the Court of Protection approval of that Court will also be required. Applications for Legal Aid can also be made by a next friend or guardian *ad litem* on behalf of an incapacitated person.

In reality the bulk of such litigation relates to compensation claims for those who have been incapacitated as a result of an accident trauma. This is looked at in more detail in Chapter 11; suffice it to say that both the Court and the Court of Protection have to approve any settlement of a claim on behalf of someone with incapacity. This ensures that even though the party may have legal representation the incapacitated party is not in any way prejudiced in the conduct or ultimate resolution of the litigation by that state of incapacity.

There is one other important area in which the Courts assist those with incapacity. That is in dealing with time periods within which those with incapacity can bring claims. For example, in an injury negligence claim, the customary period within which a claim must be commenced is 3 years (Chapter 11). However for those with incapacity that period is extended and only commences if and when they return to capacity. This does cause problems, as it can be difficult to calculate the precise expiry of the period where one has someone with lucid intervals or where a determination will have to be made of the date upon which there was a return to capacity. Clearly if there is any doubt the sooner proceedings are issued the better.

Medical decisions

As has been highlighted above, the Court of Protection cannot interfere with medical decisions nor medical treatment. It seems that it is only recently that this problem has been highlighted before other Courts. This in turn has forced the Courts to look afresh at this area and try to impose some order.

It is important to distinguish between decisions being made about the treatment for the disorder giving rise to the incapacity and decisions being made for treatment unrelated to the disorder. THORPE J made this distinction plain in the case of *B* v. *Croydon Health Authority*. This has extended even to treatment of a physical condition provided that physical condition is in consequence of a mental disorder.

When looking at decisions to be made concerning medical treatment for those under incapacity for medical matters unrelated to the incapacity the case of Re F noted above seems to be an appropriate starting point. The House of Lords held in that case that because our legal system does not allow the appointment of a substitute to take medical decisions for an incompetent patient the inherent statutory jurisdiction of the Court must be used in its declaratory capacity to fill the void. In this particular case the High Court gave a declaration to the effect that it was not unlawful to perform a sterilization operation on an adult who did lack the mental capacity to consent. The court came to this conclusion based on a 'best interest of the patient' test. Defining that test the Court relied heavily on the earlier case of *Bolam* v. *Friern Barnet Management Committee* [1957] determining that a doctor who acts in accordance with an accepted body of medical opinion is both: (i) not negligent and (ii) acting in the best interest of a patient without capacity. In a medical negligence context this test has often been called the lowest common denominator test. Certainly there seems to be little doubt that acting in a person's best interest amounts to something more than not treating that person in a negligent manner.

Judicial intervention by declaration was approved in the case of *Re S* [1993] where it was held that:

> ... the dispute as to the care of an adult patient incapable of expressing his wishes in respect of treatment or care was a judicable issue in respect of which the Courts advisory declaratory jurisdiction could probably be invoked.

Tragically the Court had to go even further in the case of *Airedale NHS Trust* v. *Bland* [1993] where it was asked to exercise declaratory jurisdiction in respect of a victim of the Hillsborough disaster whom it was accepted was in a **persistent vegetative state**. In this case there was unanimity of medical opinion of those consulted that the prognosis was that there was no hope of any improvement in the patient's condition or of recovery. The Trust here sought declarations that they might:

1. Lawfully discontinue all life-sustaining treatment and medical support measures designed to keep the patient alive in his existing persistent vegetative state including the termination of ventilation, nutrition and hydration by artificial means; and
2. Lawfully discontinue and thereafter need not furnish medical treatment to the patient except for the sole purpose of enabling the patient to end his life and die peacefully with the greatest dignity and the least pain, suffering and distress.

3. That if death should occur following such discontinuance or termination the cause of death should be attributed to the natural and other causes of the Defendant's persistent vegetative state.
4. That such discontinuance or termination and any other things done or omitted to be done in good faith in accordance with the Order of the Judge should not give rise to and would be without any civil or criminal liability on the part of the Trust or any participant whether a physician, hospital or any others.

In one of the most evocative series of judgments I have read the House of Lords unanimously held that the object of medical treatment and care was to benefit the patient and that in a case like this existence in a persistent vegetative state was not of benefit to the patient and therefore the sanctity of life was not violated by ceasing to give medical treatment and care involving invasive manipulation of the patient's body to which he had not consented and which conferred no benefit upon him. It was held that the doctors responsible for the patient's treatment were not under a duty to continue such medical care and indeed one Law Lord, Lord Browne-Wilkinson, formed the view that the doctors responsible were not entitled to continue such medical treatment.

It is a small wonder the treating doctors sought declaratory assistance from the Court as the Official Solicitor appointed to act on behalf of the patient argued that the withdrawal of the feeding regime would be murder.

The Court was clearly at great pains to heed the wishes of the treating doctors and relatives of the patient and seemed legally determined to reach their conclusion or an interpretation of the best interest test. The distinction between murder and the withdrawal of medical care and life-sustaining treatment may seem to some to be a semantic one. Lord Browne-Wilkinson was forced to question:

How can it be lawful to allow a patient to die slowly, although painlessly, over a period of weeks from lack of food but unlawful to produce his immediate death by a lethal injection thereby saving his family from yet another ordeal to add to the tragedy that has already struck them.

I find it difficult to find a moral answer to that question. But it is undoubtedly the law and nothing less save to cast out on the proposition that the doing of a positive act with the intention of ending life is and remains murder.

Lord Mustill sharing, although perhaps with a greater degree of reluctance, the views of his fellow Law Lords even managed to create a medical and moral dilemma when he said;

the distressing truth which must not be shirked is that the proposed conduct is not in the best interest of Anthony Bland for he has no best interest of any kind.

Those dealing with patients in persistent vegetative state ought also to be aware of the guidance given by the Official Solicitor to the Supreme Court in a practice note on persistent vegetative state dated March 1994.

All of the five Law Lords confirmed that in the interest of the protection of both patients and their medical advisers, in the light of the comments made above, recognizing that their interests are not to be taken lightly, and in the interest of the patient's families and the public generally it was desirable that until enough experience had been gleaned of this type of case and a standard established application should be made to the Family Division of the High Court in any case where it is considered by the medical practitioners in charge of a patient in a persistent vegetative state that continued treatment and care no longer confer benefit upon him or her. Two of the Law Lords went further and took the view that the moral, social and legal issues that this particular case raised were such that the situation should be considered by Parliament with a view to some form of statutory intervention and guidelines.

To date the matter has been taken little further than it was in the Bland ruling. Indeed the Court of Session in Edinburgh is hearing the first similar case in Scotland; a request being made to allow a hospital to stop feeding a brain-damaged patient with the inevitable consequence that she would die. Again the application was by the treating hospital trust supported by the patient's family. Similar declarations are being sought. When making submissions the Trust's legal representative highlighted the quandry whether such decisions are medical or legal ones in submitting to the Court that:

The mere fact that they can keep the vegetative existence going does not mean to say it is something in medical terms that can be justified. If it cannot be justified in medical terms, it is difficult to see how it can be justified legally.

Sadly what progress there has been made post Bland has not been by parliamentary intervention.

COPING IN ADVANCE WITH THE PROSPECT OF INCAPACITY

Airedale NHS Trust and Bland did contain certain hints from the Law Lords that their decision might have been assisted had they known what the wishes of Tony Bland would have been had he have known in advance that he would find himself in a persistent vegetative state. However Lord Mustill did temper his comments with reservations about the possible introduction of so-called 'living wills' in formulating a decision based on projection of past decisions by the patient. That said there are certain actions which can be taken by those with capacity which can assist decision-making policy in advance of any incapacity.

Enduring Powers of Attorney

The Enduring Powers of Attorney Act 1985 legislated that a person with capacity could appoint an Attorney to manage his or her affairs with such power extending even to a time where the person lost mental capacity. It is implicit in that statement that like the Court of Protection Enduring Powers of Attorney are limited to dealing with property and business matters. This limitation is imposed within the 1985 Act itself and therefore adopting the finding in *Re F & Re K* [1988] one has to conclude that Enduring Powers of Attorney do not apply to personal and medical matters.

In essence an Enduring Power of Attorney is to enable people to decide whilst they are still capable of deciding whom they would wish to deal with their affairs or part of them, not only during capacity, but after they become mentally incapable. Usually Enduring Powers of Attorney seem best suited and are most utilized in cases of gradual onset rather than sudden incapacity.

Anyone over 18 and mentally capable can grant an Enduring Power of Attorney; standard forms are published by OYEZ. It must be established that the person granting the power is still mentally capable of understanding what the Enduring Power is and what it is intended to do. If the person granting the Enduring Power cannot understand this then there is insufficient mental capacity at the time the power is being granted and the power will not be effective.

The type of decision making within the confines of the provisions that can be granted is either all encompassing or limited as the person granting the power wishes. In other words a general authority to carry out any transactions or a specific authority limited to certain decisions can be granted. It follows from this that someone may grant several Enduring Powers of Attorney to different Attornies each with different decision-making functions.

As with discharge from the Court of Protection cancellation or revocation of an Enduring Power of Attorney reverses the capacity test. There can only be cancellation or revocation if at the time of cancellation or revocation the person who granted the power is mentally capable. For the avoidance of doubt it is preferable to execute a formal **Deed of Revocation**.

For the Enduring Power of Attorney to be valid once the person granting it has become incapable the **Power of Attorney must be registered with the Court of Protection.** Until that takes place the Attorney has very limited powers.

To register an Enduring Power of Attorney the Attorney must give notice of intention to register in a set form to the person granting the Power of Attorney and to certain relations. Formal application must then be made to the Court of Protection in prescribed form accompanied by the Power of Attorney and the appropriate fee. Relatives to be notified are specified in Schedule 1 Part of the Act and notice must be given to at least three relatives. There is an order of priority which inevitably starts with spouse, children and parents. There are sometimes exceptions from this; for example, where the name or address of a person entitled to receive notice is not known and cannot reasonably to ascertained or where such people have not attained the age of 18 or are not themselves mentally capable. It is worth stressing that within each category of priority all relatives must be notified and not just sufficient to attain requisite relatives. Clearly a further exception is if there are not three living relatives. In such a case the application to the Court of Protection should simply explain this.

Provided the Court of Protection on enquiry is satisfied that the necessary notices have been served the Enduring Power of Attorney will be registered and will be stamped as being registered carrying the seal of the Court. A simple search of the Court of Protection register will indicate whether or not a Power of Attorney is registered.

Power of Attorney may be registered prior to incapacity. If that is the case and the person giving the Power of Attorney then wishes to cancel or revoke it whilst still mentally capable a formal application must be made to the Court of Protection for revocation accompanied by the original Enduring Power and any Deed of Revocation. However until the Court of Protection confirms revocation the power remains in force.

Again as with the Court of Protection it would seem that the test of incapacity is an all or nothing test. Inevitably the Enduring Powers of Attorney Act 1985 again cast into the legal spotlight the test of incapacity. The test so far as Enduring Powers of Attorney is concerned was finally established in *Re F & Re K* [1988]. The Judge in that case held that there are four pieces of information which any person creating an Enduring Power of Attorney should understand to have capacity:

1. If such be the terms of power that the Attorney will be able to assume complete authority over the donor's affairs.
2. If such be the terms of power that the Attorney will be able to do anything with the donor's property which the donor could have done.
3. That the authority will continue if the donor should be or should become mentally incapable.
4. That if he or she should be or should become mentally incapable the power will be irrevocable without confirmation by the Court of Protection.

As, until there is incapacity, the donor and the Attorney have concurrent jurisdiction over the donor's property the test ignores completely the ability of the donor to deal with his or her own property and affairs. In other words the donor may satisfy the capacity test of understanding but may not in fact have residual capacity to do the things which an Attorney is able to do under the Enduring

Powers. The test of capacity here is only whether the donor has the capacity to grant the Enduring Power of Attorney.

This was something touched upon in brief by the Judge in *Re F & Re K* [1988] who felt that in such a situation there should be immediate registration with the Court of Protection of the Enduring Power of Attorney. Given that almost half the applications for registration received by the Court of Protection are in respect of Enduring Powers made no more than 3 months prior to application one can see the importance of the test of capacity in this field. It is not surprising therefore that the medical profession may be called upon quite often to witness or approve the execution of an Enduring Power of Attorney. It must follow from this that any medical practitioner called upon in this context has to be satisfied that he or she can make that assessment and if the assessment can be made then it should be properly and accurately recorded in some form of document to be kept with the Enduring Power.

Criticism has also been made that apart from the formal registration of the enduring power with the Court of Protection the decision-making powers of the Court of Protection and those of the Attorney under an enduring power are mutually exclusive.

Living wills

This was a topic touched upon briefly in *Airedale NHS Trust* v. *Bland*. Living wills have also been the subject of much comment and documentary investigation in recent years. Often that investigation has looked at the concept in tandem with views on euthanasia. When looking at living wills in the context of incapacity one must bear in mind the fine line recited by Lord Browne-Wilkinson. It is apparent in Bland that the concept can also be looked at in situations similar to those where an Enduring Power of Attorney may be created but looking at **Personal and medical decisions** rather than the decisions to which Enduring Powers of Attorney are limited by statutory parameters.

To date there has been no statutory intervention in respect of living wills and they have not been directly tested in Court. One can only conclude from this that whilst there is much interest in such documents one can only view them now as an additional evidential factor when determining, for example in medical decisions, what represents the best interest of the patient. One can deduce from the comments of Lord Mustill in Bland that there will still be a judicial concern over the weight one should attach to the views expressed in such documents. However there can be no doubt that there will be further discussion and perhaps legislation on living wills in the foreseeable future.

To an extent certain areas of advance decision making that people already utilize may be a type of living will. There is jurisdiction of the Court to assist those who seek declaratory intervention in terms of their future treatment whilst retaining their mental capacity. *Re C* [1994] involved a case of a patient suffering chronic paranoid schizophrenia. However it was deemed that he did have sufficient mental capacity to formulate decisions on his own medical treatment at the time he appeared before the Court. He had required urgent treatment for leg ulceration. The consultant treating him had recommended that there be amputation failing which there was a strong possibility that he would not survive. The patient decided in that case he did not wish to have amputation. The consultant felt that the patient understood perfectly properly the pros and cons and did not amputate. Fortunately the patient recovered. However there was the spectra of recurrence and risk of amputation in the future. In this case the patient sought injunctive remedy from the Court to prevent future amputation without his written consent. The Court determined that as he was capable he could therefore decide what his wishes were for medical treatment in the future and it was,

therefore, perfectly proper for the Court to intervene under its inherent jurisdiction by way of injunction rather than declaration. On that basis the Court granted the patient's application.

However this case added further complication to the question of determining capacity as the patient was deemed capable enough to act without a next friend in the litigation process even though he was suffering from chronic paranoid schizophrenia. The Court did have to determine whether he was capable of deciding what was best for his future treatment and formed the view that incapacity would arise with a patient suffering this illness where he or she was so reduced by chronic mental illness that he or she 'does not sufficiently understand the nature, purpose and effects of proper treatment' If guidance is sought, and Re C by no means clarifies the issues, the Court here seemed to be particularly impressed with the detail with which the treating consultant had considered the situation and the clarity with which he was able to explain the reasons that he had deferred to the patient's wishes originally. It is perhaps, in this area too, worth remembering that those who are supposedly capable and rational frequently make decisions to accept or refuse medical procedures or treatments basing the decision on factors which are rational 'irrational, or for no reason'. One must look at the **capacity of the person making the decision** not the decision itself. In other words, as was reaffirmed in *Re T* [1993] (adult; refusal of treatment), provided that there has been a proper explanation of the treatment and that the person making the decision has capacity, that person may execute free choice.

The British Medical Association has recognized a need for consideration of advance statements of this kind and in 1995 produced a publication entitled *Advance Statements About Medical Treatment* which included a code of practice. In essence the code of practice confirms that, although not binding on health professionals, advance statements deserve thorough consideration and respect and where valid and applicable advance directives including refusals of treatment must be followed. Further guidance is given. As an appendix there is a useful suggestion on the considerations and content of written advance statements as the British Medical Association recognizes that whilst oral statements may have some effect it is plainly preferable that there should be written advance statements. The code sets out useful guidance for those who are being asked to advise a patient who is considering making an advance statement. This publication perhaps shows the current informality in terms of the validity of advance statements and living wills.

WHAT DOES THE FUTURE HOLD?

In 1995 the Law Commission produced a lengthy and detailed review of mental incapacity as part of its programme of law reform. In essence, the report concluded, that the law in this area is unnecessarily complicated and uncertain and that a greater degree of clarity is required not only for patients but also for medical practitioners who may treat or be asked to determine on incapacity. The Commission report concluded with a detailed draft bill.

Linking this report to the decisions and decision-making processes that have been considered above, and summarizing lengthy consideration given in the Law Commission report, the conclusions are that:

1. It is impossible to give an all-embracing definition of mental incapacity which represents an all-or-nothing test. Instead one should look at the definition of incapacity in relation to specific decisions that need to be made. Each time such a decision needs to be made one must look afresh at capacity, defining incapacity as the inability by reason of mental disability to make a decision for him/herself on the matter in question or being unable

to communicate a decision on that matter because of unconsciousness or other reason. However, unlike the Mental Health Act definition the proposed bill prepared by the Law Commission does define mental disability as:
(a) the inability to understand or retain the information relevant to the decision, including information about the reasonably foreseeable consequences of deciding one way or another or a failure to make the decision, or
(b) being unable to make a decision based on that information. The Mental disability or disorder of the mind or brain, whether permanent or temporary, which results in an impairment or disturbance of mental functioning. Further guidance is given in terms of degree of understanding and the fact that the decision made does not need to be rational or prudent to show capacity and the steps that have to be taken to determine whether a decision can be communicated. There is, importantly, an overriding presumption against lack of capacity, in deciding whether someone lacks capacity the decision should be made on the balance of probabilities, i.e. this is more likely than not.

2. The current system where Enduring Powers of Attorney and Court of Protection overlap but both are limited to property and affairs is unsatisfactory. The Commission suggests that an Enduring Power of Attorney be replaced by a Continuing Power of Attorney and defines how that document can be created and registered, and suggests that a Continuing Power of Attorney may extend to all or to any specified matters including personal welfare, healthcare, property, or affairs and the conduct of legal proceedings. In other words that if such a general power is

granted the Attorney can deal with more than simply property and business affairs.

3. The Commission acknowledges that the various Courts that currently have some form of jurisdiction over various elements of decision making and incapacity overlap and that eventually one Court or manager appointed by the Court to intervene is more satisfactory. Again the Commission recommends that the degree of Court intervention should be extended beyond property and affairs to include also personal welfare, health care and the conduct of legal proceedings. The recommendation continues that the Court may make any decision on behalf of a person who lacks capacity to make that decision or appoint a person to be responsible for making that decision on behalf of a person who lacks capacity to make it. Usually the report favours Court intervention and suggests that the appointment of a manager be strictly limited in scope and duration. The Commission would also wish to see the Court having powers, *inter alia*, to decide where the person concerned is to live and what contact, if any, that person is to have with other specified persons and to extend to the obtaining of statutory benefits and services.

4. Again the question of 'best interest' is very much to the fore in the consideration of the Law Commission. A draft bill put forward by the Commission would see a statutory definition of this and would require regard to be had to the following:
    (a) past and present wishes and feelings and factors which the patient would consider if able to do so, and
    (b) permitting and encouraging that person to participate or to improve his or her ability to participate as fully as possible in the decision-making process,

    (c) if practical and appropriate to consult the following people for views on:
    (i) any person named by the patient as someone to be consulted on matters,
    (ii) anyone whether spouse, relative, friend or other person engaged in caring for the patient or interested in the patient's welfare,
    (iii) the donee of any Continuing Power of Attorney granted and
    (iv) any manager appointed by the Court. It is also interesting that the Commission would wish to see some attempt at statutory protection on the basis that if anything is done or a decision is made by a person other than the Court, that person will be able to show compliance with best interest if that person can show that he or she reasonably believed that when making the decision or taking the action it was in the best interest of the patient,

5. The Law Commission drew from the various Court authorities to date, most of which have been reviewed in this chapter, some guidelines for determining when and in what capacity the Court ought to be asked to intervene in medical treatment. Court approval or consent to treatment by the donee of a Continuing Power of Attorney or manager appointed by the Court will be required under the draft Bill for any treatment or procedure:
    (a) intended or reasonably likely to render the person concerned permanently infertile except where it is for disease of the reproductive organs or for relieving existing detrimental effects of menstruation;
    (b) to facilitate the donation of non-regenerative tissue or bone marrow;
    (c) to facilitate the donation of tissue not within paragraph (b) above as may be described by the Secretary of State.

In addition to the view of the treating consultant a further registered medical practitioner will be required to confirm that the patient is without capacity to consent and that the best interests of the patient are served by the treatment or procedure recommended by the treating consultant. Beyond that, save for the exceptions set out above, the donee of a Continuing Power of Attorney or manager appointed by the Court can approve treatment.

This is all against the back drop of the proposed Bill rendering it lawful for anything to be done for the personal welfare or health care of a person who is, or is reasonably believed to be, without capacity in relation to the matter in question, if it is in all the circumstances reasonable for it to be done by the appropriate person.

This overall authority though does not override decisions which have actually been made by a person who subsequently loses capacity such as recited in *Re C*, [1994]. Indeed the proposed Bill specifically precludes the general authority extending to any treatment where there has been an advance refusal of treatment. However in the absence of an indication to the contrary the Bill envisages an assumption that the advance refusal of treatment does not apply to situations where the refusal may endanger that person's life, or if the person is a woman who is pregnant the life of the fetus. From a treater's point of view the Bill provides a statutory defence for the consequence of withholding any treatment or procedure if the treater had reasonable grounds for believing that an advance refusal of treatment by the person concerned applied or in the reverse for carrying out any treatment or procedure where there was an advance refusal unless the treater knew or had reasonable grounds for believing

that there was an advance refusal of treatment.

The Law Commission specifically looked at non-therapeutic procedures, particularly termination of life support. The Bill proposes that it shall be lawful to discontinue artificial nutritional hydration for a person who is unconscious, has no activity in his cerebral cortex and has no prospect of recovery from his condition provided that either there is approval of the Court or this consent is given within the scope of a Continuing Power of Attorney by a donee or by a manager appointed by Court or, if ultimately the Secretary of State approves it, by the provision of a certificate in writing by a registered medical practitioner appointed on behalf of the patient stating that it is appropriate for such discontinuance to take place.

CONCLUSIONS

What is patently apparent from this brief review of the decision-making process is that the area is a potential mine field for the unwary. Indeed knowledge of the whereabouts of the mines does not in itself necessarily lead to a safe path through the mine fields. There seems to be a number of different definitions of incapacity each relating to specific areas of decision making with little cross-over. The easier forums for decision making are limited and can only deal with property and affairs and even then the two major decision-making mechanisms, the Court of Protection and Enduring Powers of Attorney, overlap without much mutual assistance. In an age of seemingly increasing accountability and criticism a greater degree of clarity is required not only to protect the welfare of the patient but also those who treat. No one knowing the Official Solicitor's stance in Bland, that termination of life support may amount to murder, can take lightly the concern of the medical profession on behalf of the individual treaters.

Whilst certain elements of guidance can be gleaned from existing case law and from existing established procedures for decision making, at the moment these provide assistance but not certainty.

The key at the moment seems initially to be taking the time, where feasible, to make and record decisions on capacity and reasons for such conclusion. Only then does one move into the equally serious consideration of what constitutes best interest. Certainly when considering giving or withholding treatment which does not itself stem from the disorder, the counsel of wisdom suggests that application ought always to be made to the Court for either declaratory or injunctive remedy. In the light of judicial encouragement given in previous cases it is hard to see any Court criticizing a practitioner, authority or trust, for erring on the side of caution and passing the buck very much to the judiciary.

Perhaps the Law Commission suggestions do represent a simplified system. That said the report itself still requires daily decisions to be made on capacity, albeit looking to avoid the all-or-nothing capacity test and trying to give guidance as to how to make such a determination and having made it how best to weigh the interest of the patient. It would seem though that the truth is always that ultimately the medical profession will have to make value judgements on capacity, often in less than ideal situations, and knowing that there may ultimately be judicial intervention to examine those decisions. There seems to be no way to avoid this. I conclude with the words of Lord Gough in the House of Lords in *Airedale NHS Trust* v. *Bland* which I hope will give crumbs of comfort to those at the front line of treating and dealing with incapacity on a daily basis.

It is nevertheless the function of the Judges to state the legal principles upon which the lawfulness of the actions of doctors depend; but in the end the decisions to be made in individual cases must rest with the doctors

themselves. In these circumstances, what is required is a sensitive understanding by both the Judges and the doctors of each others respective functions, and in particular the determination by the Judges not merely to understand the problems facing the medical profession in cases of this kind, but also to regard their professional standards with respect. A mutual understanding between the doctors and the Judges is the best way to ensure the evolution of a sensitive and sensible legal framework for the treatment and care of patients, with a sound ethical basis, in the interest of the patients themselves.

REFERENCES

Airedale NHS Trust v *Bland* [1993] AC 789.
B v. *Croydon Health Authority* 20.7.94 Family Division & TLR 1.12.94.
Banks v. *Goodfellow* (1870) LR5QB549.
Bolam v. *Friern Barnet Management Committee* [1957] 2 ALL ER 118
Law Com No 231 1995.
Parker v. *Felgate* (1883) 8PD171.
Re C [1994] 1 WLR 290.
Re F [1990] 2 A.C.1.
Re F & Re K [1988] Ch 310.
Re S [1993] FAM 123.
Re T [1993] FAM 95.

It may help readers to have the following comments from the author!

Legal references are always incomprehensible, there seems to be a great stigma if one uses a rounded, rather than square bracket, or vice versa. The references in the chapter are in the correct way in which legal references ought to appear. However, by way of explanation the numbering is as follows:

Airedale NHS Trust v. *Bland* [1993]: appears in the 1993 Appeal Court Reports at page 789.
B. v. *Croydon Health Authority*: appears in the Times Law Report on December 1994.
Banks v. *Goodfellow* (1870): A Queen's Bench Division case, volume 5, page 549 from 1870.
Bolam v. *Friern Barnet Management Committee* [1957]: appears in the second edition of the ALL England Law Reports for 1957 at page 118.

Law Com No 231 1995: this is 231st Law Commission paper and its year of publication was 1995.

Parker v. *Felgate* (1883): an 1883 case that appears in the 8th edition of the Probate Division records at page 171.

Re C [1994]: appears in the 1994 Weekly Law Reports Volume 1, page 290.

Re F [1990]: appears in the second volume of the Appeal Court publications for 1990 at page 1.

Re F & Re K [1988]: appears in the 1988 Chancery Reports at page 310.

Re S [1993]: appears in the Family Reports at page 123 for 1993.

Re T [1993]: appears in the 1993 Family Reports at page 95.

If readers want to find these then the Law Commission Report can be purchased from HMSO stationery offices throughout the country. The weekly Law Reports and the All England Law Reports are kept by most Law firms but the nineteenth century cases, perhaps the Appeal Court cases and the Family Cases, will only be stocked by some firms and the likelihood is that a specialist library will be required. The Law Society library contains all these publications and, oddly enough, so do some local libraries.

11 Litigation and compensation

M.J. Powers Q.C.

INTRODUCTION

This chapter is intended to give an overview of the process of achieving compensation. It is not intended to be a legal treatise on the law so, for the sake of clarity, there are statements made which elide similar principles without further explanation or qualification. Where expression and comprehension of essential legal principles can be better achieved by an example I shall use the fictional case of a 35-year-old married man ('John') who has two dependent children. He develops a quadri-plegia as a consequence of a negligently administered anaesthetic for a routine repair of an inguinal hernia.

Each year many thousands of accidents occur in which people are injured as a consequence of the fault of others. In many of these cases solicitors will be instructed in the hope that some financial redress can be obtained from those at fault.

Compensation is not automatic. No system of **no fault liability** exists in this country. Both fault and causation of loss have to be proved. Legal **proof** means that on the evidence placed before a Judge, 'the injured party has to show, on the balance of prob-abilities, that a duty of care existed towards him, that the duty was breached and, in consequence thereof, he suffered injury'.

The prospective defendant is often an individual – such as a car driver, a workman or a medical practitioner. However, where an individual defendant is employed and the injuries sustained by the plaintiff were caused by a person in the course of his employment, the employer usually becomes the named defendant as his insurers will be in a position to meet any claim made against him.

THE LEGAL PRINCIPLES

There is no compensation available to those who suffer an inherited defect. Neither does anyone born with a deformity have any redress against anyone else – unless it can be shown that the deformity was caused by the fault of another before birth. Since the Congenital Disabilities (Civil Liability) Act 1976 came into force, there has been a statutory right to bring an action in respect of injuries sustained before birth. This right does not accrue to an unborn child until it is born and has survived. Many acquired injuries, which are not self-caused, are poten-tially compensatable by those responsible or by their insurers.

The only two legal 'causes of action' with which we need be concerned are **assault** and **negligence**. Without being too pedantic, assault is a crime, and negligence a civil wrong. The main difference is that a claim in negligence requires damage to be proved whereas damages may be claimed for

Rehabilitation of the Physically Disabled Adult. Edited by C. John Goodwill, M. Anne Chamberlain and Chris Evans. Published in 1997 by Stanley Thornes (Publishers) Ltd, Cheltenham. ISBN 0-7487-3183-0.

assault without proof of injury. Nevertheless, damages awarded for an assault either by the Criminal Injuries Compensation Board or by a civil court reflect the seriousness of the injury sustained.

In almost all circumstances in which a person suffers a non-intentional injury at the hands of another it can be said that a **duty of care** existed and was owed to the person injured by the person responsible (tortfeasor). Breach of this duty of care with consequential injury or damage is the negligence. The duty is owed to one's 'neighbour', that is anyone who is foreseeably likely to be affected by one's acts or omissions. There are many situations in which the duty of care arises. For example, one road user to another, an employer to an employee; one employee to another: the occupier of land to a visitor; the manufacturer of a product to the consumer: there are many similar examples.

The **standard** to which the duty has to be discharged is neither the highest nor the lowest. The duty is to be discharged to a reasonable standard. For example, the anaesthetist in John's case had a duty to take reasonable care for his safety in the administration of the anaesthetic. In the case of the anaesthetist, as a medical person 'professing' to have a special skill, the reasonable standard of performance is not that of the 'man on the top of the Clapham omnibus' but that of the ordinary skill of a competent person exercising that particular art. John has to show that his anaesthetist did not measure up to the level of care and/or competence of the ordinary competent anaesthetist and he will need medical expert evidence to this effect.

Having established the existence of the duty and with evidence that there was a failure properly to discharge it, the litigant then has to show that it was the breach of the duty which **caused or materially contributed to his injury**. Where a pedestrian loses his leg in a road accident, there is not likely to be any argument that the leg was lost because of the accident. However, in John's case it might be argued by the anaesthetist that although there was a close temporal association between the administration of the anaesthetic and the onset of the quadriplegia it was not any act or omission of the anaesthetist which caused it – it was 'one of those things', an Act of God, a condition of unknown aetiology, or an inherent defect awaiting opportunity to express itself.

Since the human body is a very complex machine about which much is still unknown, a defence to an action for damages may be found in the medically inexplicable.

Sometimes a defendant is prepared to accept that there has been a breach of duty of care and that some injury was caused as a consequence but may choose to contest the extent (the quantum) of the injury claimed by the plaintiff.

In respect of each element comprising negligence (duty breach, causation and quantum), the burden of proof falls on the injured party. The **standard of proof**, however, is not as high as in a criminal case where the jury has to be sure beyond reasonable doubt. The injured plaintiff in a civil claim for damages only has to show that on the **balance of probabilities**, (i.e. more likely than not) the injury is caused by the alleged negligence.

Trials of these cases are before a Judge sitting alone, either in the High Court or, for cases where the claim is worth less than £50 000, in the County Court. Claims of importance or complexity can be transferred from the County Court to the High Court for trial even though they may be claims worth less than £50 000.

So, a person can be in breach of duty of care without any ill consequence occurring and, on the other hand, adverse events can occur without any breach of duty. It is important to remember that there are very few circumstances in which the fact of the injury alone is enough to establish that it was caused by negligence. On some occasions, however, a litigant may be able simply to say the thing speaks for itself (*res ipsa loquitur*). Doubtlessly John would argue that it was enough to say he was fit when he went into the operation for his hernia repair and he has come out paralysed – something must have gone wrong for this kind of outcome does not ordinarily occur without negligence. However, it is infrequent that a plaintiff can successfully use this maxim. Where the **cause** of the injury is not known perhaps it would be unreasonable to say to a defendant it is obviously your fault. Furthermore, the maxim only places the burden of proof on the defendant to show that the injury was not the consequence of his negligence.

A plaintiff is considerably assisted in the advancement of his case (particularly where proof of what actually happened is difficult) if he is able to:

1.   use the res *ipsa loquitur* argument; or
2.   rely upon the breach by the defendant of a relevant duty imposed by an Act of Parliament; or
3.   show that the defendant has been convicted of a driving offence relevant to the accident which caused the injury about which complaint is made.

Not infrequently injuries are sustained as a consequence of a number of different factors or actions coinciding. In order to succeed the injured plaintiff does not have to prove that the defendant through his negligence **caused all** the injury/incapacity, but the plaintiff must be able to show that he materially contributed to it. It is not enough for a plaintiff simply to show that the defendant materially increased the **risk** of the injury occurring if he is not able to show the defendant actually caused the injury. If the plaintiff shows a material contribution then he can recover for the **whole** incapacity – unless it is shown that, but for the event causing the injury, there would have been some incapacity sooner or later in any event.

Contributory negligence,

Where the injured person was in breach of his duty of care to himself, that is, he failed to act as the ordinary person would have done and that failure contributed to the causation of the accident, then the defendant is entitled to say 'I should not have to pay the full compensation because you were part to blame'. In such a case the Court would apportion liability. If the plaintiff were to be found 25% liable for his injuries, he would only be awarded 75% of the full value of his claim against the defendant.

WHO CAN CLAIM?

Any person of sound mind over the age of 18 may make a claim for injuries and whether he takes the necessary steps himself or instructs a solicitor to act on his behalf at all times the injured person has the power to control what happens to his claim. He may, for example, discontinue the action, change his solicitor or accept any offer of settlement.

Chapter 10 covers powers of attorney, guardianship and related matters, and this will not be described further in any detail except to say that in respect of minors (persons under the age of 18 years) or persons who suffer from mental illness claims are brought through a 'Next Friend' (often a parent). In these claims, because of Plaintiff's incapacity, the Court has an overriding power to ensure that Justice is done between the parties and that they are bound by the decisions. Even an agreement to settle a case requires the approval of the Court.

WHEN IS THE CLAIM MADE?

If a claim is to be made, the earlier the better. Obviously there has first to be an injury and the injury has to be more than trivial (*de minimus*). The date on which the injury occurred **even if the injured person was at the time unaware of any injury** is the date on

which the cause of action accrued: that is the first date on which an action for damages for negligence could be made. There is not often much delay between the breach of duty and the injury if the breach is the cause of the injury. For example, if a workman carelessly throws a brick over a wall at the moment the brick leaves his hand he is in breach of his general duty of care but the cause of action does not accrue until someone is injured as a result. The brick may land on someone's head or it may lie in the lane until someone trips over it 2 days later. In order to achieve justice between the parties there has to be a defined period within which a plaintiff may bring his action. Without such a limitation a prospective defendant would forever have hanging over him the possibility that at some undefined time in the future an action might be brought. This would be like the prejudice to Damocles when the sword was suspended over his head at the banquet: it was suspended by a single hair and the banquet was a tantalizing torment to him. The possibility of defending an action successfully is likely to diminish with time and inevitable prejudice would be caused by the death of relevant witnesses, the faded recollection of others and the loss of critical documents.

So it is that the legal process imposes time limits within which claims have to be brought. The Court has always had the power to prevent an abuse of its process and, seeking to bring a claim many years after the relevant event may amount to an **abuse of process**. Since the time of Henry VIII, there have been a variety of pieces of legislation which have sought to define the time within which actions may be brought.

In more modern times the Limitation Act 1939 provided that actions based on contract or tort should not be brought after the expiration of 6 years from the date on which the case of action accrued. In respect of certain claims, including claims for damages for personal injuries caused by negligence, the period was subsequently reduced to only 3 years. This led to unfairness because some people were unaware that they had been injured by a defendant until it was too late to sue. However, in 1975 a new Act provided for an action to be within the limitation period if brought within 3 years of the **date of knowledge**, and a **discretion** vested in the Court to extend the 3-year limitation period was also introduced. There have been a great many legal cases reported on the subject of limitation and they may be summarized as follows:

- An action has to be brought within 3 years of either the accrual of the cause of action, or, if later, the date of knowledge.
- Actions may not be brought outside that period unless the Court is persuaded that there are good reasons for doing so and that Justice would be better served by allowing the matter to proceed than by barring it for ever.
- Those who are under disability (minority or mental) have special protection:
  (a) An infant's 3 years do not start to run until he attains his majority.
  (b) The 3 years do not start to run against a person with mental incapacity until he has recovered. This effectively means in the case of a person who is permanently mentally disabled that an action may be brought on his behalf at any time. The Courts, however, will use their inherent powers to prevent an abuse which might arise in an exceptional case when a claim is made more than 20 years late.

Since limitation is such an important topic in litigation it justifies some explanation of what amounts to sufficient 'knowledge' of a significant injury in order to start the 3-year time period running.

- The knowledge has to be of a 'significant injury'; it is significant enough if the injured person would reasonably have considered it sufficiently serious to justify his instituting proceedings for damages.

- Knowledge has to extend to the identity of the defendant.
- The injured person needs some level of awareness of the cause or attribution of the injury: he has to know in very general terms that it is capable of being attributed to some act or omission of the defendant.
- If the injury is reasonably to be considered by the plaintiff to be sufficiently serious then the clock starts ticking on the 3-year period in which the action had to be brought; the clock is not stopped even if the plaintiff believes that his injury was to have been expected or that the other party was not at fault.
- Finally, even if the injured person did not actually know, knowledge may be imputed to him from facts ascertainable by him with the help of medical or other appropriate expert advice which it would have been reasonable for him to seek: in other words the prospective plaintiff has to act reasonably.

HOW IS THE CLAIM MADE?

Usually the injured person, or someone acting on his behalf, seeks legal assistance and the most important thing is for a solicitor to be chosen who has expertise in advancing personal injury claims. In John's case a particular expertise is required and anyone who has been injured as a consequence of what they believe is negligent medical treatment or care should only go to a solicitor with expertise in medical negligence claims. Help in this respect can be obtained through the Association of Victims of Medical Accidents' or through the Law Society. A family solicitor should be prepared to advise a potential claimant on whom he should see, but help may be obtained through channels as diverse as the Injured Claimant's Union or the Automobile Association.

COST OF LEGAL ADVICE

Naturally the potential cost of litigation concerns almost everyone. However, it should be said that often the first interview with a solicitor can be obtained without charge – if only to see if the claimant is eligible for Legal Aid. There is no reason why simple enquiry should not be made soon after an accident to see what likely costs would be involved in advancing a claim. This is particularly important as, following any serious accident, time rapidly passes when there are more important matters in mind – such as recovery and how to cope with life in the presence of the limitations imposed by incapacity. It is a tragedy when a good claim for damages is lost or barred as a consequence of too long a delay.

Where there is a good claim to be advanced, even if the injured party is not eligible for Legal Aid, many solicitors will agree to a deferment in settling their fees until the case is concluded. If the case is successful the defendant not only has to pay damages, but is also responsible for the injured plaintiff's legal expenses. However, a successful claimant may not recover his full outlay on legal expenses and any shortfall then is effectively taken from the damages awarded.

STEPS THAT ARE TAKEN BEFORE PROCEEDINGS ARE COMMENCED

Before any action is considered against a potential defendant evidence has to be gathered and assessed by an experienced lawyer who will advise whether or not there is a reasonable prospect of success. The claimant and anyone else who knows about the circumstances in which the injury was sustained needs to be interviewed for the purpose of obtaining a full statement. These statements may not be in their final version for trial, but it is very important for details to be recorded whilst they are still fresh in mind. Copies of all the claimant's medical records will have to be obtained. Although this step is not always necessary as in a straightforward injury case (where there are not likely to be issues of the medical causation), if there is a suggestion from the defendant that the plaintiff had the condition before or would have had the injury in any event, analysis of the entire medical records becomes imperative. The same is so where there is an allegation of medical negligence.

Sometimes a plaintiff does not wish to have his medical records disclosed to his advisers, let alone to the defendant and his advisers. There is little that the plaintiff can do about this. As soon as a claim for injuries is advanced the plaintiff puts into issue the state of his health, the medical records often become of critical importance in relation to **causation and quantum**. In most actions **'discovery'** of documents is a stage after the commencement of the action and before trial. Occasionally, and nearly always in actions for medical negligence, it may be necessary for a prospective plaintiff to obtain **pre-action discovery** in order for his medical advisers to determine if there is a case which can be made out. John's legal advisers would require not only all the hospital medical records and X-rays but also all the earlier general practitioner records as well. These would then be submitted to one or more medical experts for opinion(s) on breach of duty and causation.

EXPERT OPINION

In all actions for personal injuries medical opinions are required. In any event there is an obligation to serve the defendant with a medical report substantiating the alleged injuries at the time of the service of **Statement of Claim** (Particulars of Claim in the County Court) in the High Court which is served either with or shortly after the service of the **Writ** (Summons in the County Court). Where the injury is complex, medical reports may have to be served from experts in different specialities. If the claim involves allegations of medical negligence against a doctor/health authority, medical expert opinions are required on breach of duty and causation. In accident cases, reports may be required from accident investigators, engineers and others who have specialist skills in order that the plaintiff can put before the court the evidence on which it is said that the defendant failed properly to discharge his duty of care. All evidence of this kind is exchanged before trial, but at a late stage.

The success or failure of litigation depends upon the quality of the evidence and the composition of expert reports is often crucial and is always important.

THE MEDICAL REPORT

Fundamental to each party's case is the evidence of the medical experts upon whom reliance is placed at trial. The defendant should be able clearly to see the case that he has to meet if the plaintiff's case has been properly pleaded in the statement of claim upon the basis of sound and corroborated medical opinions. If there has been no intimation of a willingness on the part of the defendant to settle a claim it is unlikely to follow immediately following the service of the Statement of Claim. Nevertheless, that vital pleading should be full, strong and precise, as it is through this medium that the experts' criticisms of the defendant's conduct are made. If the case has been fully and properly pleaded the medical evidence exchanged should cause the respective parties no surprises. No new issues of liability or causation should arise and, if indeed they do, amendment to the Statement of Claim will be required which is likely to occasion delay and wasted costs.

While some degree of consultation between experts and legal advisers is entirely proper, it is necessary that expert evidence presented to the court should be, and should be seen to be, the independent product of the expert, uninfluenced as to form or content by the exigencies of litigation.

An expert may be asked to amend any preliminary report in the light of the issues which emerge as central to the case and to make other adjustments to his written opinion so as to reflect more closely the weight and tenor of the opinion he has given in conference. It is commonly the case that a view formed in an early report requires extensive revision, if not an about-turn, once the expert has considered the matter more fully with the client, other experts and the lawyers.

It is for the lawyers and not the experts to assess the merits of the case. There will often be a close correlation between the view expressed by counsel and that expressed by the experts but the medical expert has to tread the difficult path between that of witness, lawyer and judge. He should not so express his expert opinion on the medical issues as to amount to a determination of the merits and above all he should not make any conclusions of fact. It is the expert's opinion on the evidence as stated, not his opinion of the facts which is required. Facts are those things which have happened. Lay witnesses can be called to say what they saw and heard happened. Where **no direct evidence** is available as to what happened, experts may be invited to draw inferences and tender an opinion as to what happened. More often expert opinion is directed at what **would** have happened and not what **should** have happened.

Finally, the expert has to avoid hyperbole. If he is experienced he will appreciate the danger of using adjectives too loosely and most importantly he should endeavour to be objective in his assessment.

Experienced solicitors and counsel have personal knowledge of experts in different specialities whose opinion is valued. Some experts, like lawyers, are better on paper than in court. This has to be borne in mind. In the early expert investigation of a case forensic ability is not essential whereas a learned, fair and objective approach is.

In a case such as John's, or where a previously fit patient dies or suffers irreversible brain damage under anaesthesia, a *prima facie* case of negligence is raised and the nature of any expert report prepared before the conference with counsel might be quite different from the medical report required at trial. Experience has shown that in a significant number of cases the early assessment of the merits, whether by doctor or lawyer, subsequently proves to be unreliable. A report which is unduly optimistic will raise hopes and may lead to a considerable waste of expenditure on legal costs before a realistic assessment of the merits is made. Of greater concern, however, is the number of inadequately researched and prepared reports leading to negative opinions. These cases may not be pursued sufficiently for their true merits ever to ascertained.

Writing an expert report on liability for the first time requires guidance. In the interest of speeding up the trial of cases not only is all evidence exchanged beforehand but the expert's report stands as that expert's **evidence 'in chief'***, so format and content are both of enormous importance. The following is an example of a medical **report on liability**[†], but the general structure of the report is appropriate for any report on liability:

- Typescript should be used, 1.5 or double-spaced on A4 paper with 1 inch margins.
- The title page should show:
  (a) The name of the plaintiff and his date of birth.
  (b) A short summary of the report, e.g. Medical Report on the circumstances surrounding the anaesthetic administered to John Doe for the repair of an inguinal hernia at St Elsewhere's General Hospital, on 1 April 1996.

---

*The first evidence given by the expert on behalf of the party calling him.
[†]That is a medical expert's criticism of the standard of care the plaintiff received.

(c) The name, qualifications and appointment of the expert making the report.

(d) The date and purpose of the report.

- A statement of on whose behalf the report has been prepared.
- A detailed list of all medical records (See 'steps that are taken before proceedings are commenced' above), reports statements and materials upon which the opinion is based.
- A chronological account of the facts as they appear from the source materials set out such that random access may be made to any particular date or time. Frequently there will be discrepancies between the dates/times given by the lay client, his witnesses, and the various entries in the medical records – most are likely to be of minor significance but ultimately these discrepancies should be reconciled if they are not to be issues at trial.
- The important events in the history should be identified and, where necessary, an account given of the relevant medical principles involved in the plaintiff's management. In John's case these would have to have included an exposition of the anaesthetic principles relevant to the standard of care John should have received. An account of the natural history of the pathological process should be given for it often proves to be of critical importance. These are perhaps the most difficult tasks for the expert. He has to reduce his great learning and experience into simple propositions which the non-expert can understand. Relevant textbook authorities and learned articles should be cited and copies appended to the report.
- Having set out the facts and the relevant fundamental medical principles, the final step is for the expert to express his opinion by formulating a conclusion on the standard and acceptability of all aspects of the care the plaintiff received. It is important for the expert to cover this ground widely. In addition he has to provide express embodiment of the opi-

nions the expert has earlier expressed. Moreover he should:

(a) Make it clear when a question or issue fell outside his expertise.

(b) State if the opinion was not properly researched because it was considered that insufficient data was available; an indication that the opinion was provisional might be necessary. In particular, if he could not assert that the report contained the truth, the whole truth and nothing but the truth then that qualification should be stated on the report.

(c) In the event of him changing his mind on a material matter (after the exchange of reports) he should communicate this change of view through the legal representatives to the other side and to the Court as soon as possible. His report will be read by the judge and it should be written in a way which is factually accurate, logical and comprehensible. A glance at a selection of expert reports is sufficient to see the range of quality of presentation and care with which they have been prepared. The lawyers' objective must be to ensure that when reference is necessary to the subject matter, the reader chooses to refer to the reports of their experts and not those of their opponents.

(c) A brief curriculum vitae, including a list of publications, should be included.

THE MEDICAL REPORT ON QUANTUM (PRESENT CONDITION AND PROGNOSIS)

As a general principle it is sensible to avoid instructing as an expert any doctor who has treated the plaintiff; such experts seem inherently unable to be other than optimistic about their efforts. On occasion, by virtue of the particular injuries suffered, this may be difficult. In any event, the expert's views should not be at odds with the plaintiff's experts on liability and causation. Obviously he should not be the professional colleague of the person alleged to be responsible, neither should he have any interest in the outcome.

No expert can properly give an opinion on the plaintiff's present condition and prognosis without the opportunity of an examination and, occasionally, some further investigation. Whilst the plaintiff usually does not object to an examination by the doctor instructed on his own behalf, it not infrequently happens that an objection is taken to the medical expert nominated by the defendants to examine the plaintiff, or, the further investigation he requires. The plaintiff is, however, under an obligation to afford the defendants' experts reasonable opportunity for examination and should he decline to submit himself for examination the defendants may make an application to the Court for an order staying the plaintiff's action until such time as he does submit to examination.

There are, amongst other factors, two fundamental rights which are cherished by the common law: the plaintiff's right to personal liberty and the right of the defendant to defend himself in the litigation as he and his advisers think fit (including the freedom to choose the witness that he will call). It is particularly important that a defendant should be able to choose his own expert witnesses if the case be one in which expert testimony is significant. The interests of justice could require one or other of the parties to have to accept an infringement of a fundamental human right cherished by the common law. The plaintiff can only be compelled, albeit indirectly, to submit to an infringement of his personal liberty if justice requires it. Similarly, the defendant can only be compelled to forgo the expert witness of his choice if justice requires it. The particular facts of the case on which the discretion has to be exercised are all important.

The general structure of the report on injury should be similar to that on liability. A short summary of the report at the beginning is helpful for the reader particularizing the data and purpose of the report (including a statement of on whose behalf the report has been prepared). Again it is important for the expert to protect his position by identifying the factual basis upon which the opinion expressed in the report has been made, to which end a detailed list of all medical records, reports, statements and materials should be provided.

The history should not be materially inconsistent with the pleaded case or with the history set out in other reports. If inconsistencies are found they must be resolved before the reports are exchanged for trial, otherwise they will provide fruitful ground for cross-examination.

The plaintiff's condition at the time of consultation must be clearly established, including the present symptoms and the effect of any disability on daily living activities, work, sport, hobbies, travelling, social and family life. It is not usual for the expert to 'lead' the plaintiff when conducting the interview but it is sometimes necessary to ask specific questions because the plaintiff does not think to mention all relevant facts.

In addition to obtaining objective evidence of physical disability, the examination offers the expert an opportunity to assess the personality of the patient and form an opinion as to whether there is any degree of exaggeration of symptoms. A qualitative assessment may be particularly important where date of knowledge and limitation issues arise.

Investigations and X-rays may be relevant and an up-to-date X-ray should be obtained if necessary. Consideration should be given to other sophisticated investigations such as CT and MRI scans. The expert should insist on seeing X-rays and must not simply rely on a radiologist's report.

It is important to establish the nature of the disability and correlate it with the plaintiff's symptoms. Factual statements should be made as to the likely cause of the disability without apportioning blame, although an expert is unlikely to be asked to prepare a report for trial if it is his view that the injuries of which complaint is made were not caused by the negligence alleged. An opinion has now to be given on prognosis and it is likely that this will have to be stated in percentage terms. From a medical expert's point of view this is an inexact science and tends to amount to guesswork. Lawyers need this information when deliberating upon the quantum of damages and a best estimate should be made. The accuracy of the prognosis should be stated and it should be mentioned if it is considered that a further review at some future date will be necessary.

Where it becomes clear that the claim is going to be resisted and steps will have to be taken to bring the case to trial the solicitor will probably wish to instruct a barrister (otherwise referred to as counsel) to advise and draft the formal legal documents setting out precisely the nature of the claim the defendant will be asked to meet.

CONFERENCE WITH COUNSEL

The one thing that barristers have in common is that they are advocates. They usually specialize in particular areas of the law. This enables the country solicitor who may have a wide-ranging practice dealing with wills, matrimonial disputes, conveyancing and commercial contracts (in addition to some personal injury work) to instruct the very best barristers in different fields of expertise and thereby provide to his client as good a service as the client could hope to get from the large firms of solicitors.

Although many solicitors are very able advocates and a few now have full rights of audience to present cases before the highest courts, it is the usual practice for a barrister to be instructed if the case is significant or if it is likely to go to trial.

Depending upon the nature of the case a conference may be convened with counsel in his chambers. In John's case, counsel experienced in medical negligence work is likely to be instructed to advise at an early stage. Very large or complex claims may need a Queen's Counsel to lead the case.

Many claims for injuries are settled between the parties without any legal proceedings being commenced, but it is not unusual for a **writ** to be issued, particularly if the limitation period is approaching or it is clear that the defendant will not admit liability. Shortly after a writ is **issued** it has to be **served** upon the defendant. Two weeks thereafter the **Statement of Claim** has to be served on the defendant. The statement of claim is a very important document. It should disclose precisely what the claim is about, the particulars of negligence which will be proved, the full extent of the injuries suffered and the consequential financial loss. This document is frequently **settled** by counsel and his/her name appears on it.

SCHEDULE OF DAMAGES

There is now an obligation for a schedule of damages to be served with the Statement of Claim. This is usually prepared by the plaintiff's solicitor and is based upon information the solicitor obtains from his client, his client's employers and experts such as occupational therapists (OTs). John has such extensive disabilities that a full assessment of his needs would be made by an OT who is often best placed to determine which other types of specialist might be needed to give opinions – such as speech therapists, physiotherapists, nurses, housing/accommodation specialists, rehabilitation experts, etc. For every item of past and prospective expenditure claimed there has to be evidence. That evidence has to withstand cross-examination. Every opinion expressed must be justifiable and it is essential for experts to be able to relate closely the said need for facilities and equipment to the injury alleged.

TRIAL

Before trial the Court gives directions as to how the case should proceed and it is customary for there to be an exchange of the written statements of lay witnesses on both sides ahead of the mutual exchange of expert evidence on liability and causation. In the larger damages claims the expert evidence on quantum is often disclosed close to trial. Where there is a changing medical condition further medical reports may be exchanged at Court.

As the case moves closer to the time of trial the minds of the parties become better focused on the strengths of their respective cases in the light of the exchanged lay and expert evidence. Unhappily, plaintiffs sometimes see a trial as a means of calling a defendant to account as there is often no other means of achieving this objective. However, as civil claims for damages have as their objective compensation, not penalty, all that can be granted by the Court is an award of damages. Therefore, a cool and objective assessment of the prospects of success and the likely recoverable damages has to be made.

A defendant may have made a **payment into Court**. If the plaintiff does not accept this sum as sufficient compensation and goes on to trial he will be liable for both sides' costs incurred after the payment in if the trial judge does not award him a greater sum in damages.

Those who are of age and of sound mind may accept a sum in settlement of their claims without going to Court. That will be an end of the matter. However, the approval of the Court is required where an action is brought on behalf of a minor or a person suffering from mental disability. The involvement of the Court in the settlement offers protection to both the plaintiff and the defendant in that the plaintiff will not be permitted to settle for a sum materially less than the claim is worth and the defendant

does not have to run the risk of a further claim (arising from the same negligence) from that plaintiff.

STRUCTURED SETTLEMENT

Structured Settlements arise as a result of a facility set up in 1987 by the Inland Revenue and the Association of British Insurers (ABI), allowing damages to be paid wholly or in part by means of instalments for the life of the plaintiff. A Structured Settlement provides a means for a defendant to pay damages in the form of a series of future annual payments rather than in the traditional lump sum. Such payments are guaranteed for the lifetime of the plaintiff and there is complete flexibility at the outset as to the proportion of the total damages which are paid by means of these instalment payments. Usually a Structured Settlement programme provides for a plaintiff to receive part of the damages in a conventional lump sum and part by means of the future annual payments. Provided the form of the Settlement complies with the agreement made between the Inland Revenue and the ABI, future payments are non-taxable. It will be seen that this would enable someone like John to save tax and the costs which would otherwise occur in managing the investment of his damages. He would also have the option of receiving his damages in a manner which is linked to his life expectancy. Thereby he could have the certainty of an increasing income guaranteed for life.

Unfortunately such settlements can **only be implemented by consent** between the parties and this gives to the defendants and their insurers the possibility of settling a very large claim at a sum appreciably lower than might otherwise have been the case. A plaintiff's lawyers should always consider a Structured Settlement, particularly where the award is likely to be over £100 000, for the successful plaintiff cannot go into the market place with his damages award and acquire a return which is paid for life and is tax-free in any alternative investment medium.

There is neither the time nor the space in which to give an account of the process of trial. Suffice to say that it is an exacting process designed to elucidate the true facts on the balance of probabilities from witnesses who are called by the respective parties to give their evidence on oath. As now all evidence is exchanged before trial most of the witness evidence which is given orally is under cross-examination. No witness should treat this lightly. Expert and lay witnesses alike are well advised to prepare themselves properly.

One of the most remarkable features of the trial is the quality of the judgment which may be expected at its conclusion. The judge provides a detailed summary of the evidence called and gives full reasons for his conclusions. Inevitably the losing party will be disappointed but neither party should feel that the judgment was unjust or unreasonable. Occasionally an injustice is done but it is to be hoped that this would be rectified on appeal.

COSTS

Whilst the Court has an absolute discretion as to who should pay the costs of an action, the usual course is for the losing party to pay the successful party's costs. When the plaintiff who is legally aided loses, the defendant cannot recover costs against him, although if the plaintiff subsequently wins the National Lottery, or any other substantial winnings, the defendant may make an application to the Court for a costs order to be enforced. If the plaintiff wins, the defendant will be ordered to pay the plaintiff's costs but often the defendant is not ordered to meet all of the expenses incurred by a plaintiff in instructing a solicitor. This shortfall is not normally very significant and can be met out of the damages the plaintiff recovers.

CONCLUSION

The process of achieving compensation is frequently prolonged, difficult and, occasionally, fruitless. Unfortunately there is too often no better way of providing money for those injured through the fault of another. Whilst money can never be a sufficient compensation, it goes some way to make more bearable the suffering and frustration of incapacity.

FURTHER READING

Medical Evidence: Guide for Doctors and Lawyers, Law Society and BMA, London.
Munkman, J. (1996) *Damages for Personal Injury and Death*, 10th edn, Butterworths, London.

USEFUL ADDRESSES

Action for Victims of Medical Accidents (AVMA)
Bank Chambers, 1 London Road, Forest Hill, London SE23 3TP, UK. Tel: 0181 291 2793.

Association of Personal Injury Lawyers (APIL)
10A Byard Lane, Nottingham, NGI 2GJ, UK. Tel: 0113 958 0585.

The Law Society
21-27 Lambs Conduit Street, London WCIN 3NJ, UK. Tel: 0171 242 1222.

12 A patient's perspective

J. Gaylor

To make a success of being disabled one needs to be a polyglot creature with the patience of Job, the persistence of Bruce's spider, the stubbornness of an ox, the hide of a rhinoceros, the memory of an elephant and the ability of a squirrel to hoard things (earlier this year I had to send a government department a photostat of a letter sent to me in 1978).

Although this book is about physically disabled adults, I feel it would be relevant at this stage to give a brief resume of my disability, which began when I was a child. In 1956, while I was at boarding school, I broke my neck in a diving accident. Being fairly near, I was fortunate to be taken to Stoke Mandeville within 8 hours. I had fractured C4, 5 and 6, and dislocated C6 and 7 vertebrae. After some weeks, movement started to return and it was expected that I would regain full use of everything: however recovery suddenly stopped and I was left with some use in my right leg and both arms. My triceps were weak and, with the exception of my right thumb, I had no use in either hand.

I was at Stoke for a year and then returned to school. I had a manual wheelchair and could get myself about to a certain extent indoors, but needed to be pushed when outside and over long distances inside. I was blessed with good friends who took me to various lessons (the classroom corridor was an eighth of a mile (200 m) long) and back to the sanatorium at the end of the school day. The only real difference my disability made to my school life was that I slept in the sanatorium and not in a dormitory. I was able to get on and off a toilet with rails on the walls, with help to begin with, and later by myself. At first there were times when I was not able to get there quickly enough but in a few years this was overcome. For my bowel I took laxatives and bulking agents, and went normally.

In the 1950s and 1960s there was very little help from either the government or the local authority – on leaving hospital one had to cope as best as one could. I left school in 1959 and from then on we were on our own. I had a wonderful Mother (a widow) and a mentally handicapped brother who was able to push me about. At that time we lived in Wales, in a cottage. We had an additional stair rail fitted, and with rails each side and my mother hauling on my trousers I got upstairs each night; morning was easier – I came down on my seat.

The only flush toilet was in the back yard. We attempted to get a grant for an inside toilet. A charity became involved and would have helped with expenses not covered by a council grant. As soon as the council realized a charity was interested they refused to do anything. The charity felt that the local council should do their part and there things

Rehabilitation of the Physically Disabled Adult. Edited by C. John Goodwill, M. Anne Chamberlain and Chris Evans. Published in 1997 by Stanley Thornes (Publishers) Ltd, Cheltenham. ISBN 0-7487-3183-0.

stayed at stalemate for the next 3 years. The council said that if my mother could not cope they would put me in an old folk's home. I was 17!

In 1962 my grandmother who lived in Cornwall had a severe stroke. She was terrified of hospitals so after some months of complicated juggling between my mother and her sisters to ensure that my grandmother was not alone we sold our house and moved to Cornwall. We lived, at first, in my grandmother's cottage, and later in a purpose-built bungalow – purchased with the money from the sale of both my mother's and grandmother's homes. At no time did my mother have any help with a partly (at first totally) paralysed mother, a physically disabled daughter and a mentally handicapped son.

Immediately after leaving school I had no job. I took a proof-reading correspondence course with the London School of Journalism. A wheelchair-bound friend who was a proof-reader with May and Baker was instrumental in getting me a job as an outside sub-editor with Pergamon Press. This was fee paying but very intermittent. When we moved to Cornwall I had an excellent Disablement Resettlement Officer who found me a job with a firm of diary manufacturers who had just moved down from Surrey. He also contacted the charity who had been interested previously and they provided me with a hand-controlled car, which opened up a new world for the whole family. I started full-time work in 1965, and after a while I was supplied with an electric wheelchair for work by the DHSS. After 5 years I changed my job and went to a small firm of jobbing printers who, in another 5 years, were taken over by the company where I am still employed.

Although both my brother and I would have been eligible for attendance allowance from when it was first introduced, the literature that was sent out at that time gave the impression that we were ineligible, and it was not until 1986 that we applied for it and were awarded it at the lower of the two rates.

Until 1987 life went on with little help from any official source. As you can tell I had not had much contact with other disabled people – both at school and at work I was the only disabled person, and other than a rail in the toilet there were no special adaptions. I was the only driver in the family and we used the car a lot. We went first on camping (tent) holidays in Southern England, and then, as my mother got older, on self-catering holidays in the north – the furthest I drove in one day was over 600 miles.

My mother died suddenly in December 1987 and it was then that we started to need outside help. By this time I was much stronger physically. I could weight bear on my left leg as well as my right and my biceps were strong. Although my hands were still paralysed I had developed trick movements and was able to do many intricate things with no problems. I needed help with dressing and undressing, and I usually started at 6.00 a.m. to be at work at 8.00 a.m. It was impossible to get any help at 6.00 a.m. and eventually I got myself up at 5.45 a.m. and a home help came for an hour from 7.00 to 8.00 a.m. to help me dress and make breakfast. At 5 p.m. we had an hour's help to make a meal. In the evening, once I was in bed, I put electrodes on my legs for an hour of functional electronic stimulation (FES). Although the home helps put on electrodes for someone else, for me the home help organizer said it was nursing, and they could not supply anyone for this task, the district nurse said it wasn't nursing and they couldn't supply anyone either. Eventually I had a private agency (for which I had to pay) who supplied an auxiliary for an hour to help me undress and put on the electrodes. One advantage of the private agency was that the time could be changed – if I wanted someone half an hour or an hour later they would send someone at that time. With a home help this was not possible. At the weekends the home helps came in from 8.30 a.m. to 10.00 or 10.30 a.m. and prepared a lunch as well as helping with dressing and getting breakfast.

After some time I had a wheel-in shower built and got up at 5.00 a.m. to shower.

I started to get a lot of pain in my arm which I was told was referred pain from my neck. The pain was one of the main reasons that I opted for an omental transposition in April 1992. This was an experimental technique pioneered by the neurosurgical department in Southampton to increase the blood supply to the spinal cord at the level of the lesion. I went in for it with a realistic hope of less pain, a bit more or stronger movement in my arms and hands, and improved bladder and bowel function. Even if there was no improvement nothing should have got worse. Sadly things did not work out as planned. After the operation there were problems with spinal fluid leakage and I returned to Cornwall a month later than was planned, and a 1- or 2-week stay in a local hospital turned into a year.

Initially, although weak, most functions returned, but then they started to go again in spite of intensive physiotherapy. I was unable to stand which meant that I could not go to the toilet by myself, nor could I get in and out of bed: therefore I could not return home under the previous arrangements.

I suppose, stemming from my time in Stoke Mandeville in the 1950s, when one of the main aims was to get rid of a catheter, to me a conventional catheter was totally unacceptable, and it really was the end of the line. Yet there was no way I could have 24-hour care. At first I hoped to get a grant from the Independent Living Fund (ILF). To be eligible for this I had to have the highest rate of attendance allowance, which the social worker felt I should have had all along. I applied for the higher rate with a letter signed by a doctor, a social worker and myself – thus covering all reasons for which the application form might have been returned. Then the ILF was closed to new applicants overnight in November 1992, instead of running until April 1993 as should have been the case. As I had not had my higher rate of attendance

allowance through I was unable to apply to the ILF and had to apply to Care in the Community.

In March 1993 I went to the Spinal Unit at Odstock (Salisbury). This was a real eye-opener, both in certain aspects of care (How had I survived? I'd been doing it all wrong for over 30 years!) and in the back-up services after leaving hospital. While at Odstock I had a supra-pubic catheter fitted and entered the esoteric world of leg and night bags (though neither are used in the way intended). In my innocence I assumed that all tubes would be of the same material, diameter, length and flexibility (they aren't), and that all taps would operate in the same way (they don't).

I could work a swing-tap that opened at 90°, and the only one that could be found was on an In-Care leg bag; however, In-Care do not make a night bag and a leg bag does not provide enough tube for my purposes. After 2 years of experimenting I have found a night bag (Simpla Trident 1000-mm tube length) which has sufficient length of tube of a suitable diameter and flexibility to need only one night bag per catheter change (not two as previously). The tube is detached from the bag and cut through about eight inches (20 cm) from the nozzle, the short piece goes into the catheter at one end and on to the smooth end of the In-Care tap at the other. The remainder fixes to the ridged end of the tap – thus I open the tap away from my body and obviate the danger of pulling too hard on the catheter, which comes up my body and out at my waist band.

When I feel that my bladder needs emptying I put the tube over the toilet and open the tap. In this way I retain what bladder tone I have and a measure of independence, as I would be unable to empty a leg bag myself if I had one.

Catheters too have their differences, primarily in material, length and flexibility. I tried Silastic and Bard Teflon coated before finding Bard Silicone Elastomer coated. The difference in comfort when I was using the latter was amazing. It also lasted longer. Unlike most people I deliberately enlarged my catheter to a size 24 and used a male one; it didn't block very often and was longer than a female catheter. It was changed every 4 weeks, and during the last week there were clear indications that change time was coming, with various types of gunge coming down the tube. Of course, once I had found something that worked well Bard stopped making it. I tried a Bard Silicone coated catheter which had to be taken out after a week – by that time I had all the symptoms of cystitis together with pain in my bladder and I was having to rush to the toilet every half hour. On removal the catheter was very mucky. Next I tried a Silastic Silicone Elastomer coated catheter – this was shorter than the Bard, but more flexible than the one just removed. This had to come out after 2 weeks as it was blocking and it too was very mucky on removal. Then I tried a Bard PTFE coated one. Unfortunately this only went up to a size 22 off the shelf, but Bard would make larger sizes to order (minimum ten). This seemed better to start with, but by the time the fifth one was in I was having to have two washouts a week. That was the change where I had a 999 dash to the local casualty department as the catheter 'hole' started bleeding profusely. It seems as though my bladder grows a skin up to the catheter.

Detective work uncovered a new Bard catheter – hydrogel coated. The reference number given to me by Bard was, according to my doctor's surgery wholesaler, something entirely different. One person at Bard said that size 24 was available off the shelf, another said it wasn't. Eventually the Gordian knot was cut by the new practice manager who ordered them direct from Bard. So far they have been worth all the trouble.

Recently I was sent a sample of an excellent new leg bag which is made by the disabled for the disabled – the Big Bendi Bag which has a choice of three outlet taps (swing, slide and tube drain) – what a simple but revolutionary idea. I wonder why no one thought of it earlier. I have described my 'Heath Robinson' bladder arrangement in some detail as it might be the answer for someone else who, like me, wants to retain at least an illusion of normality and independence.

During my time at Odstock I could see I was deteriorating further. When I arrived there in early March I was able to move my right foot a little, by the time I was due to return to Cornwall I was unable to move it. This was a worrying time as no one knew why I was deteriorating or when or if it would stop. If it had carried on to my arms it would obviously have had far-reaching effects on my whole life. Half an hour before the ambulance came to take me back to Cornwall, Southampton rang for me to go back there as they had finally found the reason for my deterioration. They felt that as I moved my head the spinal cord was rubbing on the bone of the spine at the extremes of movement. They put me in a Philadelphia collar during the day and a soft collar at night.

This was at the end of April 1993 and I am still wearing them in May 1995. I had a period in April 1994 when I tried without the hard collar for an hour or so in the evening but by May there was a small deterioration and as of now I have to carry on with the collars until June 1995 after which I can start to try without them for a short while and see what happens – very much suck it and see.

I finally returned home in June 1993 after a case conference involving 16 people. To begin with I was using a mobile hoist while I waited for the ceiling track hoist to be fitted. I had two home helps in the morning, one for an hour at teatime, and a home help and a nurse in the evening. Later this became two home helps with the nurse calling in twice a week, and now it is just one home help with a nurse calling twice a week.

While I was in hospital I was using a Chiltern ceiling track hoist. It was very easy for someone to push me to the side of the track, so that instead of hanging directly under the track I was a foot or more to the side of it. When my ceiling track hoist was being measured up I couldn't understand why the engineer kept saying that I couldn't be pushed very far to the side. It wasn't until my hoist had been installed that I realized what the reason was. The Chiltern hoist had the webbing on which the patient is suspended set parallel to the track, while the Carter's hoist, which is the one I have, has the webbing set at right angles. So obviously I would have been better with a Chiltern hoist.

This is something of which OTs and patients should be aware, because in some situations the type of hoist used can make a big difference to the patient. If I had had a Chiltern hoist I could probably have had the tract running right to the shower rather than finishing in the middle of the room as it does now. **Indeed all those who are involved in supplying anything from a catheter to a hoist should look carefully at all the minor variations, as a very small difference can make a large difference to the user's life.** If someone seems to have a problem such as mine with a catheter it is worth experimenting with different makes. It was quite by chance that we stumbled on the fact that one suited me more than another.

Providentially, I work for a firm who kept my job open for me so that I was able to return to work after I came home from hospital. They even paid me my full wage for 5 months, and they have let me alter my hours to some extent so that am still able to work my full 35 hours a week although I can no longer start at 8.00 a.m.

I now cannot drive my car (a Vauxhall Cavalier Estate with automatic transmission, power steering and various adaptions). I used to use my right foot to work the accelerator, which I can no longer do, nor can I transfer and I certainly cannot walk down the side of the garage to get to the driver's door. So I have been using a London taxi (thankfully there is one at St Ives) to get to and fro. The cost is £31 a day, £155 a week. I have to pay

this myself and then claim some of it back from the Fares to Work Scheme. They pay £95+ and I am left with about £60 to pay myself, so at the moment I am no better off financially than if I stayed at home on Invalidity Benefit. (But see later.)

Driving is very important – particularly to be able to drive oneself, as when driving one is on equal footing with able-bodied drivers; and it gives the opportunity of getting out and going wherever the fancy takes one (within reason). I have had a MAVIS assessment and drove a Eurocruiser with very fancy adaptions. I have applied to Motability for a grant for an adapted Fort Transit – the figure mentioned at the assessment was £30 000. There is a year's waiting list for grants so it looks like being a long time before there is even a chance of a vehicle. Motability have sent a list of possible charitable sources of funding and suggest that I try to obtain as much as I can in other ways, as the more I can raise independently of Motability the more likely I am to get a grant. At present I am waiting to hear from three organizations to which I have applied.

Apart from going to work I have been out of the house eight times in the 19 months I have been home from hospital. Taxi fares are too expensive to use them often and I can't get out of my chair to ride in an ordinary car. So that is one way in which my greater disability affects my life. However, I am not short of things to do, so that I can't say that I am bored. I have less time in which to do things than previously, and everything takes me longer. Indeed, it is only now that I realize just how much I was able to do before my operation. 'Before my operation' is becoming a real cut off point – rather like 'Before the flood' must have been to Noah and his family!

One of the reasons I take longer is that I drop things more easily. For months I thought I was losing strength in my hands – although a physiotherapy assessment showed otherwise – as I couldn't pick things up, and if I did they slipped out of my fingers. Eventually I realized what was happening – some of the drugs I am taking have a dry mouth listed as a side-effect. What they don't say is that it is not just saliva that dries up – mucous does, so that it is difficult to blow one's nose, and skin becomes very dry so that there is no natural moisture on the skin of the fingers and thumbs to give a purchase, hence everything slips out of my grip. A lick on finger and thumb (provided there is any moisture in my mouth) works wonders! I have also bought a pot of Tipp-Ex Fingertip, a moistener intended for office use when filing, but I have found that rubbing it over my hands enables me to hold my camera – something I have not been able to do since my operation. I also use a latex finger cot, or actually two – one on my thumb and one on my first finger. As I keep my nails long (another aid to picking up small objects) the finger cots tend not to last very long. If my hands were not paralysed surgeon's gloves would be a better solution.

One thing I find hard is that life has to be lived to a rigid timetable. At 8.20 p.m. I have to get ready for bed even if another 5 minutes would enable me to finish what I am doing. No spur-of-the-moment actions or excursions are possible. Things that can be done in bed often are, as there is no time during the hours I am up. When I have had to bring work home I have always done it in bed. The disadvantage of this is that I don't realize the time and very often it is 3 a.m. or more before I get to sleep. It's a good job the home helps wake me up!

Another thing I have found hard is the fact that I have done no standing since I came home. I was supplied with a standing frame but there was no way that the home care service could supply two people to help me up in it. So after some months it was taken away. With no means of being on my feet there is no way to strengthen the little movement that I have regained and I am afraid that it will vanish for lack of use.

The Aids to Work Scheme from the Department of Employment supplied me with a Mangar Freestyle chair – this has proved invaluable. Pre-op if couldn't reach anything I stood up, now I can't and the Mangar makes all the difference. A disadvantage is that I can't get close to anything head-on because of the foot tray, but I can get close side-on. At its highest the Mangar seat is about 3 feet (90 cm) from the ground and, of the lifting chairs that I have seen, is the highest rising, even so I could do with about 2 feet (60 cm) more when it is up, and about a foot lower when it is down.

Now that Access to Work is compulsory my taxi fares have been transferred from Fares to Work to Access to Work which is paying £135, thus leaving me with another £40 a week. This has been worked out over the 5 year period at around £35 000, well above the £21 000 ceiling, so obviously all the publicity before the introduction of Access to Work in 1994 had some effect. There has since been a directive that the £21 000 is to be adhered to strictly. Earlier this year I was sent a form to fill out stating what I required from Access to Work. I said taxi fares and an up-and-down wheelchair with maintenance. The notification I later received listed only the fares. On enquiry I found out that as my Mangar chair was supplied by Aids to Work any repairs still came from that, and not from Access to Work and so do not count against my 5 year total. Should the chair need to be replaced then that would have to come under Access to Work, which would of course cause problems with the 5 year total. Can you imagine the bureaucratic complications?

Since returning home I have noticed the stupidity of bureaucracy. Whether this is a new thing or whether I have just not encountered it before I don't know. Take the great 'Cream Controversy'. Out of the blue came an order – no home help may apply cream full stop, not even hand cream or baby oil. So the nurses had to come in each evening to apply hand cream, baby oil, Sudocrem, etc.;

things which anyone applies to a baby without a second thought. Obviously no one was happy, nurses, home helps or patients (who in some cases were being dressed by the home helps only to be undressed by the nurses half an hour later so that cream could be applied), all were upset. After a couple of months another directive was given – home helps could apply any cream/lotion that could be purchased over the counter to healthy skin – for healthy read unbroken. Surely it would not have been beyond the bounds of possibility for that to have been the original directive, saving a lot of aggravation for everyone concerned.

Obviously this is all very subjective. I am sure that my strong Christian faith has helped me to cope. With Paul I can say (most of the time) '. . . for I have learned in whatever state I am to be content'. I am not claiming in any way to be equal with Paul, nor am I saying that I never wish that things were different, but I do have an underlying peace and assurance that God is in control. He knows what I am going through and He will give me the strength to cope with each situation as it arises.

So, in conclusion, what have I learnt in over 40 years of disability?

When I was first disabled someone jokingly said to me that the first 10 years are the worst. I would amend that to the first 20 – it took me all that time to stop being self-conscious about being in a wheelchair, to stop thinking that everyone was looking at me. As a child I suffered from some of the 'Does he take sugar?' attitude. People would ask my mother, over my head, 'How is she today?' I can remember someone (unknown to us) presenting me with a bar of chocolate and another time a perfect stranger said to my mother (again over my head) 'What a pity, and so pretty, the poor dear' (the latter was definitely an exaggeration). Now I do not feel that everyone is looking at me nor do people

talk over my head. Whether this is the result of a more enlightened society or of my own attitude and outward self-confidence I do not know, but I do know that if you think of yourself as a second-class citizen you can hardly be surprised if other people do so too. I no longer feel that I have to keep proving myself.

Another thing that has changed over the years is my attitude to help. When newly disabled, I was very sensitive over assistance from other people – getting upset when anyone tried to do anything to help that I could do for myself, and I would rather have died than ask for help. As my attitude to my disability became more mature I realized that some people need to help, it makes them feel good, it doesn't hurt me – indeed it leaves me with more energy for something else more pleasurable – and it means that the helper will not be prevented from offering help to some other disabled person in the future. A brusque reaction to an offer of help may well deter that person from offering assistance to anyone else. Since my disability has worsened I have had to ask people for help and it hasn't killed me yet! Nor do I feel that it has lessened me in some way.

Having said that, no one newly disabled should accept the fact that because something has never been done it can't be done. There have been times when I have done things that were supposed not to be possible. That doesn't mean that one will be able to do anything one wants to do but there is no harm in trying; if it does prove impossible then accept it and go on to something else. Don't spoil one's own or others' lives by fretting about something that can't be changed. Even able-bodied people can't do everything they would like to do. When one is disabled everything takes longer and requires more effort – something both the disabled person and the carer/officialdom need to remember.

Any equipment that acquires a tag 'for the disabled' immediately doubles in price. I was once told by an occupational therapist that she could not order certain equipment locally, but only from a particular catalogue. She therefore had to order a shower chair (ordinary plastic type chair – not wheeled) from the catalogue when the local garden centre had a special offer on, and for the same money she could have had four similar chairs with a table thrown in. In these days of financial stringency surely it would be better for an OT to be able to purchase anything locally if it were available?

It is amazing how reliant one becomes on certain equipment, yet when it needs to be repaired often one has to wait weeks or even months for it, and life can become very difficult in consequence – even if a loan item is supplied it is not necessarily the same as that awaiting repair. Recently my chair went in to have the batteries and a switch sorted out. The switch had lost its return spring, but the chair was usable. The batteries were dealt with and the switch ordered. Although I could have used the chair then and there and it was possible to change the switch while I was in the chair, I couldn't have it back as the repairers no longer sent engineers out, only van drivers who collected and returned equipment, but couldn't repair it. I was therefore without my chair for several weeks while they waited for the switch to arrive. When I finally had the chair back it was the wrong switch, it should have been spring-loaded and wasn't – hence I have collected several spectacular bruises, and I am still waiting for the proper switch to be fitted. So often one has to fight with officialdom, and an agency which has been set up to help the disabled seems to be trying to avoid doing so by any means possible.

Last year I took out a household emergency insurance policy. I didn't use it for that year, but this year I have called them out three times in less than 2 months. So I would recommend anyone unable to do repairs for themselves to take out a policy, much as one joins the AA. Indeed the scheme is an offshoot of National Breakdown.

How can 'officialdom' help apart from finance and manpower?

Realize that different people have different perceptions of what is acceptable, a different 'bottom line' when quality of life has gone below what one feels able to accept. Often there will be a way around it, an alternative method or direction – as with my catheter. Try to give a disabled person a feeling of self-worth – if he/she can accept him or herself as still a worthwhile person in his/her own right then he or she will find it easier to accept his/her disability and feel able still to have an enjoyable life. Be sensitive to the small nuances which will probably tell you more how someone is feeling than conversation does. If a disabled person rejects your offer of help and seems offended, don't take that as a personal affront – it is themselves they are basically angry with, not you. Although it is financially better for the country if family and friends do a lot of the caring, it is harder to accept someone close to oneself performing intimate help than a stranger doing the same thing, particularly at the onset of disability.

I would like to make a plea to planners of new buildings, don't make ramps too steep, coming down can be worse than going up; make lifts large enough to take wheelchairs, remember some can be quite large, and don't combine a nappy-changing room with a toilet for the disabled for the sake of both sets of users.

Official forms have improved lately in many ways, but there is still room for further improvement. Often written initial information is not clear – sometimes one thinks one would not be eligible for a grant and one is, and vice versa. Some forms go into such fine detail that one is put off at first sight of the 'magazine' that one is required to fill out and there are still ambiguities – one sometimes wonders if they are there on purpose!

I approached this article with considerable trepidation – I am no specialist, as are the rest of the contributors, and can only speak of my own experiences of what are virtually two periods of coming to terms with disability. Although I seem to be the exception to the rule in just about everything, I hope that something relevant to others will have been found in the chapter.

PART TWO
MUSCULOSKELETAL DISABILITY

13 Osteoarthritis

M.A. Chamberlain

INTRODUCTION

Degenerative joint disease (DJD) is common. Defined radiologically it is present in a large proportion of the population in an industrialized country. Its incidence is as yet unclear, possibly 200/100 000 person years for osteoarthritis of the hip and knee in a recent US study. The prevalence of radiographic changes is easier to obtain: in the UK it is 3.8% at the knee and 1.3% at the hip, giving an overall prevalence of 23%. There is a considerable discordance between symptomatology and radiology, with probably only some 50% of those with radiological signs being symptomatic.

Osteoarthritis is the most common joint disease in the world and its impact is huge, with 80 million cases in Europe, America and Japan.

In a recent UK population survey by the OPCS (Martin et al., 1988), 20% of those aged 60–74 years and 50% of those over the age of 75 years had a locomotor disability, with the majority of these being self-reported as due to arthritis (80% of those over 70 years have some arthritis.) Some 225 000 are said to be housebound; 14 million days are lost from work annually and costs (to patient, carer and state) are in the region of a billion pounds. All societies are ageing and in many there is inequitable access to health services, usually with older persons having less access. In addition, evidence is accumulating that non-steroidal anti-inflammatory drugs, which are frequently the only medical response to osteoarthritis, are less effective than other modalities in reducing disability, whilst carrying significant risks and costs. Finally, given the large numbers of sufferers, one-to-one treatment by a therapist may well not be available. Yet, undoubtedly, the paramount task of the clinician is to decrease pain and disability and improve function.

PATHOLOGY

What is osteoarthritis? The popular concept of the disease is of 'wear and tear' with an inevitable decline into pain and dependency. But Radin (1987) stated:

'Osteoarthritis is not a condition of relentless progression. It is not a disease but rather an imbalance between the mechanical stresses on the joint and the ability of the tissues of the joint to withstand those stresses. Effective treatment is generally mechanical. In many cases the progression of the condition can be halted with appropriate intervention.'

Others consider that there are many other factors, some genetic, some biochemical (George and Dieppe, 1993). Radin's definition encourages a dynamic approach.

Rehabilitation of the Physically Disabled Adult. Edited by C. John Goodwill, M. Anne Chamberlain and Chris Evans. Published in 1997 by Stanley Thornes (Publishers) Ltd, Cheltenham. ISBN 0-7487-3183-0.

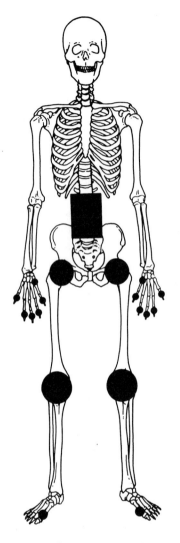

Figure 13.1 Joints affected in osteoarthritis.

results in proteoglycan loss, collagen damage, cartilage thinning and loss.

Cartilage is not the only factor in the pathogenesis of osteoarthritis. Undoubtedly, joint lubrication is of importance, as are the nature, frequency and site of joint loads and stresses.

Many situations predispose to osteoarthritis (Table 13.1). These include developmental abnormalities, for example slipped femoral epiphyses, where joint surfaces are not congruous, infections and other inflammatory processes and trauma where the joint is damaged, and inherited metabolic disorders and genetic factors leading to collagen abnormalities.

Risk factors are being identified. Obesity seems to be one for osteoarthritis of the knee or hand (but not hip), as are smoking and joint laxity; certain occupations and hobbies associated with excessive knee-bending activities are others.

The sites for osteoarthritis are shown in Figure 13.1. The radiological features are diagnostic (Table 13.2).

Patterns of disease can be identified. In particular, whilst hip and knee arthritis are both common, primary disease in the knee is often associated with osteoarthritis in the

It is perhaps best to see osteoarthritis as the final common pathway of at least several processes. This process consists of (often local) loss of articular cartilage with variable degrees of subchondral bone reaction and osteophyte formation at the joint margin. Cartilage provides a smooth surface, joint congruity and even load distribution. In the early stages of the disease its matrix is weakened, its surface damaged, and chondrocytes are activated. Later, failed repair

Table 13.1 Some causes of osteoarthritis

Primary	
Secondary	
e.g. traumatic	Mechanical damage
	Chronic (occupational injury)
	Previous joint surgery
	(meniscectomy)
e.g. anatomical	Hypermobility syndromes
	Epiphyseal dysplasias
	Congenital dislocation of hip,
	Perthes, etc.
e.g. inflammation	Inflammatory arthritis
e.g. infective	Infective arthritis
e.g. metabolic	Ochronosis, haemochromatosis,
	acromegaly, calcium crystal
	deposition

Note: there may be **normal** loading of **abnormal** tissue or **abnormal** loading of **normal** tissue.

Table 13.2 Radiological diagnosis of osteoarthritis

1. Loss of cartilage (frequently focal)
   ≡ **joint space narrowing**
2. Hypertrophic changes in subchondral bone and at periphery of joints
   ≡ **subchondral sclerosis** and **cysts**
   ≡ **marginal osteophytosis**

hand but not the hip. Osteoarthritis of the shoulders is rare unless they have been traumatized, have lost innervation or have been used for years as major weightbearing joints. Osteoarthritis is said to be less common in joints under-used because of limb paralysis.

THE NATURAL HISTORY OF OSTEOARTHRITIS

This is still unclear, but it must not be assumed that disability is inevitable or progressive.

FACTORS ASSOCIATED WITH DISABILITY

McAlindon *et al.* (1993) showed that quadriceps strength, knee pain and age are determinants of disability, although radiographic severity is not. This recognition focuses management.

CLINICAL FEATURES OF PERIPHERAL JOINT OSTEOARTHRITIS (Table 13.3)

The main complaints of patients are:

1. pain

Table 13.3 Clinical features of osteoarthritis

Symptoms	Signs
Gelling on inactivity	Local tenderness
Absent/mild early morning stiffness	Little or no synovial swelling
Pain on use/weightbearing	Soft tissue swelling
Loss of function	Bony swelling
Tenderness	Joint crepitus
Swelling	Loss of joint range
Instability	Instability
	Muscle weakness and wasting

2. loss of range of movement; instability
3. stiffness
4. loss of function; disability.

Pain

This arises from a variety of causes and structures within and around the joint. It usually lasts for many hours and is aching in character, relieved by rest and exacerbated by usage of the joint (such as by weightbearing). In the later stages, or when the joint is also inflamed or traumatized, pain may prevent the patient from sleeping. Its severity may be an indication for operation.

Stiffness

Gelling is characteristic of osteoarthritis: after a period of inactivity the joint is resistant to active movement. After a few minutes of movement the discomfort vanishes.

Loss of range and power

The muscles across the joint are weakened quickly when joint pain and swelling occur. They then atrophy and are less able to protect the joint when the patient is active so that the joint is more easily traumatized and liable to subsequent 'flare-ups' in which there may be an inflammatory element. The joint capsule may shorten and thicken.

Loss of range of movement arises early from muscle spasm in response to pain, later from loss of muscle power as well as thickening and shortening of joint capsule. Diminution in the range of movement is not always of functional importance (e.g. loss of a few degrees of elbow extension is usually of no consequence). The range required for common tasks related to the involved joint needs to be defined so that the aims of therapy are clear (e.g. all patients need 90° flexion of at least one knee to mount stairs, but only a few, perhaps those working in restricted areas, need full flexion). Joints may become unstable (particularly at the knee) leading to further trauma (Table 13.4).

Table 13.4 'Minimal' range of motion needed for functional activity

Joint	Motion	Degrees
Shoulder	Flexion	0–75
	Abduction	0–75
	Rotation	40
Elbow	Flexion	120
Hip	Flexion	0–30
	External rotation	0–25
Knee	Flexion	0–70
Ankle	Dorsiflexion	5
	Plantarflexion	15

Losses of function; disability

These arise from the above impairments. They relate to pain, diminishing range of movement and muscle weakness, so that common tasks can only be accomplished with difficulty or not at all.

Specific functional disabilities will be detailed under discussions of the specific joints involved. Impairments and disabilities can be quantified using standardized questionnaires and activities of daily living charts. For pain in the lower limbs the LeQuesne index is widely accepted; indeed, a LeQuesne index of 10–12 (out of 24, higher scores indicating greater disability) is generally felt to be indicative of the need for surgical intervention. For function, the Hospital Assessment Questionnaire (HAQ) has superseded the Steinbocker grading of disability. Function can be reliably assessed using the HAQ or the LeQuesne index of mobility; the latter being specific for weight-bearing joints whereas the former is composite. The SF36 for osteoarthritis derived from the AIMS by Meehan is validated and may be an acceptable alternative. The modified AIMS score (used as the basis of the specific osteoarthritis SF36 form) has its adherents.

Muscle power can be graded by clinicians using MRC grading. Dynamometers are rarely available but are a useful feedback to patients to encourage continued exercise. For clinical purposes range of movement is sufficiently accurately recorded with a clinical goniometer with long arms or a spirit goniometer. It is probably unnecessary to grade stiffness.

The handicaps in the six ICIDH dimensions, which relate to the person's role in society, are also worth considering. For most osteoarthritis of the lower limbs the lack of mobility which ensues will be reflected not only in the mobility dimension, but also in terms of significantly increased physical dependency, and there will be threats to occupation, social integration and economic self-sufficiency which are largely reversed by improvements in mobility.

For hand and wrist osteoarthritis handicap in all these dimensions is absent although, occasionally, economic self-sufficiency is reduced when the person depends on good hand function for his livelihood, as a musician does. For those who depend on their upper limbs for mobility, who use crutches or a wheelchair, degenerative joint disease of the shoulders is more likely to occur and will have a significant impact on mobility.

SYSTEMIC EFFECTS

Osteoarthritis has **no** systemic effects, so that the patient feels well, albeit in pain. Laboratory investigations, such as the erythrocyte sedimentation rate (ESR), C-reactive protein (CRP) and full blood count, are normal and tests for rheumatoid factor are negative.

MANAGEMENT – GENERAL

The aims of management are: (a) reduction of **impairments**, here mainly pain, stiffness, limitation of movement, reduced muscle power and mobility, (b) reduction of **disabilities** ensuing and (c) minimization of **handicap**. Engendering a positive attitude in the patient is of the greatest importance and will also help provide motivation for the prevention of further disability (e.g. by reduction in weight). Attention has to be paid to the diminution of risk factors and the secondary prevention of deformity, instability and fixed flexion, and also to physical and psychological environmental factors which can reduce the impact of the condition upon the patient's lifestyle. The areas in which the patient wishes to act (as a single individual, whether working or not, as a family member with responsibilities, as a member of local, national, even international communities) need to be addressed.

It is worth bearing in mind the Eular Measures of Efficacy for assessing drugs in osteoarthritis when evaluating the patient's status, even though these may be imperfect (Table 13.5).

Pain control

Analgesia

Where pain is **minor** patients should be encouraged to use little analgesia. They may be able to cope well if the nature and usually good prognosis of their condition are explained to them and their fears dealt with. Such analgesia as is required should be simple, with few side-effects, dispensed in containers easy for arthritic hands to open.

With **severe** intractable pain that disturbs sleep or stops weightbearing, analgesics may

Table 13.5 Eular Measures of Efficacy for Assessing Drugs in Osteoarthritis

1. Index of severity of hip and knee disease (Lequesne)
2. Investigator's overall opinion
3. Pain on VAS
4. Patient's global assessment
5. Walking time (or stair climbing time)

Eular = European League Against Rheumatism

be supplemented by tricyclic antidepressants at night, but surgery may be required. Non-steroidal anti-inflammatory drugs (NSAIDs) are often prescribed for patients with osteoarthritis, although they have not been specifically designed for this usage. Indeed, George and Dieppe (1993) ask 'is there any rationale, either clinical or experimental, for the use of (NSAIDs), and what are the potential risks and benefits of these agents in osteoarthritis?'. They answer their question, 'the answer are not yet available, but they indicate that there are both general risks and possible destruction of cartilage when these drugs are used'.

Local intra-articular steroids

These often give good relief of localized joint pain sufficient to allow the physiotherapist to begin building up muscle power across the joint. The frequency of joint injection is the subject of much argument, as is the type of corticosteroid used. In the elderly, immediate relief of pain and preservation of function will be more important than any possible delayed joint destruction arising from steroid use.

Newer drug treatment

Intra-articular polysulphated glycosaminoglycans and other substances are being tried, but none is of proven value as a chondroprotective agent as yet.

Other factors

The patient who is active, interested and engaged in life and physical activities is less vulnerable to pain and depression than the housebound, apathetic subject. Education, counselling and the teaching of pain-coping strategies are frequently ignored or not available to these patients who would benefit greatly. Their families are often not involved and may have strong negative impressions of the disease, seeing crippledom as inevitable. Often the effects of regular exercise, physical fitness and improvement in muscle power across the involved joints are not recognized and not exploited for the patient's benefit.

Restoration of function

Rehabilitation in osteoarthritis is less complex than in many neurological diseases where cognitive and other functions are impaired. It is often an easier task than in inflammatory disease as relatively few joints are involved, and the course of the disease is more predictable. Nevertheless, some patients learn only with difficulty, or are unwell with a variety of other diseases. In addition, loss of activity is usually insidious, so that numerous small restrictions of activity have been accepted.

Physiotherapy

The general aims and methods used in physiotherapy are detailed in Chapter 40. The general aims of physiotherapy in osteoarthritis are to relieve pain, mobilize stiff joints, prevent and diminish contracture, encourage correct function (e.g. gait), strengthen weak muscles related to the arthritic joint and to restore and maintain function. Therapeutic exercise is important in patients with osteoarthritis (Semple, Loeser and Wise, 1990). However, for some patients the time and energy required to attend a hospital outpatient department for repeated, regular treatments may be disproportionate to the benefit gained. The patient may be better helped by being taught exercises which can then be done at home. It is difficult for an unsupervised patient to remain enthusiastic about time-consuming, often boring exercises. Patients frequently default unless a scheme of regular recording with regular supervision is devised (Chamberlain Care and Harfield, 1982). The subject is fully reviewed by Marks (1993).

Local physical methods of treatment

Local methods (heat, cold, short-wave diathermy, transcutaneous nerve stimulation and newer modalities) relieve pain and discomfort temporarily, and allow the patient to undergo active exercise, but do not alter the course of the disease. The choice of physical modality is a matter of therapist's or patient's preference. The patient should be encouraged to improvise as necessary at home. However, they should be advised that regular exercise in osteoarthritis has been shown to decrease pain, will stabilize the joint in its functional range, may protect somewhat against repeated trauma, and will help in retaining or improving function.

Exercise

Exercises may be assisted, against gravity or resisted. Two principal groups can be distinguished: those to improve maximal strength and those to increase endurance (lower weights, more repetitions). In osteoarthritis the latter is more often required, together with exercise to increase range of movement.

Recreational exercise

Sport is useful, being a natural progression from individual exercises, and more enjoyable. There is evidence (Ekblom *et al.* 1975) that even those with inflammatory arthritis benefit from a greater level of physical fitness. It may also have a protective value, preserving the integrity of cartilage. Inappropriate sport, such as fell-walking or mountaineering, may have to be given up. Low-impact activities, such as swimming and cycling, which are non-weightbearing, are substituted. Exercise may have to be alternated with rest, or at least reduction of load on the involved joints.

Walking aids

These take a significant proportion of the load off a diseased weight-bearing joint. The load is greatest when rising from a sitting position and may be reduced by the use of high seats with arms. Walking aids are discussed elsewhere (Chapter 48).

Mobility can be preserved by using the wheelchair (for shorter excursions perhaps), by using powered outdoor chairs, mainly in suburban areas, when visiting friends and shops, and by using private instead of the less accessible public transportation systems. Transport interchanges may be difficult. Special help or transportation for disabled people may be needed and may be locally available.

Occupational therapy

Problems should be tackled according to the joints involved and the perceived priorities of the patient. The occupational therapist (OT) looks at the need for environmental modifications, such as stair rails, toilet and bathroom adaptations and kitchen alterations, if required. It is often Social Services OTs who help in obtaining ramps, equipment and wheelchairs. The therapist will consider the interaction between the patient's osteoarthritis, work and method of transport. She will frequently help in instructing the patient and family on lifestyle changes.

Patient and family education or information

This is not simple: the patient cannot be assumed to be a blank sheet awaiting information: rather, what the doctor says is filtered through the patient's belief-set and weighed against advice from other sources. Further, the giving and acceptance of information does not necessarily produce a change in behaviour. Many patients will have been subjected to outdated advice from friends and acquaintances, and even their doctors have been known to tell them 'You'll just have to live with arthritis'. This is only partly true: there is no **cure**, but there are numerous things which

can be done to make life pleasurable, and reduce the adverse effects of osteoarthritis. The enthusiastic and educated cooperation of the patient is required. One should dispel his/her fears that he/she will be helpless and, in particular, that he/she will inevitably require a wheelchair. The natural history of the condition is explained: patients with osteoarthritis have a normal lifespan and remain otherwise well. It can be explained that certain drugs, physical measures and even changes in lifestyle may be used to relieve pain and reduce stresses to affected joints. Patients also wish to know about the effect of diet, the use of exercise and rest, the impact of osteoarthritis on work and leisure, and how they are to look after joints.

The patient will probably not remember much of what is said in the anxious situation of a clinic. It is a good policy to provide the patient with a booklet on osteoarthritis (e.g. from the Arthritis and Rheumatism Council (ARC). Booklets on specific problem areas, such as the neck or lumbar spine, and the effect of arthritis on marriage, for example due to hip involvement, are also available from the ARC and are discussed in detail in the appendix to Chapter 14. It is useful for other members of the family to read these and be a party to decisions on any necessary changes in lifestyle. With good management, most patients can remain relatively independent for a long time.

Patient self-help groups are helpful and effective (Lorig, 1995). The Arthritis Foundation in the USA organizes self-management courses which patients can set up. The Primary Care Rheumatology Group in the UK produces guidelines as to when, and how, OA should be managed in general practice and when referral should be made to a hospital.

Lifestyle changes

The patient is not ill, but may be older, perhaps with concomitant disease, and may find pain and functional difficulty decrease available energy. A reasonable accommodation with disease, disability and demands arising from the environment, family and job has to be made. To maximize ability and enjoyment of life it may be necessary for the therapist, doctor, patient and family to consider items in Table 13.6, discussing which roles the patient sees as important. Then there follows a discussion of how these are to be prioritized and dealt with. For instance, a chart could be made listing objectives, ways of achieving these and target dates, perhaps leaving a copy of the charts with the patient for negotiation with the family.

Surgery in osteoarthritis

If pain remains uncontrolled and disability increases despite conservative treatment, surgery may be necessary. It should also be considered for those whose condition is less severe, but whose livelihood is threatened, or who have a dependent family or perhaps a handicapped spouse. Those who do not understand the purpose of surgery, who wish to remain dependent, or who are not prepared to work to achieve good results are less good candidates either for surgery or for other rehabilitation techniques.

Results tend to be better than in inflammatory arthritis: the hips and knees affected by osteoarthritis respond better to prosthetic surgery than those involved in rheumatoid

Table 13.6 Lifestyle decisions

Consider:
1 What is your central role?
2 What are your priorities?
3 What can you ignore, delegate, do in an easier way?
4 What must be done urgently (e.g. today) and what can be done this week, this month or this year?

arthritis, and 'bone quality' and the integrity of surrounding structures are more likely to be preserved.

MANAGEMENT – SPECIFIC OSTEOARTHRITIS

This section deals only briefly with specific disabilities, with the aim of providing the reader with a model for considering arthritis of various lower limb joints. Preservation of function in upper limb joints is dealt with in the subsequent chapter on inflammatory arthritis.

Osteoarthritis of the hip

The patient with osteoarthritis of the hip may have had an antecedent abnormality such as congenital dislocation of the hip, Perthés disease, a slipped epiphysis or perhaps inflammatory arthritis. The nature of the primary lesion may influence the siting of radiological changes.

The main complaint will be **pain** usually, at first localized to the groin or radiating to the knee, but later perhaps accompanied by backache due to fixed flexion with increased lumbar lordosis. Pain may be associated with limp and shortening of the affected leg, and is worse on weightbearing. Sleep is disturbed, energy and mobility diminished.

The patient will experience many restrictions, associated with loss of joint range and weak musculature, and usually with the fixed flexed and adducted hip; difficulty on mounting stairs, and rising from the seated position (as from an easy chair or lavatory). Kerbs and high bus steps and getting into the bath are difficult; putting on shoes, socks and tights, and cutting the toenails present problems.

Examination reveals hip deformity with the hip usually in the adducted, externally rotated and flexed position; gait is antalgic. The range of movement is limited to a variable degree and shortening is present. The intermalleolar separation is reduced: when 20 cm or less there is inability to mount high steps and kerbs and, in females, pain and difficulty with intercourse. Progressive restriction of inter-malleolar separation is an indication of the need for surgery. **Weakness** of the muscles surrounding the hip may be marked, with gluteus medius being commonly affected.

Management

The patient's **pain** is brought under control as discussed previously. Rest is interspersed with activity and there should be daily periods of prone lying to counteract the tendency towards flexion deformity.

Exercise aims to increase the power of gluteus medius, and to improve abduction and extension. Muscles are frequently so weak that exercises are done initially in sling suspension; hydrotherapy is invaluable though frequently unavailable; home exercises on a regular daily basis are necessary to maintain function. Where conservative measures cannot halt deterioration in function or pain relief, surgery has to be considered. Where surgery is imminent it is worthwhile recalling the patient for exercises preoperatively so that these can be done more effectively postoperatively.

The use of a **walking stick** is encouraged as the stick transmits half the body weight and relieves the joint load. Obese patients should be encouraged to reduce weight – often a difficult task since with decreasing mobility calorie requirements may be reduced.

Shoes: A heel raise and, later, whole shoe raise to (almost) compensate for a short leg is required on the affected side to keep the pelvis level and reduce the incidence of subsequent back pain. Shock absorption in the heel may reduce pain, particularly on walking over uneven surfaces.

Preservation of mobility Chair seats need to be high, with firm arms to assist in rising and decrease the load on the joint. Lavatory seats should be raised. Fifteen per cent of all wheelchairs are prescribed for those with osteoarthritis. A folding wheelchair, used in conjunction with a car, is helpful to many. Some require a wheelchair outside the house or even in it, but before this stage is reached, urgent consideration should be given to joint replacement. It is much easier to mobilize postoperatively a patient who has been active on a frame or crutch than one who has been in a wheelchair for a long period.

A car is the single most useful aid to the patient with mobility problems, enabling participation in a wide variety of normal social activities. Automatic transmission on the car may be helpful (Chapter 50).

Pedestrian mobility is improved by good repair and planning of paths and roadways: arthritics find it hard to negotiate slippery, unswept flagstones, uneven surfaces, wide roads with fast traffic, undropped kerbs and numerous steps. They are greatly helped by sensitive town planning which locates shopping and community facilities within range.

Preservation of normal activities Many patients cannot perform tasks in the kitchen if required to stand for a long time, but can work well when sitting at a table or on a high stool working at higher surfaces. Those who need to use a walking appliance will find difficulty in carrying (say) a cup of tea and will appreciate a trolley. Numerous aids to help pick up objects from the floor, put on tights, etc. are available and a visit to a Disabled Living Centre is recommended. (Chapter 55).

Shopping and householding will need to be modified in the light of the disability; energy can be conserved by the use of easy-care fabrics, by washing machines and tumble-driers, food can be bought in bulk, carried by a helper and stored in the fridge, freezer and cupboards. All these adaptations are helpful, but many are too expensive for arthritis subjects whose earning ability is compromised (Chapter 41).

Environmental modifications such as access rails and the installation of a shower, a downstairs toilet or stairlift are helpful in preserving the patient's independence. A bath board, seat and mat are often recommended but the patient often has to sit above the warm bath which would bring comfort. A seat, such as the Mangar, which takes the user onto the bath bottom is preferable but relatively expensive.

Osteoarthritis of the knee

The patient with osteoarthritis of the knee may have degenerative changes in any one or of all three compartments of the knee, medial (75%), lateral (26%) or patellofemoral (48%), with symptoms which are slightly different initially. Pain in the former two are mainly along the joint line on the affected side. Patellofemoral osteoarthritis is associated with pain in the front of the joint, early atrophy of the quadriceps muscle, loss of sideways mobility of the patella and loss of the last few degrees of extension. Pain is again associated with activity, with weightbearing and with a reducing flexion and extension range; it is relieved by rest. Patellofemoral osteoarthritis often presents early with pain on descending stairs.

Functional difficulties are experienced with kneeling, climbing stairs and kerbs and uneven surfaces, and in rising (as from bed, chair, lavatory, car seat). Climbing stairs becomes impossible if there is less than 90° of flexion at both knees. There is a tendency for the patient to spend increasing periods inactive in a chair, where the knee takes up the same, comfortable flexed position, the quadriceps muscle wastes further, and a fixed flexion contracture results. The patient cannot walk on flexed knees for more than the shortest of distances and becomes chair (or wheelchair) bound. The situation may become increasingly compounded by **instability**, by varus, or less often, valgus deformity that worsens on weightbearing, and is usually progressive.

Examination confirms the pain as arising from the knees with localized tenderness related to the compartment involved. The knee is seldom hot, but there is often an effusion, with or without deformity (e.g. valgus or varus, perhaps only evident on weightbearing), quadriceps muscle wasting and weakness are always present. Standing and walking are observed: on walking less time is spent with weight on the affected knee than on the good side, and there may be instability.

Management

The principles of management of osteoarthritis of the knee are similar to that of the hip. The patient is encouraged to be busy, optimistic and as fit as possible. For less severe disease, education and maintenance of muscle power may be sufficient; later analgesia is also required. Changes in lifestyle and domestic (and workplace) environment may be made to this end.

Pain is relieved, early, by active exercise and by occasional analgesics. Later, regular analgesia is required. Sometimes NSAIDs may be prescribed but these are not specific for degenerative joint disease. Intra-articular steroids may be useful and a many-pronged approach to pain may be necessary.

Rest: When the knee is rested it should be extended although splints are rarely necessary and methods such as reversed dynamic slings rarely used. **Orthoses** may be helpful where there is instability, although the knee is difficult to splint. A fabric knee support, the telescopic valgus–varus (TVS) orthosis or occasionally a more substantial knee brace, can be effective. Shock absorption in the heel brings comfort.

Exercise is of the greatest importance. Quadriceps (and hamstring) muscle exercises must be done regularly and frequently. They help in improving power, joint range, may reduce instability, may improve shock absorption and reduce micro-trauma. The aim is to increase the strength and endurance of periarticular muscles as well as the range of movement. Gerber and Hicks (1992) recommend specific stretching exercises. For strengthening, isometric exercises precede isotonic and isokinetic exercises. The presence of an effusion is a contraindication to exercise using weights. Physical modalities are used as adjuncts to exercise as required.

Load is reduced by reducing obesity, by using a stick or crutch in the opposite hand and by high seating, as with osteoarthritis of the hip. Three times the body weight is transmitted through the hip and knee on rising from a dining chair, and seven times the body weight when getting out of a low armchair (Elllis *et al.* 1979). Arms on a chair, rails beside the lavatory and access rails are helpful.

Many householding and self-care adaptations to the home can be made. These can help by ensuring that surfaces are at a correct height, that energy is conserved and used efficiently, that tasks are broken up, that loads are reduced and joints spared.

Many patients will require mobility aids, wheelchairs (for transit, outside or inside the house) and adapted cars.

Finally, some will only be spared dependency by surgery.

Osteoarthritis of the first metatarsophalangeal (MTP) joint

This is common, and causes a surprising amount of disability: body weight is normally transmitted through the joint at the end of the stance phase of gait, at push-off.

The patient complains of local pain and limps, bearing less weight for a shorter time on that area. A soft tissue bursa may develop over the first metatarsal head; the second toe may sublux or dislocate, and both the second and third MTP joints may become painful if there is an associated hallux valgus. Many patients complain more of the cosmetic deformity and have difficulty in wearing fashionable shoes.

Management

Surgery may eventually be required, but before this obesity should be controlled and the patient should obtain appropriate footwear, i.e. shoes of sufficient width and depth, particularly around the MTP joint. An outside rocker also reduces pain. The problems of the arthritic foot are further described in Chapter 14.

Osteoarthritis of the hand

Osteoarthritis of the hands is frequent; Lawrence, Bremner and Bier (1966) quoted the incidence of radiological grades 2–4 of osteoarthritis of the distal interphalangeal joints as 22% in males and 29% in females. It causes relatively mild symptoms compared with the numerous serious and complex changes seen in rheumatoid arthritis. At the first carpometacarpal joint **pain** and squaring of the 'heel' of the hand occurs. This many be helped by use of a splint for the first carpometacarpal joint only for work and for rest, by local steroid injection, by pain-relieving drugs and, occasionally, by surgery.

There are numerous minor but frustrating difficulties of grip, and it may be difficult for the patient to stabilise the thumb. Rarely, the patient's job may become impossible (e.g. the seamstress, or a craft worker), when surgery may be considered.

REFERENCES

Chamberlain, M.A., Care, G. and Harfield, B. (1982) Physiotherapy in osteoarthrosis of the knees; a controlled trial of hospital versus home exercises. *International Rehabilitation Medicine*, **4**, 101–6.

Ekbolm, B., Lovgren, O., Alderin, M. *et al.* (1975) Effect of short-term physical training on patients with rheumatoid arthritis. *Scandinavian Journal of Rheumatology* **4**, 80–6.

Ellis, M.I., Seedhom, B.B., Amis, A.A., Dowson, D. and Wright, V. (1979) Forces in the knee joint whilst rising from normal and motorised chairs. *Engineering in Medicine* **8**, 573–80.

George, E. and Dieppe, P.A. (1993) Osteoarthritis. *Hospital Update*, **19**, 450–56.

Gerber, L. and Hicks, J.E. (1992) Rehabilitation in the management of patients with osteoarthritis, in *Osteoarthritis: diagnosis and medical/surgical management*, 2nd edn (eds R.W. Moskowitz, D.S. Howell, V.M. Goldberg and H.J. Makin, WB Saunders, London.

Klippel J.H. and Dieppe P.A. (eds) (1994) *Rheumatology*, Mosby, London.

Lawrence, J.S., Bremner, J.M. and Bier, F. (1966) Osteo-arthrosis. Prevalence in the population and relationship between symptoms and X-ray changes. *Annals of the Rheumatic Diseases*, **25**, 1–24.

Lorig (1995) Patient education: treatment or nice extra. Editorial *British Journal of Rheumatology* **34**, 703–6.

Marks, R. (1993) Quadriceps strength training for osteoarthritis of the knee: a literature review and analysis. *Physiotherapy*, **79**, 13–17.

Martin, J., Meltzer, N. and Elliott, D. (1988) *The prevalence of disability among Adults*. Report No. 1 OPCS survey of disability in Great Britain, HMSO, London.

McAlindon, T.E., Cooper, C., Kirwan, J.R. and Dieppe, P.A. (1993) Determinants of disability in osteoarthritis of the knee. *Annals of the Rheumatic Diseases*, **52**, 258–62.

Radin, E.L. (1987) Osteoarthritis; what is known about prevention. *Clinical Orthopaedics and Related Research*, **222**, 60–5.

Semple, E.L., Loeser, R.F. and Wise, C.M. (1990) Therapeutic exercise for rheumatoid arthritis and osteoarthritis. *Seminars in Arthritis and Rheumatism*, **20**, 32–40.

FURTHER READING

Dickson, R.A. and Wright, V. (1984) *Integrated Clinical Science: musculo-skeletal disease*, Heinemann, London.

Banwell, B.F. and Gall, V. (eds) (1988) *Physical Therapy Management of Arthritis*, Churchill Livingstone, Edinburgh.

Wiklund, I., Romanus, B. and Hunt, S.M. (1988) Self-assessed disability in patients with arthrosis of the hip joint: reliability of the Swedish version of the Nottingham Health Profile. *International Disability Studies* **10**, 159–63.

ADVICE TO PATIENTS

Several relevant titles are available from the Arthritis and Rheumatism Council for Research, Copeman House, St Mary's Court, Chesterfield, Derbyshire S41 7TD. These include:

Driving and your Arthritis
Gardening with Arthritis
A New Hip Joint
A New Knee Joint
Osteoarthritis
Osteoarthritis of the Knees
Pain Management
Physiotherapy – What will happen?
Stairlifts
Your Home and Your Rheumatism

14 Adult rheumatoid arthritis

L. Gerber

INTRODUCTION

Arthritis is the largest cause of locomotor disability in developed countries. Rheumatoid arthritis (RA), with an incidence of 30 per 100 000 and a prevalence of 1000 per 100 000 is the most common of the inflammatory arthritides. Classically the disease presents as a symmetrical polyarthritis. The feet, hands and wrists are often involved early, but virtually any synovial joint may be affected (Figure 14.1). In addition to having articular and extra-articular manifestations, the patient may feel unwell.

The problems are protean and may include the anaemia of chronic inflammation or that secondary to treatment with inflammatory drugs, and tiredness which may be a result or due to other causes which need to be identified. Sjögren's syndrome, in which the lacrimal and salivary glands fail to secrete normally, is common. The lungs may be involved (pleural effusions, alveolitis, nodules). The heart may be diseased (pericarditis, aortic incompetence, myocarditis). Vasculitis is also seen and may cause skin lesions (rash, ulcers). Occasionally vasculitis affects the vasa nervorum leading to mononeuritis multiplex. Three other neurological complications are recognized: entrapment neuropathy, the commonest example of which is carpal tunnel syndrome, myelo-

pathy as a consequence of cervical cord instability, and rarely a symmetrical sensorimotor neuropathy. Where there is pre-existing paralysis, for example due to stroke or polio, joint disease is less severe in the affected limb(s); the reasons for this are not known.

The functional impact of this disease is substantial (Pincus *et al*, 1984). It can be measured in terms of mobility, work performance, health cost expenditures, the costs of caring, and psychosocial parameters.

During the past two decades treatment for rheumatoid arthritis has resulted in clinical improvement, but not cure (Kushner, 1989). Therefore to enhance and possibly prolong life, rehabilitation strategies should be integrated into comprehensive treatment. Outcomes sought from rehabilitation treatments are both global and specific to the disease process. Globally, patients should achieve improved function in the performance-based, psychosocial and vocational aspects of life. This population of patients also has unique needs for preservation of mechanical alignment of joints and adjustment to the metabolic impact of antirheumatic pharmaco-logical agents.

This chapter will describe the rehabilitation needs of adults with rheumatoid arthritis and the interventions and strategies effective in meeting those needs.

Rehabilitation of the Physically Disabled Adult. Edited by C. John Goodwill, M. Anne Chamberlain and Chris Evans. Published in 1997 by Stanley Thornes (Publishers) Ltd, Cheltenham. ISBN 0-7487-3183-0.

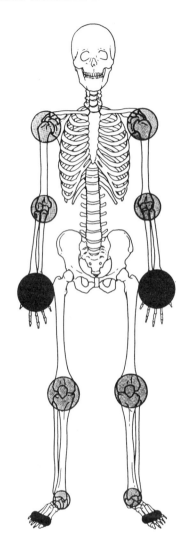

Figure 14.1 Joints affected in early rheumatoid arthritis.

EVALUATION OF THE PATIENT WITH RHEUMATOID ARTHRITIS

The history and physical examination should be comprehensive, with attention to the impairments associated with RA as well as their functional effects. The standard assessments usually include a joint count (Ritchie *et al*, 1968) which both identifies and quantifies the severity of signs and symptoms of tenderness, swelling and pain on motion. Assessments of pain (Huskisson, Jones and Scott, 1976) and fatigue (Belza *et al*, 1993) and multidimensional health status instruments (Fries *et al*, 1980; Meenan, Gertman and Mason, 1980; Pincus *et al*, 1983) should be part of initial and periodic outcome measures. These evaluations have been validated for patients with RA, and are widely used as functional outcome measures. These assessment questionnaires are referred to as the Arthritis Impact Measurement Score (AIMS), the Health Assessment Questionnaire (HAQ) and ALI (a modified form of HAQ) (Table 14.1)

Proper prescription of rehabilitation treatments require that evaluations be more detailed and have the capability of being highly individualized. Because handicap is often highly dependent upon an individual's unique needs and life activities, an attempt should be made to link specific activity with the individual's perception of his/her needs and performance. For example, it is important to understand which activities are affected and under which circumstances and for what duration of time these efforts produce fatigue, pain, stiffness or other symptoms that may interfere with performance. Identifying the causes and the conditions under which these symptoms are produced opens up opportunities for remedying them. Evaluations are available that can assist in this (Furst *et al*, 1987; Gerber and Furst, 1992)

Completion of the evaluation should give the health professional an assessment of the individual's current level of performance and capacity for performance (both physical, psychocognitive and motivational). Also, it is necessary to know the nature of symptoms that need amelioration in their order of importance to the patient, and the nature of the activities that either cause undesirable symptoms or need treatment in order to be performed. The treatment plan should derive from the assessment.

Table 14.1 Health assessment questionnaire (modified from: Fries *et al.*, 1980)

Name _____   Date _____

We are interested in learning how your illness affects your daily life. Please feel free to add any comments on the back of this page.

PLEASE **TICK** THE **ONE** RESPONSE WHICH BEST DESCRIBES YOUR USUAL ABILITIES
OVER THE PAST WEEK:

	Without **any** difficulty	With **some** difficulty	With **much** difficulty	Unable to do
1. Dressing and grooming				
— dress yourself, including tying shoelaces and doing buttons?	☐	☐	☐	☐
— shampoo your hair	☐	☐	☐	☐
2. Rising				
— stand up from an armless straight chair?	☐	☐	☐	☐
— get in and out of bed?	☐	☐	☐	☐
3. Eating				
— cut your meat?	☐	☐	☐	☐
— lift a full cup or glass to mouth?	☐	☐	☐	☐
— open a new carton of milk (or soap powder)?	☐	☐	☐	☐
4. Walking				
— walk outdoors on flat ground?	☐	☐	☐	☐
— Climb up five steps?	☐	☐	☐	☐
5. Hygiene				
— wash and dry your entire body?	☐	☐	☐	☐
— take a bath?	☐	☐	☐	☐
— get on/off the toilet?	☐	☐	☐	☐
6. Reach				
— reach and get down a 5 lb object (e.g. bag of potatoes) from just above your head?	☐	☐	☐	☐
— bend down to pick up clothing from the floor?	☐	☐	☐	☐
7. Grip				
— open car doors?	☐	☐	☐	☐
— open jars which have been previously opened?	☐	☐	☐	☐
— turn taps on/off?	☐	☐	☐	☐
8. Activities				
— Run errands and shop?	☐	☐	☐	☐
— get in/out of a car?	☐	☐	☐	☐
— do chores; e.g. vacuuming, housework or light gardening	☐	☐	☐	☐

Domains of evaluation:

- level of performance – physical, phychocognitive, motivational;
- capacity for performance – physical, phychocognitive, motivational;
- symptoms in need of amelioration;
- activities associated with undesirable symptoms.

Specific evaluation needed for problem identification and treatment planning:

- fatigue;
- joint pain and stiffness;
- mobility and daily activity;
- psychosocial dysfunction;
- environmental obstacles to function;
- soft tissue/bony malalignment

Typically, for adults with RA, rehabilitation evaluations should identify the following problems and point to the organ or system to target for therapeutic intervention:

1. **Fatigue** and its potential causes (unrefreshed sleep, decreased aerobic capacity, muscle weakness and depression or lack of motivation).
2. **Joint pain and stiffness** and its potential causes (joint swelling and pain, loss of range of motion, gel phenomenon, mechanical malalignment).
3. **Mobility and daily activity** and its potential causes (inability to ambulate, transfer, perform self-care, vocational or avocational activity).
4. **Psychosocial dysfunction** and its potential causes (depression, social isolation, economic dependence, lack of motivation, initiation or participation in care).
5. **Environmental obstacles** to function (architectural, emotional barriers).
6. **Orthopaedic problem** that may promote malalignment (to identify joint malalignment, soft tissue changes that contribute to this).

Once evaluation is completed and treatment goals agreed with the patient, a therapeutic plan is devised. It should be dynamic and will require input from patient and family as well as professionals. The more involved the patient's family are with the programme, the more likely it is to be followed and effective.

MEDICAL TREATMENTS

Patients with active disease with evidence of joint inflammation, raised acute phase reactants and progressive joint damage require recognizing by a joint activity scoring such as the Ritchie Articular Index. Their global functional activity needs to be known. Knowing both specific and global deficits allows treatment to be better targeted.

Previously many patients would be maintained for long periods of time on non-steroidal anti-inflammatory drugs (NSAID), for example, ibuprofen, indomethacin. Such drugs reduce pain and stiffness but do not modify the course of the disease. It is increasingly recognized that best practice consists of preventing joint damage and functional deterioration and that early decline in functional status carries a bad prognosis, as do nodules. Patients who begin to manifest objective signs of joint damage (however early) should be offered disease-modifying drugs. Sulphasalazine will often be used, but methotrexate is being prescribed earlier. Gold and penicillamine are perhaps less commonly used than previously.

All these drugs require regular monitoring for side-effects, usually with monthly blood and urine tests (details vary and can be obtained from National Pharmacopeia), principally for bone marrow depression, rise in liver function tests and proteinuria. Response to treatment is often delayed some 3 months and patients usually need to stay on medication for many years.

Those whose disease is very aggressive, or unresponsive to methotrexate and whose work is in jeopardy, may need more experimental treatments, such as repeated immunoglobulin injections. Patients who are unable or unwilling to cooperate, have disease limited to a single joint, or who are very elderly are probably not best treated with these drugs.

Elderly patients often respond to relatively small doses of steroid (prednisolone up to 7.5 mg per day).

It is good policy to supply patients with record cards noting their current drug therapy so that the interchange of information between hospital and general practice is facilitated. Patients as well as general practitioners should be informed about the toxic effects these drugs can produce. Many patients will be unable to open childproof containers and the formulation of any medication for arthritic people needs to take account of their poor grip.

PHYSICAL TREATMENTS

Adults recently diagnosed with RA are often overwhelmed by the diagnosis and what it may entail. Conversely, many are in a state of denial. However, often they are suffering from a functional status change which includes pain, fatigue and to some degree loss of ability to maintain life routines. They often fear dependence and disability from work and are depressed. Pain is more intense and disability greater in depressed patients (Afflect *et al*, 1991; Beckham *et al*, 1992). Each day may seem quite different from the last or the next, and hence strategies designed to plan for a variety of eventualities are useful. Early rehabilitation interventions should include efforts to control pain, preserve sleep and reduce fear of work disability and conserve energy.

Pain management

Rehabilitation treatments are often non-pharmacological and consist of cold, heat, electricity, hydrotherapy, light (low intensity laser) and, most recently, acupuncture.

Cold packs, gels and frozen pellets (such as peas) have been demonstrated to be good analgesic agents, as effective as heat in increasing shoulder range of movement (ROM) in adhesive capsulitis, and help reduce muscle spasm (Michlovitz, 1990). These packs should be applied for 10 minutes to swollen, stiff or painful joints and periarticular structures. Reduction of pain and swelling occur through reduction in metabolic rate. Cold has been demonstrated to exacerbate Raynaud's syndrome, decrease tissue elasticity, and blood viscosity. It should not be used for patients with vascular insufficiency or compromise.

Heat may be administered in the form of hot packs (moist or dry), paraffin or warm baths, all of which deliver heat superficially. Hydrotherapy is also a form of superficial heat and is effective in delivering sedation, relaxation, analgesia as well as buoyancy. Ultrasound can deliver a form of heat that is able to penetrate the skin to a depth of 5 cm. Both forms are good analgesic agents and can increase distensibility and elasticity of tissue. Hot packs should be applied for 15–20 minutes, longer durations may increase intra-articular temperature and result in increased metabolic rates and cellular infiltration (Harris and McCroskery, 1974). Hydrotherapy should be given in a body tank or therapeutic pool in which the temperature is 37–40°C. Because of its ability to increase the metabolic rate, deep heat should not be used for acute synovitis or for joints that have substantial effusions. Heat treatment is best used for subacute or stiff joints.

Table 14.2 summarizes the influences of heat and cold in arthritic joints. This table

Table 14.2 Effects of temperature on arthritic joints

Heat	Use for warm, or stiff contracted, painful, subacute/chronic joints
Cold	Use for hot, swollen, painful, acute joints

may help in the selection of treatment modalities for RA patients.

Electric current has been demonstrated to be clinically useful in reducing pain and muscle spasm. It is suggested (Melzack and Wall, 1965) that the electrical stimulus bombards large diameter nerve fibres which then pass through the gate, blocking transmission of signals from smaller fibres which are transmitters of painful sensations. Transcutaneous nerve stimulators (TENS) deliver such stimuli and have been shown to reduce pain associated with peripheral neuropathy and reduce wrist pain in RA (Mannheimer, Lard and Carlsson, 1978). Pain reduction was associated with a functional improvement. Other forms of electrical stimuli have been used to re-educate muscle. Few clinical trials have been done to support this and most of the evidence is anecdotal.

Low intensity, (cold) light amplification by stimulated emission radiation (LASER) has been used to relieve pain in arthritis (Basford *et al*, 1987). No improvement of functional parameters was noted. Approval for use of this treatment has not yet been granted by the FDA in the USA.

Acupuncture has been used as an adjunctive therapy for pain in musculoskeletal syndromes for hundreds of years. Several studies report the efficacy of acupuncture in the relief of joint pain in RA patients (Sanders, 1985). Some studies suggest that acupuncture influences cellular and cytokine production in RA (Xinlian *et al*, 1993). This treatment must be administered by a certified acupuncturist who uses good aseptic techniques, otherwise transmission of HIV, hepatitis and other potentially harmful pathogens is possible.

Educational and behavioural interventions

Education of patients about how to solve problems and devise appropriate routines for exercise, among other interventions, have been shown to be important in enhancing participation and improving clinical outcomes for the RA patient (Perlman, Connel and Albert 1987; Lorig *et al*, 1989)

Energy conservation

Teaching patients with RA how to pace their activities and plan their days to include rest periods results in increased ability. When patients are taught to take rest breaks designed to interrupt physically demanding activity, they are then able to sustain a higher level of performance than if they did not do that (Gerber *et al*, 1987).

Joint protection

The application of principles designed to use larger, more proximal joints to lift objects and stabilize limb positions is thought to be more energy efficient and protects small joints from deforming forces. Similarly, physical activity that does not result in post exercise fatigue or pain lasting more than 1 hour after completion is acceptable. More than that may result in disease flare or muscle injury. These principles are referred to as joint protection and energy conservation techniques that are often used in patient educational programmes (Brattstrom, 1987)

Deformity occurs in rheumatoid joints for at least three reasons: the joint itself becomes misshapen; the ligaments and capsule around the joint become lax; and associated muscles become weak. The relative importance of these factors varies from one joint to another and from patient to patient.

'Joint protection' is based on the hypothesis that if a joint is used in a way which minimizes strains on the ligaments and the capsule, and if muscle power is maintained, the risk of long-term damage and deformity is reduced. If this hypothesis is correct, teaching a patient techniques to minimize load or strain on inflamed joints, encouraging the use of appropriate aids and teaching exercises to maintain range of movement and muscle strength should reduce long-term disability.

The following paragraphs describe application of joint protection principles to specific joints. Over the course of many years the joints bearing the brunt of the disease will vary, and thus the components of joint protection will be continuously varying. Regular assessment by the occupational therapist and physiotherapist is therefore necessary so that the patient can be taught the relevant aspects of joint protection.

Hands and wrist

The 'pinch' grip used when gripping small objects (e.g. turning keys and taps) increases the risk of subluxation of the metacarpophalangeal (MCP) joints and derangement of the interphalangeal (IP) joint of the thumb, both common deformities in RA (Figure 14.2). Provision of such things as tap- or key-turners, which either use a lever principle to reduce the effort needed, or have a large grip, can reduce the strain on the MCP joints and hence the tendency for these to sublux. Scissors with a spring handle rather than a two-finger grip are also helpful.

Patients should avoid load-bearing with the involved hands, and should not use knuckles when rising from a chair. This stresses the finger PIP and MCP joints and wrists. Whenever heavy objects are carried **both** hands should be used, and where possible the weight should be supported on the forearm. Provision of aids such as long-sleeved oven gloves, so that the heavy pans can be carried on the forearm, will help this. A working wrist splint which holds the **wrist** in slight ulnar deviation (5 in, 13 cm) will also reduce the strain and tendency to radial deviation at this joint. A rigid splint (usually made of a low-temperature thermoplastic) can also be supplied to maintain this position whilst the patient is resting at night.

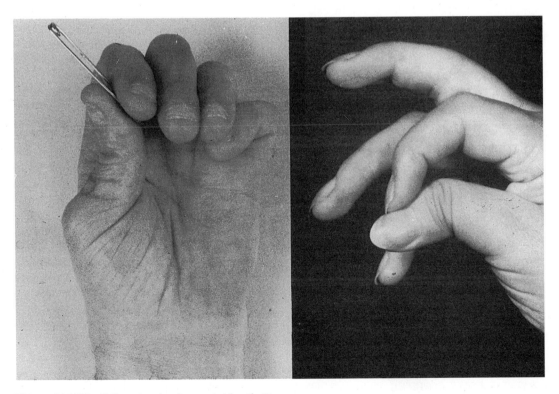

Figure 14.2 Hand function in rheumatoid arthritis.

The patient should be encouraged to practise ulnar deviation of this wrist with a slightly clenched fist, or maximal abduction of the thumb, which exercises extensor carpiulnaris. Weakness of this muscle is said to increase the likelihood of radial deviation at the wrist which occurs with ulnar deviation at the MCP joint.

Elbows

Maintenance of range of movement, and avoiding heavy loads on the joints are both important. Loss of extension can be tolerated in one elbow, and results in little functional disability, but when both elbows have fixed flexion over 45° the patient will have several problems, including driving a car; during eating, drinking, dressing; and in particular in reaching the perineum and carrying out personal hygiene. The embarrassment that this causes can be avoided by providing appropriate aids, but if the problem can be prevented by regular exercises to maintain elbow movement, this of course is preferable.

Flexion of >100° is essential for bringing the hand to the head/mouth. Small losses of pronation and supination can cause significant disability. This movement is required for basic household tasks such as opening jars, turning keys, etc. Pronation is also vital for those whose work involves the operation of a keyboard. One of our young patients was obliged to reconsider a career in computing when she found operating the computer keyboard impossible because both elbows were fixed in a 'neutral' position.

Shoulders

These joints are particularly likely to lose range of movement, and the patient must be encouraged to put the shoulders through a full range each day. Patients often believe they should struggle on with a difficult task which they can just manage, such as carrying a heavy shopping bag, whereas it would be better to use a shopping trolley or a spouse! A trolley within the house for transporting heavy objects can also be invaluable. Where shoulder movement has already become restricted, provision of aids such as a long-handled comb can do much to preserve independence and self-respect.

Spine

Attention needs to be drawn to **sitting and resting positions**, particularly when doing close work such as sewing, other handiwork or reading. The patient may need to wear a collar to maintain a correct neck position and a head restraint is desirable in the car to prevent neck injury in an accident.

Hips and knees

The knees are usually involved early in the course of RA. Quadriceps weakness and wasting are a rapid, almost inevitable consequence, and destruction of cartilage may ensue later. This, together with damage to the joint capsule and associated ligaments, can lead to an unstable knee joint which usually adopts a valgus position. During weight-bearing on such an unstable joint, some of the load may be transmitted to non-bony structures rather than along the long axes of the bones. Since ligaments are not designed to support body weight they may rupture. The instability and deformity is therefore increased and the destructive process is accelerated.

Fixed flexion is often seen in the badly damaged knee. Left untreated this leads to flexion deformity in the hip and may prevent the patient standing. The other important consequence of hip involvement in RA is loss of abduction, which leads to difficulties in intercourse and childbirth in women.

To avoid these problems the principles of joint protection need to be applied by the patient. This means:

1. Putting hip and knee joints through a full range of movement each day. Swimming

(using breast stroke) should be encouraged, since this uses a wide range of joint positions with reduced weightbearing.

2. A daily period of resting or sleeping prone, to encourage extension at the hip and knee. A pillow may be placed under the chest to make this more comfortable.

3. Encouraging exercises to strengthen adjacent muscles. Quadriceps strengthening exercises are easy to perform and vital, since knee instability is low if this muscle becomes weak.

4. The treatment of obesity to reduce the load on weightbearing joints. However, the position of the joints at the time of weightbearing is also important. For example, rising from a chair where the seat is raised and the hip is in a semi-flexed rather than a fully flexed position is considerably easier than rising from a 'bucket-seat'. The ARC booklet *Are You Sitting Comfortably* is helpful when choosing chairs for arthritics (see Appendix; see also Chapter 45).

Strategically placed supports, such as grab-rails in bathrooms, toilets and on stairs, serve the same purpose. Unfortunately, similar features are seldom incorporated into car design. It is a common sight to see the arthritic patient struggling to pull him/herself out of a car by grabbing the edge of a swinging car door.

Resting positions for knees and hips should not be those which encourage deformity. Patients may choose to rest with a pillow under the knees, but this encourages flexion of hips and knees. It is preferable to provide resting splints for the knees which restrict the degree of flexion.

Even where the patient and clinician have been diligent in managing the disease, treatment of established deformities may have to be undertaken. Where flexion deformity of the knee has developed, serial splinting with progressively straighter plaster splints may reduce the deformity, but it usually returns rapidly unless the treatment is backed up by physiotherapy. Prosthetic surgery for the knees may eventually be required. Hip flexion may also require surgical intervention. Total hip replacement is usually the appropriate procedure in the adult with severe RA. 'Anterior release' of the hip is occasionally performed, but is more relevant to the treatment of juvenile chronic arthritis than RA. The latter operation will only produce lasting improvement if it is reinforced by persistent and intensive physiotherapy and adequate relief of pain. Reversed dynamic slings to maintain extension can be useful prior to, and after, surgery.

Where lateral instability in the knee is a problem an orthosis with steel struts hinged at the knee, such as the Cinch, Cam-Am etc., can be used; this may help to relieve weightbearing pain (Chapter 47). The more active patient probably requires intensive active physiotherapy coupled with prosthetic surgical treatment.

Walking aids may be used to increase stability and reduce the load borne by the legs, but the patient and therapist must remember that the increased loads borne by the arms when sticks or crutches are used can accelerate damage to these joints. Axillary or elbow crutches are seldom suitable for the rheumatoid patient. When walking sticks are used, the handle should be broad or be moulded to conform to the patient's hand, as does the handle of the Fischer stick. Sometimes supplementing this with a wrist splint is helpful. Where crutches or a walking frame are necessary the 'gutter' type should be chosen for their more even distribution of load (Chapter 48)

In more severely affected patients, where walking or standing requires considerable effort it is often helpful to provide a wheel chair at least for outdoor use. This avoids the situation where the patient expends all his or her energy in getting from 'A' to 'B' and is then unable to carry out any useful activity at 'B' (Chapter 44)

Modification of the environment can do much to ease the strain on damaged hips and knees. For example, the kitchen layout should take account of the fact that the sink is the most-used piece of equipment; it should be central and have adjacent work surfaces at a convenient height. Some work may be done seated, and storage should be carefully planned to minimize difficulties of reaching and carrying, and to conserve energy. These principles can be applied to all tasks by those who understand the principles of joint protection.

Ground floor accommodation with easy access is ideal, but other factors such as helpful neighbours or family nearby should be taken into consideration before moving patients away from 'unsuitable accommodation'. Even for the severely disabled, major housing modifications such as stairlift installations (Chapter 46) and provision of ramps may be cheaper and more convenient than moving house (Chapter 54)

Ankle and foot

Ankle stability depends on the integrity of ligaments holding the tibia and fibula together and connecting these two bones to the talus and calcaneum. If these ligaments become stretched or eroded by the rheumatoid process, pronation and eversion of the foot tends to develop. Rarely Achilles tendon rupture may occur, particularly at the site of nodules within the tendon. These features only occur in more severe disease. Subtalar joint involvement with valgus deformity occurs more frequently, and leads to loss of inversion and eversion. This causes difficulty and pain when walking on uneven ground.

Involvement of metatarsophalangeal (MTP) joints occurs in the majority of RA patients, and pain arising from these joints is often a presenting feature of the disease. The common deformities which occur are separation and downwards subluxation of the

metatarsal heads, with associated claw-toe deformities, hallux valgus and bunion formation. As a consequence, the metatarsal heads no longer rest on protective fat pads and ulcers can develop at pressure points under the metatarsal heads. (Figure 14.3).

Protection of the ankles and feet in RA inevitably depends on weight reduction and load reduction. In addition, the patient usually needs altered footwear and must recognize this as an ongoing problem. Initially all that most patients need is a broader shoe with thicker soles and lower heels. Full-length metatarsal supports can be fitted into the patient's shoes. Wedges or heel cups should be tried for hindfoot symptoms. Unfortunately patients often have difficulty finding footwear that is broad or deep enough to accommodate these orthoses. These patients, and those with more severe deformities, need made-to-measure shoes. These can be purchased in a variety of available styles and colours; ready-made 'comfort' shoes and training shoes designed to take orthoses are also now available. Where ankle problems exist a boot will give additional support. Whatever footwear is used, fastenings must be straightforward (e.g. Velcro) so that patients can manage despite hand involvement. Ankle–foot orthoses are available for those with ankle or subtalar instability causing pain on weightbearing, but many patients prefer to use foot supports only (Chapter 48).

As stressed earlier, both doctor and patient must recognize not only that adequate footwear will prevent calluses and pressure ulcers developing, but also that the foot shape is likely to alter from year to year and footwear will need regular adjustment. This is particularly important in those few patients who also have a sensory neuropathy.

Many patients with RA have difficulty with cutting their toenails, and referral to a chiropodist is useful, particularly when the patient lives alone and grip is poor.

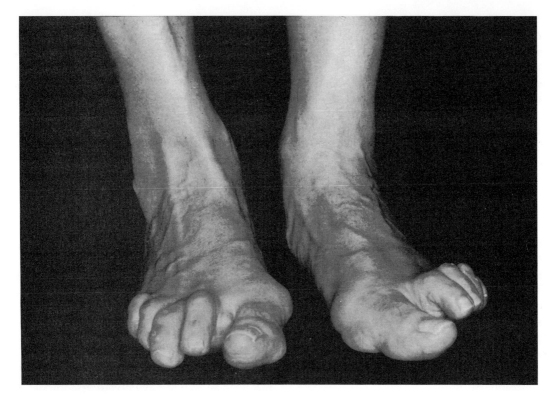

Figure 14.3 Feet showing the effects of rheumatoid arthritis.

EDUCATIONAL ASPECTS

Perhaps the most interesting aspect of educational techniques has been in the use of biofeedback and guided imagery in the amelioration of symptoms and enhancement of well-being. Biofeedback has been used to raise skin temperature and alleviate symptoms of Raynaud's. Relaxation using guided imagery, deep breathing, meditation and self-hypnosis have all been used with some degree of success in reducing chronic pain associated with arthritis. Few scientifically controlled trials have been done, but at least one review suggests that we should not be unduly sceptical about the adjunctive use of these techniques (Blackmore, 1991). The mechanisms by which these techniques work have not been described. Current theories attempt to dispel the notion of the mind and body being totally separate and describe the interrelationships as probably being dependent upon feedback loops that relate hormonal-releasing factors with cytokine activity. And further, in RA (at least in animal models of adjuvant-induced arthritis) there are abnormal stress reactions that contribute to the progression of the disease (Sternberg *et al*, 1989) which may be modulated by behavioural changes. These can be taught through biofeedback, hypnotherapy, guided imagery and other similar techniques.

Education for patients with inflammatory arthritis is of the greatest importance. The rheumatologist or rehabilitation specialist will usually need the help of others to deliver this to patients and their families effectively. Several models exist: educational courses may be given when (and if) the patient is admitted for inpatient treatment and many professionals are often involved in this programme. The multidisciplinary team in the unit frequently provides a focus for enquiries and support when the patient goes home.

Most education has to be delivered on an outpatient basis. The occupational therapy department may take on the responsibility of running a series of sessions in which there is discussion on joint protection and energy conservation. Usually there will be liaison with the nurse practitioner. The latter may run his/her own clinic alongside the doctor and may be the focus for monitoring drugs, which provides an excellent opportunity for sustained contact and education. Liaison work my fall to any of the professionals who may visit the patient at home whichever model is used, the essential features are that communication is of agreed material (supplemented by written information) and is effective, not only with the patient but between professionals.

EXERCISE

Fatigue is a prevalent complaint which is often ignored by doctors; data from women with RA show that their maximal oxygen uptake was reduced by 30% and their strength was reduced by 30–50% (Ekblom *et al*, 1974). These women responded to a programme that was designed to increase strength and improve fitness. Much data have been accumulated on the benefits of exercise in RA, supporting the view that exercise improves range of movement, strength, aerobic capacity, improves function and helps modulate pain (Harkcom *et al*, 1985). Exercise has been shown to reduce cholesterol, aid in weight reduction, reduce bone demineralization, and improve mood, sleep patterns and socialization.

The reasons for prescribing exercise for RA patients are varied, and may include all the above-mentioned benefits. Hence the goals

should be carefully considered before the exercise prescription is written. Also the patient with RA may have cardiac disease; they may also have pulmonary complications secondary to the rheumatoid arthritis, and signs of vasculitis or neuropathy; all of which may require adjustments to exercise regimens. Nonetheless, people with arthritis are able to participate in most forms of moderate training.

In general, when first prescribing exercise a range of movement exercise is recommended to actively restore functional range and to achieve as pain-free a range as possible. Clinically derived functional ranges of motion have been described, and should be the goals of such an exercise programme (Gerber, 1981).

Isometric techniques are recommended for the patient with acute synovitis or active disease (Minor *et al*, 1989). Isometric exercise has been the treatment of choice for patients with RA because it is so well tolerated and has been shown to have no adverse impact on joint erosion. Recent data, however, show that dynamic training is more effective than static in strengthening muscles of RA patients (Ekdahl *et al*, 1990). Isokinetic exercise, a dynamic form of exercise that uses a constant angular velocity, has also been shown to be effective and well tolerated in RA (Lyngberg *et al*, 1994). Methods for training have been described for each of the types of exercise described above.

Isometric exercise is usually recommended initially when patients are just starting a strengthening programme and when there are inflamed joints. Isometrics can be performed at home and require no equipment. A 6-second maximal contraction performed daily can increase strength by 5% weekly. Submaximal contractions are also effective in increasing strength, although they are not as effective as maximal and there is little improvement in motor performance. The prescription is for several sets of from three to six submaximal or maximal contractions daily, if possible. The exercise should be performed at an angle at which there is no pain.

Isotonic exercise is more effective than isometric exercise in strength training and will improve motor performance and muscle endurance. Resistance is used throughout the range and exercise may be either eccentric or concentric. Eccentric training is often associated with significant muscle soreness and is poorly tolerated in RA. Most isotonic programmes involve the use of free weights, fixed or variable resistance machines or elastic devices. We suggest this form of training start with low resistance and frequent repetitions, with slowly increasing weights. The routine should be performed at least three times per week, with the patient doing his/her optimal under the supervision of the therapist. Both eccentric and concentric contractions should be done. This type of training, while most effective for increasing strength, should not be done in patients with effusions, synovitis or active joint symptoms.

Isokinetic exercise is tolerated in arthritic patients when the angular velocities are high ($120° \text{ s}^{-1}$ and above) because the forces across the joints are lower. Lower speeds produce significant joint pain, and may result in articular or periarticular effusion (Wessel and Quinney, 1984). This type of exercise should be performed using a limited arc of motion, and probably should not be done at all in the presence of significant popliteal cyst or joint instability. Strength gained at fast speeds seems to be useful at either slow or fast speeds. Isokinetic strengthening techniques result in improved motor performance and provide multi-joint strength improvement.

Endurance training is designed to improve the ability of a muscle to sustain contractions over time. Endurance requires local muscle endurance, which is determined by muscle strength, and aerobic capacity. Endurance will increase with an aerobic training programme whose requirements are frequent repetition and low intensity and when large muscle groups are used. Stamina improvement has been documented in patients whose programmes are 15 minutes, three times weekly at 60% VO_2 (Harkcom *et al*, 1985; Depie Zhongyi and Zoulu 1992). Many studies report that aerobic programmes are well tolerated and are effective in increasing aerobic capacity in patients with RA. Aquatic programmes are very effective for improving fitness and are particularly well suited for the RA patient because of the buoyance, relaxation and benefits in ROM from the activity. Data shows there is an added strengthing effect, in addition to the aerobic benefit (Danneskjold-Samsoe *et al*, 1987)

Avocational and enjoyable physical activity should not be overlooked. Recommendations about when to begin or discontinue exercise should be based on disease activity, level of fitness and previous experience doing the activity. When the arthritis is in an acute phase, only limited recreational activity should be permitted and this of the low impact type, such as swimming and walking. When the arthritis enters a subacute phase, bicycling (including stationary), gardening with adapted seating and possibly cross-country skiing and brisk walking may be recommended. High impact recreational activity such as basketball, volleyball, running and gymnastics, is not usually recommended.

A summary of exercise recommendations is presented in Table 14.3.

ORTHOSES

Most patients with RA have involvement of many joints, typically involving the soft tissues as well as the articular structure. Management of this requires coordination between rheumatologist, orthopaedist, rehabilitation specialist and orthotist. The hope is that with multidisciplinary treatments there will be good management of inflammation,

Table 14.3 Exercise recommendations for patients with rheumatoid arthritis

Stage of arthritis	Type of exercise				
	Isometric	Isotonic[1]	Isokinetic[2]	Active ROM	Aerobic[3]
Acute	+	–	–	+	+
Subacute	+	±	+	+	+
Inactive	+	+	+	+	+

[1] Limited arc of motion.
[2] High angular velocity.
[3] Low impact.

preservation of mechanical alignment and relief of symptoms while function is preserved. Some critical ranges of motion are needed for self-care and mobility (Table 14.4).

Orthotic devices provide adjunctive, but important treatment for preservation of joint alignment, although there is no conclusive data supporting the belief that splints prevent deformity and such would be difficult to obtain. Orthoses are prescribed to support or immobilize body parts in functional positions, or substitute for lost function. These splints can be either static or dynamic. They have been demonstrated to reduce pain and swelling without reducing the ROM (Gault and Spyker, 1969).

Table 14.4 Critical ranges of motion for function

Joint	Range of motion
Hip	0–30° flexion
Knee	0–70° flexion
Ankle	10° dorsiflexion to 20° plantar flexion
Shoulder	45° flexion, 90° abduction, 20° external rotation, 15° internal rotation
Elbow	120° flexion
CMC	30° internal rotation
MCP	45° flexion
PIP	50° flexion

CMC = carpometacarpal; MCP = metacarpophalangeal; proximal interphalangeal joints.
Note: these depend on range of movement in adjacent joints.

Upper limb

Splinting for the upper extremity is usually confined to the hand and wrist, although post operative elbow splints and shoulder slings are often used. The abnormalities seen in the hands of persons with RA are quite characteristic and often there is loss of one or more of the four types of grip (Figure 14.4):

A. **Power** in which the wrist is extended and MCPs and IPs flexed.
B. **Pinch grip** where the tip of the thumb makes contact with the tip of the index finger.
C. **Key grip** in which the thumb is opposed to the side of the index finger.
D. **Hook grip** involving flexion of the MCPs and IPs with the wrist in neutral position, without thumb involvement.

There may be fusiform swelling of the digits, with prominence of the MCP joints and a slightly flexed position in which the hand is held. Stretching of the intrinsic muscles of the hands with active extension is recommended. As the disease persists or progresses additional changes occur. The intrinsic muscles tighten, pulling down the lateral bands of the muscles and causing deformities of the fingers in which the proximal interphalangeal joints (PIP) becomes hyperrextended and the distal interphalangeal joints (DIP) are flexed causing

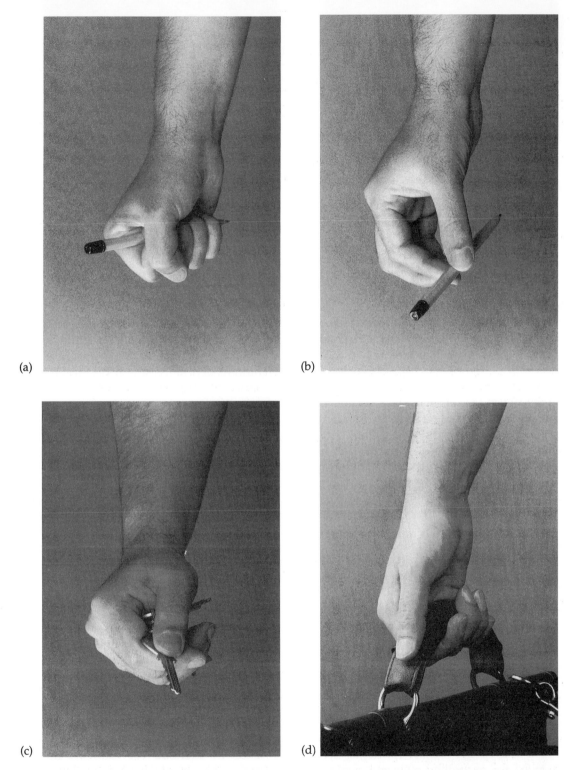

Figure 14.4 Variants of normal grip in hand function: (a), power grip; (b), pinch grip; (c), key grip; (d), lockgrip.

a swan-neck deformity. The reverse can also occur in which the PIP is fixed in flexion and the DIP is hyperextended, the so-called boutonnière deformity. The thumb undergoes a similar deforming process in which the IP joint is extended and the MCP joint is flexed. This poses a significant functional problem for pinch or key grip because it renders the thumb unable to successfully oppose the index finger (Figure 14.2).

Tendon and tendon sheath involvement cause triggering and rupture. The hand may also undergo additional changes as a result of joint subluxation and other mechanical malalignments. Ulnar deviation of the fingers occurs as a result of the combination of intrinsic tightness, MCP subluxation, radial deviation of the wrist and the ulnarward slippage of the extensor tendons. Dynamically, this results in the inability to make a power grip, and possibly tip pinch of thumb to index or middle finger. Subluxation of the carpal bones can result in wrist flexion. Wrist flexion contractures render the hand unusable, because the fingers cannot extend. Proper wrist positioning is essential for hand function. When preservation of alignment is desired splints should be prescribed. Surgery may be needed for wrist or small hand joints.

Fortunately, there are lightweight, low temperature mouldable plastic materials available for splinting. Many ready-to-wear, hand splints are available, which are useful but not ideal for this population. Often patients need custom-moulded splints for proper fitting. The most frequently prescribed splints for the hand/wrist in RA include the functional wrist splint, the finger ring splint and the thumb stabilizing splint.

The **resting hand splint** may be useful for full wrist and finger immobilization. It renders the hand(s) unavailable for functional activity and so cannot be worn during the day.

The **functional wrist splint** is recommended for controlling pain and swelling in the wrist and for relieving carpal tunnel symptoms through its control of wrist position. This splint allows free movement of all digits and hence can be tolerated during waking hours. It permits the user to perform most daily routines.

Finger ring splints which may be fabricated from thermoplastic materials or metals control motion at a single joint. These are effective in reducing hyperextension at the PIP joint, as seen in swan-neck deformities or limiting flexion in the PIP, as seen in boutonnière deformities.

The *thumb post splint* is used to relieve pain in the carpometacarpal (CMC) joint, and the first MCP joint or to stabilize the first MCP.

Dynamic splinting of the hand has been used mainly in the postoperative period to assist in extension of the digits, but this type of dynamic splinting has also been used to align digits and to assist patients with mononeuritis who may have weak finger extensors (Melvin, 1982).

Lower limb

Knee orthoses in RA are used primarily for immobilization; that is, to stabilize the joint and reduce frontal plane deformity or keep the knee in extension. An ankle–foot orthosis can control knee flexion by positioning the ankle. Eliminating plantarflexion will maintain knee flexion; maintaining the foot in plantarflexion will favour knee extension.

Foot and ankle deformities are frequently seen in the arthritic patient. These include painful, swollen, subluxed MTP joints, cocked-toe deformities with corns and callous formation, hallux valgus, subtalar pain and collapse of the medial arch into a pes planus deformity with the calcaneus everted. These anatomical abnormalities are frequently associated with deviations in gait, either due to pain or deficits in critical ROMs or levels of strength. For example, muscle strength below the 3+ level is inadequate to put a limb through full range and would result in an observable gait deviation. Similarly, if the foot is unable to come to neutral, the toes may seem to drag. Abnormalities often spawn compensatory movement patterns that are not energy efficient.

The first therapeutic step is to help the patient accept a properly fitting, mechanically appropriate shoe. This is no simple matter because the combination of a cosmetically acceptable and comfortable shoe that will accommodate an orthosis is indeed rare! The shoe must be wide enough to accommodate the forefoot, deep enough to clear the toes and have adequate support of the medial column (arch) and the heel. A soft, cushioned sole and heel are often helpful in reducing the ground reaction forces. The heel may need support to control valgus deformity.

New materials of lightweight, heat-formable plastics and closed cell and microcellular rubbers, have rendered fabrication of foot orthotics convenient and affordable. Foot orthotic devices that go into the shoe, in conjunction with shoe modifications, or ankle–foot orthoses that come above the ankle are available to provide relief. The inserts commonly used are microcellular rubber MTP joint pads that are placed proximal to the joint and unload the weight from the subluxed metatarsal heads. A scaphoid pad or felt pad can be placed under the medial arch to prevent pes planus and relieve the navicular from bearing weight. Occasionally, the collapse of the medial arch is so profound and the subtalar joint pain is so disabling that the deformity must be treated with a rigid orthotic device that immobilizes the hindfoot (Gerber and Hunt, 1985). Weight on the involved lower limb can be reduced by using walking aids.

The neck

Neck pain arising from the upper rather than lower cervical spine synovial joints and the serious condition of C1–2 instability also needs to be addressed. Heat and TENS to the area of pain may be therapeutic. Seating should be in a chair with a supportive back that comes up to the level of the scapula and the head should be held in neutral with the chin slightly forward flexed and the neck retracted to provide a stretch to the extensor muscles of the neck. Sleeping posture is important and soft or contoured pillows with an occipital depression and a narrow foam band are recommended.

When the problem is atlanto-axial instability and flexion radiographs show more than 8 mm of subluxation of C1–2, spinal stabiliation may need to be considered. Occasionally there is also vertical displacement.

A cervical orthotic device is often required for activities that are associated with rapid flexion/extension. A SOMI type brace, which consists of a rigid neck brace with a chin attached, is recommended. Both the anterior and posterior portions are supported by struts. The Philadelphia collar is less cumbersome, better tolerated, but less restrictive of flexion/extension. This will reduce motion by 70%. The SOMI will reduce it by 90%. It is difficult for patients to don and doff these orthoses. They are prominent and often not cosmetically acceptable to patients. The four poster is usually rejected as too difficult to put on and whilst the soft collar frequently gives symptomatic relief of neck pain it needs to be recognized that it does not immobilize the neck.

Careful attention should be given to neck problems because of the potential for cervical cord damage or nerve root compression. Patients with RA have muscle atrophy and peripheral nerves are at increased risk of compression; for example carpal tunnel syndrome.

SURGERY

Surgery has a considerable part to play in maximizing function, though it is not used alone. The long-term aim of surgery is not only to reduce pain but to prevent malignment which in weightbearing joints will eventually produce premature osteoarthritis in joints distal to the involved one (and often pain in proximal ones including the back). Similarly in the hands prevention of further joint and tendon damage may be a legitimate aim of surgery. To maximize the benefits of surgery, the RA should be as inactive as possible.

Arthrodesis of the wrist is a worthwhile procedure for the above reasons, arthrodesis elsewhere is less often undertaken and it has been largely superceded by joint replacement surgery. Hip joint replacements are highly effective in increasing the range of functional hip movement and decreasing pain: knee, shoulder and elbow replacements are increasingly available and should not be delayed too long: the person in a wheelchair has much more difficulty in resuming a normal life than the person who has not given up working. The adult whose job is threatened may need surgery rapidly, as may the young person who requires access to training, leisure and social activities to establish his/her adult identity. Often the surgeon will have in mind a 'fall back' position should the joint replacement later fail and the gains in the years given by the surgery will be agreed by all as having been worthwhile.

ENVIRONMENTAL ADAPTATIONS

The individual with RA has to adapt to new physical and emotional challenges. Those advising the patient should take the information that was gathered from the rehabilitation evaluation and mesh that with the patient's goals. It is critical to support all the key roles in an individual's life. This is a complex situation, often requiring the use of adaptive equipment, environmental adjustment and strategies for utilizing social and vocational services.

The daily life routines of bathing, grooming, dressing, eating, food preparation and domestic chores have to be addressed.

Some, such as domestic activities, may be delegated or paid for. For those which **have** to be done adaptive devices are available. These may extend reach, save energy, reduce joint stress or increase grip strength (Arthritis Foundation, 1988). They range from raised toilet seats, grab bars and bath seats, to reachers, utensils and writing implements with built-up handles. Mobility aids such as canes, crutches and walkers, motorized scooters and adapted mobility aids (i.e. with forearm supports) are often most useful during the course of RA. General principles for the use of these are to provide pain-free functional activity, reduce energy expenditure and limit fatigue, and to promote independence in performing tasks beyond the patient's reach.

SOCIAL EFFECTS

Appearance may be altered by medication and the joint deformity. Clothing, make-up and hair management may present serious obstacles to an individual who may already be depressed or frightened. Adapted clothing, workshops for fashion and adaptive equipment for grooming may be helpful, but it must be recognized that the problem is perceived as major by many.

Intimate sexual relationships, as well as normal social interchanges, may be affected by the disease. Sexual intercourse may be painful due to joint pain, especially from the hips and may be unwanted because of mood, fatigue or alteration in libido. These changes may be secondary to medication. In addition there may be poor self esteem and poor body image. These problems can be helped (ARC publication Arthritis: Sexual aspects and parenthood; see Appendix).

Gainful employment, whether inside or outside of the home, is desirable and necessary for most people. Newer legislation in the USA has changed the standards for the workplace and improved accessibility. In the

USA vocational counselling is generally available and work-site modification and/or retraining is often the outcome of this kind of activity. The Social Security Act in the USA provides both disability insurance and supplemental income for those who meet criteria for disability. This act also assures medical coverage for the qualified. In the UK, an individual may be referred to the Department of Employment's Placement, Assessment and Counselling Team (PACT) for evaluation (Chapter 52)

UNPROVEN REMEDIES

People who have a chronic systemic illness that has significant impact on life activity seek help from many sources, often dictated by ethnic and social background, peer influence, information networking and idiosyncratic responses. The Arthritis Foundation has found that American adults spend $10 billion per year on 'alternative' treatment. An excellent review of the scope and variety of these therapies is available (Champion, 1994). These therapies often give the individual some rationale as to the cause of their disease and some apparent control over its development. It is important for the well-being of many to have a measure of control over their life rather than being blown where the disease takes them. More formal programmes developed by the Arthritis Foundation in the USA and by Arthritis Care in the UK aim to give the patient back some of this control over their lives, reducing the impact of disease on it to a manageable level.

REFERENCES

Affelct, G., Tennen, H., Urrows, S. *et al.* (1991) Individual differences in the day-to-day experience of chronic pain: a prospective daily study of rheumatoid arthritis patients. *Health Psychol*, **10**, 419–26.

Basford, J.R., Sheffield, C.G., Mair, S.D. and Ilstrup, D.M. (1987) Low energy helium neon laser treatment of thumb osteoarthritis. *Archives of Physical Medicine and Rehabilitation*, **68**, 794–7.

Beckham, J.C., D'Amico, C.J., Rice, JR, *et al.* (1992) Depression and level of functioning in patients with rheumatoid arthritis. *Canadian Journal of Psychiatry*, **37**, 539–43.

Belza, B.L., Henke, C.L., Yelin, E.H. *et al.* (1993) Correlation of fatigue in older adults with rheumatoid arthritis. *Nursing Research*, **42**, 93–9.

Blackmore, S. (1991) Is meditation good for you? *New Scientist*, **131**, 24–7.

Brattstrom, M. (1987) *Joint Protection and Rehabilitation in Chronic Rheumatic Disorders*, Wolfe Medical, London.

Champion, D.G. (1994) Unproven remedies: alternative and complementary medicine, in *Rheumatology*, vol. 8 P.A. (eds J.H. Klippel and P.A. Dieppe). Mosby, London, pp. 1–15.

Danneskjold-Samsoe, B., Lyngberg, K., Risum, T. *et al.* (1987) The effect of water exercise therapy given to patients with rheumatoid arthritis. *Scandanavian Journal of Rehabilitation*, **19**, 31–5.

Depie, X., Zhongyi, Z. and Zuolu, S. (1992) Acupuncture treatment of rheumatoid arthritis and exploration of acupuncture manipulations. *Journal of Chinese Traditional Medicine*, **12**, 35–40.

Ekblom, B., Lorgren, O., Alderin, M. *et al.* (1974) Physical performance in patients with rheumatoid arthritis. *Scandinavian Journal of Rheumatology*, **3**, 121–7.

Ekdahl, C., Andersson, S.I., Mortiz, U. *et al.* (1990) Dynamic versus static training in patients with rheumatoid arthritis. *Scandinavian Journal of Rheumatology*, **19**, 17–26.

Fries, J.F., Spitz, P., Kraines, R.G. and Holman, H. (1980) Measurement of patient outcome in arthritis. *Arthritis and Rheumatism* **23**, 137–45.

Furst, G.P., Gerber, L.H., Smith CC. *et al.* (1987) A program for improving energy conservation behaviours in adults with rheumatoid arthritis. *American Journal of Occupational Therapy* **41**, 102–11.

Gault, S.J. and Spyker, J.M. (1969) Beneficial effects of immobilization of joints in rheumatoid arthritis and related arthritides. *Arthritis and Rheumatism* **12**, 34–9.

Gerber, L.H. (1981) Principles in the rehabilitation of patients with rheumatic diseases, In *Textbook of Rheumatology*, 1st edn (eds W.N. Kelley *et al.*). Saunders, Philadelphia, chap. 12.

Gerber, L.H. and Hunt, G.C. (1985) Evaluation and management of the rheumatoid foot. *Bulletin of the New York Academy of Medicine*, **61**, 359–68.

Gerber, L.H., Furst, G., Shulman, B. *et al.* (1987) Patient education program to teach energy conservation behaviours to patients with rheumatoid arthritis: a pilot study *Archives of Physical Medicine and Rehabilitation*, **68**, 442–5.

Gerber, L.H. and Furst, G.P. (1992) Validation of the NIH activity record for patients with musculoskeletal disorders. *Arthritis Care and Research*, **5**, 151–6.

Arthritis Foundation (1988) *Guide to Independent Living: for people with arthritis*, Arthritis Foundation, Atlanta.

Harkcom, TM., Lampman, R.M., Banwell, B.F. and Castor, C.W. (1985) Therapeutic value of graded aerobic exercise training in rheumatoid arthritis. *Arthritis and Rheumatism*, **28**, 32–39.

Harris Jr, E.D. and McCroskery, P.A. (1974) The influence of temperature and fibril stability on degradation of cartilage collagen by rheumatoid synovial collagenase. *New England Journal of Medicine*, **290**, 1–6.

Huskisson, E.C., Jones, J. and Scott, P.J. (1976) Application of visual analog scales to the measurement of functional capacity. *Rheumatology and Rehabilitation*, **15**, 185–7.

Kushner, I. (1989) Does aggressive therapy of rheumatoid arthritis affect outcome? *Journal of Rheumatology*, **16**, 1–3.

Lorig, K., Chastain, R.L., Ung, E. *et al.* (1989) Development and evaluation of a scale to measure perceived self-efficacy in people with arthritis. *Arthritis and Rheumatism*, **32**, 37–44.

Lyngberg, K.K., Ramsing, B.U., Nawrocki, A. *et al.* (1994) Safe and effective isokinetic knee extension training in rheumatoid arthritis. *Arthritis and Rheumatism*, **37**, 623–8.

Mannheimer, C., Lard, S. and Carlsson, C.A. (1978) The effect of transcutaneous electrical nerve stimulation (TENS) on joint pain in patients with rheumatoid arthritis. *Scandinavian Journal of Rheumatology*, **7**, 13.

Meenan, R.F., Gertman, P.M. and Mason, J.H. (1980) Measuring health status in arthritis: the arthritis impact measurement scales. *Arthritis and Rheumatism*, **23**, 146–52.

Melvin, J.L. (1982) *Rheumatic Disease: occupational therapy and rehabilitation*, 3rd edn, Davis, Philadelphia.

Melzack, R. and Wall, P.D. (1965) Pain mechanisms: a new theory. *Science*, **150**, 971–9.

Michlovitz, S.L. (1990) The use of heat and cold in the management of rheumatic diseases, in *Thermal Agents in Rehabilitation*, 2nd edn (ed. S. Michlovitz), Davis, Philadelphia, pp. 158–74.

Minor, M.M., Hewett, J.E., Webel, R.R. *et al.* (1989) Efficacy of physical conditioning in patients with rheumatoid arthritis and osteoarthritis. *Arthritis and Rheumatism*, **32**, 1396–405.

Perlman, S.G., Connel, K. and Albert, J. (1987) Synergistic effects of exercise and problem solving education for RA patients. *Arthritis and Rheumatism*, **13**, 305.

Pincus, T., Summey, J.A., Soraci Jr, S.A. *et al.* (1983) Assessment of patient satisfaction in activities of daily living using a modified Stanford health assessment questionnaire. *Arthritis and Rheumatism*, **26**, 1346–53.

Pincus, T., Callaghan, L.F., Sale, W.G. *et al.* (1984) Severe functional declines, work disability, and increased mortality in seventy-five rheumatoid arthritis patients studied over nine years. *Arthritis and Rheumatism*, **27**, 864–72.

Ritchie, D.M., Boyle, J.A., McInnes, J.M. *et al.* (1968) A measurement of arthritic joints. *Quality Journal of Medicine*, **37**, 393–6.

Sanders, D.B. (1985) Acupuncture for rheumatoid arthritis: an analysis of the literature. *Seminars in Arthritis and Rheumatism*, **14**, 225–31.

Sternberg, E.M., Hill, J.M., Chrousos, G.P. *et al.* (1989) Inflammatory mediator induced hypothalamic-pituitary-adrenal axis activation is defective in streptococcus cell wall arthritis in susceptible Lewis rats. *Proceedings of the National Academy of Sciences USA*, **86**, 2374–8.

Wessel, J. and Quinney, H.A. (1984) Pain experienced by persons with rheumatoid arthritis during isometric and isokinetic exercise. *Physiotherapy Canada*, **36**, 131–143.

Xinlian, L., Shuying, Y., Chenggui, L, *et al.* (1993) Effect of acupunctuure and point injection treatment on immunological function in rheumatoid arthritis. *Journal of Traditional Chinese Medicine*, **13**, 174–8.

Companies (USA only) supplying adaptive equipment, splints and splinting materials, and instruments for testing hand function.

North Coast Medical, Inc.
187 Stauffer Boulevard
San Jose
CA 95125
USA

Smith & Nephew Rehabilitation
One Quality Drive
PO Box 1005
Germantown
WI 53022
USA

Sammons Preston
PO Box 5071
Bolingbrook
IL 60440
USA

Appendix

THE ARTHRITIS & RHEUMATISM COUNCIL

A New Hip Joint ......   Polymyalgia Rheumatica (PMR) ......
A New Knee Joint ......   Psoriatic Arthritis ......
Alternative Medicine ......   Reactive Arthritis ......
Ankylosing Spondylitis ......   Rheumatoid Arthritis ......
Are You Sitting Comfortably? ......   Scleroderma ......
Arthritis: Sports Injuries ......
   sexual aspects & parenthood ......   Stairlifts ......
Backache ......   Student Handbook
Choosing Shoes ......   (NB: FOR STUDENTS) ......
Diet & Arthritis ......   Tennis Elbow ......
Dermatomyositis/ Polymositis ......   The Painful Shoulder ......
Driving & Your Arthritis ......   When a Young Person has Arthritis
Fibromyalgia ......   (N.B. FOR TEACHERS) ......
Gardening with Arthritis ......   When Your Child has Arthritis ......
Gout ......   Work Related Rheumatic
Introducing Arthritis ......   Complaints ......
Joint Hypermobility ......   Your Home & Your Rheumatism ......
Knee Pain in Young Adults ......
Lupus (SLE) ......   INFORMATION SHEETS
Osteoarthritis ......   Allergy ......
Osteoarthritis of the Knee ......   Drugs & Arthritis ......
Osteoporosis ......   Exercise ......
Pain in the Neck ......   Weather ......

15 Amputation

R. Luff

INTRODUCTION

It may seem simplistic to describe amputation as an operation which cannot be undone. However, for a full understanding of care of the amputee, it must be appreciated that the irreversible nature of the surgery means that the patient, carers and health care professionals must look forward to the development of new skills and abilities. This is very different from the typical concepts about limb loss which are essentially negative in outlook. Too often, emphasis is placed on the loss of ability resulting from the 'failure' of accepted medical and surgical treatment. Limb ablation, apart from the unusual (in the UK) cases in which limb loss results immediately from trauma, entails the removal of an appendage which is no longer of any functional value and may be actively life threatening.

SCOPE

This chapter addresses all clinicians who work with adults with limb deficiency. Passing reference will be made to the small but important group of adults with congenital limb deficiency but the text concentrates on those with acquired deficiency. For those with a special interest in amputee care a further reading list is provided. The rehabilitation practices described relate to those current in the UK; there may be differences, minor and major, in aetiology and prosthetic practice elsewhere in the world. Basic principles of the surgery, assessment and rehabilitation however will not differ.

HISTORICAL PERSPECTIVE

Limb ablation as a therapeutic procedure has an extremely long history. A review of the history of amputation surgery, prosthetics and rehabilitation is given by Wilson (1992). Much of the surgery has been in the literature for centuries – the myocutaneous transtibial amputation for instance, described in 1695 by Verdyun – as have the prostheses. The author has recently withdrawn a prosthesis from an elderly user which is virtually identical to that supplied to the Marquis of Anglesey in 1815.

EPIDEMIOLOGY

The pathology giving rise to amputation has a marked influence on the rehabilitation goals for an amputee. It is only in the last century that amputation has become a treatment option for anything other than life-threatening complications of trauma. Regrettably, limb ablation is still undertaken as an emergency procedure; more commonly it is an elective procedure made necessary by irreversible change – necrosis, loss of function or malignant change. In the developed world, it is an

Rehabilitation of the Physically Disabled Adult. Edited by C. John Goodwill, M. Anne Chamberlain and Chris Evans. Published in 1997 by Stanley Thornes (Publishers) Ltd, Cheltenham. ISBN 0-7487-3183-0.

operation of the middle or later years of life with active survivors in the ninth decade being by no means the exception. The most common pathological processes are end-stage obliterative arterial disease and the microangiopathic and neurological consequences of diabetes. In the developing world, the modal age is substantially younger and the aetiology is much more concerned with trauma and infection.

Major risk factors in the developed world are those for arterial disease – hypertension, obesity, diabetes, hyperlipidaemia, tobacco smoking; the expected downturn in amputation arising from end-stage arterial disease as the population changes its smoking habit has yet to be clearly seen. Tobacco consumption is increasing in the developing world and this may substantially alter current aetiological patterns. The impact of the armaments industry on limb loss, particularly of distal lower limb loss, is marked in countries where very large numbers of antipersonnel mines have been deployed.

It is difficult to provide accurate estimates of the prevalence of limb loss and the incidence of amputation since data is collected incompletely in the UK. Approximately 10 000 amputations are performed per annum (Dormandy and Thomas 1988), of whom some 5000 are referred for prosthetic treatment annually. There is evidence that the impact of modern vascular surgery may reduce the incidence of amputation (Gutteridge, Torrie and Galland, 1994).

Table 15.1

Amputation level	No.	% of total
Hemipelvectomy	10	0.2
Disarticulation, hip	35	0.8
Transfemoral	2077	45.4
Disarticulation, knee	156	3.4
Transtibial	2174	47.5
Distal	124	2.7
Total amputations	4576	100.0

Data in Tables 15–15.3 are abstracted from *Amputation Statistics for England, Wales and Northern Ireland* (1987). Totals differ since some tables refer to amputees and others to amputations. Miscellaneous entries have not been included for clarity.

Table 15.2

Aetiology	Affected limb(s) (no.)			
	One leg	Both legs	One arm	Both arms
Trauma	296	10	100	0
Vascular	2917	110	20	2
Diabetes	992	41	0	0
Infection	92	3	4	0
Malignancy	157	0	37	0

See note to Table 15.1.

Tables 15.1–15.3 show extracts from the data set for England for 1987, giving information about aetiology, age and lower limb amputation level. Analysis of two 10-year cohorts of amputees in Scotland indicates that survival is improving (Stewart, Jain and Ogston, 1992), suggesting that the amputee

Table 15.3

Aetiology	Age (years)					
	0–9	10–19	20–39	40–59	60–79	80+
Trauma	1	33	158	93	41	7
Vascular	2	0	17	294	1563	323
Diabetic	2	0	5	140	507	68
Infection	1	0	13	13	28	2
Malignancy	0	11	26	28	37	10

See note to Table 15.1.

population may increase from this cause as it decreases following the impact of vascular reconstruction. An excellent discussion of the factors affecting the incidence of amputation is given by Barbsy *et al.* (1995).

The prevalence in the UK equates to 1.3 amputees per 1000, with similar figures quoted for the USA (Sanders and May, 1986). Individuals with limb deficiency but with no other concurrent, major pathology will have an almost normal survival expectation. Although amputations from trauma and congenital limb deficiency are in themselves rare in the UK, they will give rise to relatively large proportions of the amputee population. Limb loss from the more common aetiologies – obliterative arterial disease and diabetes – is associated with a relatively poor prognosis (Stewart, Jain and Ogston, 1992) and thus smaller component parts of the overall population.

AMPUTEE CARE TEAMS

Much amputee care is provided by groups of professionals orientated towards the specific needs of this patient group. The ideal team size is relatively small and large numbers of professionals are better employed in two or more complementary teams as described below. Rehabilitation begins as soon as amputation is considered; valuable opportunities are lost if the processes begin post-amputation.

The surgical phase

The team acting during the surgical phase comprises the potential amputee and carer(s), surgeon, counsellor, physiotherapist, occupational therapist, nurse, consultant in pain relief and consultant in rehabilitation medicine. This order does not reflect either sequence of involvement or importance to the amputee.

The discharge planning phase

At the stage at which discharge planning is taking place, the team extends to include the primary care physician and social work input. There is substantial overlap with the team undertaking later phases of the rehabilitation process; the prosthetist may be involved at preamputation consultation or later, as may a specialist physiotherapist and chiropodist. The latter may well have been involved in the individual's care long before amputation was considered. All major lower limb amputees will need a wheelchair in the early stages as described below. A significant proportion of the elderly lower limb amputation population will use wheelchair mobility for at least part of every day as one of the final rehabilitation goals.

The community phase

These teams will in turn overlap with the community-based team who will supervise the long-term care. From the rehabilitation standpoint, the amputee requires lifelong care, although the frequency of review decreases markedly once the amputee's condition and abilities have stabilized. This team will include the patient and any carer(s), the primary care physician, community-based therapists and nurses and an outpatient amputee care team – consultant in rehabilitation medicine, prosthetist, therapists, counsellor, chiropodist and orthotist.

Preamputation consultations

The ease with which preamputation consultations can take place varies considerably depending on local circumstances. Time should always be made available to listen and to inform any individual approaching amputation unless limb ablation is needed as an emergency. An informed and sympathetic surgeon together with a physiotherapist and nurse trained in amputee care can provide appropriate information and counselling. In the presence of uncertainty about rehabilitation outcome or of perceived need for high-level counselling, specialist help should be sought from an amputee care centre.

INFORMING THE POTENTIAL AMPUTEE

The patient and any carer(s) will need to know whether there is any alternative to amputation and what is involved in the procedure. Presurgical, surgical and postsurgical care and activities must be described in terms accessible to the lay persons involved. It is reasonable to give a realistic but guarded opinion on likely outcomes following amputation and to demonstrate the mechanism of force transmission through the residual limb. If time permits, and if the individual so wishes, access to a stabilized amputee of similar age, aetiology and amputation level should be offered. Self-help groups such as the Limbless Association (see Useful addresses) can help in this respect.

Phantom limb pain

Many potential amputees express considerable concern about phantom pain. This is an important element of information which must be made comprehensible to the patient and carers. It is valuable, for the reasons outlined below, to distinguish between phantom limb sensation and phantom pain (Jensen *et al.* 1983). The reported incidence of phantom pain has varied widely; it is reasonable to assume that most if not all amputees experience some phantom pain and to counsel them accordingly. The patient should be reassured that this is a natural phenomenon arising from amputation and that it is a temporary phase for the great majority.

Phantom limb sensation

Phantom limb sensation can be an extraordinarily real experience which results in an appreciable hazard to the new amputee since the individual may literally forget that the limb has been ablated. In the first few weeks after amputation, falls are not infrequent and occur when an attempt to stand to transfer or walk is made before safe transfers and prosthetic use are established. Reflex activity on falling results in damage to the amputation site causing bruising at the least and occasionally wound breakdown. This risk can be minimized by advising as early as possible that the risk exists and to raise self-awareness of the absence of the limb before any movement is made in the early post-amputation phase.

MULTIDISCIPLINARY PREAMPUTATION CONSULTATION

An amputating surgeon may seek a joint consultation preoperatively with the specialist amputee care team; issues discussed may include the advisability of amputation, level and technical options, aspects of postoperative care and likely outcomes. Clearly, the level of ablation has a major effect on realistic rehabilitation goals and the chances of achieving and sustaining them. It follows that surgical decisions and actions will in effect determine the nature of the discharge plan and the ease of its execution.

PREAMPUTATION CARE

Recent investigations into mental states of amputees (Hanspal and Fisher, 1991) indicate significant levels of anxiety. Early contact with rehabilitation services is thus beneficial in providing both counselling skills and information. Many of the conditions resulting in limb loss cause severe and sometimes disabling degrees of pain for which adequate and sustained pain relief should be provided. Complete pain relief for 72 hours before amputation results in reduced symptomatology from phantom pain (Bach, Norenz and Tjellden, 1988); epidural anaesthesia is of value in achieving this. After clear explanation of the procedure and its effects, epidural anaesthesia should be established for at least 24 hours before surgery and maintained for 45 hours postamputation. This relatively straightforward and safe technique is a short-term humane intervention with the valuable long-term benefit indicated above. In contrast, allowing distress in an individual after amputation as a result of inadequate analgesia represents mismanagement and puts the rehabilitation programme at risk. The advice of the local pain management team should be sought to facilitate the transfer to effective oral analgesia.

The general health of the amputee

Repeated courses of antibiotics and prolonged high-dose analgesia are frequent concomitants of the preamputation phase. Toxaemia together with the side-effects of drug treatment can result in prolonged malnutrition with the risk of infection, delayed wound healing and slowing of rehabilitation. Body index, plasma albumin and ferritin are useful indices. Dietetic advice should be sought if there is any doubt about nutritional status. Increase in body weight, often to a considerable extent, can be expected after amputation; this arises from the relief of pain, reduction in analgesic needs and elimination of toxaemia. Relative immobility and comfort eating may cause further weight increase.

EARLY POSTOPERATIVE MOBILITY

Mobility will be substantially reduced in the presence of rest pain whilst neuropathic ulceration may have necessitated prolonged periods of non-weightbearing. Attention to pain relief, nutrition and motivation will often restore a useful degree of mobility with appropriate aids (Figure 15.1) before amputation. This will expedite further rehabilitation. A chiropodist should treat the remaining foot and ensure, in collaboration with medical staff, that correct footwear is available. It is useful to remind the potential amputee that it is the remaining foot which requires correct footwear; the artificial foot can be adjusted to fit any shoe and it is an error to buy shoes to fit the artificial rather than the biological foot. Proximal amputation levels and intercurrent pathology may require use of a wheelchair for at least part of every day. A supportive stump board (Figure 15.2) should be fitted to the wheelchair for any amputation level distal to the transfemoral. Bilateral amputees, very proximal non-limb-wearing amputees and those at risk of early contralateral amputation should use wheelchairs having added stability, which is usually obtained by extending the wheelbase rearwards. Recent designs (e.g. see Figure 15.3) have variable rear axle mounts which permit very easy adjustment of stability.

Fitness training

Early mobilization of amputees requires sufficient strength to transfer and stand for long enough to permit casting, measurement and fitting of an artificial limb. Freedom of movement and dexterity to enable donning and doffing of the limb, upper limb strength to facilitate transfer and sit-to-stand and the exercise tolerance to work effectively under physiotherapy direction must be developed. A recent text (Burgess and Rappaport, undated) describes fitness regimes appropriate to the amputee athlete. Techniques which entail use of flexed joints, particularly the knee, should be avoided, as should hopping, since this places extreme loading on the – vulnerable and valuable – remaining foot.

GENERAL ISSUES IN AMPUTATION SURGERY

Confusion arises, especially amongst non-specialists, in the use of the terms **level** and **length** when discussing where to amputate –

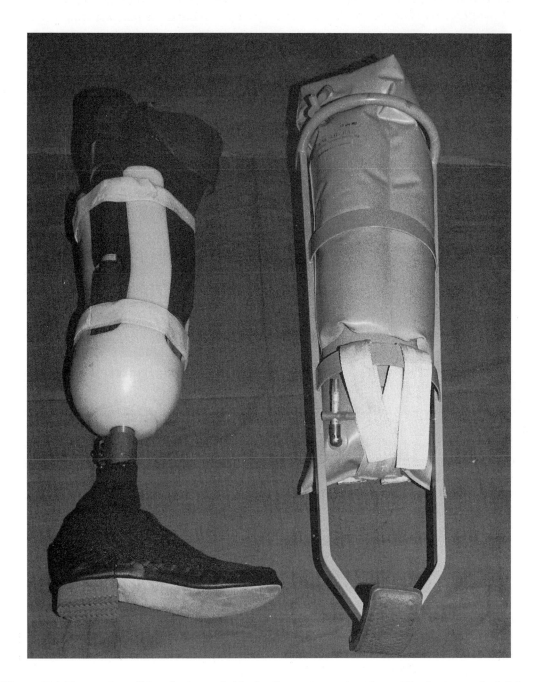

Figure 15.1 Two early walking devices suitable for the postoperative phase. The device on the left is a Tulip Limb and that on the right is the Pneumatic Post-Amputation Mobility Aid (PPAM aid or 'pamaid'). The Tulip is of use with stable transtibial stumps while the PPAM aid may be used for knee disarticulation and transfemoral stumps with the addition of further soft suspension (Figure 15.11).

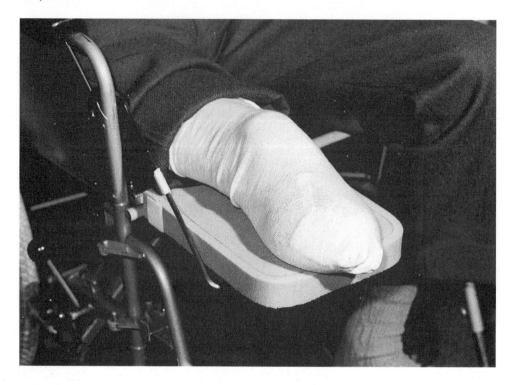

Figure 15.2 An adjustable stump support board suitable for a right limb amputee. The design allows the stump board to fold away in a similar fashion to the leg rest used for an intact limb.

the level – and how to reconstruct the residual limb – to determine its length. The amputation level can now be accurately described, except for cases of congenital deficiency, using internationally recognized descriptors (British Standard, 1993). These use the major bone transected, or the disarticulated joint and the site descriptor. The most common lower limb levels are thus **transtibial** and **transfemoral** (in place of 'below knee' and 'above knee'). Similarly, in the upper limb the most common sites of major loss are described as **transradial** and **transhumeral** (in place of 'below elbow' and 'above elbow'). Amputation through the knee joint carries the descriptor **knee disarticulation**. The complete standard contains internationally accepted descriptors for every aspect of acquired residual limb description. Congenital limb

deficiency is described by a separate standard descriptor set (International Standards Organisation, 1989).

Impact of site on outcome

It has long been accepted that in the lower limb preservation of a functioning knee joint is of substantial benefit to the individual in terms of resumption of independent walking and reduced energy cost of walking (Waters and Yakura, 1990). It follows that, with every more proximal amputation level, the likelihood of achieving independent walking decreases and for those who do walk the energy cost increases. There is an energy cost for any lower limb amputation proximal to the metatarsophalangeal joints; such amputees will walk slower and fatigue faster than a

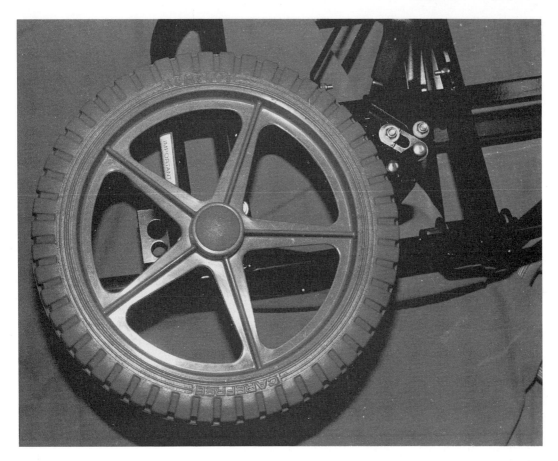

Figure 15.3 The axle mounting block for the rear wheel has several positions, the rearward offering increased stability whereas the forward position offers greater manoeuvrability (Access wheelchair manufactured by Remploy UK. Attendant-propelled model shown but self-propelled version is readily available.)

non-amputee matched for age, gender, equivalent medical condition and fitness.

Similar considerations with regard to the level of limb loss apply in the upper limb. Whilst the energy consumption issues are less marked, the functional loss increases dramatically with more proximal sites. It is axiomatic that loss of the functioning hand severely impairs the function of the residual limb, since replacement can at best provide only a grasping and positioning tool with very limited sensory feedback via socket and appendages.

Impact of residual limb length on outcome

The residual limb permits force transmission and provides sensory input. The design and construction of the residual limb will determine the interactions between the residual limb and the prosthesis; the prosthetic prescription will thus be markedly influenced by surgical decisions and procedures. It follows that for a given amputation level, there will be an ideal compromise between stump length, increase in which will increase lever arm length and surface area, and clearance from the end of the stump to allow for prosthetic components. As a **general** rule, amputation between the middle and distal thirds of the thigh will be appropriate for a transfemoral amputation and between the proximal and middle thirds of the tibia will be appropriate for the transtibial level. It is clear therefore that disarticulation levels, although providing great potential for force transmission (the knee disarticulation can be full weightbearing through its termination), will cause great difficulty in terms of prosthetic prescription especially artificial joint placement (Redhead *et al.* 1991).

Amputees whose rehabilitation goals are based on wheelchair use **will not benefit** from preservation of the knee and comprise a group for whom knee disarticulation or Gritti–Stokes amputations will be of greater value.

Length of the residual upper limb

The ideal length for amputation at any given level in the upper limb is more complex and consultation with an amputee rehabilitation centre is recommended. In general, preservation of any functional, sensate partial hand with digital remnants is worthwhile since reconstruction may be possible. Whilst a good cosmetic restoration is possible for transverse complete partial hand amputations (transmetacarpal, transcarpal), function may be poor. If grasp and carry functions are essential requirements, a more proximal transdiaphyseal amputation may be necessary.

Skin in the residual limb

In any residual limb, skin forms the immediate interface between outside forces and the amputee. Although amputation through insensate or grafted skin should be avoided if possible, modern prosthetic interface techniques (see below) can allow successful transmission of the necessary forces through such skin. Skin flaps should be designed to ensure successful healing in the first instance and ideally to avoid scar adherence to bone or divided nerves. The means of skin closure is immaterial to the quality of the mature scar.

Skin flap design

Flap design for the transfemoral level is not controversial, most surgeons using anterior and posterior equal flaps although a long anterior flap has theoretical advantages. Knee disarticulation is best closed to provide an anteroposterior scar in the midline. At the transtibial level there is no clear advantage of the well-established long posterior flap technique (Burgess *et al*, 1971) and the skew flap technique (Robinson, Haile and Coddington, 1982). The latter technique has the theoretical advantage of complying with the pattern of the microcirculation around the knee and the practical advantage of moving the terminal scar away from any risk of adherence to bone.

Muscle in the residual limb

Any amputation proximal to the digital level will require the section of some muscle. Two important considerations which affect subsequent rehabilitation are the length of muscle groups and their bulk. In general terms, any divided muscle should be re-attached at its physiological length. This is particularly important at the transfemoral level where the value of a well-constructed myoplasty (Neff, 1988) is increased by careful attention to the reattachment of the adductor muscles (Gottschalk, 1992).

At the transtibial level, muscle reattachment improves blood flow and healing and also results in improved protection of the bone ends and thus greater eventual function. It is crucial that the bulk of the muscle flap is reduced by excision of the soleus muscle, otherwise the resultant stump becomes divergent in shape and causes considerable difficulty   in   satisfactory   socket   design.

Occasionally, such stumps have to be refashioned.

Bone in the residual limb

Analysis of pressure experienced over curved surfaces shows that pressure is inversely proportional to the radius of curvature – the more acute the curve, the greater the local pressure. The 90° angle edge produced by transection of a long bone may result in very high local pressure. It is thus essential that **any** transected bone has the resulting sharp edges rounded off. This is nowhere more important than at the transtibial level where the traditional 'bevel' formed at the transected end of the tibia should be followed by careful rounding of every edge. Periosteum should not be stripped back.

Nerves in the residual limb

Every transected nerve will form a neuroma; the essence of nerve handling in amputations is to ensure that the resulting neuromas form in areas subject to minimal trauma and away from risk of adhesion to scar or bone. The simplest management – gentle traction and clean section allowing the nerve stump to retract into muscle – works well.

Avoidance of haematoma formation

All amputation stumps are constructed with large areas of tissue which may produce serosanguinous exudate and contain potential spaces where such exudates may collect. Suction drainage for 48 hours postamputation is valuable and does not delay rehabilitation.

Residual limbs – special cases

Almost all amputation stumps are ready for force transmission as soon as the wound has achieved stability with evidence of skin healing. Complete wound healing is not always necessary although consultation with an amputee care service is recommended in such cases. A few unusual levels require care, however. The Gritti–Stokes amputation is a modified knee disarticulation in which the articular surfaces of the patella and femoral condyles are excised and the exposed cancellous bone surfaces opposed. This stump has effectively a fracture in its construction and thus should not end bear for 6 weeks.

Modern prosthetic techniques have allowed much more successful fitting of partial foot amputation stumps including the Syme amputation but at such distal levels the skin wound is vulnerable and most surgeons wait for 6 weeks before weightbearing.

CARE OF THE RESIDUAL LIMB

Any healing amputation wound is susceptible to trauma, oedema and infection and any of these may give rise to distress to the patient and delay rehabilitation. The environment of the residual limb is thus of importance in setting the scene for effective rehabilitation. In centres where the necessary resources are available, a **carefully fashioned** plaster of Paris dressing may be applied (Burgess, Traub and Wilson, 1967). This may be combined with either immediate or early postoperative prosthetic fitting. Most centres in the UK perform too few amputations to make this technique appropriate and find that removal of the surgical dressing on the third postoperative day, with subsequent application of a two-layered sheath of one-way stretch Tubifast over dry dressings, is effective. This allows easy wound inspection and mobilization and does not require extensive specialist resources. Early walking aids are used as detailed below.

THE THERAPISTS' ROLES

The role of therapists, especially the physiotherapist, in amputee care is complex. This has recently been described in detail (Engstrom and Van de Ven 1993). In

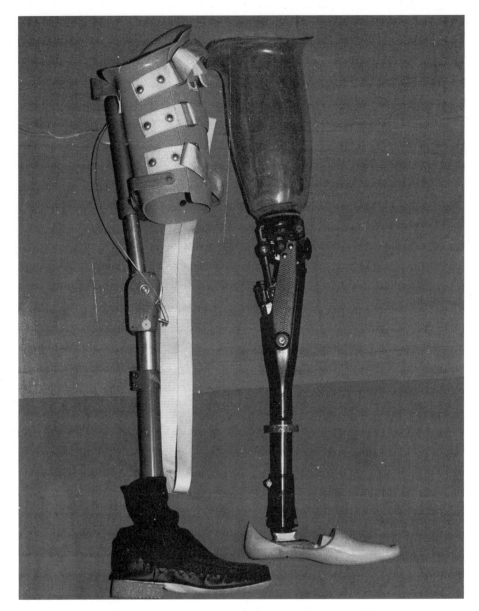

Figure 15.4 Early walking and assessment devices suitable for the transfemoral stump. The device on the right is a modular (Blatchford Endolite) assessment prosthesis with a clear thermoplastic (Northplex) diagnostic socket. The device on the left is the Femuret, again with volume adjustable socket. This device employs an adjustable shoulder strap for suspension and incorporates a therapist-controlled optional knee lock, but can also be used with a soft suspension (see Figure 15.11).

essence, the physiotherapist takes a pivotal role in ensuring pain-free early mobilization of the whole patient, building on the fitness training mentioned above. At the appropriate time, an early walking aid (Figures 15.1 and 15.4) will be introduced. In conjunction with an occupational therapist, assessment of the amputee will allow prescription of the correct wheelchair which should always have some form of stump support for any amputation at or distal to the knee disarticulation. This will minimize dependent oedema formation and reduce stump pain.

EARLY WALKING AIDS

Early walking aids (Figures 15.1 and 15.4), of which the pneumatic postamputation mobility aid (the PPAM aid or 'pamaid') is the best known in the UK, provide three-fold function – assessment of the patient, treatment of the residual limb and treatment of the whole patient. Proven benefits include oedema reduction and promotion of healing.

Various forms of early walking aids are in use in the UK. Their use is often delayed as a result of unnecessary caution, since they may be safely used from the seventh postoperative day given normal tissue nutrition or from the tenth postoperative day in dysvascular cases. Introduction to force transmission is gradual, progressing through acceptance of the necessary pressure, weight transfer, and partial weight bearing to walking within parallel bars. Some devices such as the Femuret can be fully weightbearing.

Early walking aids are more cumbersome than the equivalent prosthesis and it can be assumed that the ability to stand and walk at this stage is a good prognostic sign for benefit from subsequent prosthetic treatment. This assessment role is a valuable extension of the treatment aspects of this phase of amputee care. The physiotherapy opinion after an early walking aid assessment is frequently the determining factor in the development of definitive rehabilitation plans. The author's practice in situations of doubt after early walking assessment is to proceed to an assessment prosthesis (e.g. see Figure 15.4); a pair of such prostheses is used for goal setting for bilateral transfemoral amputees before any prescription is made.

CARE OF THE REMAINING LIMB

Every amputee, upper or lower limb deficient, is heavily dependent on the remaining limb. The issues for the upper limb are straightforward and require sensible care and adequate insurance against further limb loss. In the lower limb, pathological processes are frequently bilateral and the remaining limb must be protected as actively as possible. The contralateral limb requires full assessment, concentrating particularly on its circulation, nutrition and innervation. Foot care including chiropody is of the utmost importance; appropriate footwear should be provided as a matter of course if there is any doubt about the suitability of the amputee's own footwear.

POSTAMPUTATION CARE

Assessment of the amputee is a continuous process which starts from the moment that amputation is first considered until the final treatment plan has been executed and stabilized. All members of the care teams outlined above take part in the process and the outcome of assessment must be owned by all those concerned, particularly the amputee and the carers. Exchange of information and views is essential and some elements of the assessment such as early walking aid trials may need to be repeated at intervals. Many amputations take place at the end of heroic attempts to preserve a limb and leave the patient physically and emotionally exhausted. Assessment too early can thus be misleading and a reasonable period must be given to await the return of optimal health.

Planning appropriate goals

Rehabilitation goals are specific to the individual amputee. Making the amputee less dependent in transfers may be just as important for one as is return to full-time employment or to vigorous sport for another. This should be remembered when some forms of outcome measure are quoted. Assessment must be holistic and consider not only the amputation but also the individual in physical, mental and social terms in their own environment(s). This will permit the first stage of rehabilitation programming which aims to develop the competencies needed for safe and sustained discharge from hospital. The relevant goals must be determined and agreed and a timetable established. This will involve a prosthetic stage for all those deemed likely to benefit; all amputating services remote from an amputee care service will need to be particularly careful about communication and liaison.

Timing of prosthetic treatment

Prescription, casting and measurement should be possible on the fourteenth postoperative day when skin circulation and nutrition is normal (trauma, malignancy) and on the twenty-first day in the presence of circulatory deficiency or diabetes. Ideal stump configuration and minimal oedema may shorten these intervals by 3–5 days. Modular systems are used from the very first prescription. Temporary cosmetic covers shorten delivery times but their use must be explained to the amputee who may otherwise find the cosmetic deficit unacceptable.

Gait re-education with the first prosthesis follows a sequence common to all lower limb levels of amputation:

- full weightbearing and weight transfer;
- walking within parallel bars, turning by stepping;
- walking with sticks between parallel bars;
- walking with one stick between parallel bars;
- walking with aids out of the bars;
- optimal gait with minimal walking aids.

Some amputees may need to work through a walking frame stage initially. Crutches – elbow, Canadian and axillary – are best avoided in elderly amputees for the reasons

mentioned above. The younger patient may find crutches allow more rapid movement but such use should be carefully monitored since it is energetically inefficient and may delay rehabilitation.

FOLLOWING UP THE AMPUTEE

Amputation aetiology usually gives rise to the need for follow up by the hospital care team. Amputees whose discharge plans are based on wheelchair use will required follow up by community disability teams as well. Where prosthetic treatment is continued, amputee care services will arrange continued care. In the UK, this is by direct access since it is recognized that there is a need for continual maintenance of amputees in the community without repeated reference to primary care physicians. Such access often includes continued chiropody care and footwear provision.

PROSTHETIC PRESCRIPTION IN GENERAL

All prostheses which act as artificial limbs have certain features in common and may be prescribed for cosmetic, everyday or specialized use. The common features are:

- an interface with the residual limb;
- a socket structure;
- a skeletal structure;
- articular structures;
- terminal structures;
- a cosmetic covering;
- a suspension.

It is convenient to describe prostheses as being exo-skeletal in which the external skin is both the skeletal structure and the cosmetic covering, and endo-skeletal (often called 'modular') in which the internal components form an internal force-transmitting structure and there is a separate external cosmetic covering. The great majority of modern prosthetic designs fall into this latter category.

THE INTERFACE BETWEEN STUMP AND SOCKET

In pressure differential socket designs, the stump skin is in direct contact with the material of the inner surface of the socket. An intimate and stable fit is essential to ensure retention of the prosthesis (see below) and the design must be optimal to protect the vulnerable proximal skin ('surface matching', B. Klasson, personal communication). The interface material can be chosen from flexible or rigid thermoplastics, laminate, metal or wood. The amputee must be able to draw the stump into the socket to ensure accurate and effective donning.

Suction/adhesion designs use varieties of silicone (Figure 15.5) as the interface. Despite its (justified) reputation for causing transient increases in perspiration, this is the interface of choice when dealing with a stump covered with substantial areas of skin graft. Owing to elastic stretching of the silicone during swing phase, it is less satisfactory in active transfemoral amputees. Some of the newer materials in use provide excellent interface properties with the ability to 'creep' to allow for small changes in stump volume.

All other socket designs use some form of stump sheath (sometimes called stump socks) as the interface. Nylon sheaths are used to provide a degree of relief from shear although silicone-lined sheaths, such as those produced by Otto Bock, are more successful. Cotton sheaths come in various thicknesses and weave types and have the great advantage of being hot washable. The traditional stump sheath is wool and the typical delivery standard for this type of socket is 'a one wool sock fit'. The advantage of the various sheath materials and thicknesses, particularly for the amputee with an immature stump or who is subject to rapid volume fluctuation, is that fit can be easily adjusted by using combinations of sheaths. Such self-adjustment can be potentially hazardous and the amputee must clearly understand the technique before permission is given to vary fit independent of the prosthetist.

PROSTHETIC PRESCRIPTION FOR THE UPPER LIMB

The only obligate users of upper limb prostheses are bilateral amputees who are unable to substitute missing abilities by lower limb function. Unilateral arm amputees have a relatively low uptake and continued use of prostheses which must be regarded as poor substitutes for the ablated limb. A summary of UK practice in prosthetic prescribing may be found in Day, Kulkarni and Datta (1993).

Cosmetic prostheses can be made for any level of limb ablation including transpectoral. These can be exo- or endo-skeletal, the former being substantially lighter (Figure 15.6) but more difficult to adjust if an alternative finger position is required. Complete ablation of the upper limb including the pectoral girdle is usually replaced with a simple shoulder cap to restore the shoulder contour, although full 'functional' restorations can be prescribed.

Functional prostheses may be fabricated to a variety of specifications depending on desired use and may be body powered or externally powered. A prosthesis for body-powered function for a transradial amputee is shown in Figure 15.7, together with an externally powered prosthesis for a similar level of limb loss. This prosthesis has electrodes to permit control of the battery-powered electric hand by selective contraction of the flexor and extensor muscle groups in the residual limb (myoelectric control; Datta and Brain, 1992). Every articulation – shoulder, elbow, wrist and hand – can be externally powered as in the Boston arm but the resultant function rarely merits the very substantial resource implications.

The aspect of arm prostheses most often on view is the terminal device. The most effective of these in replacing function – although of very poor aesthetic appeal – is the split hook (Figure 15.8), of which there are several

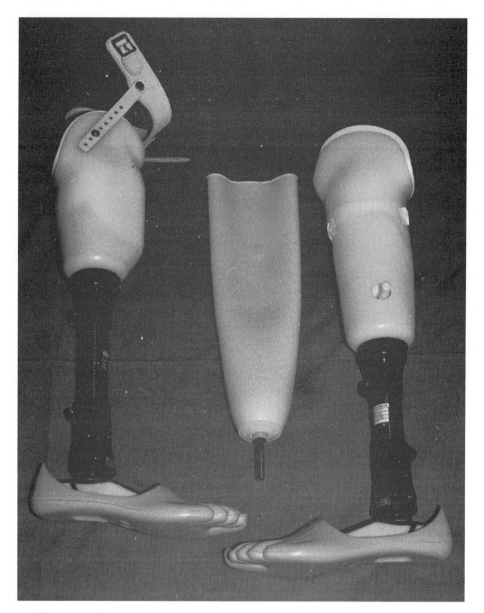

Figure 15.5 These endoskeletal prostheses (shown without cosmetic coverings) for the transtibial level show a traditional form of suspension – the leather cuff with adjustable tabs – and a recent development, the silicone suspension sleeve (Iceross manufactured by Ossur, Iceland). The shuttle pin is clearly seen on the closed end of the sleeve, whilst the shutter lock release button is visible on the socket shell.

externally powered versions. Many prescriptions will include a disconnection interface to allow exchange with other terminal devices such as body-powered hands or cosmetic (non-functioning) hands. Figure 15.7 shows both externally powered and body-powered hands. The wide range of socket design, articulations, terminal devices and control

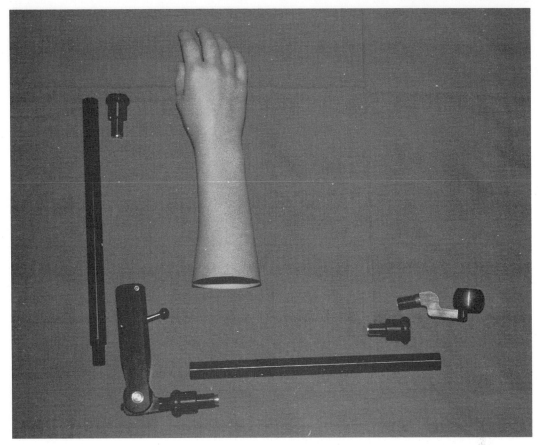

Figure 15.6 Two approaches to lightweight cosmetic prostheses for upper limb loss. The one-piece cosmetic forearm unit (manufactured by Hosmer USA) is a plastic shell comprising forearm and hand; finger position may be adjusted by warming. This may be combined with a laminate socket to form a very lightweight cosmetic forearm prosthesis. The unit is shown without the high-definition silicone covering normally used. Disassembled components of a modular prosthesis (manufactured by Vessa UK) for a shoulder disarticulation are shown. The assembled endoskeleton is covered with a foam fairing, an appropriate hand fitted – cosmetic foam or shell hands or externally powered units may be used – and a high definition silicone hand covering fitted.

systems available are beyond the scope of this chapter but may be pursued in the appropriate texts given in the bibliography.

PROSTHETIC PRESCRIPTION FOR THE LOWER LIMB

Design issues

Prostheses for lower limb replacement, unless purely cosmetic in use, must be able to resist the forces transmitted during stance and gait over a reasonable period without risk of hazardous failure. All systems prescribed in the UK must comply with minimum standards determined by the Department of Health. They must comply with the Medical Devices Directive issued by the European Community and legally enforced from 1997. The necessary safety margins result in durable prostheses which

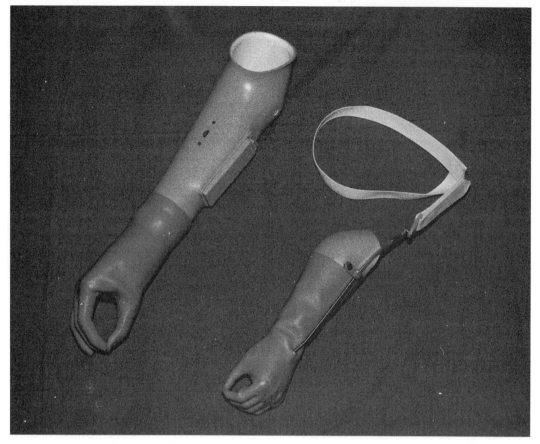

Figure 15.7 Two prostheses for forearm deficiencies. The prosthesis on the left has an externally powered hand and uses two site myoelectric control of the hand. The closing electrode can be seen where the cosmetic cover has been rolled back. In this small user, a remote battery pack with a belt clip is necessary. The prosthesis on the right has a body-powered hand. The operating cord leading to the axillary loop for the contralateral shoulder is shown.

have appreciable subjective and objective weights.

Cosmetic prostheses

Purely cosmetic lower limb prostheses are prescribed occasionally, usually in cases of bilateral transfemoral ablation. Such prostheses are made from lightweight foam and are pre-flexed to be used in the sitting position, most frequently in a wheelchair. They are not designed to permit any weight-bearing and may thus hinder wheelchair

transfers. This issue should be carefully explored with the amputee and involved therapists before prescription.

Power for lower limb prostheses

Unlike the arm prostheses described above, functional lower limb prostheses are entirely body powered although electrically powered design features are becoming more common (Figure 15.9), The driving force and sensory feedback come from the residual part of the limb; the efficacy of this is determined by

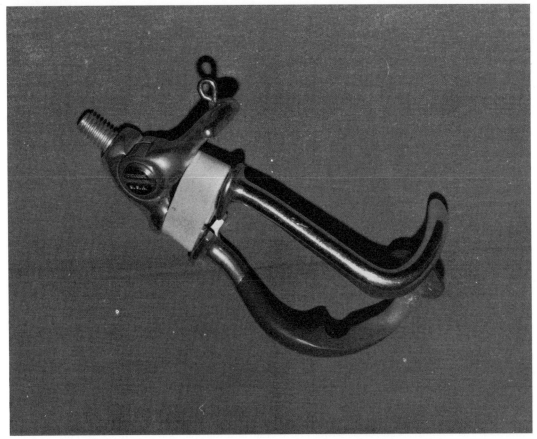

Figure 15.8 The alloy split hook terminal device. This is body powered using shoulder movement and an operating cord (as in Figure 15.7). Variation in the number of elastic bands fitted to the device provides variable grip; this device works as a voluntary opening hook, although voluntary closing units are available. (The jaws are held open by a small coin.)

socket design and fit and stability by the interactions between the musculoskeletal system and the prosthesis.

SOCKET PRESCRIPTION

Transfemoral

Socket prescription reflects assessment of the configuration of the stump and the quality of the soft tissues. Although the socket and its interface with the skin must replace the interface between the foot and the ground, the actual interface and socket shape vary considerably depending on the level of amputation. All levels proximal to the knee disarticulation use the structure of the true pelvis to ultimately transmit forces, the ipsilateral ischial tuberosity being employed except for transpelvic amputation when the contralateral structure is used. The tuberosity can provide support via a posterior shelf at the proximal brim – the quadrilateral socket – or by inclusion within the proximal part of the socket, the ischial containment socket. There is much discussion about the design of the latter socket and much variability in its execution.

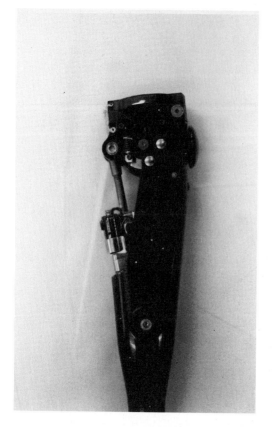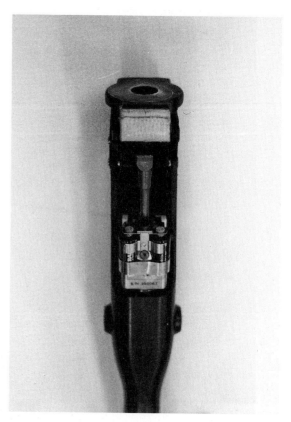

Figure 15.9 The computer-controlled swing phase unit for a transfemoral prosthesis (IP Plus manufactured by Blatchford). The knee joint is uniaxial, has a stance phase stabilizer and a stance phase shock absorber – the shock-absorbing pad can be seen in the lateral view, posterior to the knee pivot.

Overall support of the stump is best achieved by total surface contact with the socket interface. Suspension of the socket and thus the whole prosthesis is optimal in pressure differential ('suction') designs (Figure 15.10), but can also be provided by suction/adhesion (silicon sleeves, e.g. Iceross, or polyurethane, e.g. TEC), elastic support (TES (Figure 15.11); Otto Bock Elastic Support), Silesian belt or rigid pelvic band (the 'RPB').

Disarticulation

The knee disarticulation and modified ankle disarticulation (Syme's amputation) are com-

pletely end-bearing stumps capable of transmitting full body weight. Socket designs make use of this feature and frequently use the proximal waist of the stump to allow, by incorporating a self-retaining liner, self-suspension of the limb.

Transtibial

The transtibial level traditionally uses a variation of the patellar tendon bearing design (the 'PTB'), which is in fact a complex three-dimensional surface which exploits all the load-tolerant areas of the stump to transmit forces whilst protecting vulnerable areas. There are several techni-

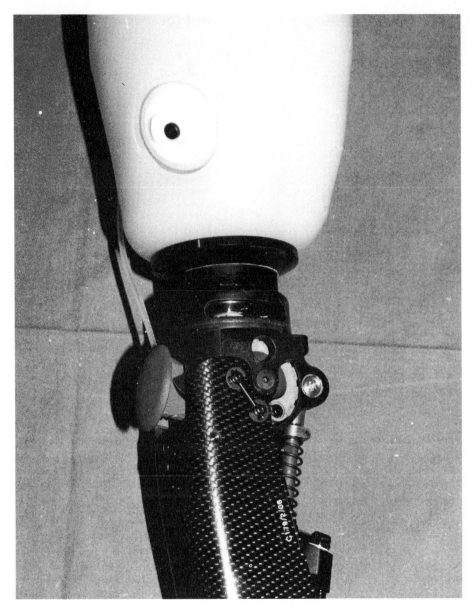

Figure 15.10 A suction socket forming part of a transfemoral prosthesis. The suction valve is seen in the distal zone of the socket. The user draws the stump fully into the socket with a sock or bandage through the valve aperture which is then occluded with the valve.

ques to achieve satisfactory sockets, each having particular usefulness for some stump configurations, and texts of prosthetics should be consulted for details (see Further reading). The recent re-introduction of positive pressure casting techniques but using very high pressure has all but eliminated cast modification and the

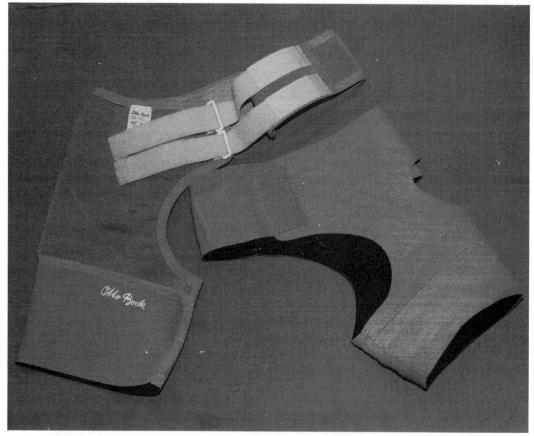

Figure 15.11 Soft suspensions used with transfemoral prostheses (from Otto Buck on the left and from Blatchford on the right).

concept of the PTB socket may need to be revised (O. Krissenson, personal communication).

Suspension for transtibial prostheses

There is a large variety of suspension options for the transtibial level from the traditional leather cuff and tabs through self-suspending designs to the silicon sleeve suction/adhesion designs (Figure 15.5). Again, suspension selection is a matter of prescription according to patient need and interacts with the socket design and the other components of the prosthesis.

Articulations

Ankle

The artificial ankle joint is unusual in prosthetic terms in needing to be polyaxial, although for decades amputees in the UK had to be content with a single axis design! Three distinct forms of ankle are in widespread use, the solid ankle, cushion heel (the 'SACH' or 'sash') foot, polyaxial ankles (e.g. the Blatchford Endolite Multiflex) and carbon fibre based foot/ankle/shin unitary systems (Springlite, Flex Foot; see Figure 15.12). An example of the SACH foot is seen on the waterproof limb shown in Figure 15.13. There

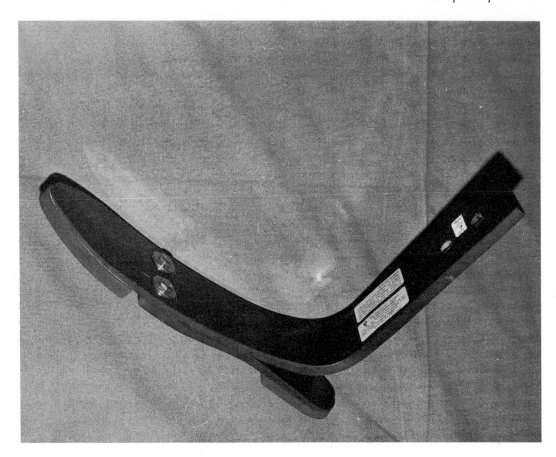

Figure 15.12 A high activity ankle/foot carbon fibre unit suitable for ankle disarticulation (manufactured by Flex Foot USA). The unit may be supplied with a complete cosmetic fairing.

are also various transitional types which combine solid ankle concepts with a variety of active heel and forefoot components (e.g. Blatchford Endolite Dynamic, Vessa Quantum, Carbon Copy 2). It is possible to combine some of the options to achieve particular desirable effects as in the poly-axial/SACH arrangement using Multiflex and Seattle components.

Knee

Knee joints may be unicentric or poly-centric but will only have one plane of movement. Minimal function but maximum stability and minimum weight can be achieved by a design which automatically locks when fully extended (the 'semi-auto-matic knee' or SAKL). This may be unlocked to provide knee flexion on sitting but will lock on standing. Free knee gait is more efficient and requires the additional prosthetic functions of stance phase stability and swing phase control. Stance phase stability can be produced by deliberate alignment, by specific knee joint design ('stabilized' knees) or by a combina-tion of the two. An optional knee lock can be prescribed to supplement these for occasional absolute stance stability.

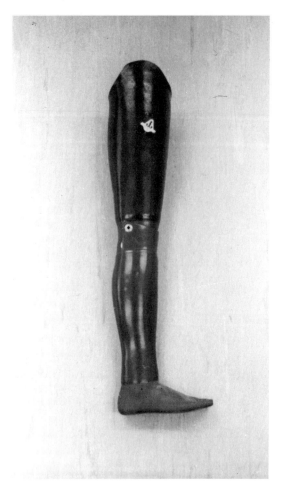

Figure 15.13 A waterproof (beach activity) prosthesis for the transfemoral level (Otto Bock). A suction socket provides suspension and the knee lock is optional. Note the basic SACH foot.

Swing phase control   Swing phase control is an important element in allowing a free knee walker to achieve an efficient and responsive gait. Increase in walking velocity requires control of swing phase time, which in turn entails limitation of knee flexion in the swing phase and acceleration of the distal limb segment into extension ready for the next heel strike (Chapter 8 provides more detail). Conventional swing phase control devices, pneumatic or hydraulic, can be adjusted for different gait velocities but will only work efficiently at that set velocity. The amputee is thus controlled by the prosthesis. It is now possible to prescribe a swing phase control (Blatchford Endolite I.P. Plus; (Figure 15.9) in which a sensor responds to change in the rate of knee flexion, causing the microprocessor to adjust the swing phase characteristics of the prosthesis.

Hip

The hip joint may similarly be uni- or polycentric but always moves through a single plane. A variety of types exist to provide free or lockable hip motion, stride length limitation and alternatives in joint position in sitting. The details may be obtained from specialist prosthetic texts (see Further reading).

Foot prescription

It is not possible to separate foot design from ankle design in modern prosthetics. The SACH design, of which the Seattle foot is a high performance version, has been mentioned above. Modern feet have reasonable cosmetic finishing with toes and can be prescribed with a separated hallux for sandal wear. The genuine running style of shin/ankle/foot unit is typified by Figure 15.14; here the whole unit deflects during the stance phase and the stored energy released to provide acceleration at the toe-off point. Amputee athletes have recorded remarkable achievements using adaptations of this design and acceptance of such designs is good (Alaranta *et al.* 1994).

The partial foot prosthesis

The modern prostheses for partial foot amputations, both transverse (transmetatarsal, transtarsal) and longitudinal (ray amputations) are a further special case of prosthetic foot design. Here, silicone materials are used

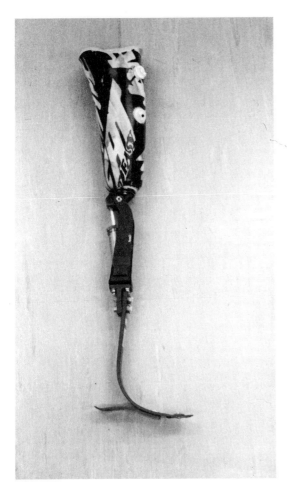

orthopaedic – and carbon fibre insoles, excellent function can be achieved. These prostheses can allow active full weightbearing on grafted plantar surfaces when only partial thickness skin graft has been used.

The importance of footwear heel height

A finished prosthesis can really only be considered in terms of the amputee/prosthesis/footwear complex and the final alignment will reflect every component of the complex, including the footwear. Should this be changed such that the effective heel height is altered, the entire alignment of the prosthesis will be affected and thus the comfort, stability and efficiency. Unfortunately, only the Masterstep design (Ossur) provides ready adjustment to allow for heel height adjustment by the amputee (apart from the obsolescent single axis ankle), yet **alignment error because of footwear change** is perhaps the commonest problem encountered in amputee clinics after changes of fit.

Special needs

Cosmesis

The final appearance of a prosthesis reflects the interactions of a number of factors:

- the stump configuration;
- the presence of joint deformity;
- the limb system in use;
- the cosmetic cover in use;
- prosthetic and technician skills.

As a consequence, the cosmetic result can be less than ideal for reasons beyond the control of a prosthetic service. The socket has to surround the stump and to prevent unsightly narrowing, the subsequent shaping has to blend in with this so further limiting scope for cosmetic improvement. Very high definition finishes are available using silicone materials

Figure 15.14 A prosthesis built for a transfemoral amputee who runs competitively. The suction socket has a further modification, seen as the white control device near the socket brim. This controls inflation/deflation of air sacs within the socket, placing the amputee in charge of minute to minute volume adjustment of the socket. The shin/ankle/foot unit is a carbon fibre high activity unit (Modular III Plex Foot with Split Toe, manufactured by Flex Foot USA).

to reconstruct the ablated foot (Kulkarni *et al.*, 1995) to provide interface, socket, structure and cosmesis as an entity (Figure 15.15). In combination with footwear – standard or

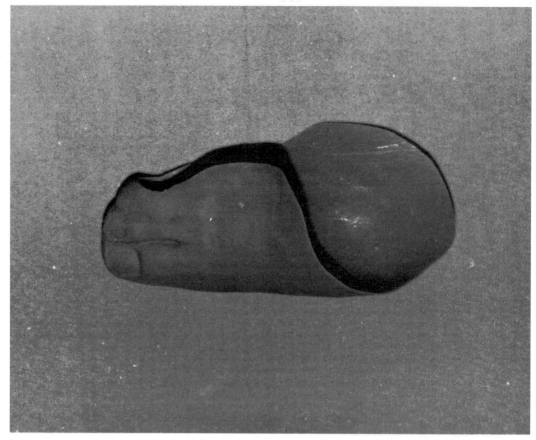

Figure 15.15 A custom-made silicone partial foot prosthesis (manufactured by Rehabilitation Services Limited UK) for a patient with distal loss affecting the first, second and third rays of the right foot.

but sometimes at a resource cost beyond the NHS provision.

Water resistance

Both exo- and endo-skeletal prostheses are not usually water resistant, so getting into water for showers or recreation using crutches or hopping can be hazardous. Where an amputee has a valid reason for regular access to wet environments, the provision of a specifically waterproof limb (Figure 15.15) is reasonable. These can be prescribed as such. For occasional protection from water, a protective sleeve as used for plaster cast protection is useful.

Heavy duty

The standard specification for prostheses is, as described above, aimed at reasonable everyday use. Amputees, both upper and lower limb, who are known to place very heavy demands on prostheses may be prescribed heavy-duty components. An example for the transfemoral level is shown in Figure 15.16.

Sports

This category is appropriate for lower limb amputees and refers principally to those taking part in high activity sports. Here a heavy-duty build needs to be combined with

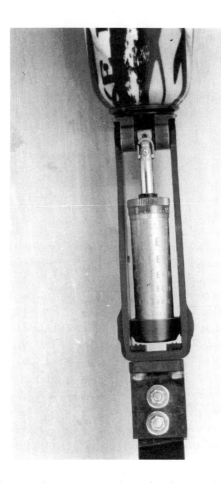

Figure 15.16 A heavy-duty performance prosthesis for the transfemoral level (manufactured by Blatchfords UK). The single axis knee and modular components are built to enhanced lamination and metallurgical specifications. The swing phase control is a durable hydraulic design (CaTech, USA).

components affording adjustment and extreme durability; for example, hydraulic swing phase controls and energy storing/releasing shin/ankle/foot systems (Figure 15.14).

Cultural needs

The importance of full assessment of the individual in appropriate environments was mentioned above. In addition to sporting requirements, cultural needs must be considered (Qureshi, 1994). Thus an alignment to allow barefoot walking may be necessary.

Similarly, floor-sitting societies require socket design which permits easy access to a comfortable position at floor level. For transfemoral or more proximal levels, an axial rotation device may be needed. Very vigorous walkers, those with shear problems in force transmitting skin and golfers find an axial torque absorbing device helpful.

DRIVING

It is unreasonable to bar any amputee from driving simply as a result of limb loss. Frequently, intercurrent disease is the determining factor. Upper limb amputees require a steering knob together with appropriate power assistance and usually automatic transmission. Lower limb amputees, even bilateral distal amputees, can drive standard vehicles with manual gearboxes. Unilateral proximal (transfemoral) amputees may require an additional accelerator pedal on the side of the remaining limb combined with automatic transmission. Bilateral proximal amputees need hand controls (Chapter 50).

OUTCOMES

Because of the very individualized nature of rehabilitation of amputees, development of a comprehensive outcome measure has proved difficult. The mobility measures currently used in the UK comprise the Harold Wood/ Stanmore scale (Hanspal and Fisher, 1991) and the Guys scale (Houghton *et al.* 1992). The Grise (Grise, Gauthier-Gagners and Martineau, 1993, 1994) scale is validated as a general outcome scale for amputees but is insensitive to change. Any presentation discussing outcomes should be analysed in terms of the amputee population and the forms of rehabilitation employed. Diversity in the field of amputee care makes interpretation of the literature difficult.

SUMMARY

This chapter surveys the care of adult amputees from the time when amputation is first considered through to the stage of the established and stabilized individual. It can be no more than a survey, however, and the interested reader is referred to the appropriate major texts and to specialist centres for more information. This is an exciting period for amputee rehabilitation during which microprocessor control has entered the field and shows signs of further and important development. For a proportion of the amputee population, perhaps the most exciting medium term prospect is the development of direct interfacing of the prosthesis with the skeleton – so

called osseointegration. Some aspects of amputee care and the consequent outcomes will change considerably in the near future.

REFERENCES

Alaranta, H., Kinnunen, A., Karkkainen, M., Pohjolainen, T. and Heliovaara, M. (1994) Practical benefits of Flex-Foot in below knee amputees. Journal of Prosthetics and Orthotics 3, 179–81.

Amputation Statistics for England, Wales and Northern Ireland (1987) Department of Health and Social Security.

Bach, S., Norenz, M.F. and Tjellden, N.U. (1988) Phantom limb pain in amputees during the first twelve months following limb amputation after pre-operative lumbar epidural seventy two hours pre-operation. Pain, 33, 297–301.

Barsby, P., Ham, R., Lumley, C. and Roberts, V.C. (1995) *Amputee Management: a handbook*, Kings College School of Medicine and Dentistry, London.

British Standard (1993) Prosthetics and Orthotics. Part 3. Method of describing lower limb amputation stumps. BS 7313: Part 3: ISO 8548–2: 1993, 1–16.

Burgess, M.D. and Rappaport, C.P. (undated) Physical fitness: a guide for individuals with limb loss. USA Veterans Administration Research and Development.

Burgess, E.M., Romano, R.L., Zettl, J.H. and Schrock R.D. (1971) Amputation of the leg for peripheral vascular insufficiency. *Journal of Bone and Joint Surgery* 53A, 874–89

Burgess, E.M., Traub, J.E. and Wilson, A.B. (1967) *Immediate Post-surgical Prostheses in the Management of Lower Extremity Amputees*, Published for the Prosthetic and Sensory Aids Service, Veterans Administration, Washington.

Datta, D. and Brain, N.D. (1992) Clinical applications of myoelectrically controlled prostheses. *Critical Reviews in Physical and Rehabilitation Medicine*, 4, 215–39.

Day, H.J.B., Kulkarni, J.R. and Datta, D. (1993) *Prescribing Upper Limb Prostheses*, Amputee Medical Rehabilitation Society, London.

Dormandy, J.A. and Thomas, P.R.S. (1988) What is the natural history of a critical ischaemic patient with and without his leg? in *Limb Salvage and Amputation for Vascular Disease*? (eds R.M. Greenhalgh, C.W. Jamieson and A.N. Nicolaides), W B Saunders Harcourt Brace Jovanovich, Philadelphia, pp. 11–26.

Engstrom, B. and Van de Ven, C. (1993) *Physiotherapy for Amputees – the Roehampton approach*, 2nd, edn, Churchill Livingstone, London.

Gottschalk, F. (1992) Transfemoral Amputation, in *Atlas of Limb Prosthetics: prosthetic and rehabilitation principles*, 2nd edn (eds J.M. Bowker and J.W. Michale),

Grise, M.C., Gauthier-Gagny, C. and Martineau, G.G. (1993) Prosthetic profile of people with lower extremity amputation: conception and design of a follow-up questionnaire. *Archives of Physical Medicine and Rehabilitation* **74**, 862–70.

Grise, M.C., Gauthier-Gagnon, C. and Martineau, G.G. (1994) Prosthetic profile of the amputee validity and reliability. *Archives of Physical Medicine and Rehabilitation,* **75**, 1309–14.

Gutteridge, W., Torrie, P. and Galland, R. (1994) Trends on arterial reconstruction, angioplasty and amputation. *Health Trends,* **26**, 88–91.

Hanspal, R.S. and Fisher, K. (1991) Assessment of cognitive and psychomotor function and rehabilitation of elderly people with prosthesis. *British Medical Journal,* **302**, 940.

Houghton, A.D., Taylor, P.R., Thurlow, S., Rootes, E. and McColl, I. (1992) Success rates for rehabilitation of vascular amputees: implications fore pre-operative assessment and amputation level. *British Journal of Surgery,* **79**, 753–5.

International Standards Organisation (1989) *ISO 8548–1: Prosthetics and Orthotics – limb deficiencies – Part 1: Method of describing limb deficiencies present at birth,* ISO Central Secretariat, Geneva.

Jensen, T., Krebs, B., Nielson, J. and Rasmussen, P. (1983) Phantom limb, phantom pain and stump pain in amputees during the first 6 months following limb amputation. *Pain,* **17**, 243–56.

Kulkarni, J., Curran, B., Ebdon-Parry, M. and Harrison, D. (1995) Total contact silicone partial foot prostheses for partial foot amputations. *Foot,* **5**, 32–5.

Neff, G. (1988) Surgery (of above knee amputation), in *Amputation Surgery and Lower Limb Prosthetics* (ed. G. Murdoch), Blackwell Scientific, Oxford.

Qureshi, B. (1994) *Transcultural Medicine,* 2nd edn, Kluwer Academic, Dordrecht.

Redhead, R., Day, H.J.B., Marks, L. and Lachman, S. (1991) *Prescribing Lower Limb Prostheses,* Disablement Services Authority.

Robinson, K.P., Hoile, R. and Coddington, T. (1982) Skew flap myoplastic below knee amputation: a preliminary report. *British Journal of Surgery,* **69**, 554–7. 1982.

Sanders, G.T. and May, B.J. (1986) *Lower Limb Amputations: a guide to rehabilitation,* F.A. Davis, Philadelphia.

Stewart, C.P.U., Jain, A.S. and Ogston, S.A. (1992) Lower Limb Amputee Survival. *Prosthetics and Orthotics International,* **16**, 11–18.

Wilson Jr, A.B. (1992) History of amputation surgery and prosthetics, in *Atlas of Limb Prosthetics: Surgical, Prosthetic and Rehabilitation Principles* (ed. J.H. Bowker and J.W. Michael), Mosby, St Louis.

Waters, R. and Yakura, J. (1990) Energy expenditure of normal and abnormal ambulation, in *Gait in Rehabilitation* (ed. G.L. Smidt), Churchill Livingstone, London.

FURTHER READING

Atkins, D.J. and Meier, R. (eds) 1989) *Comprehensive Management of the Upper Limb Amputee,* Springer-Verlag.

Bowker, J.H. and Michael, J.W. (eds) (1992) *Atlas of Limb Prosthetics,* Mosby Year Books, London.

Bowker, J.H. and Michael, J.W. (1992) *Atlas of Limb Prosthetics: surgical, prosthetic and rehabilitation principles,* CV Mosby, St Louis.

Levy, W.S. and Warren, H. (1983) *Skin Problems of the Amputee,* Green Inc., St Louis.

Smidt, G.L. (ed.) (1990) *Gait in Rehabilitation,* Churchill Livingstone, London.

USEFUL ADDRESSES

Amputee Medical Rehabilitation Society:
The Royal College of Physicians, St Andrews Place, London, UK

British Amputee Sports Association and Les Autres Federation:
30 Greaves Close, Arnold, Nottingham NG5 6RS, UK

British Association of Chartered Physiotherapists in Amputee Rehabilitation:
The Secretary, The Oak Tree Lane Centre, Selly Oak, Birmingham, UK

British Association of Prosthetists and Orthotists
Dunnon & District General Hospital, Ben Corrumbrae, Dunoon, PA23 8HU, Argyll

British Limbless Ex-Service Men's Association:
The General Secretary, 185–187 High Street, Chadwell Heath, Romford, Essex RM6 6NA, UK

Clinical Interest Group in Orthotics, Prosthetics and Wheelchairs:
Occupational Therapy Department, Arrowe Park Hospital, Upton, Wirral, Merseyside, UK

International Society for Prosthetics and Orthotics:
Borgervaenget – 5,2100 Copenhagen 0, Denmark

Limbless Association:
31 The Mall, Ealing, London W5 2PX, UK

16 Chronic low back pain

P. Helliwell

INTRODUCTION

Back pain is a symptom and not a disease. Most of us are likely to experience an episode of back pain during our lives. For about 30–40% of us back pain will be a recurrent phenomenon. Age-related changes are commonly seen in the lumbar spine on radiography, but the relationship between these structural changes and the symptom of back pain is not straightforward and theories based on a causal link between the two may have retarded research and treatment for back pain sufferers. In this chapter the orthodox medical model of an illness will be acknowledged, although it will be emphasized that alternative models may be more suitable, particularly in cases of chronic back pain.

EPIDEMIOLOGY

Age and sex prevalence data

Generally, if people are asked whether they have had back pain in the last 12 months, the peak prevalence (about 40%) will occur in the age group 45–54 years, with the number of females slightly more than the number of males (Figure 16.1). There is a reduction in prevalence either side of this decade, although a significant annual prevalence in children under 15 years of age does occur (30% in Finland) (Salminen Pentti and Jerho, 1992). It

is likely that different aetiological factors occur at different ages. These will be discussed under 'causes of back pain' below.

Heavy lifting

There is a well-established relationship between heavy lifting and back pain in industry. Miners have more back pain than clerical workers (Lawrence, 1977). Chaffin (1974) was able to show that a mis-match between lifting capacity and job-specific lifting requirement was much more likely to lead to episodes of back pain. Nurses have a high prevalence of work-related back pain, thought to be related to lifting heavy and potentially unstable weights (i.e. patients).

Vibration

Vibration is potentially harmful to the body. Damage may occur as a result of the energy delivered to the tissues during the passage and attenuation of the accelerations though the body. Damage may also result from ischaemia as a result of vibration-induced vasospasm. Where employees work on vibrating platforms, a high prevalence of accelerated radiographic spinal degeneration is seen. Prolonged exposure to commonly experienced vibration, such as that experienced whilst riding in vehicles, is associated

Rehabilitation of the Physically Disabled Adult. Edited by C. John Goodwill, M. Anne Chamberlain and Chris Evans. Published in 1997 by Stanley Thornes (Publishers) Ltd, Cheltenham. ISBN 0-7487-3183-0.

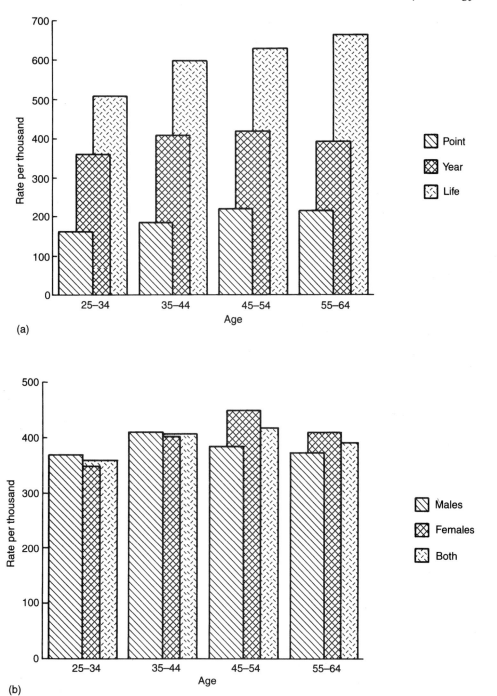

Figure 16.1 (a) Point, annual and lifetime prevalence of low back pain, by decade; (b) age and sex specific annual prevalence of low back pain. (Figures adjusted for bias. Data from a postal survey of 1 in 5 households in Bradford, West Yorkshire. Hillman *et al*, 1996.)

with back pain and prolapsed intervertebral disc, presumably through mechanisms described above (Smeathers and Helliwell, 1993).

Anthropometric

Back pain is commoner in taller people because most work stations are designed for the average person, thus constraining the taller individual to work in a potentially abnormal posture. There are conflicting opinions on the association between back pain and obesity, although we have found a positive association. There may well be other, as yet unrecorded, anthropometric variables which are important, for example, subtle differences in the biochemistry of collagen. An extreme example of this is the hypermobile patient who has excessively lax ligaments and in whom back pain is a common feature.

Leg-length inequality greater than 1.5 cm is regarded by some as an important risk factor but this remains controversial (Figure 16.2)

Prolonged abnormal posture

Moving from the recumbent position to standing upright will result in a few millimetres loss of height, largely due to loss of fluid from the intervertebral discs. Leaning forward at 30° from the vertical will produce creep in the tensioned posterior elements of the spine with subsequent abnormal loading of the spinal tissues. The high prevalence of back pain in dentists may result from such postural constraints (Figure 16.3) (Zakaria, Smeathers and Helliwell, 1994).

Pregnancy

In pregnancy ligaments are more extensible as a result of hormonal changes, thus accentuating creep effects. A further significant factor is the abnormal load carried anterior to the lumbar spine.

Other factors

Job satisfaction, socioeconomic influences and psychosocial factors, are related to episodes of back pain in the workplace but it may be that these factors are associated with the presentation of symptoms and the amount of sickness absence rather than be directly related to the causation of back pain. Indeed, it is likely that potential physical triggers have declined (as a result of ergonomic and workplace awareness) in the last two decades yet claims for sickness benefit due to back pain continue to increase (Waddell, 1992). Smoking cigarettes may be causally linked by a vasospastic effect on blood vessels and by inhibition of fibrinolysis.

CAUSES OF BACK PAIN

Mechanical

In simple or mechanical back pain the source of the pain is often not clearly defined. Anatomically, studies of innervation have shown most spinal tissues to be potential causes of pain but the presence of widespread anatomical abnormalities in asymptomatic people obscures the relationship between pathology and pain. Even the use of diagnostic blocks using local anaesthetic may be misleading because of diffusion of anaesthetic away from the area under examination. Discography, with reproduction of pain, is thought by some to fulfil necessary criteria for identification of the painful tissue but the neurological mechanisms surrounding pain perception, both at local, spinal and subcortical level, make simple interpretation of such techniques hazardous.

The putative painful tissue in acute low back pain remains to be identified. It is likely that there are a number of structures which may give rise to pain in the acute situation, including ligament, muscle, disc and joint. If nerve roots are involved then the anatomical localization becomes more precise. In chronic back pain, more complex neurological

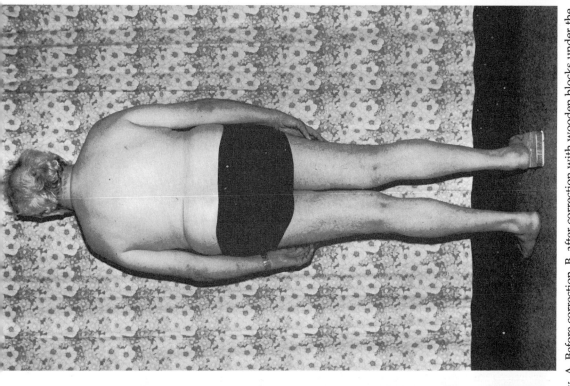

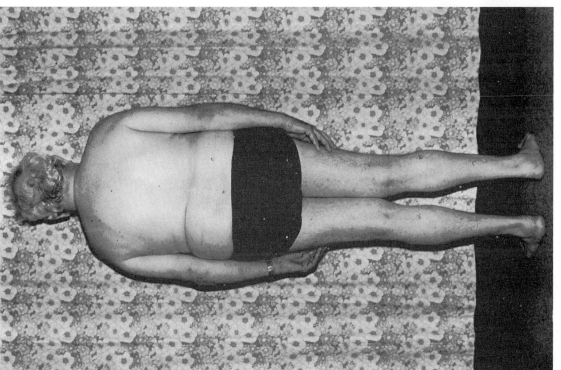

Figure 16.2 Pelvic tilt and spinal curvature due to leg-length inequality. A, Before correction, B, after correction with wooden blocks under the foot. Note the asymmetrical lumbar roll of fat.

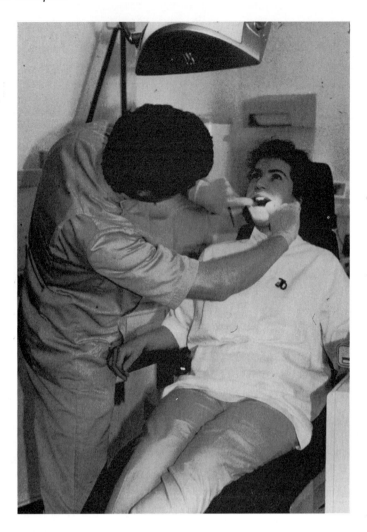

Figure 16.3 The prolonged leaning/twisting postures adopted by dentists may contribute to the high prevalence of back pain in this group.

mechanisms may be operating, such that merely identifying an abnormality on, for example, a computerized tomograph of the spine, is not sufficient; this may have been the source of the pain originally but may no longer be playing a part in the continuation of pain (Harvey, 1987). In this situation a procedure designed to remove (or inject or sclerose or liquify) this abnormality may provide little improvement for the patient.

A number of mechanisms may contribute to persistent pain – in some cases the original physical insult may have been resolved satisfactorily. Neural pain networks may be established which, because of resulting abnormal movement patterns, are never abolished. Descending influences on spinal pain perception may also be important, thus providing a link to psychosocial factors. The Manchester Group has published on the possible role of abnormal fibrinolysis with consequent perineurial fibrosis and persistence of pain. Local biochemical effects may also be prominent because of the relatively avascular nature of the disc and the production of inflammatory cytokines in these tissues (Jayson, 1994).

Other causes

It is important to recognize that there are many other causes of back pain and that to a certain extent the diagnosis of simple mechanical back pain is one of exclusion. Generally speaking, other diagnoses group by age and it is this criterion that is used in the simple classification noted in Table 16.1 discussed below.

Children less that 16 years

Persistent back pain in children should always be taken seriously and investigated by plain radiology and, if necessary, isotope bone scan and magnetic resonance imaging.

Young adults 16–40 years

Marked early morning back stiffness, especially in young males, should suggest the possibility of ankylosing spondylitis. The pain and stiffness in this condition often responds to exercise, which is usually not the case with mechanical low back pain. Restriction of spinal mobility, chest expansion and the presence of sacroiliitis confirm the diagnosis.

Older adults 40–65 years

Spinal stenosis or spinal claudication may become apparent at this age when age-related disc prolapse critically compromises a congenitally narrow or trefoil-shaped spinal canal. The typical symptoms of spinal stenosis are exercise-related symptoms in the legs which may also come on after standing for some time, and are relieved by sitting, lying or bending forward. Unlike intermittent clau-

Table 16.1 Conditions to exclude, by age group. Note: the commonest cause of back pain at all ages is 'mechanical', i.e. pain arising from the soft tissues of the spine as the disc, joint capsule, ligament, muscle and associated neural tissue such as the dura mater. The conditions listed below are uncommon but must be excluded because of their morbidity and potentially different treatment strategy

Age range	Diagnoses to exclude
Children <16 years	Tumour, e.g. osteoid osteome Infection, e.g. pyogenic abscess Discitis Spondylolysis/spondylolisthesis Hypermobility syndrome Osteochondritis (Scheuermann's disease)
Young adults 16–40 years	Infection, e.g. pyogenic abscess, tuberculosis Ankylosing spondylitis Osteochondritis (Scheuermann's disease) Hypermobility syndrome
Older adults 40–65 years	Osteoporosis – fracture Tumour: secondary (e.g. to breast, stomach, lung, kidney, thyroid, prostate) primary (e.g. multiple myeloma) Infection, e.g. abscess Spinal stenosis
Elderly >65 years	Osteoporosis – fracture Osteomalacia Paget's disease Tumour: secondary (e.g. to breast, stomach, lung, kidney, thyroid, prostate) primary (e.g. multiple myeloma)

dication due to arterial insufficiency, the symptoms of this disorder are usually worse when walking downhill (when the spine is relatively extended) rather than uphill.

Over 65 years

Osteoporosis per se is not painful but may become painful when fracture ensues and may remain painful following a fracture because of compression of adjacent spinal elements. Paget's disease may present with neurological problems or spinal claudication and very rarely with spinal cord compression.

At all ages it is important to be aware of the fact that tumour (either primary or secondary) and infection may be the cause of the back pain. Unremitting pain, particularly at night, weight loss and night sweats are of serious importance. Deyo, Rainville and Kent (1992) have noted the following historical features to be most sensitive for spinal tumour: age > 50 years, previous history of tumour elsewhere, unexplained weight loss, no relief with bed rest and pain for longer than a month. The commonest sites from which bony second-aries originate are breast, prostate, lung, stomach and kidney.

Visceral disorders

Uncommonly, pain is referred to the back from the abdomen. Possible sites are the retroperitoneum where fibrosis or lymphade-nopathy may cause pain and where aortic aneurysms may dissect, leak or rupture. It is possible that cyclical back pain in females originates from the reproductive system but chronic persistent back pain is occasionally due to pathological change such as an ovarian tumour, pelvic inflammatory disease or endo-metriosis. Neoplastic disease within the peri-toneal cavity (e.g. pancreatic carcinoma, rectal carcinoma and biliary disease) may also present with back pain.

ASSESSMENT OF THE BACK PAIN PATIENT

A thorough evaluation of the back pain patient takes time and a lot of effort. Often this time is not available in the routine clinic and further steps must be taken to complete the evaluation. Some short cuts may be taken by administering self-completed question-naires prior to attending, and during, the clinic appointment. The following comments apply mostly to the assessment of a patient

with chronic simple back pain, but minimal criteria required for a complete assessment are also included.

A further problem in the assessment of a patient with chronic simple back pain lies in the question of taxonomy. Whereas the author accepts that there are certain well-defined conditions with a typical presenta-tion, clinical findings and radiological abnormality (e.g. radicular pain with disc herniation), the majority of cases of back pain do not fit into such a pattern and, until a meaningful taxonomy based on clinical presentation, natural history and treatment can be found, then much of the clinical examination will be empirical. Furthermore, Nelson *et al.,* (1979) has shown that many of the historical features and physical signs are unreliable and subject to interobserver var-iation. What follows is a simple procedure used by the author which can be carried out relatively easily within the time allowed in the clinic.

History

Define the site of the pain: a pain drawing provides a permanent record of this. Note the character, periodicity, aggravating and relieving factors and radiation of the pain: these will provide many helpful clues about the patient's experience and their reaction to it. Seek other historical features, particularly symptoms of systemic disease such as fever, anorexia, weight loss, night sweats and generalized symptoms such as fatigue, sleep disturbance, headache and dizziness. Ask about mood and work, particularly work status, job tasks and any modifications that may have been necessary, and beliefs about the cause of the pain. Bladder symptoms should be asked for, if not volunteered.

Disability resulting from back pain can be catalogued; a number of instruments are available (Helliwell, Moll and Wright, 1992). The author finds the Oswestry Disability

Index (Baker, Pinsent and Fairbank, 1990) useful and the patients find the questionnaire easy to complete, although the question on sexual function is often neglected.

Enquire about the effect of previous physiotherapy and the use of heterodox therapy such as osteopathy, chiropractic, aromatherapy and reflexology.

Examination

Examine the patient standing and note the shape of the thoracolumbar spine and neck, any pelvic tilt (Figure 16.2), range of movement in the spine, the presence of positional pain and any tenderness. Examine the patient prone and supine, checking leg length, stressing the sacroiliac joints, examining mobility of spinal segments and pain provocation. Neurological examination should include Laségues test, femoral stretch test and lower limb neurology including sensory loss in the saddle area.

If indicated, examine breasts, neck and abdomen for abnormal lumps and perform a rectal examination to examine the prostate. Briefly inspect the rest of the musculoskeletal system for signs of osteoarthritis or an inflammatory arthritis. Look for hypermobility in the peripheral joints.

NON-ORGANIC SYMPTOMS AND SIGNS

Waddell *et al.*, (1984) detailed a group of seven symptoms and eight physical signs deemed medically inappropriate and a clue to distress and illness behaviour in the patient (Table 16.2). It is important to recognize that if these symptoms/signs are present this does not necessarily mean the patient is malingering. When present, they should provide the physician with a reminder that there is another dimension to the patient's illness requiring attention before improvement can be obtained.

Table 16.2 Non-organic (inappropriate) symptoms and signs (Waddell *et al.*, 1984)

Inappropriate symptoms
Tailbone pain
Whole leg pain
Whole leg numbness
Whole leg giving way
No pain-free spells
Intolerance of treatments
Emergency admissions

Inappropriate signs
Superficial tenderness
Non-anatomical tenderness
Axial loading of vertex resulting in back pain
Passive rotation of shoulders with pelvis causing back pain (simulated rotation)
Straight-leg raise positive when supine, negative when sitting (distracted straight-leg raising)
Regional weakness
Regional sensory loss
Over-reaction to examination (excessive verbalization, grimacing or collapsing)

INVESTIGATION

The minimal requirements are a full blood count, plasma viscosity (or erythrocyte sedimentation rate), calcium, phosphate and alkaline phosphatase. Where necessary, check the serum prostatic specific antigen and protein electrophoresis.

Radiological examination is not recommended in cases of acute back pain of less than 6 weeks duration unless there are features suggesting serious spinal pathology. A plain radiograph of the lumbar spine after 6 weeks will often show age-related changes but will rarely show a significant spinal pathology. The poor correlation between age-related changes and clinical findings is mirrored by the frequent finding of disc prolapse found in asymptomatic individuals on magnetic resonance imaging (MRI) (Jensen *et al.*, 1994)

Radiological techniques such as computerized axial tomography (CT) or MRI able to show surgically correctable lesions are not usually done unless it has been decided that surgery is an option. Electromyography may be useful to confirm nerve root involvement. In some centres, discography is used to both image and provoke suspected pathological intervertebral discs. If necessary the surgeon may proceed to chemonucleolysis.

MANAGEMENT OF BACK PAIN

A simple algorithm for the management of back pain is shown in Figure 16.4. Such decision trees are useful for agreeing treatment and referral guidelines between for example, community and hospital practice, but local negotiation is essential.

Unsubstantiated claims abound for specific treatments. Confusion arises because of several factors, notably:

- the good outcome of most acute episodes of back pain;
- poorly controlled trials;
- the use of a medical model when a bio-psycho-social model is more appropriate (Waddell, 1992);
- the poor taxonomy of back pain syndromes and inappropriate outcome measures in controlled trials.

Acute back pain

The prognosis for most people with acute back pain is favourable. Manipulation may result in more rapid resolution of symptoms but makes no difference to the final outcome. The optimum period of bed rest is 2 days. Simple analgesics are recommended but patients often prefer something stronger such as non-steroidal anti-inflammatory drugs (NSAIDs), occasionally by injection. Severe acute back pain can be treated by epidural injection of local anaesthetic. At this stage it is helpful to give a back exercise regime which the patient can begin as soon as the pain improves. Ergonomics, posture and workplace advice are recommended to prevent further episodes.

Chronic simple back pain

Deyo (1983) has shown that many trials of conservative therapy are flawed by inadequate descriptions of patients, the interventions used and related outcome measures. The Quebec Task Force on back pain (Spitzer, LeBlanc and Dupuis, 1987) concluded that most conservative therapies were unproven. In the following discussion where uncertainty exists about a particular therapy this will be indicated.

TREATMENT OF BACK PAIN

Drug therapy

Simple analgesics are recommended although most patients find them inadequate for pain relief. Compound analgesics or NSAIDs are often substituted. Muscle relaxant drugs are advocated by some on the basis that muscle spasm is contributing to the pain but this treatment remains empirical. Narcotic analgesics should be avoided because of the risk of dependency. Low dose tricyclic antidepressant therapy may be useful adjunctive therapy where distress is a feature of the presentation.

Exercises

There are advocates of different regimes. Maitland favours extension exercises to increase strength and range but others favour strengthening of muscles anterior to the spine including the abdominal wall. Muscle wasting and dysfunction does occur in chronic back pain and restoration of function will depend on successful rehabilitation: some advocate the use of isokinetic devices to help with functional restoration (Helliwell, Moll and Wright, 1992). It seems sensible to include arm and leg muscles in aerobic exercise training because patients with chronic pain are often de-conditioned and because of the beneficial effect of aerobic conditioning on pain in general. In practice,

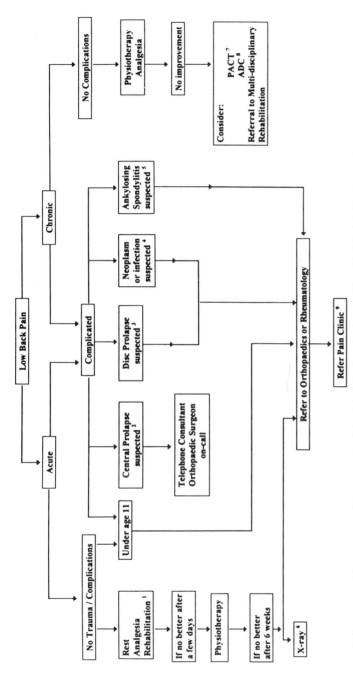

Low Back Pain

Acute

No Trauma / Complications

Rest
Analgesia
Rehabilitation [1]

If no better after
a few days

Physiotherapy

If no better
after 6 weeks

X-ray [6]

Under age 11

Complicated

Central Prolapse suspected [2]

Telephone Consultant
Orthopaedic Surgeon
on-call

Disc Prolapse suspected [3]

Neoplasm or infection suspected [4]

Chronic

Ankylosing Spondylitis suspected [5]

No Complications

Physiotherapy
Analgesia

No improvement

Consider:
PACT [7]
ADC [8]
Referral to Multi-disciplinary
Rehabilitation

Refer to Orthopaedics or Rheumatology

Refer Pain Clinic [9]

1. Rest means avoiding strenuous activity, no more than 2 days in bed. Simple analgesics preferable to NSAID's. Rehabilitation exercise sheets available from the Rheumatology Department.
2. Central disc prolapse suggested by bi-lateral leg symptoms/signs, bladder symptoms and saddle anaesthesia.
3. Disc prolapse suggested by back pain with sciatica extending below the knee, + neurological signs (weakness, anaesthesia, loss of reflex)
4. Infection or neoplasm suggested by fever, weight loss, unremitting 24 hour per day pain.
5. Ankylosing Spondylitis suggested by morning stiffness, pain and stiffness relieved by exercise, family history, iritis, associated inflammatory bowel disease or psoriasis
6. Lumbar spine X-ray's are often not necessary and involve a very significant radiation dose. It may be more appropriate to X-ray a patient who is over 50 years old. Young patients with unremitting problems are likely to need more extensive investigation than a straight X-ray.
7. PACT - Placement, Assessment and Counselling Team.
8. ADC - Abilities Development Centre
9. The Pain Clinic is a tertiary referral centre for treatment only and is not able to accept patients for investigation, or patients who have not yet been referred to Orthopaedics or Rheumatology

Figure 16.4 Simple algorithm for back pain useful for agreeing treatment and referral guidelines between community and secondary care.

promoting exercise will also help the patient take control of their illness.

Traction

Continuous pelvic traction would seem to serve no other purpose than to keep the patient immobile and this in itself is probably counterproductive beyond a 2–3 day period. Intermittent lumbar traction to 80 kg using an hydraulic device may have more local effects on the lumbar spine: Cyriax (1984) claimed reduction of some disc protrusions, but the evidence was anecdotal.

Manipulation

Manipulation may terminate an acute attack of back pain but the role of manipulation in chronic simple back pain is less clear. The Medical Research Council study reported in 1991 suggested medium-term benefit for manipulative therapy of the chiropractic type (Meade *et al*, 1990).

Transcutaneous electrical nerve stimulation

This is widely used for managing chronic spinal pain, although a recent controlled trial found no objective benefit (Deyo *et al.*, 1990).

Injections

Epidural injections of local anaesthetic may help in the management of an acute episode of back pain but their role in chronic back pain, with or without sciatica, is less clear and certainly the addition of corticosteroid to the local anaesthetic solution appears to make no difference to the outcome. Corticosteroid injection into the zygapophyseal joints, although widely practised, is also unproven (Deyo, 1990).

Hydrotherapy

Hydrotherapy continues to be popular in the treatment of chronic back pain because,

firstly, the heat relieves pain and, secondly, it allows patients to perform exercises they would be unable to perform on dry land. Spa water may have additional benefits (Guillemin *et al.*, 1994).

Corsets

Corsets, both rigid and semi-rigid, are often prescribed but most probably fail in their intended function. Lumbar supports do not reduce spinal movement unless very rigid and are unable to transmit a significant load (Helliwell and Wright, 1991).

Surgery

Laminectomy and removal of the disc is historically the operation of choice for presumed disc disorders but the frequency of this operation is falling. There are several reasons for this:

- recent evidence suggesting that disc prolapses are commonly asymptomatic;
- the introduction of new surgical techniques, e.g. chemonucleolysis, laser micro-surgery;
- the finding that outcome could be predicted on the basis of psychological criteria (Roberts *et al.*, 1984).

Clear indications for surgical intervention remain the cauda equina syndrome due to a central disc prolapse and severe spinal claudication. Less clear indications are: disc prolapse resulting in sciatica, since with or without surgery the functional outcome at 6 months is similar (Hakelius, 1970), spinal fusion for severe degenerative and possibly unstable spinal segments, and microdiscectomy for disc abnormalities found on provocation discography.

Multidisciplinary rehabilitation

For most patients with chronic simple back pain treatment for the spine should be supplemented by an approach which encompasses psychosocial and workplace factors. This requires a multidisciplinary team of physician, physiotherapist, occupational therapist, psychologist and ergonomist but may incorporate other team members according to local requirements and availability. Within the rehabilitation programme are elements of education (including anatomy, physiology, biomechanics and function), ergonomics, personal psychosocial and general psychosocial (e.g. stress management) and strength/fitness. Improvement in back strength and range of movement may be aided by the use of a computer-linked isokinetic device which also provides objective data on work endurance, time to peak torque and fatigue. Such systems enable a gradual increase in effort and range of movement to a level which matches that required during the work environment. Such expensive technology is not mandatory, however, and the same result may be achieved, albeit at the expense of prolonged therapist involvement, in the gym.

There are reports of impressive results with such rehabilitation programmes (Mayer *et al.*, 1985). It seems important that such programmes are linked to the workplace, although there are difficulties engaging the interest of employers. If the patient has lost their job then in the UK the Placement Assessment and Counselling Team provides a channel back into the workplace. If the patient is still in employment then it may be possible to make modifications at the workplace with the help of Employment Medical Advisory Service. Recurrence of back pain may be predicted by work dissatisfaction and disempowerment: modern managerial methods which empower the worker may help in this respect.

RISK FACTORS FOR CHRONICITY

For primary and secondary prevention of back pain (see below) risk factors for chronicity must be identified even though they may

not be amenable to modification. Significant risk factors may be summarized as:

- the concept of injury and the possibility of compensation;
- poor socioeconomic status;
- psychological distress at presentation;
- previous episodes of pain;
- employment dissatisfaction and requirements of the job.

PREVENTION OF CHRONICITY

Primary prevention

The value of pre-employment screening remains controversial. The work of Chaffin (1974) suggests that matching the strength of the worker to the job may reduce episodes of back pain. Education within the workplace in the form of a back school is widely practised in Scandinavia. Although correct lifting techniques may be taught, this does not mean that they will be practised (Kuorinka, Lortie and Gautreau, 1994) but it has been shown that training of patient handling skills may reduce the risk of subsequent back pain in nurses (Videmann *et al.*, 1989). The introduction of manual handling regulations (Manual Handling Operations Regulations, 1992 under the Health and Safety at Work Act, 1974) in the UK may help reduce back pain in industry but as yet no data is available.

Acute sufferers prefer to lie on a firm surface. A considerable amount of money is spent on 'recommended' beds and mattresses but there is no evidence that they have any role in prevention. Similar remarks also apply to seating. Although intradiscal pressure measurements have shown the optimal seating angle (20° backwards from the vertical), similar work on pelvic tilt, and thigh and arm support is lacking. The spine functions as a shock absorber and reduction of both workplace and domestic vibration will play a role in primary prevention. Improved road surfaces and shock-absorbing insoles in shoes are two ways in which this might be effected (Helliwell, Smeathers and Wright, 1989).

Secondary prevention

Back schools are widely advocated but their benefit is unproven. Most authors suggest that the programme needs to be developed with care and with adequate fiscal support and staff to carry out the programme. Recently a focused programme was shown to reduce the length but not the incidence of absenteeism due to back pain (Versloot *et al.*, 1992). Most exercise regimes given to back pain patients by physiotherapists are designed not to help the current episode but to prevent the recurrence of acute episodes of back pain.

Tertiary prevention

Workplace modification may be required for a back pain patient to return to work. In the UK this can be done with the help of the Placement and Counselling Teams. Adaptations such as the introduction of lifting aids may, however, be argued as part of the primary and secondary prevention programme. The philosophy of treatment of back pain emphasizes active intervention and continuing aerobic fitness and the introduction of adaptations or aids, which in other musculoskeletal diseases may be seen as necessary, may be thought to be counterproductive: in effect the aim is to remove excessive loads from the lumbar spine while enabling the patient to continue in employment.

SUMMARY

Back pain is such a common problem that it might almost be regarded as a normal phenomenon. Most episodes resolve spontaneously. Of those that persist a few have serious and potentially remedial causes, a few have surgically treatable back pain and a few have inflammatory rheumatic disease. The remainder constitute patients with chronic simple back pain in whom the majority of resources should be concentrated. For this group it is important to recognize that rehabilitation measures focusing on multiple aspects of the patient are the best available treatments at the present time.

Future research should be concentrated on exposing the reasons for the increase in disability due to back pain which has occurred over the last 10 years. It is possible that this is a social rather than a medical issue and therefore appropriate sociological approaches may be required. With established chronic simple back pain research efforts should move away from identifying the putative painful structure towards elucidating the pathophysiology of back pain. Pathophysiological research might also encompass the neurophysiology and psychology of pain.

REFERENCES

Baker, D., Pinsent, P.B. and Fairbank, J.C.T. (1989). The Oswestry disability index revisited: its reliability, repeatability and validity and a comparison with the St Thomas's disability index, in *Back Pain New Approaches to Rehabilitation and Education* (eds M. Rowland and J.R. Jenner), Manchester University Press, pp. 174–86.

Chaffin, B.B. (1974) Human strength capability and low back pain. *Journal of Occupational Medicine*, **16**, 248-54.

Cyriax, J. (1984) *Textbook of Orthopaedic Medicine*, vol. II, 11th edn, Baillière Tindall, London.

Deyo, R. (1983) Conservative therapy for low back pain – distinguishing useful from useless therapy. *Journal of the American Medical Association*, **250**, 1057–62.

Deyo, R. (1991) Fads in the treatment of low back pain. *New England Journal of Medicine*, **325**, 1039–40.

Deyo, R., Rainville, J. and Kent, D.L. (1992) What can the history and physical examination tell us about low back pain? *Journal of the American Medical Association*, **268**, 760–5.

Deyo, R., Walsh, N.E., Martin, D.C., Schoenfeld, L.S. and Ramamurthy, S. (1990) A controlled trial of transcutaneous electrical stimulation (TENS) and exercise for chronic low back pain. *New England Journal of Medicine*, **322**, 1627–34.

Guillemin, F., Constant, F., Collin, J.F. and Boulange, M. (1994) Short and long-term effect of spa therapy in chronic low back pain. *British Journal of Rheumatology*, **33**, 148–51.

Hakelius, A. (1970) Prognosis in sciatica: a clinical follow-up of surgical and non-surgical treatment. *Acta Orthopaedica Scandinavica Supplementum*, 129.

Harvey, A.H. (1987) Neurophysiology of rheumatic pain, in *Pain* (V. Wright, ed.); *Baillière's Clinical Rheumatology*, **1**, 1–26.

Helliwell, P.S., Moll, J.M.H. and Wright, V. (1992) Measurement of spinal movement and function, in *The Lumbar Spine and Back Pain*, 4th edn (ed. M.I.V. Jayson), Churchill Livingstone, Edinburgh.

Helliwell, P.S., Smeathers, J., and Wright, V. (1989) The measurement of shock absorption in the spinal column in normals and in ankylosing spondylitis. *Proceedings of the Institute of Mechanical Engineers, part H, Journal of Engineering in Medicine*, **203**, 187–90.

Helliwell, P.S. and Wright, V. (1991) Low back pain, indications for use of a lumbar corset. *British Journal of Rheumatology*, **30**, 62.

Hillman, M., Wright, H., Rajaratnam, G., Tennant, A. and Chamberlain, M.A. (1996) *J. Epid. Comm. Health*, **50**, 347–52.

Jayson, M.I.V. (1994) Mechanisms underlying chronic back pain. *British Medical Journal*, **309**, 681–2.

Jensen, M.C., Brant-Zawadzki, M.N., Obuchowski, N., Modic, M.T., Malkasian, D. and Ross, J.R. (1994) Magnetic resonance imaging of the lumbar spine in people without back pain. *New England Journal of Medicine*, **331**, 69–73.

Kourinka, I., Lortie, M., and Gautreau, M. (1994) Manual handling in warehouses: the illusion of correct working postures. *Ergonomics*, **37**, 655–61.

Lawrence, J.S. (1977) *Rheumatism in Populations*, Heinemann, London.

Mayer, T.G., Gatchel, R.J., Kisheno, N., Keeley, J., Capra, P., Mayer, H., Barnett, J. and Mooney V. (1985) Objective assessment of spine function following industrial injury – a prospective study with comparison group and one year follow-up. *Spine*, **10**, 482–93.

Meade, T.W., Dyer, S., Browne, W., Townsend, J. and Frank, A.O. (1990) Low back pain of mechanical origin: randomised comparison of chiropractic and hospital outpatient treatment. *British Medical Journal*, **300**, 1431–7.

Nelson, M.A., Allen, P., Clamp, S. and De Dombal, F. (1979) Reliability and reproducibility of clinical findings in low back pain. *Spine*, **4**, 97–101.

Roberts, N., Smith, R., Bennett, S., Cape, J., Norton, R. and Kilburn, P. (1984) Health beliefs and rehabilitation after lumbar disc surgery. *Journal of Psychosomatic Research*, **28**, 139–44.

Salminen, J.J., Pentti, J. and Jerho, P. (1992) Low back pain and disability in 14-year-old schoolchildren. *Acta Paediatrica*, **81**, 1035–9.

Smeathers, J.E. and Helliwell, P.S. (1993) Effect of vibration, in *Mechanics of Human Joints* (eds V. Wright and E. Radin), Marcel Dekker: New York, pp. 313–39.

Spitzer, W.O., LeBlanc, F.E., and Dupuis, M. (1987) Scientific approach to the assessment and management of activity-related spinal disorders. *Spine*, **12**, 51–9.

Versloot, J.M., Rozeman, A., Van Son, A.M., van Akkerveekan, F. (1992) The cost effectiveness of a back school programme in industry. *Spine*, **17**, 22–7.

Videmann, T., Rauhala, H., Asp, S., Lindstrom, K., Cedercreutz, G., Kamppi, M., Tola, S. and Troup, J.D.G. (1989) Patient handling skill, back injuries and back pain – an intervention study in nursing. *Spine*, **14**, 148–56.

Waddell, G. (1992) Bio-psychosocial analysis of low back pain. In: M. Nordin, T.L. Vischer (Eds). Common low back pain: prevention of chronicity. *Baillière's Clinical Rheumatology*, **6**, 523–59.

Waddell, G., Bircher, M., Finlayson, D. and Main, C.J. (1984) Symptoms and signs: physical disease or illness behaviour? *British Medical Journal*, **289**, 739–41.

Zakaria, A., Smeathers, J.E. and Helliwell, P.S. (1994) Relationship between working posture and back pain in dentists. *British Journal of Rheumatology*, **333**, (suppl. 1), 118.

FURTHER READING

Jayson, M.I.V. (ed.) (1992) *The Lumbar Spine and Back Pain*, 4th edn, Churchill Livingstone, Edinburgh.

Nordin, M. and Vischer, T.L. (eds) (1992) Common low back pain – prevention of chronicity. *Baillière's Clinical Rheumatology*, **6**, (3).

Wright, V. (ed.) (1987) Pain. *Baillière's Clinical Rheumatology*, **1**, (1).

ADVICE FOR PATIENTS/USEFUL ADDRESSES

Arthritis and Rheumatism Council (ARC)

Backache and Disc ('Slipped Disc') Disorders, a handbook for patients, ARC, London.

Manual Handling Regulations (1992) HMSO, London.

Parker, H. and Main, C. (1990) *Living with Back Pain*, Manchester University Press.

USEFUL ADDRESSES

Arthritis and Rheumatism Council, Copeman House, St Mary's Court, St Mary's Gate, Chesterfield S41 7TD, UK.

National Back Pain Association, 16 Elmtree Road, Teddington, Middlesex TW11 8ST, UK.

PART THREE

ENERGY-RESTRICTING DISABILITY

17 Respiratory rehabilitation

J. Moxham

INTRODUCTION

In the UK respiratory diseases account for one in five deaths, one in three working days lost through illness and a quarter of medical admissions to hospital. Respiratory disorders are frequently chronic and disabling. Rehabilitation can seldom restore normal health, but much can be done to improve respiratory function and exercise capacity. Rehabilitation may halt or slow the otherwise inevitable decline in pulmonary function and enable the patient to tolerate his or her symptoms of breathlessness and exercise limitation. Disability is most commonly due to chronic bronchitis and emphysema. It is largely as a consequence of cigarette smoking and imposes a huge social and economic burden on society. In the UK 10% of absence from work and 10% of the occupancy of medical hospital beds are the result of these diseases, and it is estimated that up to a quarter of males aged 50–59 have chronic bronchitis. Worldwide the increase in smoking will substantially add to the global burden of respiratory disability.

In patients with chronic bronchitis and emphysema, and many individuals with other chronic chest diseases, restoration of normal function is not possible and the aim of therapy is to reduce disability by treating the interrelated problems of recurrent infections, airways obstruction, breathlessness, hypoxia and poor exercise tolerance. Factors aggravating chronic bronchitis and other lung disorders, particularly cigarette smoking, must be avoided.

OXYGEN THERAPY

Many patients with chronic lung disease are hypoxic and benefit from oxygen therapy. In those with hypercapnia, oxygen must be given with care and at low concentrations to avoid a dangerous increase in CO_2. As an aid to rehabilitation, oxygen therapy is most common in patients with chronic obstructive pulmonary disease (COPD). Studies suggest that long-term controlled oxygen therapy (LTOT) can benefit patients with severe chronic airways obstruction, who have an FEV_1 of less than 1.2 litres, severe hypoxia (PO_2 less than 7.5 kPa) and who do not smoke cigarettes. Not only is smoking and oxygen therapy dangerous, it also mitigates against the beneficial effect of treatment. A Medical Research Council (MRC) study looked at 87 patients with COPD and associated hypoxia, hypercapnia, pulmonary hypertension and secondary polycythaemia. Half of the patients were treated with oxygen (2 litres per min by nasal prongs) for 15 hours each day for 5 years, the other half did not receive oxygen. Those not treated with oxygen fared badly, with a 5-year survival of 30%, but those treated with oxygen did better, and their

Rehabilitation of the Physically Disabled Adult. Edited by C. John Goodwill, M. Anne Chamberlain and Chris Evans. Published in 1997 by Stanley Thornes (Publishers) Ltd, Cheltenham. ISBN 0-7487-3183-0.

survival was almost double (Medical Research Council Working, Party, 1981). A similar American study compared oxygen therapy for 12 hours a day with oxygen for 18 hours each day, both groups having oxygen therapy throughout the night. Oxygen for 12 hours daily produced results similar to oxygen for 15 hours each day, reported in the MRC study, but oxygen for 18 hours each day further prolonged survival and reduced the frequency and duration of hospital admissions (Nocturnal Oxygen Therapy Trial Group, 1980). The physiological evaluation of the patients in those studies suggested that oxygen therapy reversed secondary polycythaemia, and slowed the progressive increase in pulmonary vascular resistance and pulmonary artery pressure, that occurs without oxygen therapy.

A more recent study in patients with severe COPD (FEV_1 0.78 litres, PaO_2 6.1 kPa, $PaCO_2$ 6.9 kPa) showed that LTOT may be even more beneficial than previously thought, with a 5-year survival of 62% and, in males an increase in average life expectancy from 4 to 9 years (Cooper, Waterhouse and Howard, 1987). However, after 9 or 10 years the survival advantage was rapidly lost as progression of the underlying pathological process led to severe hypoxia, pulmonary hypertension and terminal cor pulmonale. On the basis of these studies, it is likely that LTOT is most beneficial when started relatively early.

In patients with cor pulmonale the treatment of peripheral oedema can be difficult. Oxygen therapy is helpful in removing oedema, in part by improving renal blood flow and function (Baudouin et al., 1992).

Although LTOT is most often prescribed in COPD, it is possible that patients with other conditions causing severe chronic hypoxaemia (bronchiectasis, cystic fibrosis) could also benefit.

The administration of continuous oxygen presents formidable practical and financial difficulties. In the past oxygen was supplied in cylinders in the UK and continuous oxygen therapy for up to 15 hours each day required 15–20 large oxygen cylinders each week, at an annual cost of several thousand pounds. A more satisfactory alternative is the oxygen concentrator, now routinely available in the UK and many other countries. The present system of prescribing domiciliary oxygen is often unsatisfactory. Many patients receive oxygen without careful assessment and conversely patients who could benefit from oxygen therapy do not receive it. Oxygen is a difficult and expensive drug to administer, and in most cases should only be prescribed after careful clinical and physiological assessment by a respiratory physician.

Short-term and portable oxygen therapy

In practice much oxygen used by patients in their homes is for a few minutes and often only on a few occasions each week. Patients report that they take oxygen in this way for relief of breathlessness. This may be correct because oxygen therapy reduces respiratory rate and therefore the work of breathing, but the effect of short bursts of oxygen therapy on the sensation of breathlessness has been little studied and remains of unproven benefit. Waterhouse and Howard, 1983, Evans et al., 1986; Liss and Grant, 1988.

The purpose of portable oxygen is to relieve hypoxia during exercise and hopefully to increase exercise capacity. Small cylinders are available which weigh 2 kg and have sufficient oxygen to last approximately 30 minutes. In patients with COPD cylinders require appropriate reducing valves to facilitate a flow rate of 2 l/min^{-1} and they can be refilled from a larger oxygen cylinder in the patient's home. However, the process of refilling is rather difficult and is frequently unsatisfactory. In appropriate patients, it is possible to administer oxygen at a flow rate (0.5–1 l/min^{-1}) directly into the trachea via an indwelling fine catheter (Shneerson, 1992). This technique may be more acceptable to some patients and may also be more efficient, thereby prolonging the life of oxygen cylinders. In some countries, particularly North America, liquid oxygen is used to provide a portable supply, substantially increasing the duration of oxygen availability. Oxygen use can be made more economical by a range of oxygen-conserving delivery devices (Moore-Gillon, 1989). Most techniques limit oxygen delivery to the inspiratory phase of each breath. Controlled trials of portable oxygen therapy have demonstrated a small benefit in terms of exercise capacity (Cotes, 1960; Bradley *et al.*, 1994), but some patients report a reduction in breathlessness, even though they do not walk further. Further studies of portable oxygen therapy are required, but it should not be forgotten that when patients claim benefit from portable oxygen they may well be correct, and the inability of physicians to document objective improvement may reflect the lack of precision of current techniques for evaluating exercise tolerance and breathlessness.

Hypoxia and oxygen therapy during sleep

Patients with severe COPD can have profound nocturnal hypoxaemia, particularly during rapid eye movement (REM) sleep (Figure 17.1) (Flick and Block, 1977; Douglas and Flenley, 1990). Nocturnal hypoxaemia is

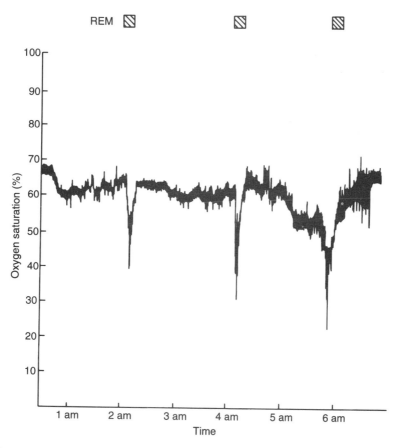

Figure 17.1 Oxygen saturation throughout the night in a patient with COPD (shaded areas represent rapid eye movement sleep). (Redrawn with permission from Douglas and Flenley, 1990.)

much more severe in the 'blue bloater' than the 'pink puffer'; normal subjects and pink puffers do have minor nocturnal hypoxaemia, but the oxygen saturation reached is much lower in the already hypoxic chronic bronchitic. Similar, profound nocturnal hypoxaemia occurs in patients with other diseases causing ventilatory failure (e.g. kyphoscoliosis). In patients with respiratory muscle weakness, nocturnal desaturation may be the first evidence of ventilatory failure. Much of the hypoxia is caused by hypoventilation and irregular breathing patterns during REM sleep, or increased ventilation–perfusion mismatch, and is not due to obstructive sleep apnoea. Oxygen therapy during the night (2 l/min^{-1} by nasal prongs) can alleviate hypoxaemia and make hypoxic dips much less severe. Studies of nocturnal oxygen saturation and carbon dioxide levels (by transcutaneous electrodes) are often important to confirm that oxygen therapy avoids hypoxic dips and does not cause severe hypercapnia.

MANAGEMENT OF AIRWAYS OBSTRUCTION

The large number of disabled patients with chronic bronchitis, emphysema, chronic asthma, bronchiectasis and cystic fibrosis, make airways obstruction a common cause of breathlessness and exercise limitation. In COPD airflow limitation is due to reduced elastic recoil of the lung, hypertrophy and oedema of the bronchial wall mucus membrane, excess mucus within the airways and contraction of bronchial wall smooth muscle. The increased resistance of gas flow within the bronchial tree increases the work of breathing and overall oxygen consumption. As a consequence of airways obstruction there is excess gas trapping in the lungs, hyperinflation and disordered rib cage geometry, all of which shorten the respiratory muscles, make the diaphragm less curved and greatly reduce ventilatory capacity. Airways obstruc-

tion therefore increases ventilatory work at the same time as reducing ventilatory capacity. This leads to breathlessness, exercise limitation and ventilatory failure (Figure 17.2). Successful treatment of airways obstruction reduces the work of breathing, as well as increasing the capacity of the thorax to achieve the ventilation required. This improvement reduces breathlessness, reduces ventilatory failure and improves exercise capacity.

Conventionally the airways obstruction of COPD is regarded as being irreversible. However the majority of patients show a small improvement in lung function with therapy aimed at relaxing bronchial wall smooth muscle, and in the rehabilitation of severely disabled patients every effort must be made to provide optimum treatment for airways obstruction, whatever the underlying cause. The relatively small response with bronchodilators may, nevertheless, depend on dosage and higher doses than conventionally used may be appropriate (Figure 17.3) (Jenkins and Moxham, 1987). Demonstration of a bronchodilator response is best achieved by measuring the 'slow' vital capacity. The most important agents are selective **beta-adrenergic-agonists** (salbutamol, terbutaline) best administered as an aerosol. Careful instruction in the use of metered dose inhalers is of critical importance and a variety of modifications to basic inhaler design are available to help patients who have difficulty in mastering the correct inhaler technique. Breath-activated inhalers and large volume spacer devices can be helpful. Drug in powder form, administered by a rotahaler device, may be an effective alternative to pressurized aerosols.

For those patients who find it impossible to successfully use a metered dose inhaler, beta-2-agonists can be administered by a nebulizer driven by an air compressor. Using a nebulizer the conventional dose of beta-2-agonist is large, for example 2.5 or 5.0 mg of salbutamol, and this therapy

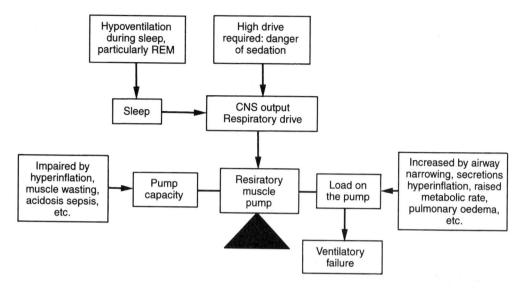

Figure 17.2 COPD increases the load imposed on the respiratory muscles and reduces their capacity. To sustain ventilation a high respiratory drive is required. As the load increases patients develop breathlessness and eventually ventilatory failure. (Redrawn with permission from Moxham 1995.)

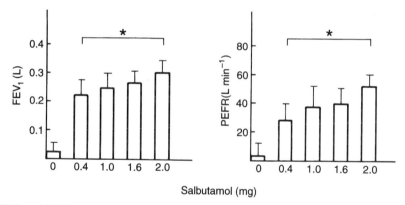

Figure 17.3 FEV and PEFR response at 30 minutes following salbutamol and placebo in 10 patients (mean $\pm$ SEM). $P < 0.05$. (Redrawn from Jenkins and Moxham, 1987.)

should not be administered without specialist assessment. As a consequence of the large drug dosage, patients with COPD frequently report that nebulizer therapy is superior to that from metered dose inhalers. However, if metered dose inhaler therapy is increased to achieve maximum bronchodilation, from four to six 100-µg inhalations being taken rather than the standard dose of 200 µg, many patients are helped equally by the two methods of drug administration (Jenkins *et al.*, 1987).

Inhaled atropine analogues (ipratropium bromide) can be helpful instead of, or in addition to, beta-2-agonists, and can be administered either by metered dose inhaler, or nebulizer. It is important to establish optimum dosage.

Oral theophyllines available in slow-release formulation, are of undoubted value in chronic asthma, particularly when nocturnal symptoms are severe, but they are of marginal usefulness in chronic bronchitis and emphysema (Cochrane, 1984). They should not be prescribed long term without critical review. Therapeutic and toxic drug levels are close, side-effects can be serious, and it is frequently necessary to monitor blood theophylline levels. In addition to a bronchodilator action, it is possible that theophyllines have a small beneficial action on the contractility of skeletal muscle, including the respiratory muscles, but the clinical importance of this remains uncertain (Moxham, 1988).

All patients with severe airways obstruction should have a **therapeutic trial of steroids**, for example oral prednisolone 30 mg daily for a period of 2 or 3 weeks, providing there is no contraindication to this drug. If respiratory function unequivocally improves then inhaled steroids should be tried. Long-term oral steroids will not be indicated in most patients; such therapy requires regular assessment and long-term dosage should seldom exceed 7.5–10 mg daily, thereby reducing drug complications. It is possible that long-term oral steroids produce respiratory muscle weakness, and thereby intensify respiratory problems, even at a dose of less than 10 mg daily (Decramer *et al.*, 1994). Careful clinical judgement is required in cases where there is subjective improvement in symptoms, but no objective change in lung function, or exercise capacity. The value of long-term inhaled steroids in COPD remains uncertain and is the subject of large clinical trials.

Mucolytic agents (e.g. bromhexine) reduce sputum viscosity, but are of unproven value in chronic bronchitis. Occasional patients report substantial benefits from mucolytic agents, and when sputum retention is a major problem a therapeutic trial is justified. In advanced cystic fibrosis nebulized DNase, an enzyme which breaks down the long polymerized chains of DNA in bronchial secretions, reduces the viscosity of sputum and may be helpful in carefully selected patients (Shak *et al.*, 1990).

Chronic hypoxia eventually causes secondary polycythaemia, possibly with increased risk of vascular thrombosis. Relief of hypoxia by treatment of the underlying pulmonary disease, or by long-term oxygen therapy, represents the most satisfactory way to reverse polycythaemia. Venesection, or erythropheresis, is only effective in the short term, but alleviates the symptoms and avoids the complications of hyperviscosity (Harrison and Stokes, 1982).

In acute exacerbations of chronic bronchitis an infective viral or bacterial pathogen is isolated in less than 50% of cases. However, viral infections are frequently complicated by bacterial overgrowth and the majority of patients develop purulent sputum. **Antibacterial therapy** is therefore of the greatest importance. Whereas minor exacerbations are associated with increased airways obstruction and breathlessness, severe exacerbations are characterized by worsening hypercapnic ventilatory failure and up to 25% mortality (Warren *et al.*, 1980). For most patients long-term chemoprophylaxis is not helpful, not reducing the number of exacerbations, but if intermittent treatment fails a trial of continuous rotating antibiotic therapy is justified. Prompt therapy of infection is important, and patients should always have available appropriate antibiotics, to be taken when symptoms first develop. In patients with bronchiectasis, particularly those with cystic fibrosis, long-term nebulized antibiotics can be beneficial. Antibiotics are selected according to the organisms cultured from sputum, and their sensitivities. Occasional patients require repeated courses of intravenous antibiotics and systems for permanent venous access are necessary.

Immunization against *Haemophilus influenzae*, *Staphylococcus aureus* and *Streptococcus pneumoniae* have not been shown to be effective. Immunization against the common cold virus is similarly ineffective, but annual immunization against influenza virus, using killed vaccine, is of value and should be considered in the severely disabled patient with frequent infections.

THERAPY FOR BREATHLESSNESS

Although severe hypoxia can contribute to breathlessness, the major cause of this distressing symptom is an excessive load on the respiratory system relative to ventilatory capacity (Figure 17.2). In some cases breathlessness reflects primarily excess load (e.g. lung fibrosis), in some load is increased and capacity is reduced (e.g. COPD) and in others the main problem is reduced ventilatory capacity (e.g. neuromuscular disease). The best treatment for breathlessness, whenever possible, is a reduction in ventilatory load (e.g. bronchodilatation) or an increase in capacity (e.g. improved nutrition, the treatment of myasthenia). In patients with airways obstruction it is the pink puffers with normal CO_2 values and mild hypoxia who are characteristically severely breathless (the problem being a large respiratory load, reduced ventilatory capacity and a high respiratory drive). However, blue bloaters with hypoxia, hypercapnia and CO_2 retention may be equally incapacited and dyspnoea can be particularly disabling in patients with pulmonary fibrosis. There is evidence that diazepam, promethazine and dihydrocodeine

can reduce breathlessness in pink puffers, and the careful use of such therapy is justified in severe cases (Woodcock *et al.*, 1981).

For the devasting dyspnoea which is frequently a feature of terminal respiratory failure morphine is helpful (e.g. oral morphine sulphate solution 10 mg 4 hourly). Drugs that reduce breathlessness reduce respiratory drive and therefore the ventilatory load on the system. They may also reduce anxiety and alter the central perception of breathlessness. Drugs must be used with great care in hypercapnic patients, the relief of breathlessness may cause worsening ventilatory failure. In some patients depression aggravates breathlessness (Morgan *et al.*, 1983) and appropriate therapy (e.g. amitriptyline, up to 150 mg daily, usually at nights for a minimum of 4 weeks) improves symptoms.

NUTRITION AND BODY WEIGHT

With increasing disability many patients exercise less and gain weight, thereby increasing respiratory work. Severe obesity adversely affects chest wall mechanics and may also predispose to obstructive sleep apnoea. Even modest obesity reduces lung function (Jenkins and Moxham, 1991) (Table 17.1). Many patients with chronic airways obstruction are depressed and some eat excessively as an expression of their psychiatric state. Appetite may be further stimulated if patients are successful in stopping smoking, or treated with oral steroids. Depression is

Table 17.1 Effect of mild obesity on lung function. (Adapted from Jenkins and Moxham, 1991)

	Grade 0 (n = 28)	Grade I (n = 91)	Grade II (n = 25)
BMI	20–24.9	25–29.9	30–40
Weight (kg)	70.8 (8.9)	81.1 (9.0)**	90.1 (8.8)**
FRC (% Predicted)	99.7 (17.9)	90.6 (18.3)*	78.4 (19.9)**
PaO_2	11.05 (1.34)	10.47 (0.99)*	9.99 (0.96)**
A-aPO_2 (kPa)	2.47 (1.30)	3.14 (0.99)*	3.88 (1.06)*

FRC = functional residual capacity; PaO_2 arterial oxygen tensions; A-aPO_2 = alveolar-arterial oxygen difference.
Values are means with standard deviations in parentheses.
Statistical significance as compared with Grade 0 patients: *$P < 0.05$; **$P < 0.01$.

positively correlated with the severity of breathlessness (Morgan *el al.*, 1983) and the treatment of depression, as well as reduction in body weight, may be helpful, although such therapy is frequently difficult. In contrast, with advanced respiratory disease weight loss and muscle wasting is common, the respiratory muscles sharing in this atrophy. In part, weight loss is due to the increased energy consumed by breathing, oxygen consumption is raised by up to 20% in advanced COPD (Lanigan, Moxham and Ponte, 1990).

Inadequate nutrition, common in these patients, accelerates the wasting process and further diminishes respiratory reserve (Arora and Rochester, 1982). This reduction of respiratory muscle capacity contributes to breathlessness. The clinical picture therefore of advanced COPD, particularly emphysema, is progressive relentless weight loss and breathlessness. It is not yet clear whether supplementary high calorie and high protein diets can improve respiratory muscle bulk and pulmonary function. In practice it is very difficult to achieve weight gain (Muers and Green, 1993).

OBSTRUCTIVE SLEEP APNOEA – CONTINUOUS POSITIVE AIRWAY PRESSURE (CPAP) THERAPY

Obstructive sleep apnoea is a common cause of respiratory disability that frequently goes unrecognized. It may complicate other disabling conditions; for example, severe obesity or neuromuscular diseases. Obstructive sleep apnoea affects approximately 1% of the adult male population, particularly those who are middle-aged or elderly and obese, and those who snore. It is made worse by alcohol, sedatives and hypnotics (Saunders and Sullivan, 1984; Phillipson, 1993). When asleep the patients exhibit periodic breathing with episodes of apnoea, during which strong inspiratory efforts are made against an occluded upper airway. Profound hypoxia occurs and

sleep is disrupted. The major daytime symptom is somnolence and patients eventually develop respiratory failure and cor pulmonale. Appropriate therapy can reverse these changes. Anatomical abnormalities frequently contribute; narrowing of the upper airway results in more negative intrapharyngeal pressures during inspiration and a greater tendency to pharyngeal collapse. Obstruction is relieved when the upper airway muscles are sufficiently activated and this is frequently only possible by the recruitment of the higher nervous system and therefore the interruption of sleep.

In the management of obstructive sleep apnoea, **weight reduction** is helpful, but difficult to achieve. **Tracheostomy** is effective, but presents management difficulties, and many patients are reluctant to agree to this line of treatment. Nasal **continuous positive airway pressure (CPAP)** is highly effective (Sullivan *et al.*, 1984) and for most patients is the treatment of choice.

Surgery to correct abnormalities of facial anatomy and to enlarge the pharyngeal airway is occasionally appropriate, but nocturnal CPAP remains, for the present, the mainstay of therapy.

DOMICILIARY VENTILATION

Patients with severe scoliosis, or rib cage deformity from thoracoplasty, eventually develop hypercapnic ventilatory failure and cor pulmonale. These patients can be helped by ventilatory assistance using negative pressure tank, cuirass or jacket ventilation (Sawicka, Branthwaite and Spencer, 1983; Hoeppner *et al.*, 1984). However, in recent years most patients in need of nocturnal ventilatory support have been treated with non-invasive positive pressure ventilation via a nasal mask (Ellis *et al.*, 1987; Elliott and Moxham, 1994). Patients with respiratory failure secondary to chronic respiratory muscle weakness can be treated in the same way, although some may be better managed with positive pressure ventilation via a tracheostomy. The advent of non-invasive nasal ventilation has substantially increased the number of patients received domiciliary ventilatory support. For many patients ventilatory support is required for short periods, and in practice nocturnal ventilation is frequently both convenient and effective. It is of note that such ventilatory support produces long-term improvement in ambulatory blood gas tensions. For patients with scoliosis, and some cases of chronic, stable or slowly progressive respiratory muscle weakness, the results of assisted ventilation treatment have been excellent, with enhanced quality of life for many years.

The key to the success of non-invasive ventilation is that it unloads the hard-pressed respiratory muscle pump, and avoids nocturnal hypoventilation and hypercapnia. This restores normal daytime ventilatory control. By supporting ventilation every night the improvement by day can be sustained (Figure 17.4). Non-invasive ventilation also reduces breathlessness, and may have a role in the palliative care of patients with advanced respiratory muscle weakness (e.g. motor neurone disease). The value of non-invasive ventilation in stable COPD is less clear, although some benefit has been reported (Elliott *et al.*, 1991). Controlled clinical trials are needed, particularly to establish whether nocturnal nasal ventilation is superior to long-term oxygen therapy. In acute exacerbations of COPD non-invasive ventilation can reduce breathlessness, reverse hypercapnia and reduce mortality (Bott *et al.*, 1993).

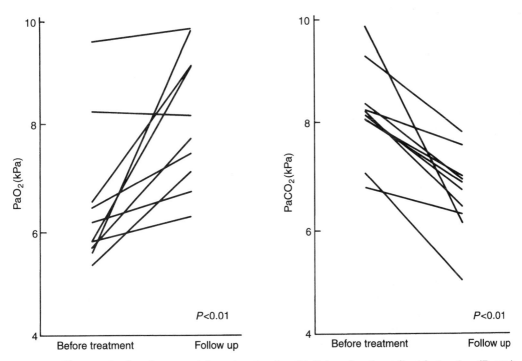

Figure 17.4 Changes in day-time arterial oxygen tension (PaO_2) and carbon dioxide tension ($PaCO_2$), sampled when breathing air, before and 6 months after initiating nocturnal nasal ventilation (Redrawn from Carroll and Braithwaite, 1988.)

DIAPHRAGM PACING

Diaphragm pacing involves repetitive electrical stimulation by electrodes implanted around the phrenic nerves in the thorax or in the neck (Glenn and Sairenji, 1985; Moxham and Shneerson, 1993). The electrodes are stimulated by a receiver implanted in the soft tissues of the thorax, which is activated by an external power source. Diaphragm pacing has been available for more than 30 years, and about 1000 patients have been treated.

Patients most suitable for diaphragm pacing are those with a high cervical cord injury. A smaller group who are sometimes suitable are those with central alveolar hypoventilation. The major advantage of diaphragm pacing is that it can achieve adequate ventilation without any apparatus being applied to the patient's airway. Patients are therefore more independent and mobile.

For diaphragm pacing to be successful it is crucial that phrenic nerve, diaphragm and lung function are good. Patients with lower motor neurone lesions of the phrenic nerves, or diaphragm myopathy are not suitable. Diaphragm pacing is a highly specialized treatment and choice of pacing systems, surgical technique and pacing schedules require skill and experience. Unilateral pacing can provide adequate ventilation in many adults, but most patients are bilaterally paced and providing appropriate stimulation schedules are developed diaphragm fatigue can usually be avoided.

Failure of pacing precipitates ventilatory failure and can be due to surgical damage to the phrenic nerves at the time of electrode implantation, incorrect pacing schedules or mechanical problems. Upper airways obstruction is a common problem, and frequently a tracheostomy is necessary. Pacing failure also occurs if the demands on the respiratory system are increased as, for example, in pneumonia.

Over the years diaphragm pacing has been most commonly undertaken in children and in young adults with quadriplegia. This group does well with a 10-year survival of 90%. Pacing equipment is generally reliable, but back-up systems are needed. The procedure is costly. Most quadriplegics do not receive diaphragm pacing and are managed satisfactorily in their own homes with positive pressure ventilation via a tracheostomy. For many the advantages of diaphragm pacing are relatively few and not worth the cost. Totally implantable systems, capable of being triggered, would increase the independence and mobility of quadriplegic patients and would be a significant advance.

TRACHEOSTOMY

Long-term tracheostomy is most commonly required for domiciliary positive pressure ventilation, to avoid aspiration in patients unable to protect the upper airway, to bypass upper airway obstruction and for the suctioning of excessive bronchial secretions. In some patients who are managed in intensive care for prolonged periods, and in whom weaning from mechanical ventilation is difficult a tracheostomy may continue to be needed for several weeks or months, to reduce dead space, and facilitate the suction of secretions. Nocturnal negative pressure ventilation can precipitate upper airway obstruction and tracheostomy may therefore be necessary. Occasional patients with obstructive sleep apnoea are unable to tolerate CPAP and are not appropriate for alternative therapies, and therefore require tracheostomy.

Prolonged treatment with a tracheostomy can cause both psychological and physical problems. However, patients eventually learn to speak well with a speaking tube, and many become expert at tracheostomy care. Although complications are relatively unusual a few patients develop serious problems.

Complications of tracheostomy

1. During surgery:
   (a) haemorrhage
   (b) pneumothorax
   (c) pneumomediastinum
   (d) subcutaneous emphysema.
2. Early:
   (a) aspiration past deflated cuff
   (b) stomal haemorrhage.
3. Late:
   (a) swallowing dysfunction
   (b) obstruction of tracheostomy tube
   (c) stomal infection
   (d) erosion into oesophagus
   (e) erosion into innominate artery
   (f) tracheal stenosis
   (g) bronchial/pulmonary infections.

The advent of mini-tracheostomy for suctioning excessive secretions, non-invasive nasal and face mask ventilation for domiciliary management of ventilatory failure, and endoscopically placed feeding tubes to feed patients who aspirate when eating and drinking, have reduced the number of patients who require long-term tracheostomy.

Some patients may eventually no longer need their tracheostomy. Following removal of a tracheostomy tube tracheal stenosis and tracheal collapse can be important problems, sometimes most evident when the neck is flexed. Careful bronchoscopy before removing the tracheostomy tube is helpful, and bronchoscopy plus respiratory function tests, especially flow volume loops, are required to assess tracheal structure and function if there are any problems following removal of the tracheostomy tube.

CHEST PHYSIOTHERAPY

Studies of the long-term effects of chest physiotherapy aimed at improving breathing patterns have been few and have been reviewed by Sutton and co-workers (1982). Slow purse-lipped breathing can improve blood gases. Abdominal (diaphragmatic) breathing leads to deeper and slower respiration, but probably does not alter the distribution of ventilation. The aim of instruction in such breathing techniques is to produce a more relaxed breathing pattern and thereby reduce the work of ventilation and oxygen consumption of the respiratory muscles. This hypothesis remains untested. Although altered breathing patterns can be adopted in the short term, they do not persist. Overall there is little convincing data that breathing training is beneficial (Sergysels *et al.*, 1991) and controlled clinical studies are urgently needed. Postural drainage is of undoubted benefit in patients with excessive bronchial secretions. It enhances mucociliary clearance, sputum volumes are increased, and some studies have documented improved lung function (Cochrane, Webber and Clarke, 1977). The effectiveness of postural drainage is increased by coughing or forced expiratory manoeuvres. Forced expiratory 'huffs' increase the efficacy of postural drainage in cystic fibrosis. In patients with excessive secretions cough clears sputum from central and intermediate regions of the lungs, but there is doubt about its efficiency in clearing peripheral airways. Most clinical studies have shown little immediate effect of physiotherapy on arterial blood gas tensions.

In asthma vigorous physiotherapy, especially forced expiratory manoeuvres, can increase bronchospasm. During acute exacerbations of bronchitis, and in pneumonia, studies have shown no benefit from physiotherapy, and in the absence of excessive secretions it is difficult to justify physiotherapy for these patients. Mucociliary clearance is decreased and basal collapse increased during general anaesthesia and surgery, particularly surgery to the upper abdomen. However, the case for routine physiotherapy in patients with chronic airflow limitation is not proven, except for high risk cases. Following coronary artery bypass grafting, recovery of blood gases and lung function is just as rapid with mobilization, as with specific physiotherapy (Jenkins *et al.*, 1989).

Overall, with the exception of sputum clearance in cystic fibrosis and bronchiectasis, it is difficult to see a specific role for chest physiotherapy in respiratory rehabilitation (Cornudella and Sangenis, 1991).

REHABILITATION PROGRAMMES

Pulmonary rehabilitation is of considerable current interest (Donner and Howard, 1991; Belman, 1993; Petty, 1993). The scope of rehabilitation can include long-term oxygen therapy, general exercise training, specific respiratory muscle training, nutritional supplementation, as well as patient education and support. In North America the key elements of rehabilitation are considered to be: patient and family education, pharmacological agents, breathing training and exercises, systemic exercise, oxygen therapy and patient support groups. It is the provision of all of these forms of therapy together, within the context of a rehabilitation programme, facilitated by a multidisciplinary team that makes rehabilitation distinct from conventional management.

Over and above the benefits of drug therapy, oxygen therapy and stopping smoking, there may be substantial benefit from rehabilitation programmes, education, physical training and patient support. Such programmes have been widely used in the USA for many years, but are relatively little used in the UK and Europe. The usual pattern is for small groups of patients to take part in a particular programme, working together, and for them to be treated over a period of approximately 8 weeks. Education about medical problems and discussion of therapy is followed by breathing training and exercises. General exercise training to recondition muscle and other systems is considered to be of central importance. In most rehabilitation programmes, walking is considered the most appropriate general exercise, and it is possible

that regular general training may reduce lactate production by exercising muscle, and therefore reduce ventilatory requirements (Casaburi *et al.*, 1991).

The deconditioned limb muscles of patients with severe respiratory disease have abnormal biochemistry and histology (Thompson *et al.*, 1993). However, most patients with COPD are limited by breathlessness and this limits their capacity to perform general training, and therefore reduces any possible beneficial effect that might otherwise follow cardiovascular and muscle reconditioning. In addition to breathlessness there are many patients whose exercise capacity is limited by leg fatigue (Killian *et al.*, 1992).

A number of uncontrolled clinical studies of general exercise training have indicated improved performance (Guthrie and Petty, 1970; Belman, 1986), but this improvement reflects many different factors including increased skill at performing the task that is being assessed, reduced breathlessness as a consequence of reduced anxiety, increased motivation because of the support received, or an increase in the metabolic efficiency and performance of muscle. No studies have demonstrated any improvement in lung function. It remains unclear whether improved motivation, enhanced skills and any reduction in breathlessness, in response to general exercise training, translates into reduced disability or improvement in quality of life. Rehabilitation programmes produce physical, psychological and placebo responses. In the small number of available controlled studies, relatively minor increases in 12-minute walking distance have been demonstrated (McGavin *et at.*, 1977; Cockcroft and Berry, 1981.). In a more recent and larger controlled study, 119 patients with COPD were randomized to receive either a full rehabilitation programme, or simple education alone (Toshima, Kaplan and Ries, 1990). There was an increase in treadmill walking time in patients who received the full rehabilitation programme, compared to those receiving education alone, although the mechanism for the improvement remained unclear. More controlled clinical studies are required to answer the fundamental questions as to whether rehabilitation programmes are effective and, if so, what are the mechanisms whereby improvement is produced. A key question is also whether any improvement in exercise performance translates into reduced breathlessness, improved performance in everyday activities and enhanced quality of life. Until these central questions are answered it is probably not sensible to invest scarce health care resources into respiratory rehabilitation.

RESPIRATORY MUSCLE TRAINING

In patients with airways obstruction or pulmonary fibrosis, the work of breathing is increased and this excessive load is borne predominantly by the muscles of inspiration. With suitable training programmes limb muscle performance can be improved, and a large number of studies have been undertaken to assess the value of specific respiratory muscle training. In normal subjects Leith and Bradley (1976) documented substantial improvement in the strength and endurance of the respiratory muscles following training. Some studies in patients with chronic airflow limitation, cystic fibrosis and quadriplegia, have shown benefit in terms of respiratory muscle strength, endurance and exercise tolerance. However other studies have shown little or no objective improvement, and as part of a general rehabilitation programme it remains doubtful whether specific training of the respiratory muscles is useful. A recent meta-analysis of the 17 controlled studies available in the literature concluded that there was little evidence of clinically important benefit of respiratory muscle training in patients with chronic airflow limitation (Smith *et al.*, 1992).

SMOKING

Smoking is an important aetiological factor in chronic bronchitis, emphysema, lung cancer and ischaemic heart disease, as well as causing, cough, aggravating asthma and increasing susceptibility to pulmonary infection. All patients with chronic lung disease should stop smoking, If patients with chronic bronchitis and emphysema can stop smoking, particularly in the earlier stages of their disease, airways obstruction is improved. The problem for both patients and physicians is how this is to be achieved (Higenbottam and Chamberlain, 1984; Samet and Coultas, 1991; Worth 1991; Austoker, Sanders and Fowler, 1994). A powerful influence on successfully stopping smoking is whether a patient's spouse or cohabitant continues to smoke, and the physician needs to involve the patient's family in the task. It is as well to remember that up to 20% of patients falsely claim to have stopped smoking.

Nicotine is the most active pharmacological agent in cigarette smoke, exerting a powerful effect on the autonomic nervous system, and nicotine-containing compounds have been widely used as cigarette substitutes. The most extensively studied has been nicotine chewing gum, which has been shown to help those patients who ask for it and who are therefore highly motivated to stop smoking (Jarvis *et al.*, 1982). In patients with smoking-related diseases randomly allocated between nicotine gum, placebo and advice only, long-term abstinence is less than 10% with no difference between the three treatment groups. Transdermal nicotine replacement therapy is more effective than gum (Abelin *et al.*, 1989), and has an important place in any comprehensive strategy to help patients quit smoking. The place of nicotine nasal spray therapy has yet to be fully evaluated. Results from anti-smoking clinics offering advice and guidance show them to be relatively ineffective, with less than 15% long-term abstinence if biochemical verification of non-smoking is demanded. A physician's advice, particularly to the symptomatic patient, is more effective, as may be the advice of nurses and other health staff. The opportunity to advise patients to stop smoking should therefore never be let pass. Controlled studies suggest that hypnosis and acupuncture have little effect and aversion therapy is seldom successful.

The majority of patients will continue to smoke despite all available measures to persuade them to stop. If smokers are not able to quit, they should be encouraged to smoke fewer cigarettes, switch to low tar brands, not to over smoke low tar cigarettes, take fewer puffs, and inhale less. When cigarette smokers switch to cigars and pipes, they usually continue to inhale, and can therefore achieve similar or increased tobacco smoke exposure.

REFERENCES

Abelin, T., Muller, P., Buchler, A. *et al.* (1989) Controlled trial of transdermal nicotine patches in smoking cesssation. Lancet, **1**, 7-9.

Arora, N.S. and Rochester, D.F. (1982) Ventilatory muscle strength and maximum voluntary ventilation in undernourished patients *American Review of Respiratory Disease*, **126**, 5–8.

Austoker, J., Sanders, D. and Fowler, G. (1994) Smoking and cancer: smoking cessation. *British Medical Journal*, **308**, 1478–82.

Baudouin, S.V., Bott, J., Ward, A., Deane, C. and Moxham, J. (1992) Short-term effect of oxygen on renal haemodynamics in patients with hypoxaemic chronic obstructive airways disease *Thorax*, **47**, 550–4.

Belman, J.M. (1993) Exercise in patients with chronic obstructive pulmonary disease. *Thorax*, **48**, 936–46.

Belman, M.J. (1986) Exercise in chronic obstructive pulmonary disease. *Clinics in Chest Medicine*, **7**, 585–97.

Bott, J., Carrol, M.P., Conway, J.H., Keilty, S.E.J., Ward, E.M., Brown, A.M., Paul, E.A., Elliott, M.W., Godfrey, R.C., Wedzicha, J.A. and Moxham, J. (1993) Randomised controlled trial of nasal ventilation in acute ventilatory failure due to chronic obstructive airways disease. *Lancet*, **341**, 1555–7.

Bradley, B.L., Garner, A.E., Billiu, D., Mestas, J.M. and Forman, J. (1978) Oxygen-assisted exercise in chronic obstructive lung disease. *American Review of Respiratory Disease*, **118**, 239–43.

Carroll, N. and Branthwaite, M.A. (1988) Control of nocturnal hypoventilation by nasal intermittent positive pressure ventilation. *Thorax*, **43**, 349–53.

Casaburi, R.R., Patession, A., Ioli, F., Zanaboni, S., Donner, C.G. and Wasserman, K. (1991) Reductions in exercise lactic acidosis and ventilation as a result of exercise training in patients with obstructive lung disease. *American Review of Respiratory Disease*, **143**, 9–18.

Cochrane, G.M. (1984) Editorial: show-release theophyllines and chronic bronchitis. *British Medical Journal*, **289**, 1643–4.

Cochrane, G.M., Webber, B.A. and Clarke, S.W. (1977) Effects of sputum on pulmonary function. *British Medical Journal*, **2**, 1181–3.

Cockcroft, A.E. and Berry, G. (1981) Randomised controlled trial of rehabilitation in chronic respiratory disability. *Thorax*, **36**, 200–03.

Cooper, C.B., Waterhouse, J. and Howard, P. (1987) Twelve year clinical study of patients with hypoxic cor pulmonale given long-term domiciliary oxygen therapy. *Thorax*, **42**, 105–10.

Cornudella, R. and Sangenis, M. (1991) Chest physical therapy. *European Respiratory Review*, **1**, 503–6.

Cotes, J.E. (1960) Respiratory function and portable oxygen therapy in chronic non-specific lung disease in relation to prognosis. *Thorax*, **15**, 244–51.

Decramer, M, Lacque, L.M., Fagard, R. and Rogiers, P. (1994) Corticosteroids contribute to muscle weakness in chronic airflow obstruction. *American Journal of Respiratory and Critical Care Medicine*, **150**, 11–16.

Douglas, N.J. and Flenley, D.C. (1990) Breathing during sleep in patients with obstructive lung disease. *American Review of Respiratory Disease*, **141**, 1055–70.

Donner, C.F. and Howard, P. (eds) (1991) Pulmonary rehabilitation in chronic obstructive pulmonary disease (COPD) with recommendations for its use. *European Respiratory Review*, **1**, 463–568.

Elliott, M. and Moxham, J. (1994) Non-invasive mechanical ventilation by nasal or face mask, in *Principles and Practice of Mechanical Ventilation*, (ed. M.J. Tobin), McGraw-Hill, New York, pp. 427–453.

Elliott, M.W., Mulvey, D.A., Moxham, J, Green, M. and Branthwaite, M.A. (1991) Domiciliary nocturnal nasal intermittent positive pressure ventilation in COPD: mechanisms underlying changes in arterial blood gas tensions. *European Respiratory Journal*, **4**, 1044–52.

Ellis, E.R., Bye, P.T.D., Bruderer, J.W. and Sullivan, C.E. (1987) Treatment of respiratory failure during sleep in patients with neuromuscular disease. *Americal Review of Respiratory Disease*, **135**, 148–2.

Evans, T.W., Waterhouse, J.C., Carter, A., Nicholl, J.F. and Howard, P. (1986) Short burst oxygen treatment for breathlessness in chronic obstructive airways disease. *Thorax*, **41**, 611–15.

Flick, M.R. and Block, A.J. (1977) Continuous in-vivo monitoring of arterial oxygenation in chronic obstructive lung disease. *Annals of Internal Medicine*, **86**, 725–30.

Glenn, W.W.L. and Sairenji, H. (1985) Diaphragm pacing in the treatment of chronic ventilatory insufficiency, in *The Thorax: lung biology in health and disease*, vol. 29 (eds C. Roussos and P.T. Macklem), Marcel Dekker, New York, pp. 1407–40.

Guthrie, A.G. and Petty, T.L. (1970) Improved exercise tolerance in patients with chronic airway obstruction. *Physical Therapy*, **50**, 1333–7.

Harris-Eze, A.O., Sridhar, G., Clemens, R.E., Gallagher, C.G. and Marciniuk, D.D. (1994) Oxygen improves maximal exercise performance in interstitial lung disease. *American Journal of Respiration and Critical Care Medicine*, **150**, 1616–22.

Harrison, B.D.W. and Stokes, T.C. (1982) Secondary polycythaemia: its causes, effects and treatment. *British Journal of Diseases of the Chest*, **76**, 313–40.

Higenbottam, T. and Chamberlain, A. (1984) Editorial: giving up smoking. *Thorax*, **39**, 641–6.

Hoeppner, V.H., Cockcroft, D.W., Dosman, J.A. and Cotton, D.J. (1984) Nighttime ventilation improves respiratory failure in secondary kyphoscoliosis. *American Review of Respiratory Disease*, **135**, 1049–55.

Jarvis, M.J., Raw, M., Russell, M.A.H. and Feyerabend, C. (1982) Randomised controlled trial of nicotine chewing gum. *British Medical Journal*, **285**, 537–48.

Jenkins, S.C., Heaton, R.W., Fulton, T.J. and Moxham, J. (1987) Comparison of domiciliary nebulised salbutamol and salbutamol from a metered dose inhaler in stable chronic airflow limitation. *Chest*, **91**, 804–7.

Jenkins, S.C., Soutar, S.A., Loukola, J.M., Johnson, L.C. and Moxham, J. (1989) Physiotherapy after coronary surgery: are breathing exercises necessary? *Thorax*, **44**, 634–9.

Jenkins, S.C. and Moxham, J. (1987) High dose salbutamol in chronic bronchitis: comparison of 400 µg, 1 mg, 1.6 mg, 2 mg and placebo delivered by rotahaler. *British Journal of Diseases of the Chest*, **81**, 242–7.

Jenkins, S.C. and Moxham, J. (1991) The effects of mild obesity on lung function. *Respiratory Medicine*, **85**, 309–11.

Killian, K.J., LeBlanc, P., Martin, D.H., Summers, E., Jones, N.L. and Campbell, E.J.M. (1992) Exercise capacity and ventilatory, circulatory, and symptom limitation in patients with chronic airflow limitation. *American Review of Respiratory Disease*, **146**, 935–40.

Lanigan, C., Moxham, J., and Ponte, J. (1990) Effect of chronic airflow limitation on resting oxygen consumption. *Thorax*, **45**, 388–90.

Leith, D.E. and Bradley, M. (1976) Ventilatory muscle strength and endurance training. *Journal of Applied Physiology*, **41**, 508–16.

Liss, H.P. and Grant, B.J. (1988) The effect of nasal flow on breathlessness in patients with chronic obstructive pulmonary disease. *American Review of Respiratory Disease*, **137**, 1285–8.

McGavin, C.R., Gupta, S.P., Lloyd, E.L. and McHardy, G.J.R. (1977) Physical rehabilitation for the chronic bronchitic: results of a controlled trial of exercises in the home. *Thorax*, **32**, 307–11.

Medical Research Council Working Party (1981) Long-term domiciliary oxygen therapy in chronic hypoxic cor pulmonale complicating bronchitis and emphysema. *Lancet*, **i**, 681–6.

Moore-Gillon, J. (1989) Oxygen-conserving delivery devices. *Respiratory Medicine*, **83**, 263–4.

Morgan, A.D., Peck, D.F., Buchanan, R and McHardy, G.J.R. (1983) Effect of attitudes and beliefs on exercise tolerance in chronic bronchitis. *British Medical Journal*, **286**, 171–3.

Moxham, J. (1988) Theophylline and the respiratory muscles: an alternative view: *Clinics in Chest Medicine*, **9**, 352–6.

Moxham, J. (1995) The management of chronic respiratory failure and cor pulmonale, in *Oxford Textbook of Medicine*, 3rd edn (eds D. Weatherall, J.G.G. Ledinghan and D.A. Warrell), Oxford University Press, Oxford.

Moxham, J. and Shneerson, J. M. (1993) Diaphragmatic pacing. *American Review of Respiratory Disease*, **148**, 533–6.

Muers, M.F. and Green, J.H. (1993) Weight loss in chronic obstructive pulmonary disease. *European Respiratory Journal*, **6**, 729–34.

Nocturnal Oxygen Therapy Trial Group (1980) Continuous or nocturnal therapy in hypoxemic chronic obstructive lung disease. A clinical trial. *Annals of Internal Medicine*, **93**, 391–8.

Petty, T.L. (1993) Pulmonary rehabilitation in perspective: historical roots, present status and future projections. *Thorax*, **48**, 855–62.

Phillipson, E.A. (1993) Sleep apnoeal – a major public health problem. *New England Journal of Medicine*, **328**, 1271–3.

Samet, J.M. and Coultas, D.B. (eds) (!991) Smoking cessation. *Clinics in Chest Medicine*, **12**, (4).

Saunders, N.A. and Sullivan, C.E. (1984) Sleep and breathing, in *Lung biology in health and disease*, vol. 21 (ed. C. Lenfant), Marcel Dekker, New York: pp. 299,363.

Sawicka, E.H., Branthwaite, M.A. and Spencer, G.T. (1983) Respiratory failure after thoracoplasty: treatment by intermitent negative-pressure ventilation. *Thorax*, **38**, 433–5.

Sergysels, R., Lachman, A., Sanna, A. and Thys, P. (1991) Breathing retraining. *European Respiratory Review*, **1**, 498–502.

Shak, S., Capon, D.J., Helmis, R., Marsters, S.A. and Baker, C.L. (1990) Recombinant human DNase I reduces the viscosity of cystic fibrosis sputum. *Proceedings of the National Academy of Sciences, USA*, **87**, 9188–92.

Shneerson, J. (1992) Transtracheal oxygen delivery. *Thorax*, **47**, 57–9.

Smith, K., Cook, D., Guyatt, G.H., Madhavan, J. and Oxman, A.D. (1992) Respiratory muscle training in chronic airflow limitation: a meta-analysis. *American Review of Respiratory Disease*, **145**, 533–9.

Sullivan, C.E., Issa, F.G., Berthon-Jones, M., McAnley, V.B. and Costas, L.J.V. (1984) Home treatment of obstructive sleep apnoea with continuous positive airway pressure applied through a nose mask. *Clinical Respiratory Physiology*, **20**, 49–54.

Sutton, P.P., Pavia, D., Bateman, J.R.M. and Clarke S.W. (1982) Chest physiotherapy: a review. *European Journal of Respiratory Disease*, **63**, 188–201.

Swinburn, C.R., Wakefield, J.M. and Jones, P.W. (1984) Relationship between ventilation and breathlessness during exercise in chronic obstructive airways disease is not altered by prevention of hypoxemia. *Clinical Science*, **67**, 515–19.

Thompson, C.H., Davies, R.J.O., Kemp, G.J., Gaylor, D.J., Radda, G.K. and Rajagopalan, B. (1993) Skeletal muscle metabolism during exercise and recovery in patients with respiratory failure. *Thorax*, **48**, 486–90.

Toshima, M.T., Kaplan, R.M. and Ries, A.L. (1990) Experimental evaluation of rehabilitation in chronic obstructive pulmonary disease: short-term effects on exercise endurance and health status. *Health Psychology*, **9**, 237–52.

Warren, P.M., Flenley, D.C., Millar, J.S. and Avery, A. (1980) Respiratory failure revisited: acute exacerbations of chronic bronchitis between 1961–1968 and 1970–1976. *Lancet*, **i**, 467–71.

Waterhouse, J.C. and Howard, P. (1983) Breathlessness and portable oxygen in chronic obstructive airways disease. *Thorax*, **38**, 302–6.

Woodcock, A.A., Gross, E.R., Gellert, A., Shah, S., Johnson, M. and Geddes, D.M. (1981) Effects of dihydrocodeine, alcohol, and caffeine on breathlessness and exercise tolerance in patients with chronic obstructive lung disease and normal blood gases. *New England Journal of Medicine*, **305**, 1611–16.

Worth, H. (1991) Smoking cessation. *European Respiratory Review*, **1**, 507–10.

18 *Cardiac rehabilitation*

G. Jackson

BACKGROUND

Coronary artery disease (CAD) is the single greatest cause of disability and mortality for men and women. Each year in the UK it is estimated that 320 000 people consult for angina and 300 000 experience a myocardial infarct. Furthermore, 80 000 men and 70 000 women die from CAD each year. The predicted need for coronary artery bypass grafting (CABG) is 400–500 per million of the population, with a similar estimated need for percutaneous transluminal coronary angioplasty (PTCA). There are a substantial number of patients with symptomatic CAD, a growing number of patients post CABG and PTCA and the likelihood that the numbers will increase as the population ages (Fourth Report of a Joint Cardiology Committee, 1992).

Though CAD remains the principle cause of premature disability it is important not to overlook the needs of those with specific heart muscle disease (cardiomyopathy) or with degenerative valve disease who may need surgery. This is likely to be an increasing problem with an ageing population. Cardiomyopathies most often present as heart failure. Heart failure increases in incidence with age (Figure 18.1) and most often reflects underlying CAD (Kannel and Belanger, 1991).

The indirect costs of CAD are substantial. In 1989 the estimated annual cost to the NHS was £500 million with only £10 million being spent on prevention. Lost production and earnings annually represent a loss of £1800 million and CAD accounts for 11.6% of all sick leave (Tunstall-Pedoe, 1991).

The running cost of a cardiac rehabilitation session is at most £20 per patient (1995 prices) and often substantially less – in other words its a cheap form of therapy (Horgan, Bethell and Carson, 1992).

Cardiac rehabilitation should be widely available. It is inexpensive and improves both quality and quantity of life (Chua and Lipkin, 1993). Studies of quality-adjusted life years (QALYS) have shown a favourable comparison with lipid-lowering therapy and CABG (Oldridge, Furlong and Feeny, 1993).

DEFINITION

Cardiac rehabilitation is about restoring patients with cardiac disease – usually CAD – to their optimal physical, psychological, emotional and vocational status. Though an exercise programme is the focal point, it is also essential to develop a strategy for long-term lifestyle changes to reduce cardiovascular risk factors such as smoking and hyperlipidaemia.

Does it reduce mortality?

Preoccupation with length of life rather than quality of life is not always in the best interest

Rehabilitation of the Physically Disabled Adult. Edited by C. John Goodwill, M. Anne Chamberlain and Chris Evans. Published in 1997 by Stanley Thornes (Publishers) Ltd, Cheltenham. ISBN 0-7487-3183-0.

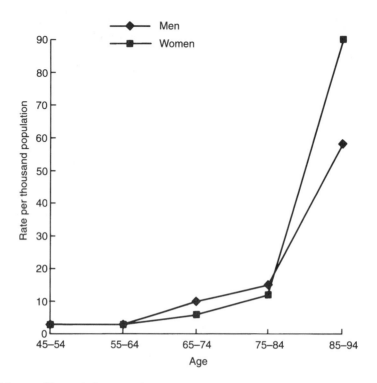

Figure 18.1 Incidence of heart failure. By the year 2001, 22% of people will be over 75 years of age and there will be a 70% increase in those over 85 years of age. Successful therapy at an early stage increases the quality and quantity of life, increasing the need for, and value of, rehabilitation programmes.

of the patient; ideally any treatment should make the patient feel better **and** live longer.

Though meta-analyses have certain limitations, an overview of 22 trials of exercise-based rehabilitation allowed the evaluation of 4500 post infarction patients (O'Connor, Buring and Yusuf 1989). This study identified a 20%–25% reduction in overall and cardiovascular mortality over 3 years comparing those who participated in a cardiac rehabilitation programme with those who did not. There appeared to be no reduction in non-fatal infarction. Only 3% of those evaluated were women and only 4 of the 22 studies included women.

These programmes also included risk factor advice and increased patient supervision so that exercise training was only a part of a multidisciplinary approach. Trials of exercise alone, without other risk factor modification, are small in number and though showing favourable trends are not statistically significant.

Exercise-based cardiac rehabilitation programmes therefore have prognostic benefits as part of an overall comprehensive risk factor reduction programme for the post–myocardial infarction patient. Whilst women form only a small number of those evaluated (3% of 4500) there is no reason to assume they will not benefit as much as men.

Does it improve quality of life?

In 1772 Heberden described a patient with angina who 'set himself a task of sawing wood for half an hour every day, and was clearly cured' over a 6-month period. Paul

Dudley-White, the great American cardiologist and pioneer of preventive and rehabilitation cardiology, advocated exercise in the early part of this century for its physical and psychological benefits in normal people and those with cardiac disease (Curfman, 1993).

We are however, generally unfit and cardiac patients more so (Paffenbarger, Hyde and Wing, 1993). After a heart attack physical fitness improves by about 10% as the heart recovers but a course of exercise can increase this to 25–30% (Haskell and De Busk, 1979). This increase has been shown to make people feel better (physical fitness leading to mental fitness) and more confident in their ability to return to manual jobs or partake in more physically demanding leisure activities (e.g. brisk walking, cycling). The only limitation on improving exercise ability post infarction is the extent of myocardial damage. Large infarcts lead to cardiac failure where management is more difficult though benefits remain possible.

Exercise promotes beneficial changes in the cardiovascular system leading to a reduced heart rate and blood pressure at rest and on exercise, thereby reducing oxygen demand. In the short term after infarction exercise reduces sympathetic tone and improves peripheral circulatory efficiency whereas in the longer term with more sustained exercise there will be an improvement centrally leading to an increased stroke volume and ejection fraction.

Regular exercise post infarction therefore has been shown to improve functional work capacity. Patients with angina benefit in a similar fashion, developing less ischaemia at a greater exercise ability. Exercise tests demonstrate less ST segment depression and thallium scans show improved perfusion. This implies that exercise on a regular basis can improve collateral blood supply (Franklin, 1991).

Exercise training can also reduce the incidence of ventricular extra-systoles in the post infarct patient. This is probably secondary to decreasing sympathetic tone as ventricular extra-systoles are increased in the presence of increased sympathetic activity and decreased parasympathetic activity. Recent studies have identified an increased mortality in post infarction and heart failure patients who demonstrate a reduction in heart rate variability, reflecting sympathetic and parasympathetic effects on the heart, and it is possible that exercise training may also be beneficial in this situation (American College of Cardiovascular Technology Assessment Committee, 1993).

Many members of the community are quite happy leading a slothful existence, making the minimum effort and enjoying activities such as television and public houses. The problem we face in rehabilitation is restoring the person to where he/she was before the illness, and then convincing him/her that by various lifestyle changes a further illness may be prevented, while remembering that the personality of each patient is so different. Exercise training is only part of the story and no aspect of risk factor reduction or rehabilitation can be viewed in isolation:

- Exercise-based rehabilitation as part of a secondary prevention programme post infarction improves prognosis.
- Quality of life is improved by exercise training post infarction and for those with angina and cardiac failure. Similar benefits can be obtained after cardiac surgery.

MYOCARDIAL INFARCTION

This condition gives rise to much morbidity, so it is not surprising that most cardiac rehabilitation is orientated towards it. There are other conditions, such as angina, post surgery and after coronary heart disease (CHD), in which rehabilitation may also be helpful. It is useful, however, to use myocardial infarction (MI) as the model.

Rehabilitation begins at the onset of the illness with as much communication as possible between the medical professions and the patient, spouse and family. The outcome will be related to personality (coping ability and comprehension of the illness) and social background (work, housing, finances and family responsibilities). It will also be modified by family strengths and weaknesses.

Normal reactions to an infarct are denial, anxiety and depression. The degree of the reactions is usually mild from 'why me' to a temporary bout of 'the blues'. Occasionally the reaction is pathological, usually because of a preceding problem either recognized or not; profound depression, or rarely a psychotic episode may follow. Emotional disturbances can be expected in about 60% of people admitted to a coronary care unit.

The onset of myocardial infarction is painful and frightening. In many ways how the patient copes depends on how he/she is dealt with initially. The immediate relief of pain with intravenous diamorphine with the antiemetic cyclizine helps to alleviate the patient's and families' immediate fears which revolve around death. The family are relieved to be in a 'safe' environment (hospital) and the immediate alleviation of the major symptom reinforces the idea that whatever has or is happening the patient is 'in the right hands'.

Coronary care unit

Initially the patient is anxious, tired and may still be in pain (Table 18.1). At this point the diagnosis should be explained in simple terms to both the patient and spouse at the same interview, so each knows what the other knows, saying the heart is bruised and sore and needs to rest, and the best thing the patient can do to help for the first day is to rest in bed. Even at this stage the patient learns that he/she is helping him/herself. Monitors are explained as routine protection and the patient is to be seen as the most important individual of a team.

Denial is a common problem, especially with professionals, particularly doctors.

Table 18.1 Patients' thoughts

What is wrong with me?
Am I going to die?
How can I stop this happening again?
Why can't my children visit?
I'm bored in hospital.
I'm lonely at night.
Why is my wife/husband so anxious?
What about my job?
Should I cancel my holiday?

Resorting to antacids, anything to avoid the obvious, leads to its own problems, for in the first 6 hours the greatest mortality occurs and the greatest potential for restoring patency by thrombolysis or PTCA and reducing mortality. Denial usually gives away to reality, but often in the Type A personality (aggressive, ambitious, impatient) it persists, and though this may be useful in the short term with regard to a positive approach to recovery, in the long term it may be detrimental. It is estimated that 20% of people 2 weeks after an infarct still doubt it happened. Men exhibit more denial than women, and it is invariably men who take their own discharge against advice.

Anxiety is universal. What is wrong with me? Am I going to die? The patient may see and be distressed by the death of other patients in the unit. When the patient is transferred to a general ward, the loss of high staffing level and the 'high-tech' equipment gives a sense of vulnerability. Whenever questions arise, the opportunity to ask must be available and the questions should not be avoided. The doctor or nurse must talk to the patient taking time and giving eye contact. Ideally they should sit with the patient. Patients with poor understanding need more patience, not less time. Moving to the ward is accompanied by stating how good the progress is and 'you don't need to be here any more'. At this point a plan for the patient should evolve now that the patient and family are more able to absorb the meaning of the illness and plan for the future. The future can be seen as a series of two's:

Two weeks (or less) – in hospital for healing and gradual mobilization;

Two weeks – at home gradually increasing activity;

Two weeks – at home accelerating back to normal with a positive approach to the future and a 6-week medical assessment to deal with problems or advise the patient on return to work. Keeping it simple and straightforward is the key to recovery. Those who remain anxious may benefit from a short course of diazepam.

Depression may not be a problem but, if it is, it usually presents on the third day after leaving the coronary care unit (Leng, 1994). There may be concern over jobs in the current economic climate, especially for heavy goods vehicle or public service vehicle drivers; guilt, invariably because of heavy smoking, and helplessness are paramount. The male feels his 'manhood' is challenged – especially the younger male. Women may be concerned for their family, often placing others before themselves, and feel especially guilty (Jackson, 1994). With a positive approach to the future this is less of a problem. Talking of the future and planning rehabilitation circumvents many of the problems without recourse to specific antidepressant therapy. If depression persists psychiatric assessment should be undertaken before prescribing drugs because there may have been a preceding problem which needs specialist evaluation (Thompson, 1994).

Booklets

No matter how clearly the doctor or nurse feels they have expressed themselves, with the background of stress and anxiety the patient and family may misinterpret or become confused by the information given. Providing written information for the patient and spouse as soon as possible answers many of the asked and unasked questions which preoccupy all concerned. There is a far greater understanding of the illness, and a more satisfactory recovery in those given written as well as oral information. Booklets are not a substitute for talking, but complement and often enhance the interviews by prompting the patient to ask relevant and sometimes awkward but important questions (Jackson, 1978). Sources include The British Heart Foundation and Zeneca Pharmaceuticals.

The general ward

Physical rehabilitation commences here. The rehabilitation programme should be run by specially trained physiotherapists and a designated rehabilitation nurse who acts as a coordinator. Where necessary patients with difficulties can be seen by a psychiatrist, who may enrol them in group counselling sessions where concerns can be freely discussed and mutual reassurance given.

Education will help to alleviate fear and anxiety. If the doctor really 'doesn't have time' to talk he/she should say so, but emphatically make the point that he/she is going to come back. Simple, accurate information is all that is needed initially. From the general ward and into convalescence recommendations on management and prevention must be given to the patient. Table 18.2 illustrates the inpatient programme in the author's hospital.

After discharge

The hospital environment is controlled and protective; some anxiety may occur upon discharge. Feelings of fatigue usually follow the environmental change, but can also reflect

Table 18.2 Inpatient exercise programme, coronary/CABG

Days 1 and 2 in CCU or ITU		
	(i)	Routine breathing exercises
	(ii)	Foot exercises and knee flexion
Days 3–4 to ward		
	If patient is pain free for 24 hours, then:	
Day 3	(iii)	Sit over side of bed
	(iv)	Shoulder elevation
	(v)	Shoulder shrugging
Day 3/4	(vi)	Sit in chair
Day 4/5	(vii)	Walk in ward and to toilet
Day 5/6	(viii)	Straight-leg raising in long sitting
	(ix)	Lifting technique
Day 6/7	(x)	Stairs, gradually increasing amount
	(xi)	Introduce home exercise programme

Patients are usually discharged from day 7 onwards and should be given a home exercise sheet and the leaflet on coronary heart disease.

too much physical activity. The patient should be told to anticipate this and not overdo things initially. Aches and pains previously discounted may assume greater importance. The patient should have the difference between cardiac and non-cardiac pain carefully explained (Table 18.3).

Table 18.3 Chest pain characteristics

Cardiac	Non-cardiac
Tightness	Sharp (not severe)
Pressure	Knife-like
Weight	Stabbing
Constriction	'Like a stitch'
Ache	'Like a needle'
Dull	Pricking feeling
Squeezing feeling	Shooting
Soreness	Reproduced by pressure or position
Crushing	Can walk around with it
'Like a band'	Continuous: 'It's there all day, Doc.'
Breathlessness	

Getting back to normal

For most patients prolonged rest and convalescence are unnecessary. Those who have a positive treadmill test will have an increased morbidity and mortality at 1 year. For them elective bypass surgery or PTCA may be able to prevent subsequent infarction and death. By combining the treadmill test with the rehabilitation process it is possible to reinforce the recovery of the patient. Early ambulation reduces problems such as deep vein thrombosis, as well as anxiety and depression. Enrolment into a cardiac rehabilitation programme at this stage is of considerable help. The programme is two pronged, with an exercise programme supported by group activities.

The exercise programme has to be tailored to the individual. Originally such programmes were developed for middle-aged males; women and older men did not attend. Poor attendance may be associated with the fact that the women experience more depression, anxiety and guilt about their illness (Jackson, 1994).

A typical support programme may consist of monthly meetings in which a variety of issues are addressed such as smoking, diet and general health. Medical information about bypass surgery and angioplasty can be given. The meetings provide the opportunity to discuss and teach relaxation techniques. The Royal College of Physicians advice that 'a crucial aspect of rehabilitation is the appointment of a person with special responsibility for the programmes' is sound. Patients may be given a long-term exercise programme supplemented by literature and tapes to promote healthy living.

Treadmill ECG

All patients under the age of 70 who have sustained an uncomplicated myocardial infarct should undergo routine treadmill testing to their maximum ability from 2 to 4 weeks after infarct. If this is combined with a programme of rehabilitation it helps to encourage maximum recovery.

Work

Most people (up to 90%) in employment before their heart attack can return to work and may do so after 3–6 months. Trials showing the effects of rehabilitation on speed of returning to work have variable results, probably reflecting the economic (job) climate (Horgan, Betrell and Carson, 1992). Those in more physically demanding jobs may benefit from a more vigorous exercise programme whilst others by virtue of the nature of their previous occupation may not be able to return and early retirement may be the most sensible option. It is important to make clear to the patient that other alternatives may be available and early retirement does not equate with 'failure'.

Returning to work was previously the yardstick by which successful rehabilitation was judged. This is less appropriate now as employers use illness as grounds for 'medical retirement' in the presence of high employment and increased redundancy.

Travel and driving

Air travel (in commercial pressurized aircraft) is safe from 6 weeks but may be undertaken earlier if essential. Ordinarily non-vocational car driving may be resumed from 4 weeks. It is not necessary to inform the DVLA but it is essential to inform the car insurance company of the illness. However, when driving is part of the occupation the DVLA has introduced clear and practical guideliness covering all aspects of cardiovascular problems. Group 1 is the ordinary driving licence whereas Group 2 is the Large Goods Vehicle Licence (LGV) – previously HGV/PSV.

Sexual activity

Following a heart attack fears by the patient and/or partner that sex may 'damage the heart' or 'bring about another attack' can increase anxiety and reduce sexual interest and activity. Fear about performance and post infarction depression may also reduce the desire to make love.

Fortunately several studies are available which can be used as a basis for giving advice and guidelines to cardiac patients. Nemec, Mansfield and Ward Kennedy, (1976) studied 10 normal males aged 24–40 years, recording heart rate on a portable (Holter) ECG recorder, and blood pressure with an automatic Doppler device. This study was conducted in the home environment with their wives. The average resting heart rate was 60 ± 8 beats per minute rising to 92 ± 13 at intromission and achieving a maximal rate of 114 ± 14 at orgasm. At 120 seconds of resolution the rate had already fallen to 69 ± 12 beats per minute. Similar responses occurred whether the male was on top or underneath. Blood pressure rose from a mean of 112/66 mmHg at rest to 148/79 at intromission and a maximum of 163/81 at orgasm. Resting levels were achieved 120 seconds into resolution. Position made no significant difference.

Hellerstein and Friedman (1970), evaluating middle-aged (mean 47 years) patients with ischaemic heart disease, reported an average maximal heart rate of 117 beats per minute (range 90–114) during sex, in comparison to 120 (range 107–130) during other activities. Similar findings were reported in patients with angina pectoris who were studied in the UK, with heart rates during sex at 122 ± 7.1 beats per minute and 124 ± 7.2 during other activities. Larson *et al.* (1980) compared the cardiovascular response to sex with stair climbing. The stair test involved walking for 10 minutes then climbing 22 stairs in 10 seconds (the average English flight is 12–13 stairs). In the control subjects the mean maximal heart rate was 123 ± 8 during sex and 122 ± 5 on the stairs, whilst in the patients who had suffered coronaries it was 118 ± 6 and 115 ± 7 respectively. The systolic blood pressure rose modestly to 146 ± 2 mmHg in the controls for both stresses, but in the coronary patients it was actually less during sex (144 ± 6 mmHg) than on the stairs (164 ± 7 mmHg) ($P < 0.01$).

A pattern of cardiovascular responses emerges. For those married or cohabiting for a long time the heart rate and blood pressure response is modest, achieving its maximum at orgasm. For middle-aged couples this occurs on average twice a week, with a maximal response representing only 15 seconds or so of the 16 minutes' average duration of sexual intercourse.

Sex is part of a normal lifestyle of an individual, whether he or she has coronary disease or not. As in any form of exercise, myocardial demand (heart rate and blood pressure) will increase. With appropriate background information the physician or nurse can place the demand in its appropriate context, reassure the needlessly concerned and by simple tests (e.g. climbing two flights of stairs) enable individuals to lead full and satisfactory lives. The subject may not be raised by the patient, but a failure to advise on a resumption of sex can lead to frustration and marital conflict, especially if one of the partners is much younger than the other. Masturbation helps some regain their confidence because it does not involve such a vigorous cardiac response and it can ease the transition to intercourse. Oral sex places no undue stress on the heart. Anal intercourse may lead to cardiac arrhythmias but the data is sparse and should not cause concern to cohabiting homosexuals.

Death during sex is rare but more common with extramarital sex when it usually follows a meal and drink and takes place in an unfamiliar and stressful environment – 'hotel sex'. Sex between couples in a long-term relationship who are comfortable with each other has no increased risk of death or infarction compared with other similar degrees of physical stress on the heart.

Reducing risk factors

Stopping smoking

Cigarette smoking alone is responsible for 25% of coronary deaths in those under 65 years and 80% for men below 45 years. The risk of a future infarct can be halved within 5 years of stopping smoking. All smokers are at risk but especially those with additional risk factors such as hypertension or diabetes. Therefore, a most important part of cardiac rehabilitation is to help people stop smoking.

Stress

Stress cannot be easily defined; it is an individual's perception of life. It is a particular problem if other risk factors are present. Emotionally demanding aspects of an individual's lifestyle, whether at home or work, can provoke stress. Regular holidays, non-stressful lunchtimes and restful home activities (e.g. gardening, walking, reading) may help to make a lifestyle change. This may be easier for the patient to follow than expected. No one on his death bed wished that he had spent more time at the office!

Diet

Obesity increases blood pressure and can be associated with abnormal glucose tolerance and hyperlipidaemia. Weight loss will reduce cardiac load. A weight-reducing, low saturated fat diet is, therefore, an important part of rehabilitation. Hyperlipidaemia found after the development of CAD should be treated. In the Scandinavian Simvastatin Survival Study Group (1994) simvastatin significantly reduced overall mortality, coronary mortality, PTCA and CABG events when compared with placebo. It is thought that this was due to a direct effect of lowering cholesterol (Table 18.4).

Cardiologists have recently been rebuked for failing to involve themselves with the metabolic components of CAD (Stevenson *et*

Table 18.4 Result of the Scandinavian Simvastatin Survival Study

End-point	Effect of simvastatin
Overall risk of death	30% reduction
Risk of coronary death	42% reduction
Risk of major coronary events	34% reduction
Risk of revascularization procedures	37% reduction
Event-free survival	26% increase
LDL cholesterol reduction[a]	35%
HDL cholesterol elevation[a]	8%
Total cholesterol reduction[a]	25%

[a]Over the whole course of the study.

al, 1994) The truth is a mixture, with some fully involved and some totally uninterested. The facts, however, are clear.

All patients with CAD should have a full lipid profile. Exercise will lower total cholesterol and increase the protective HDL (high density lipoprotein) cholesterol but the effects are not usually enough and need to be supplemented by diet and drugs in most cases. Angiographic benefits in regressing atheroma and delaying progression of atheroma are compelling on their own (MAAS Investigators, 1994), but combined with significantly improved mortality and morbidity end-points it is now essential to fully evaluate and normalize the lipid status of all those with proven CAD, working towards a target LDL cholesterol of 3.4 mmol l^{-1} or less and an ideal of 3.0 mmol l^{-1}. Lipids may be falsely normal or low for 2 months after infarction and 1 month after CABG.

Blood pressure

Controlling blood pressure significantly reduces the incidence of stroke and to a lesser extent (though not significant) cardiac events. Immediately post infarction or CABG the blood pressure may be normal, rising to hypertensive levels over 2–3 weeks. Hypertension can be managed initially by weight loss, reduced salt and alcohol intake (Alderman, 1994). This should be part of routine advice on the rehabilitation course. Annual blood pressure monitoring for normotensive patients as a means of screening for hypertension is worthwhile because treatment reduces the incidence of stroke.

ANGINA

Angina is chest pain brought on by effort or emotion and relieved by rest and/or sublingual glyceryl trinitrate. The extent of obstructive CAD which may induce anginal chest pain varies widely between individuals. Identifying those at risk of infarction and death whose prognosis may be substantially improved by coronary bypass surgery is not difficult. Too many people are confined to unacceptable limitations because of too great an emphasis on conservative medical treatment. Mild symptoms are easily accepted by patient and physician but neither knows whether the underlying anatomical problem is potentially dangerous. All patients under 70 years of age should undergo treadmill exercise testing to establish their risk status. If positive for ischaemia, angiography may identify a pattern of coronary lesions which, independent of symptoms, adversely affects prognosis, a prognosis which surgery will improve (Jackson, 1995).

For the patient angina means heart disease and the possibility of infarction and death. Counselling the patient on risk factor modification is essential and weight reduction, blood pressure control and stopping smoking are essential. A frank discussion with patient and spouse is strongly advised. The patient must be encouraged to volunteer any difficulties he or she may have. It is easy to prescribe beta blocking drugs which help to reduce anginal attacks and increase exercise performance. Particularly with everyday life they preserve the spontaneity of events, whereas nitrates sublingually at the wrong time can emphasize the underlying problem. Many hypotensive drugs may produce impotence, including beta blockers in up to 15% (this is rarely mentioned).

An exercise programme may improve well-being and it should be pleasurable. It is no use jogging if it is hated; better to walk in the countryside, swim, dance or play tennis. Some prefer golf, others would sooner sit and fish. There has to be enjoyment, otherwise stress will be all that follows. Booklets should be used to supplement the advice given at consultation.

HEART FAILURE

This is one of the more difficult aspects of cardiac disease to rehabilitate, though careful regular exercise can be helpful. If the failure reflects valvar damage and medical therapy is unsuccessful, valve replacement can be dramatically beneficial. When the problem is heart muscle disease, from whatever cause, then controlling symptoms at the same time as maintaining activity requires the early use of angiotensin converting enzyme (ACE) inhibitors (McMurray and Rankin, 1994).

Conventional therapy of heart failure involves diuretics and digoxin in appropriate cases. Diuretics are excellent in removing volume and relieving breathlessness. However, as the need for diuretics increases so the volume decreases, until the critical balance between blood returning to the heart and blood leaving it is reduced too far. Breathlessness will be resolved but cardiac output will not be increased and a dry-skinned, dehydrated, tired and lethargic individual will result.

By the early use of ACE inhibitors the blood returning to the heart (preload) can be reduced and the blood leaving the heart have the resistance reduced (afterload), thereby facilitating cardiac output. A 25–30% improvement in performance can be achieved without the social inconvenience and debility of excessive diuresis. The

quality of life improves for a substantial number of patients. Importantly, ACE inhibitors not only improve well-being but lengthen life and are an essential component of heart failure management (Jackson, 1993).

CARDIAC SURGERY

After surgery the immediate problem is musculoskeletal pain from the thoracic spine and anterior chest wall. There may be pain from the leg scars as a result of vein dissection after CABG. The patient needs to be warned that this is going to happen and booklets can supplement the advice given by doctors and nursing staff. The pain normally resolves slowly, though in a small but significant number it persists and interferes with mobilization. Here a 2- to 4-week course of a non-steroidal anti-inflammatory drug may help.

Surgical patients are in hospital an average of 8 days and on discharge are mobile, climbing stairs, etc. It is important to emphasize to the patient and spouse that they have not had an illness but had one prevented or corrected. They cannot undo the good of the operation – it will not fall apart. Sexual relations can be resumed as so desired but the sternal pain may be limiting. The side-to-side position or mutual masturbation will usually circumvent these problems. The male hair may grow back 'prickly like a hedgehog' and be painful to the female. A soft cushion between partners is helpful.

With the emphasis on resuming normal life, a return to walking or swimming should begin as early as possible. Car driving can usually be resumed after 1 month (see above), with a return to work at approximately 8–10 weeks. If progress at 6 weeks is not as quick as expected the reason may be a lack of confidence. A rehabilitation programme can help.

CONGENITAL HEART DISEASE

With successful surgery in childhood many adolescents now live much longer, but have persisting symptoms and handicap. The problems of heart failure, pulmonary hypertension and arrhythmias are compounded by the normal problems of growing up. The problems of the young disabled adult are discussed elsewhere (Chapter 51). Heart transplantation may be an option, but is only palliative and may need repeating in 5–6 years. There is a need for the paediatric cardiologist to supervise into adult life to maintain continuity of care and expertise.

PROBLEMS ENCOUNTERED BY WOMEN

The problems of the woman with cardiac illness are sometimes forgotten. In many homes women still do much of the housework. Following a heart attack the patient comes home after 8–10 days and should have time before resuming full household activities. She needs help from her husband, children or other relatives and friends; firm medical advice may help this to be forthcoming.

Whilst women are in general older and with more advanced disease at presentation a significant number of younger women are developing CAD and their needs are substantially different. There is increasing evidence that hormone replacement therapy (HRT) can reduce cardiovascular events by 50% so advice on HRT should now be available as part of a cardiac rehabilitation programme (Rich-Edwards *et al*, 1995). Women may need a more specifically designed rehabilitation programme or single sex programme.

SAFETY

People may be concerned that physical exercise might bring about sudden death, but it is extremely rare as part of a properly structured and supervised rehabilitation programme. The risks are reduced by using the treadmill ECG as a means of screening those

especially at risk and beginning the exercise regime gradually, avoiding over-exercise and carefully monitoring patients for exercise-induced symptoms. Staff need to be fully trained in resuscitation techniques and a defibrillator and appropriate resuscitation drugs should be readily available.

AUDIT

The treatment programme should be audited for physical progress, psychological and social outcome, and reduction of risk factors to ensure that it fulfills the needs of the patients.

SUMMARY

Cardiac illness is a family problem. All members need advice about what is going on, what will happen and how everyone, including the patient, can contribute to a quick recovery and a healthy future. We need to know more about the effects on children when a parent suffers cardiac disease and we should provide a comprehensive family approach to rehabilitation. Cardiac rehabilitation is an essential aspect of the care we provide for patients with CAD, especially post infarction or after CABG. It is cheap, safe and effective and should be available to all who may benefit.

REFERENCES

Alderman, M.H. (1994) Non-pharmacological treatment of hypertension. *Lancet*, **344**, 307–11.

American College of Cardiovascular Technology Assessment Committee (1993) Heart rate variability for risk stratification of life-threatening arrhythmias. *Journal of the American College of Cardiology*, **22**, 948–50.

Chua, T.P. and Lipkin, D.P. (1993). Cardiac rehabilitation: should be available to all who would benefit. *British Medical Journal*, **306**, 731–2.

Curfman, G.D. (1993) The health benefits of exercise: a critical reappraisal. *New England Journal of Medicine*, **328**, 574–576.

Fourth Report of a Joint Cardiology Committee of the Royal College of Physicians of London and the Royal College of Surgeons of England (1992) Provision of services for the diagnosis and treatment of heart disease *British Heart Journal*, **67**, 106–16.

Franklin, B. (1991) Exercise training and coronary collateral circulation. *Medicine and Science in Sports and Exercises*, **23**, 648–53.

Haskell, W. and De Busk, R. (1979) Cardiovascular responses to repeated treadmill exercise testing soon after myocardial infarction. *Circulation*, **60**, 1247–51.

Hellerstein, J.H. and Friedman, E.H. (1970) Sexual activity in the post coronary patient. *Archives of Internal Medicine*, **125**, 987–99.

Horgan, J. Bethell, H. and Carson, P. (1992) Working party report on cardiac rehabilitation. *British Heart Journal*, **67**, 412–8.

Jackson, G. (1978) Sexual intercourse and angina pectoris. *British Medical Journal*, **2**, 16.

Jackson, G. (1993) *Heart Failure*, 2nd edn, Martin Dunitz, London.

Jackson, G. (1994) Coronary artery disease and women. *British Medical Journal*, **309**, 555–7.

Jackson, G. (1995) *Angina*, 2nd edn, Martin Dunitz, London.

Kannel, W.B. and Belanger, A.J. (1991) Epidemiology of heart failure. *American Heart Journal* **121**, 951–7.

Larson, J.L., McNaughton, M.W., Ward Kennedy, J. and Mansfield, L.W. (1980) Heart rate and blood pressure response to sexual activity and a stair climbing test. *Heart and Lung*, **9**, 1025–30.

Leng, G.C. (1994) Depression following myocardial infarction. *Lancet*, **343**, 2–3.

McMurray, J. and Rankin, A. (1994) Cardiology – II: treatment of heart failure and artrial fibrillation and arrhythmias. *British Medical Journal*, **309**, 1631–5.

MAAS Investigators (1994) Effect of simvastatin on coronary atheroma: the multicentre anti-atheroma study (MAAS). *Lancet*, **344**, 633–8.

Nemec, E.D., Mansfield, L. and Ward Kennedy, J. (1976) Heart rate and blood pressure responses during sexual activity in normal males. *American Heart Journal*, **92**, 274–7.

O'Connor, G.T., Buring, J.E. and Yusuf, S. (1989) An overview of randomised trials of rehabilitation with exercise after myocardial infarction. *Circulation*, **80**, 234–44.

Oldridge, N., Furlong, W. and Feeny, D. (1993) Economic evaluation of cardiac rehabilitation soon after acute myocardial infarction. *American Journal of Cardiology*, **72**, 154–61.

Paffenbarger, R., Hyde, R. and Wing, A. (1993) The association of changes in physical activity level and other lifestyle characteristics with mortality among men. *New England Journal of Medicine*, **328**, 538–545.

Rich-Edwards, J.W., Manson, J.E., Hennekens, C.H. and Buring, J.E. (1995) The primary prevention of coronary heart disease in women. *New England Journal of Medicine*, **322**, 1758–66.

Scandinavian Simvastatin Survival Study Group (1994) Randomised trial of cholesterol lowering in 4444 patients with coronary heart disease: The Scandinavian Simvastatin Survival Study (4S). *Lancet*, **344**, 1383–9.

Stevenson, J.C., Godsland, I.F. and Wynn, V. (1994) Cardiologists rebuked. *Lancet*, **344**, 1557.

Thompson, D.R. (1994) Cardiac rehabilitation services: the need to develop guidelines. *Quality in Health Care*, **33**, 169–72.

Tunstall-Pedoe, H. (1991) The Health of the Nation: responses. Coronary heart disease. *British Medical Journal*, **303**, 701–4.

FURTHER READING

Taylor, J.F. (ed.) (1995) *Medical Aspects of Fitness to Drive: a guide for medical practitioners*, Medical Commission on Accident Prevention, London.

PART FOUR
SENSORY AND COMMUNICATION DISABILITY

19 Auditory disability

S.D.G. Stephens

INTRODUCTION

The OPCS Survey (Martin, Metzler and Elliott, 1988) indicated that the prevalence of hearing disability was second only to musculoskeletal disability. Furthermore, the National Study of Hearing (Davis, 1989) has indicated that even the OPCS figures were an underestimate of the true situation. In addition, both tinnitus and balance disorders arising from inner ear damage, disease or degeneration can add markedly to the individual's handicap. Within this chapter the role of tinnitus, in addition to hearing loss, will be considered. Balance disorders will not be discussed as these would cover too wide a range of additional problems.

DEFINITIONS

The World Health Organization (WHO) classification of disablements (WHO, 1980) will be used in the context of hearing loss and tinnitus, with an amendment regarding tinnitus as a discomfort, analogous to chronic pain. Tinnitus is broadly defined as a noise or noises arising in the head of an individual, in the absence of any external stimulus, and which is experienced as being heard either in one or both ears or the head. Most tinnitus arises from disorders affecting the inner ear.

Within these definitions the aetiology (e.g.

noise exposure) will result in pathological changes (e.g. hair cell damage) which, in turn, results in a measurable hearing **impairment** (elevation of the audiometric threshold at high frequencies). Other impairments will include poor frequency resolution and poor measured speech discrimination in the presence of background noise.

This impairment will subsequently impinge on the individual's listening abilities; for example, difficulty hearing the telephone bell when the television is on, needing the television turned up louder, and causing the punch lines of jokes to be missed, etc. These are the **disabilities.**

In turn these disabilities may lead to **handicaps** (the non-auditory effects of the hearing loss on the individual's life). These may include social withdrawal with consequent isolation and depression, marital problems and reduction in the person's employability. The individual's spouse, children, workmates, carer, etc. will play a major role, both positive and negative, in the determination of the degree and types of handicap experienced.

As mentioned above, the pathology may give rise to tinnitus. This may increase the disability of hearing in noisy places and may result in handicaps, particularly sleep disturbance, irritability and difficulty in concentration. These interactions are shown in Figure 19.1.

Rehabilitation of the Physically Disabled Adult. Edited by C. John Goodwill, M. Anne Chamberlain and Chris Evans. Published in 1997 by Stanley Thornes (Publishers) Ltd, Cheltenham. ISBN 0-7487-3183-0.

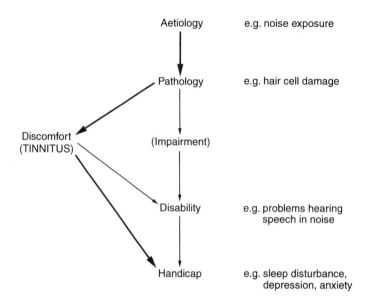

Figure 19.1 Tinnitus in relation to the WHO classification of disablements.

CAUSES OF HEARING DISABILITY

The National Study of Hearing has shown that the vast majority of hearing losses affecting the better hearing ear are related to inner ear causes. In the worse ear, however, a conductive hearing loss may contribute to 50% of the causes.

Conductive hearing losses are caused by abnormalities and disorders of the outer and middle ears. Once wax has been excluded or removed as a cause, by far the most common causes are chronic otitis media and otosclerosis. The former is a consequence of upper respiratory tract infection and may result in fibrosis of the middle ear or even destruction of the ossicles. Otosclerosis is an autosomal dominant hereditary condition of low penetrance which may be triggered by an immunological response to the measles virus. Hearing loss in this condition usually develops in the mid twenties age group in women and the mid thirties in men and results in ankylosis of the stapedial footplate

interfering with the transmission of sound from the ossicular chain into the cochlea. Both otosclerosis and chronic otitis media are frequently associated with an additional hearing loss component from damage to the cochlea.

Cochlear hearing loss has a plethora of causes but the main group is generally referred to as 'age-related hearing loss'. This is rarely due only to ageing; additional influences come from late-onset genetic hearing loss, vascular and metabolic problems, ototoxicity and social noise exposure. Many of these may also have some effect on the cochlear nerve.

Cochlear hearing loss, occurring at the transducer stage of the hearing mechanism, results in distortions of the auditory input, rather than a simple attenuation which occurs with middle ear disorders. The pattern of hearing disabilities experienced by the individual thus differs, and the handicap is often enhanced by the concomitant tinnitus. One of the more straightforward causes of cochlear hearing loss is noise exposure, whether occupationally related, from gunfire or from social noise. Noise-induced permanent hearing loss is usually preceded by episodes of temporary loss and tinnitus, which become permanent as the noise exposure is repeated.

Severe/profound congenital hearing loss occurs in only 1 per 1000 of the population, so while qualitatively important, quantitatively it is not a major problem. Most of such hearing loss is genetically determined and there are a number of conditions in which the hearing loss begins in middle age or later. A mitochondrial disorder may result in the individual being particularly sensitive to ototoxic hearing loss, especially related to streptomycin.

Drug-induced hearing loss: Streptomycin and other aminoglyocides often result in permanent inner ear damage, although certain of these drugs (e.g. streptomycin, gentamicin) affect predominantly the vestibular labyrinth while others (e.g. kanamycin, neomycin) the cochlea. Certain antimitotic drugs, particularly cis-platinum, also have permanent effects on the cochlea, as may some of the heavy metals, such as gold. Other drugs such as aspirin, NSAIDs, loop diuretics and quinine may have reversible effects on hearing, but this can occasionally be permanent. Loop diuretics can potentiate the effects of the aminoglycosides which, in their turn, can potentiate the effects of noise exposure.

Menière's disorder is an idiopathic endolymphatic hydrops, with a build up of endolymph in the scala media of the cochlea. Classically it results in episodic vertigo, fluctuant low frequency hearing loss, tinnitus and a feeling of pressure in the ear. However, many patients do not show all this classical group of symptoms. Frequently the condition is stress related. It may also be paralleled by a stress-related secondary endolymphatic hydrops aggravating the impairment in previously damaged ears.

Hearing loss is rarely caused by disorders affecting the central auditory pathways, such as multiple sclerosis, and the disabilities resulting are usually relatively minor compared with conditions affecting the middle and inner ears.

PREVALENCE OF HEARING DISABILITY

All estimates of hearing disability indicate it is very common and increases with age. In the Cardiff Health Survey respondents were asked : 'Do you have any difficulties with your hearing? If yes, please write down the most troublesome problem you have'. In a random sample of 4266 individuals, 14.7% responded that they had difficulty, the prevalence increasing markedly as a function of age (Figure 19.2). Those with hearing disability were more likely to report chronic physical disability. There was also a strong relationship between hearing disability and reported falls in elderly individuals (Stephens *et al.*, 1991).

Hearing disability was 1.3 times more common in manual workers, but gender effects were not significant. The specific difficulties listed by the individuals are shown in Table 19.1, which reflects the disabilities reported by clinic populations (Stephens, Lewis and Charny, 1990).

Significant tinnitus is found in 12–14% of the adult population with a peak prevalence in the 50–70 age group. The strongest predictor of the presence of tinnitus is the

Table 19.1 Main hearing problems listed in a community survey

Problem	%
Television/radio	22
General conversation	20
Speech in background noise	8
Hearing from one side	7
Group conversation	6
Tinnitus	4
Telephone bell/doorbell	2
Telephone conversation	1

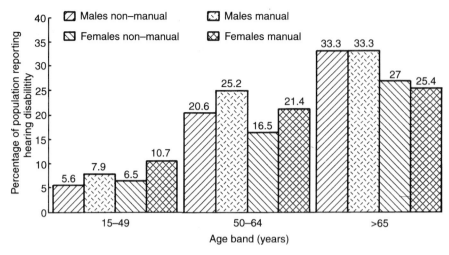

Figure 19.2 Prevalence of hearing disability in the Cardiff Health Survey.

level of hearing loss in the worse hearing ear at the higher frequencies (Coles, Davis and Smith, 1991).

CONSEQUENCES OF HEARING DISABILITY

Hearing disability may result in various types of handicap. While many studies have failed to find marked effects on employment and marital relationships in terms of unemployment and divorce, there is increasing evidence of under-employment with hearing disabled individuals failing to achieve the grade of employment which they might otherwise be expected to reach. Furthermore, while relationships do not usually breakdown altogether, they are frequently more strained and require more effort on the part of both partners to maintain them. This will depend very much on the attitude and approach of the spouses. This has been the topic of increasing study over the last few years (Hétu, Jones and Getty, 1993). Effects on the partner include stress, the need for effort and the consequent fatigue, as well as frustration, anger, resentment and guilt.

Difficulty hearing in noisy places and group situations results in social withdrawal and subsequent loneliness which is one of the most common consequences of hearing loss. Many individuals with hearing loss, even those working in noisy industries, indicate that they know no one else with hearing problems despite the fact that a sizeable proportion of their workmates have hearing losses themselves. This attitude, related in part to the stigma involved, leads to increased feeling of loneliness.

Many studies have indicated that depression is the most common psychological consequence of hearing loss. It may be made worse in many patients who also have tinnitus which, in itself, frequently results in either depression or anxiety-related symptoms. Relationships between hearing loss and suspiciousness or paranoia are less clearly documented although frequently suggested in the past. It may be that the hearing loss merely exacerbates or increases such feelings in those with an existing tendency.

The relationship between hearing loss and dementia is equally uncertain. While early evidence was at best ambivalent, some recent studies have suggested that hearing loss in those with organic brain syndromes increases the cognitive deficit, but that it does not lead to cognitive decline in the otherwise normal elderly.

MEDICAL AND SURGICAL TREATMENT

Medical and surgical treatment has only a limited role in those with hearing disabilities. As mentioned earlier, the vast majority of individuals with hearing disability have sensorineural hearing losses for which there is little evidence for improved hearing following pharmacological or surgical intervention. In those with conductive hearing loss surgery may be helpful but the patient is often left with a residual hearing disability after surgery. The two causes of permanent conductive hearing loss most amenable to surgery are otosclerosis and chronic otitis media.

The main mechanism of **otosclerosis** is a fixation of the stapes footplate causing a conductive hearing loss. However, in many individuals there may also be some cochlear hearing loss as well. Surgery entails drilling out the stapes footplate and either replacing the stapes completely with a metal or Teflon piston as a stapedectomy, or by repositioning part of the stapes as a stapedotomy. Results in terms of overcoming the conductive hearing loss are good in experienced hands but there remains a risk that the procedure may result in a more severe inner ear loss, even a dead ear, in certain cases.

In **chronic otitis media,** repair of perforations (myringoplasty) or repair of perforation with some reconstruction of the ossicular chain (tympanoplasty) may be indicated. These procedures rarely result in much improvement in hearing, but if the perforation is closed it would be easier to fit a hearing aid without complications.

Pharmacological treatment has been suggested as a means of improving hearing in certain individuals with immunological disorders, congenital syphilis, dyslipidaemias, metabolic disorders and Menières disorder. In some conditions the hearing loss may be reversible if the intervention takes place early, but once the condition is established, it is unusual for there to be a significant improvement in the hearing. At such a stage, pharmacological treatment may, however, prevent progression of the condition and relieve related symptoms such as tinnitus, vertigo or pressure sensations.

Various surgical and pharmacological treatments have been proposed for tinnitus. However, the only approach shown to cause a reduction or abolition of the symptom in properly controlled studies is intravenous lignocaine. The effects of this are of short duration so it cannot be used on a general therapeutic basis. Other drugs have been useful only in reducing other symptoms secondary to the tinnitus such as depression, anxiety and insomnia.

REHABILITATION

Like any other type of rehabilitation, audiological rehabilitation may be described as a 'problem-solving process aimed at minimizing disability and reducing or avoiding handicap'. It should be focused on the individual with his or her specific set of problems.

Often in the past approaches to audiological rehabilitation have either concentrated almost entirely on hearing aids or, alternatively, almost ignored them altogether. What must be done is to take a broad perspective of the individual's needs and how they can best be met within their particular environment.

In the early 1980s a comprehensive management model was developed for audiological rehabilitation (Goldstein and Stephens, 1981) which is widely applicable. The principle behind the model is that all components of the process should be considered in all individuals even if, for a certain individual, they may be immediately dismissed as irrelevant. The depth to which any particular element will be pursued, either in evaluation or remediation, will depend on the specific individual's needs and the facilities available to meet these needs.

Figure 19.3 shows the four components. In 'Evaluation' the individual's needs are defined. The different elements of this are drawn together in the 'Decision Making', together with relevant decision being made about the broad approach necessary for the individual concerned. 'Short-Term Management' covers the different aspects of the remediation process that can be dealt with in two or three clinic sessions, but 'On-Going

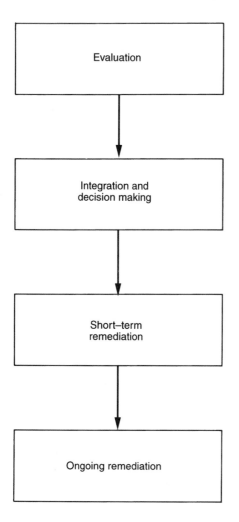

Figure 19.3 Major components of audiological rehabilitation.

Management', while brief in most individuals, in others can continue over days, weeks or even years.

Evaluation

This comprises four components: disability and handicap, communication status, associated variables and related conditions.

Within **disability and handicap** it is endeavoured to determine the real problems which the individual is facing in his/her daily environment. These may be determined by direct questioning, by the use of structured questionnaires, and by open-ended questionnaires. In the last, which may be sent to the patient with their appointment letter, they are asked to list the problems which they have because of their hearing loss. Sending it to them prior to their appointment enables them to focus on their problems and discuss them with their family and friends. The clinician can then use such a questionnaire during the clinic appointment as a basis for further probing of the individual's problems and as a starting point for quantitative assessment. Similar questionnaires may also be given to family and friends to describe their perception of the patient's difficulties and also to probe for the effects of the patient's hearing loss on them.

Communication status entails evaluating existing communication skills of the individual, so providing the 'raw material' for the rehabilitation programme. It entails assessing the auditory and visual abilities of the individual, their speech production skills, their knowledge and abilities in manual communication and non-verbal communication, an integration of all means of communication and an enquiry as to any previous rehabilitation. Its main components are shown in Table 19.2.

The auditory status entails evaluating the main aspects of auditory function relevant to the rehabilitation process. These entail threshold sensitivity, dynamic range and

Table 19.2 Communication status

1. Auditory
2. Visual:
   (a) acuity
   (b) speechreading (lipreading)
3. Speech and language production
4. Manual communication
5. Non-verbal communication
6. Overall
7. Previous rehabilitation

speech discrimination, together with other relevant psychoacoustical characteristics which may relate to signal processing hearing aids.

Visual status, which includes both visual acuity and whether it is appropriately corrected, will have an important bearing on speechreading (lipreading) skills. The degree of emphasis on speechreading will depend on the nature and severity of the individual's hearing loss. Speechreading tests may range from simple clinical tests to computer-generated audiovisual stimuli. They may also range from simple vowel or consonant confusions (e.g. HID/HEAD or ABA/APA) through to sentences and connected discourse tracking. In the last the patient is required to repeat the words of a text read by the tester with repeats and simplifications where necessary. The type of spectacles and how often they are worn may influence the type of hearing aid to be fitted.

Speech and language production problems are generally associated with prelingual or congenital hearing loss. An acquired profound hearing loss with lack of feedback to the individual of the sound of their own voice may also lead to a breakdown of intonation patterns and the control of loudness. High frequency hearing losses may also lead to problems with production of certain consonants such as 's' or 'sh'.

Manual communication (signing), likewise, is relevant largely to the prelingually deaf people, although a few people with profound acquired hearing loss may learn it and find it useful. It is unusual, however, for those with acquired deafness to want to or to be able to fully integrate into the deaf society. Various simplified elements of sign language may be used, and finger spelling can be helpful to supplement speechreading.

Most people have a general subconscious understanding of non-verbal communication (facial expression, body movements, behavioural idiosyncrasies), but in certain people with severe hearing losses it may be necessary to support this understanding as a way of improving their communication skills.

Finally, it is important to define what has already been done in the way of rehabilitation by whatever means. The therapist can then build on the positive aspects of previous experience and overcome negative aspects, such as inappropriate hearing aid fitting.

Associated variables are the psychosocial factors which affect the person's attitude and approach to their disability and any steps to overcome this.

Psychological factors include the individual's attitude to disability in general, hearing disability in particular, and whether they perceive it as a stigma. Personality factors, in particular the individual's mental and emotional state, can have a major bearing on this.

Probably the biggest sociological factor is the role of those closest to the person. A number of recent studies have highlighted the impact their attitudes can have on the hearing-impaired individual. It is worth noting that amongst individuals presenting to a rehabilitation/hearing aid clinic for the first time, about twice as many individuals admit to coming because of pressure from family members than from self-motivation.

In addition, the attitudes within the society in which the individual lives will have a major bearing on the individual's attitude to his/her own disabilities. It may also be true of his/her place of work or education. In some, the atmosphere may be positive and supportive, in others so negative that the individual seeks to hide or deny their disabilities.

Related conditions are factors which will have a bearing on what is to be done. Thus the patient's mobility (whether bedbound, housebound or fully mobile) will influence how much emphasis is put on environmental aids (television, telephone, doorbell, devices, etc.) as opposed to or in addition to wearable hearing aids. Upper limb function (tactile sensitivity and fine manipulative skills) will affect the choice of particular hearing aids and earmoulds which are easy for the individual to fit and control.

Other aural pathology (tinnitus, ear discharge, feeling of pressure) will influence the earmould and the type of hearing aid. Intractable ear discharge may necessitate the fitting of a bone-anchored hearing aid, which is linked to the head via a titanium screw put into the skull behind the ear.

Decision making

All the information gathered during the evaluation process needs to be collated and then decisions can be made about the management. We divide the patients into four main categories.

Some patients have a straightforward problem and are well motivated. For them fitting the appropriate hearing aid, giving advice on environmental aid provision and discussing hearing aid tactics with them and their relatives is likely to be all that is required. Follow-up is needed to identify and deal with any minor problems.

Some patients, though positively motivated, have complicating factors such as disturbing tinnitus, discharging ears, profound hearing loss or limited manipulative skills. They will require more intensive follow-up and rehabilitation, possibly for a long period of time. Such sessions may range from learning to manipulate the hearing aid and earmould, through to developing new communicative skills with a cochlear implant.

The third group of patients who want some help may be very negative about hearing aids. Alternatively they may expect hearing aids to solve all their psychosocial problems which may have little to do with their hearing loss. They require an indirect, often lengthy approach to introduce the relevant part of the rehabilitation process in a non-threatening way.

Finally there are those who deny any hearing disability and come to the clinic as a result of pressure from their long-suffering family. It is generally unhelpful to intervene in such cases, but leave the door open for them to return if they wish. However, indirect help can be provided by offering advice in communication tactics and environmental aids to the family and friends.

Short-term management

Instrumental approaches can be divided into wearable instruments worn by the individual and general instruments or environmental aids which may also be used by others.

The range of personal instruments is shown in Table 19.3. The vast majority of those fitted are air conduction hearing aids (mainly BTE, ITE and ITC aids in the UK), with about half a million being fitted a year. There are about 100–200 cochlear implants and 100 BAHAs. Similar numbers of vibrotactile aids are also fitted.

Thus the vast majority of patients for whom personal instrumentation is considered will be candidates for air conduction hearing aids. Acoustical devices are generally restricted to small numbers of individuals in residential homes for the elderly.

Most hearing aids are simple analogue amplifiers comprising a microphone, amplifier circuit and output transducer which feeds the sound to the external ear, either via tubing and a earmould or directly, as in the case of ITCs and ITEs. Various approaches to more sophisticated signal processing, ranging from compression circuits to digital processing,

Table 19.3 Personal instruments

Acoustical devices
   Ear trumpets
   Listening tubes

Air conduction hearing aids
   In the canal (ITC)
   In the ear (ITE)
   Behind the ear with spectacle (BTE)
   Body worn (BW)

Bone conduction hearing aids
   Spring-loaded vibrators
   Headband or spectacle
   Bone-anchored hearing aids (BAHA)

Cochlear implants
   Single-channel
   Multi-channel

Tactile aids Vibrotactile
     Electrotactile

have been tried in recent years but so far the results have shown little or no increased benefit as compared with simple amplification circuits for most hearing aid users.

Apart from cosmetic factors, in-the-ear aids (ITEs and ITCs) have the advantage of avoiding the acoustical resonances inherent in connecting the BTE to the ear via tubing, but the disadvantages of increased liability to feedback and small controls which many elderly people find difficult. The ITCs have the additional benefit of being able to take full advantage of the pinna echo effects.

Binaural hearing aid fitting (fitting hearing aids to both ears) has a number of advantages, particularly in individuals with approximately equal hearing loss in the two ears. They provide localization ability, and hence are very important in people with severe visual disabilities, improved speech in noise discrimination and added loudness. The disadvantages are cosmetic, additional difficulties with adjusting the aids and cost.

For patients with bilaterally absent external meati or meati which are grossly deformed, or those with chronically discharging ears resis-tant to control by medical and surgical techniques, bone conduction hearing aids may be considered. These bypass the outer and middle ear, stimulating the cochlea directly. Traditional approaches have used a bodyworn hearing aid linked to a vibrator held against the skull by a headband or spectacle frame. More recently an approach has been used with good results by which a vibrator hearing aid is attached directly to the skull via a titanium screw inserted into the skull behind the pinna (BAHA). In patients with absent or grossly deformed pinnas this may be combined with the insertion of similar screws to which an artificial pinna may be attached, usually giving a much more realistic result than reconstructions with plastic surgery.

While BAHAs bypass the outer and middle ears, the aim of cochlear implant is to bypass the hair cells of the cochlea, stimulating the cochlear nerve directly. Cochlear implants, which are indicated for people with no useful hearing with the best hearing aids, comprise three main components. There is a microphone which is usually located on a hearing aid case on the ear, leading to a speech processor, the output of which goes, directly or indirectly, to the implanted electrode. The speech processor may be incorporated in the hearing aid case in single-channel electrodes or in a box attached to the chest or waist in multi-channel electrodes. A great variety of signal processing techniques are available in these boxes with different implant systems. The output of the speech processor may either be taken through a direct transcutaneous plug behind the ear to the electrode or to a small radiofrequency transmitter fixed magnetically to the receiver of the electrode under the skin behind the ear.

A variety of types of cochlear implant exist, although the most commonly used fall into two groups; a multi-channel or single-channel implant.

A multi-channel implant which is inserted through the round window into the cochlea with different electrodes is used for various frequency bands following the tonotopic organization of the cochlea. With these devices most patients are able to discriminate some speech without speechreading. Following some conditions, often bacterial meningitis or cochlear otosclerosis, there may be ossification of the cochlea so that it is impossible to insert a multi-channel implant. In these cases a single-channel implant may be used providing gross stimulation of the surviving cochlear nerve fibres. This electrode is usually placed on the round window. With such a device, the patient rarely has any purely auditory discrimination of speech but it will facilitate speechreading, enable the person to monitor their own speech and make them aware of environmental sounds.

Some profoundly deaf patients choose not to have implants, may not be well enough to have them or may be judged to be unlikely to benefit from them. In such cases a variety of tactile aids may be considered. These again range from single- to multi-channel devices and stimulate the individual's hands or arms by vibrotactile or electrical stimuli. The results with such devices are inferior to those obtained with most implants. In general the patients need far more training to benefit from them. They do, however, help patients to monitor their own voices, in speechreading and in hearing environmental sounds.

General instruments covering environmental aids or assistive listening devices are aimed at facilitating electronic communication or the recognition of alerting/warning signals. They are summarized in Tables 19.4 and 19.5.

One of the simplest ways of facilitating TV/video listening, in addition to the use of hearing aids, is the use of a good quality external loudspeaker near the listener's chair to replace the poor quality speakers normally found in television sets. Doorbells may be improved by using a low frequency buzzer instead of the normal bell, as most hearing-

Table 19.4 General instrumentation: electronic speech

	Improving signal/noise ratio		
	Loops/infra-red	Additional amplifiers/speaker	Use of written text
TV/video	+	+	+
Telephone	+	+	+
PA systems	+	+	+
Radio	+	+	−

Table 19.5 General instrumentation: alerting/warning systems

	Different signals	Extension bells	Use of visual and tactile signals
Telephone bells	−	+	+
Doorbells	+	+	+
Smoke alarms	+	−	+
Baby alarms	+	−	+

impaired people have predominantly high frequency hearing losses with better hearing at the low frequencies.

Hearing tactics constitute a means of facilitating communication by improving the individual's physical and human environment. The individual's personality and attitudes of family and friends need to be taken into account in defining specific goals to be targeted in this respect.

Hearing tactics may be divided into three categories: manipulating social interaction, manipulating the physical environment and observation.

The first category entails ensuring that the speaker faces you, speaks slowly and clearly without his/her face obscured, provides contextual cues and gives feedback with non-verbal gestures. It is obviously important that the hearing-impaired person makes such a speaker aware of their hearing problems for this to happen.

Manipulating the physical environment entails choosing a level of minimal background noise and optimal illumination, particularly of the speaker's face: such communication is also facilitated by a non-reverberant environment.

Observation entails the listener observing the face and non-verbal communication of the speaker, filling in gaps from background knowledge and avoiding getting tense and flustered if they do not catch everything.

Other professionals who are not an integral part of the audiological rehabilitation team may be recruited to meet specific needs. These may include disability employment advisors, specialist social workers, physicians, psychologists, opticians, educationalists, etc.

Social workers may act as interpreters for profoundly deaf individuals and are also responsible for providing aids when indicated under the terms of the Chronically Sick and Disabled Persons' Act. Opticians have an important role both in providing optimal correction for visual abnormalities and so improving the patient's potential for speechreading, and also for helping with the integration of hearing aids and spectacle frames when these may be in conflict.

Long-term management

All the steps in the rehabilitation programme so far described, apart from the training of those people receiving cochlear implants or tactile aids, can generally be achieved quickly. Long-term rehabilitation has four components: information provision, skill building, instrument modification and counselling.

Information provision may range from explanation of the causes and mechanisms of the disabilities to what can be expected from a particular instrument and how to make optimal use of it. It is often as important for the family to have this knowledge as well. It allows them to reinforce the information given to the patient.

This last factor is important in the **skill-building** process, particularly when it comes to helping the patient to fit and adjust their hearing aid and to use an implant or tactile aid optimally. Even with developing better communication skills – speechreading and listening abilities – and also appropriate hearing tactics, the support and understanding of the significant other can be essential.

Instrumentation modification comes after the initial fitting. Several studies have shown that a patient may initially prefer to listen to sounds with a frequency pattern similar to that caused by their hearing loss. Putting in a more ideal configuration may lead to them rejecting the hearing aid(s), however, as they may need to have more high frequencies included (they may need to be 'weaned' onto the ideal over a period of months).

At the time of the initial fitting it should be noted that the individual's ability to hear the doorbell/telephone bell while listening to the television is not going to be helped by a hearing aid, so attention to extension bells, etc. should be considered at that stage. However, it is only after the person has tried the hearing aid for listening to the television in a family environment over a period of time that we can define whether other devices will be necessary.

Most patients will experience some difficulties. They may react badly to failures, improvements may not come sufficiently quickly, or they may experience new situations with which they do not know how to cope. All these can be covered in **counselling** sessions with the patient and family.

This overall process of communication training should continue until the patient and therapist are happy that the best rehabilitation has been achieved, leaving the facility for the patient to return should new problems arise.

It is important at this stage for the professional to consider appropriate outcome measures, for example satisfaction based on changes in disability/handicap, to audit the process and improve provisions.

REFERENCES

Coles, R., Davies, A. and Smith, P. (1991) Tinnitus: its epidemiology and management, in *Presbyacusis* (ed. J. Hartvig-Hensen) Danavox, Copenhagen, pp. 377–402.

Davis, A.C. (1989) The prevalence of hearing impairment and reported hearing disability among adults in Great Britain. *Int. J. Epidemiol* **18**, 911–17.

Goldstein, D.P. and Stephens, S.D.G. (1981) Audiological rehabilitation: management model I. Audiology **20**, 432–452.

Hétu, R., Jones, L. and Getty, L. (1993) The impact of acquired hearing impairment on intimate relationships: implications for rehabilitation. *Audiology*, **32**, 363–81.

Martin, J., Meltzer, H. and Elliott, D. (1988) OPCS Surveys of disability in Great Britain, Report 1, the prevalence of disability among adults, HMSO, London.

Stephens, S.D.G., Lewis, P.A., Charny, M.C., Farrow, S.C. and Francis, M. (1990) Characteristics of self-reported hearing problems in a community survey. *Audiology*, **29**, 93–100.

Stephens, S.D.G., Lewis, P.A. and Charny, M.C. (1991) Assessing hearing problems within a community survey. *British Journal of Audiology*, **25**, 337–43.

WHO (1980) *International Classification of Impairments, Disabilities and Handicaps*, World Health Organization, Geneva.

ORGANIZATIONS

British Deaf Association – concerned essentially with individuals with prelingual deafness and using sign language
38 Victoria Place, Carlisle CA1 1HU, UK.

British Tinnitus Association – for people whose main problem is tinnitus
14–18 West Bar Green, Sheffield S1 ZDA, UK.

Hearing Concern (formerly British Association for the Hard of Hearing) – for people with acquired hearing loss or less severe congenital loss managing well with hearing aids; has a youth section
7/11 Armstrong Road, London W3 7JL, UK.

National Association of Deafened People – for those with an acquired profound hearing loss
103 Heath Road, Widnes WA8 7NU, UK.

National Deaf Children's Society – mainly for the parents of deaf children
24 Wakefield Road, Rothwell Haigh, Leeds LS26 0SF, UK.

Royal National Institute for Deaf People – concerned with various aspects of hearing-impaired people
19–23 Featherstone Street, London EC17 8SL, UK.

20 Visual disability

R.L. Coakes

INTRODUCTION

The normally sighted adult who loses vision may face formidable social, economic and emotional problems. Help in overcoming these problems is available from a variety of agencies, but there is no clear-cut pathway for the rehabilitation of the visually handicapped. Indeed, it would be surprising if there were, for individual requirements vary considerably depending on the extent of the handicap, age, adaptability, emotional resilience and so on.

The aim of this chapter is to outline the causes of visual handicap, the practical steps that can be taken to maximize use of residual vision and the help that can be obtained from the various agencies concerned with the welfare of the blind and the partially sighted.

THE NATURE OF VISUAL HANDICAP

Visual handicap may result from loss of central vision, loss of peripheral vision or both. Less commonly it can be caused by a disorder of ocular motility and, very occasionally, there may be a psychogenic basis.

The macular area of the retina is responsible for the fine, discriminating vision necessary for reading and other detailed close work, and the visual acuity is a measure of this function of central vision. Colour vision is also predominantly a function of the central retina where the concentration of cone photoreceptors is greatest.

The outer part of the visual field is essential for full awareness of the immediate environment and, in particular, for navigation. The peripheral retina contains mainly rod photoreceptors which function more efficiently than the cone photoreceptors at low levels of illumination, and dark adaptation, essential for good night vision, is a function of the peripheral retina.

Few people registered as blind are totally without sight; that is unable to differentiate between light and dark (Table 20.1). Generally speaking a person is eligible for blind registration if the visual acuity with both eyes together is less than 3/60, but a person with better, or even normal, visual acuity may be eligible if the field of vision is severely contracted. The definition of blindness is therefore deliberately vague, and for registration in the UK a person must be considered 'so blind as to be unable to perform any work for which eyesight is essential'.

Table 20.1 The vision of those registered as blind. (Sources: Sorsby, 1966)

Level of vision	% of total
Total blindness	3.4
Perception of light only	10.4
Hand movements to 3/60	58.8
Visual acuity better than 3/60	27.4

Rehabilitation of the Physically Disabled Adult. Edited by C. John Goodwill, M. Anne Chamberlain and Chris Evans. Published in 1997 by Stanley Thornes (Publishers) Ltd, Cheltenham. ISBN 0-7487-3183-0.

There is no statutory definition of partial sight, but for registration purposes those with visual acuity between 3/60 and 6/60 are eligible, as are those with better visual acuity but whose visual fields are contracted. It should be noted that loss of vision in one eye, even if total, does not by itself constitute partial sight for registration purposes.

THE INCIDENCE AND PREVALENCE OF VISUAL DISABILITY

Approximately 12 000 individuals are registered as blind in England and Wales each year, of whom 72% are over the age of 70 (Sorsby, 1972).

The prevalence of visual disability has been steadily rising as the population has aged, and approximately 340 per 100 000 of the population are now registered as blind or partially sighted. In 1980 there were officially 120 000 blind and 40 000 partially sighted individuals in England and Wales (DHSS, 1980).

These figures do not give a complete picture of the extent of visual disability in the community, for many, especially the elderly, have vision that is poor but still too good for the purpose of registration. Cullinan (1977), in a community-based survey, found that 520 adults per 100 000 had a visual acuity of less than 6/18 when examined in their own homes, but less than one-third would have been eligible for blind or partial-sighted registration on the grounds of visual acuity alone. He also showed that visual acuity measured at home was considerably worse than when measured in the hospital clinic, and Silver and colleagues (1978), in a subsequent study, concluded that if hospital conditions of illumination existed at home the number of adults functioning as visually disabled would be substantially reduced.

THE CAUSES OF VISUAL DISABILITY

The leading causes of blindness in the UK are given by age in Table 20.2.

Table 20.2 Leading causes of blindness. (Source: Ghafour *et al.*, 1983)

Age group and cause of blindness	%
20–44 years	
Diabetic retinopathy	20
Myopic degeneration	20
Optic atrophy	20
Uveitis	10
Glaucoma	7
All others	23
Total	100
45–64 years	
Diabetic retinopathy	19
Macular degeneration	14
Glaucoma	13
Myopic degeneration	9
Optic atrophy	9
All others	36
Total	100
65+ years	
Macular degeneration	39
Glaucoma	17
Cataract	13
Diabetic retinopathy	7
Myopic degeneration	5
All others	19
Total	100
All ages	
Macular degeneration	30
Glaucoma	15
Cataract	10
Diabetic retinopathy	9
Myopic degeneration	6
All others	30
Total	100

Senile macular degeneration

This is the commonest cause of blindness among persons over the age of 65. Distortion of central vision progresses to the development of a dense central scotoma and a fall in visual acuity to less than 6/60, but peripheral vision is retained. A small number of patients may benefit from laser photocoagulation but for the majority the condition is untreatable.

Diabetic retinopathy

The is now the commonest cause of blindness in adults under the age of 65, affecting mainly diabetics who have been dependent on insulin for many years. Vision may be affected either through involvement of the macula with gradual loss of visual acuity, or from the development of new blood vessels on the surface of the optic disc and retina. Bleeding from these new vessels gives rise to repeated vitreous haemorrhage and leads eventually to retinal detachment and blindness. Laser photocoagulation of the retina and microsurgical techniques for repairing damaged retinae have greatly improved the visual prognosis of patients with diabetic eye disease.

Glaucoma

The hallmark of this prevalent eye disease is gradual loss of the peripheral visual field with preservation of central vision, until the late stages of the disease, giving rise to 'tunnel vision'. Vision that has been lost cannot be regained, but lowering the intraocular pressure by drug, laser or surgical treatment can arrest or significantly slow the progress of the disease.

Cataract

This is a very common cause of deteriorating vision in the elderly, but with few exceptions, it can be successfully treated, even in the very old and infirm. The modern practice of implanting an acrylic lens in the eye at the time of surgery has eliminated the optical distortion caused by thick postcataract spectacles, and has encouraged the earlier treatment of cataract. Most patients with cataract who are registered as blind have coexisting untreatable ocular disease such as senile macular degeneration.

Degenerative myopia

The highly myopic eye is frequently unhealthy and prone to develop retinal detachment and chronic glaucoma. Atrophy of the choroid and retina, especially in the region of the macula, is the most common cause of disabling loss of vision in this condition, and is untreatable.

Other, less common, causes of visual disability

These include retinitis pigmentosa, an inheritable condition causing night blindness and 'tunnel vision', chronic ocular inflammation and neurological disease. Stroke may result in extensive visual field loss if the visual pathway or occipital cortex are involved, and repeated attacks of optic neuritis in multiple sclerosis lead to optic atrophy and progressive loss of visual acuity.

THE ROLE OF THE OPHTHALMOLOGIST

The majority of elderly patients with visual handicap are referred by their general practitioner for specialist assessment, often after a sight test by an ophthalmic optician has revealed an abnormality that cannot be corrected by spectacles. Other sources of referral include social workers, geriatricians, diabetic physicians and physicians concerned with rehabilitation of the physically disabled.

The role of the ophthalmologist in the care of the visually handicapped is threefold. Firstly, where possible, to improve or restore sight and prevent further deterioration. Secondly, to ensure maximum use of the remaining vision by the provision of low vision aids and thirdly, where indicated, to initiate rehabilitation by clarifying the medical situation and registering the patient as blind or partially sighted.

LOW-VISION AIDS

A low-vision aid is any appliance which may be used to augment residual vision. The provision of one or more of these aids can dramatically improve the quality of life for the user and may allow a return to economic and social independence. A consultant ophthalmologist can prescribe an aid, refer the patient to the low-vision clinic within the hospital eye service or send him to a private optician.

The simplest type of low-vision aid is the single-lens, hand-held magnifier which is readily available from opticians and a variety of retail outlets. These have the advantage of being relatively cheap and easy to use but, being hand held, they restrict manual tasks. Stand magnifiers may include an illumination system and variable focusing and are generally more satisfactory, especially for the elderly who often find it difficult to hold a magnifier steady in front of a book or newspaper.

Spectacle- and head-borne magnifiers increase magnification by reducing the working distance between observer and object. The Keeler spectacle mounted Redifit series gives magnification ranging from $2 \times$ and $8 \times$ with corresponding working distances of 14 to 4 cm and can be dispensed by any high street optician stocking the product.

If the observer to object distance is fixed a telescopic system, usually Galilean, can be employed. Telescopic aids may be hand held or spectacle mounted and designed for near or distance vision, but they tend to be heavy and rather difficult to use since they permit only a restricted field of view.

Closed circuit television (CCTV) systems allow a variable degree of distortion-free magnification up to 60 times on monochrome or colour monitors (Figure 20.1). Some systems incorporate automatic focusing and portable versions are available. Although expensive, CCTV systems allow many visually handicapped individuals to work in a variety of desk jobs or at home. In Britain their prescription is limited to certain approved low-vision aid centres but when required for work the Employment Service provides the equipment.

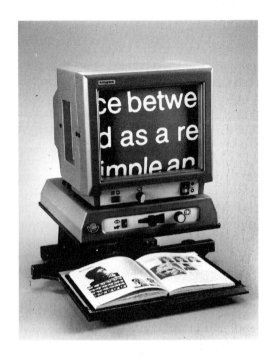

Figure 20.1 Magnilink 409 CCTV. (Courtesy of LVI Low-Vision International.)

The majority of patients referred to a low-vision aid clinic have macular disease, but this group has less success than those with diseases of the optic nerve or media, possibly because the average age of the patients is older, and the importance of adequate levels of illumination for the elderly with macular disease has been emphasized by Humphry and Thompson (1986).

REGISTRATION OF THE PARTIALLY SIGHTED AND BLIND

In England and Wales this is carried out by a consultant ophthalmologist who completes the Form BD8. One part of this form, containing information relating to the cause of blindness or partial sight, is used for the central collation of statistical data on visual disability; another part is forwarded to the local authority.

AGENCIES PROVIDING HELP FOR THE VISUALLY HANDICAPPED

Local authority social services

Each local social services department has a statutory responsibility to provide services for the partially sighted and blind. Rehabilitation workers for the visually impaired, trained at schools run by the Royal National Institute for the Blind (RNIB) and Guide Dogs for the Blind, teach communication, mobility and daily living skills and are supported by social workers who assist with benefits and general advice.

Department of Education and Employment

The Employment Services division of the Government Department has responsibility for assisting the disabled obtain and hold work. Access to help provided by this agency is through local job centres and, for the visually handicapped, is not necessarily restricted to those registered partially sighted or blind.

Voluntary agencies

The visually handicapped may be referred directly to the voluntary agencies by an ophthalmologist or social worker. The largest and best known is the RNIB which provides a wide range of services. Other national agencies include the Partially Sighted Society and St Dunstan's Organisation, which cares for those blinded during war service. There are also local voluntary societies and self-help groups in most areas. In recent years a number of social services department have contracted out responsibility for the provision of services to the partially sighted and blind to voluntary agencies.

British Broadcasting Corporation

The weekly BBC Radio 4 programme 'In Touch' has broadcast news and information for the visually handicapped since 1961 and a quarterly bulletin summarizing the information broadcast during the previous 3 months is published. The handbook *In Touch* (Ford and Heschel 1996) details aids and services for the partially sighted and blind.

ASPECTS OF REHABILITATION OF THE VISUALLY HANDICAPPED

Psychological adjustment to visual loss

The emotional reaction to visual loss and its implications varies from one individual to another and depends to a large extent on the degree to which normal life has been disrupted. Resolution of the emotional problems is a necessary first step before the practical problems of visual handicap can be tackled.

The psychological reaction to loss is grief, and the gradual realization of the fact and implications of loss has been termed the 'grief syndrome'. Its applicability to visual loss has been demonstrated by Fitzgerald (1970), and Hicks (1978) has outlined the phases of the syndrome which must be worked through to resolution. It is a gradually unfolding process in which there must be acceptance of the visual loss and its implications, followed by rejection of unhelpful attitudes and emotions. Once these stages have been passed new patterns of behaviour and new relationships can be acquired.

At least one-third of patients registered blind under the age of 60 are in need of immediate counselling or psychotherapy (Todd, 1988). This applies particularly to those whose blindness is traumatic or genetic, where there is severe illness or multihandicap and when the individual is mentally or socially unstable.

It is important that all patients are given a clear explanation of their visual impairment at an early stage, and this is the role of the ophthalmologist. The possibility or probability of blindness, if this has not already occurred, should be discussed and any false hope for return of vision should be avoided as this may impair or retard successful rehabilitation.

The role of counsellor usually falls on the social worker, who is also responsible for assessing the patient's needs, planning a treatment programme and mobilizing resources. There is unfortunately little or no specialist training in counselling related to visual loss, though generic social workers usually have skills in problem-oriented counselling.

Social implications of visual loss.

For most newly registered blind and partially sighted persons there are also social implications of their visual handicap which are intertwined with the emotional and psychological reactions outlined above. Social isolation and loss of self-esteem, frequently compounded by stereotyped attitudes and increased dependence on others, are accentuated by restricted mobility and lack of information about rehabilitation and available benefits. Discussion and support groups set up by voluntary societies, adult education centres and some social services department play a valuable part in restoring social confidences and facilitating the establishment of new relationships.

COMMUNICATION – READING, WRITING AND LISTENING

Reading

Of all the limitations imposed by failing sight the one most often resented is the inability to read. If the loss of central vision is not too severe the individual may be able to read large-print books with the use of reading glasses and a good light, or a low-vision aid may be required. There are now over 1300 titles, both fiction and non-fiction, in the original Ulverscroft series which can be obtained from public libraries, but there are other large-print publishers and a list of these can be obtained from the Library Association.

For the blind, and those unable to use residual vision, there are two systems of embossed script read by the fingertips, the best known of which is Braille. The English version consists of 63 symbols which are variations on the dots of a domino six. There are a great number of Braille publications – between 500 and 800 per year – including the *Radio Times*. The other system is Moon, which consists of simplified Roman letters. It is easier for the elderly to learn but there is less literature available and, unlike Braille, it cannot be written. Teaching of both systems is the responsibility of the local authority, but the service provided varies considerably from area to area.

Two different types of reading machine are available. The more widely used and cheaper is the Optacon, which converts the printed word to a tactile stimulus which is read by the user's forefinger. Training programmes for the use of these machines are run by the RNIB and Electronic Aids for the Blind.

The other type of reading machine uses optical character recognition and converts the printed word into synthetic speech. Rapid technological development has resulted in easy to use but still expensive equipment. Examples are The Reading Edge (Sight and Sound Technology) and An Open Book (Dolphin Systems).

Writing

Many people with low visual acuity are able to write and this is made easier if the contrast between ink and paper is improved by suitable choice of writing materials. For those able to type, large-print typewriters can be used but these are being superceded by PC-based systems. Software which allows enlargement of text and graphics acts like a magnifying glass between other software and the screen, and computer speech systems using screen access software (screen reader) and speech synthesizing software further enhance the value of PC systems for the visually handicapped. Braille terminals, Braille translation software and Braille embossers are also available.

Listening

Registered blind people over the age of 16 are eligible for a radio set on free permanent loan from either the local Social Services Department or local voluntary society, and a sound-only television set which requires no licence can be purchased from the RNIB. Blind people who have an ordinary television set are entitled to a small reduction in the licence fee. Talking book machines are issued to the registered blind and to any visually handicapped person with defective reading vision (generally N12 or worse) whose application is supported by an ophthalmologist. There are several thousand titles recorded onto cassettes which can be played back only on these machines, which are available from the British Talking Book Service.

MOBILITY

To the newly blind loss of free movement is an additional handicap which saps self-confidence and increases the sense of isolation from the outside world. Mobility training is an essential early step in rehabilitation, and this is usually undertaken by the mobility officer employed by the local authority.

Moving about safely in the home is not usually a problem for the blind, with the exception of the very elderly, but lighting improvements may help the partially sighted. Outside the home the blind individual has to be taught ways of moving about safely and effectively using a variety of aids

The white stick

There are several types of white stick, all available through the RNIB. The 'symbol cane', a collapsible stick made of sections of white tubing, can be used as a probe, but more useful in this respect is the long cane which has a special grip and is tailored to the user's height. It is swung in an arc roughly the width of the body to check the ground ahead. These sticks cannot be used for support, and the infirm may need a crook-handled white wooden walking stick that they can lean on.

Sonic aids

A variety of hand-held and spectacle-mounted devices are available which transmit a beam of high-frequency sound, some of which is reflected back by obstacles in the beam's path and converted into an audible or vibratory warning signal. These tend to be expensive but hand-held sonic aids may be borrowed for use under the supervision of a mobility officer.

Guide dogs

Registered blind persons over the age of 17 can apply to the Guide Dogs for the Blind Association for a guide dog. A doctor's certificate of fitness is required as is the endorsement of the local blind welfare authority. If accepted by the Association the trainee attends one of its centres which are in Exeter, Leamington Spa, Bolton, Wokingham and Forfar.

Travel concessions

The mobile blind or partially sighted are entitled to a variety of local authority concessions, which may include free bus and underground passes, a taxi service and disabled person's railcard. Free escorts are available from the British Red Cross, and the train company (helpline no. 0345 484950) will arrange for blind persons to be accompanied to trains.

DAILY LIVING SKILLS

Instruction in daily living skills, such as housekeeping, cooking and personal care, is normally given by rehabilitation workers who are qualified to teach technical and mobility skills. Other important aspects of their work are adaptation of the home to provide the best possible environment for the visually handicapped person, and the provision of household aids. For the elderly and infirm a wider range of services is often required and the district nurse, health visitor, meals-on-wheels and home helps may be called upon to provide support.

EMPLOYMENT

The Employment Services division of the Department of Education and Employment is charged with providing help and assistance to the disabled in obtaining work and holding a job. Throughout the country there are some 65 Placing, Assessment and Counselling Teams (PACTs) and access to these is through job centres. The disabled employment advisors (DEAs) who make up these teams are often based in job centres and are readily accessible. The role of the PACT is to make an initial assessment through interview and, where appropriate, tests and then to assist with training, rehabilitation and securing employment. Where necessary 'access to work' is facilitated; in the case of the visually handicapped this may, for example, mean the provision of suitable low-vision aids or computer software.

Training courses run by employment services and voluntary agencies include light engineering, shorthand and audio typing, telephony, computer programming, piano tuning and physiotherapy. In the professional field, apart from physiotherapy, there are no special training schemes but many visually handicapped people are able to follow the same courses as sighted students and qualify as teachers, solicitors, musicians and social workers.

HOUSING

The majority of the visually handicapped are elderly and many live alone or have a spouse who is infirm. For those who are unable to maintain an independent life, even with the help of support services, sheltered accommodation with a warden and some communal facilities are often a satisfactory alternative, but the pressure on local authority sheltered accommodation is great. The local authority is, however, obliged to provide accommodation for those 'in need of care and attention which is not otherwise available to them' and does so in the form of residential homes. Occasionally local authorities run residential homes specifically for the blind.

Housing for the blind and partially sighted is also provided by voluntary housing associations and private charities, and the RNIB publishes a list of homes for the adult blind.

ADULT EDUCATION AND LEISURE

Participation in further education can play an important part in the rehabilitation of the visually handicapped person. Local education authorities often run special courses for the blind and partially sighted in subjects such as Braille, tailoring, dressmaking, cookery, sports activities and dancing, which not only teach useful skills but increase confidence and self-esteem, and lead to social integration and further study. Many visually handicapped people join normal adult education classes, and some have graduated through the Open University, which offers special facilities including a weekend preparatory study course at which help and advice is given by counsellors and blind graduates.

The range of leisure activities in which the visually handicapped can participate is now large. Some, with the use of special equipment or techniques, such as Braille playing cards and Braille music, allow the blind to participate with the sighted, while other activities, particularly team sports, are of necessity so modified that they are more specifically for the visually handicapped. The popularity of sport is such that in cricket and five-a-side football national leagues have been formed.

The *In Touch* book lists the facilities available in the wide range of recreational activities for the visually handicapped, and the RNIB's sport and recreation officer can supply information about the provision made for any particular sport or hobby.

ADDITIONAL HANDICAP

Sixty per cent of those persons registered as blind have at least one additional handicap (DHSS, 1976), and of these diabetes, deafness and physical disability pose particular problems.

Diabetes

Most visually handicapped diabetics are insulin dependent and they experience increasing difficulty with self-injection as their sight deteriorates. Good illumination, and the use of a magnifier which leaves both hands free, help distinguish the calibrations on the syringe, but when magnification is no longer sufficient a pre-set syringe or, if mixed doses are used, a click-count syringe is needed. Inserting the needle into the insulin bottle is aided by the use of a funnel-shaped needle guide, which fits over the cap of the bottle, or by the plastic location tray, manufactured by Hypoguard, which holds both syringe and bottle in correct alignment. The same firm also produce an audio urine meter which allows self-monitoring of the urine glucose level.

The British Diabetic Association publishes a bimonthly newspaper which is also recorded on cassette for the visually handicapped.

Deafness

Most deaf-blind patients have acquired their disabilities in old age, and many can be helped by a combination of hearing and low-vision aids. The problems of the profoundly deaf-blind, usually younger people suffering from congenital rubella or Usher's or Norrey's syndrome, are of a different order of magnitude. Communication is the greatest problem and a number of different techniques are used to overcome it. Some employ the tracing of letters on the deaf-blind person's palm, but if Braille or Moon can be read other methods are more effective. The RNIB's communicator disc, which has a moving pointer and Braille or Moon letters, and the more sophisticated Tellatouch, a 'type-writer' which forms Braille letters one at a time on a touch cell, allow the sighted and deaf-blind to communicate.

Various aids employing tactile stimuli as warning signals are helpful to the deaf-blind, for example an alarm clock with an attached vibrator which is placed beneath the pillow, and the RNIB supplies a white stick with two red bands denoting deaf-blindness. Rehabilitation facilities are available through several blind associations and the National Deaf/Blind Helpers League.

Physical disability

Loss of manual dexterity – from arthritis, stroke, multiple sclerosis or other neurological disorder – limits the use of touch and the ability to use many of the aids designed for the visually handicapped. Modified switches and controls on domestic and electrical appliances, which can be operated by the forearm, can be fitted, and the Talking Book can be modified to incorporate a semi-automatic cassette changer. Stand- or spectacle-mounted low-vision aids are generally easier to manage than a hand-held magnifier, and at times an advantage can be obtained by the construction of a frame, incorporating the low-vision aid, that can be attached to the patient's chair or bed. For the recumbent, bedridden patient prismatic glasses can allow a book to be read, or television watched, at 90% from the direction of gaze. Unfortunately. there is usually little that can be done to help the patient whose reading difficulties stem from grossly defective ocular motility or homonymous hemianopia following stroke.

Multi-handicap

This term is generally used to imply a combination of visual, physical and mental handicaps, and is applied to the young rather than the elderly. Most have spent their childhood in residential centres, though a number of adults fall into this category following severe trauma or neurological disease. The range of disability is wide, from those who live at home and work in sheltered schemes to those who, through lack of suitable residential facilities, become long-term residents of hospitals for the mentally handicapped. There are a very small number of specialist residential homes for the blind and partially sighted, with additional severe handicaps, the largest of which is the Royal School for the Blind at Leatherhead.

ACKNOWLEDGEMENTS

In preparing this Chapter I am grateful for the advice of Mrs Mary Todd, past advisor to the visually handicapped at King's College Hospital, London.

REFERENCES

Cullinan, T.R. (1977) *Visually Disabled People in the community. Health Services Research Unit Report No. 28*, University of Kent, Canterbury.

DHSS (1976) *An Investigation into Some Aspects of Visual Handicap. Statistical and research report series No. 14*, HMSO, London.

DHSS (1980) *Registered Blind and Partially Sighted Persons. Year ending March 31st 1980*, HMSO, London.

Fitzgerald, R. (1970) Reactions to blindness: an exploratory study of adults with recent loss of sight *Archives of General Psychiatry*, **22**, 370–9.

Ford and Heschel (1996) *In Touch* 12th edn, In Touch Publishing.

Ghafour, I.M., Allan, D. and Foulds, W.S. (1983) Common causes of blindness and visual handicap in the west of Scotland, British Journal of Ophthalmology, **67**, 209.

Hicks, S. (1978) Psycho-social and rehabilitation aspects of acquired visual handicap. *Transactions of the Ophthalmological Society of the UK*, **98**, 252–61.

Humphry, R.C. and Thompson, G.M. (1986) Low vision aids – evaluation in a general eye department. *Transactions of the Ophthalmological Society of the UK*, **105**, 296–8.

Seebohm Report (1968) *Report of the Committee on Local Authority and Allied Personal Social Services*, Cmnd 3703, HMSO, London.

Silver, J.H., Gould, E.S., Irvine, D. and Cullinan, T.R. (1978) Visual acuity at home and in eye clinics. *Transactions of the Ophthalmological Society of the UK*, **98**, 262–6.

Sorsby, A. (1966) *The Incidence and Causes of Blindness in England and Wales, 1948–62*, HMSO, London.

Sorsby, A. (1972) *Incidence and Causes of blindness in England and Wales, 1963–68*, HMSO, London.

Todd, M. (1988) *Working with People with Loss or Threatened Loss of Vision*. King's Fund Publication, London.

USEFUL ADDRESSES

British Diabetic Association
10 Queen Anne Street, London W1M 0BD, UK.

British Talking Book Service for the Blind
Mount Pleasant, Alperton, Wembly, Middlesex HA0 1RR, UK.

Guide Dogs for the Blind Association
Alexandra House, 9–11 Part Street, Windsor, Berkshire SL4 1JR, UK.

Hypoguard Ltd
Dock Lane, Melton, Woodbridge, Suffolk TP12 1PE, UK.

In Touch
Room 6113, BBC, London W1A 1AA, UK.

In Touch Publishing
37 Charles Street, Cardiff CF1 4EB, UK.

Library Association
7 Ridgmount, London WC1E 7AE, UK.

National Deaf/Blind Helpers League
18 Rainbow Court, Paston Ridings, Peterborough PE4 6UP, UK.

Partially Sighted Society
Secretariat Office: Breaston, Derby DE7 3UE, UK.
Publications and aids: 40 Wordsworth Street, Hove East Sussex BN3 5BH, UK.

Royal National Institute for the Blind
224/6/8 Great Portland Street, London W1N 6AA, UK.

St Dunstan's Organisation for Men and Women Blinded on War Service
191 Old Marylebone Road, London NW1 5QN, UK.

Ulverscroft Large-Print Books
The Green, Bradgate Road, Anstey, Leicester LE7 7FU, UK.

A comprehensive list of organizations for the blind is contained in the Directory of Agencies for the Blind, published by the RNIB.

21 Orthoptics in rehabilitation

A. Buller and F. Struthers

INTRODUCTION

Orthoptics is a profession allied to medicine which is more usually known for work with children. In this role they diagnose, measure and undertake non-surgical treatment of squint (strabismus). The aim of this chapter is to explain the role that orthoptists can play as a member of the multidisciplinary team involved in the rehabilitation of the physically disabled adult.

The training in the UK is a degree course of 3 year's duration in one of three universities, with clinical placements totalling a minimum of 30 weeks in orthoptic departments which have been validated by the Council For Professions Supplementary to Medicine. As a member of the ophthalmic team and involved with a wide variety of ophthalmic cases, the orthoptist's knowledge of when referral to an optometrist or consultant ophthalmologist is indicated saves time and hastens the rehabilitation process.

ROLE OF THE ORTHOPTIST

An orthoptist can provide detailed and helpful information regarding the state of a patient's visual system. This includes diagnosis of visual loss (bilaterally or uniocular), diplopia (double vision) and visual field defects. For example, the existence of diplopia will make it very difficult not only for a patient to relearn walking skills, but will also affect depth perception and hand–eye coordination. Orthoptists test visual acuity using various methods explained in this chapter, many of which do not rely on communication and are therefore helpful with patients who have dysphasia or language difficulties. Recognition of visual loss is important in planning a care programme, and may help in the understanding of the extent of cerebral damage in certain conditions.

DOUBLE VISION

The orthoptist is often used in the diagnosis and treatment of diplopia. After stroke or head injury a patient may experience diplopia. It may be transient, but in some patients can be longstanding and require treatment. Elimination of diplopia produces immediate relief in a short period of time, and the effect of this can be dramatic in promoting both physical and psychological recovery. In addition, appreciation of the presence and nature of diplopia is helpful to other members of the rehabilitation team in planning treatment; for example, a patient who appreciates diplopia only when looking to the left can respond more easily to instructions when material is presented from the right-hand side where no diplopia is present.

Recording of the area of visual field provides similar useful information, particu-

Rehabilitation of the Physically Disabled Adult. Edited by C. John Goodwill, M. Anne Chamberlain and Chris Evans. Published in 1997 by Stanley Thornes (Publishers) Ltd, Cheltenham. ISBN 0-7487-3183-0.

larly where there is a large area of field loss as in homonymous hemianopia (half of the area of vision is absent or significantly reduced in clarity). Measuring the visual field can be done by simple confrontational methods, or by utilizing one of the modern manual or automated field analysers. Charting of a visual field loss over a period of time can show where improvement or deterioration is occurring. In the course of the next three sections more detail will be given on the above topics.

VISUAL ACUITY

Visual acuity may be assessed by several methods, the one chosen will depend on the patient's current ability to communicate. The quality of vision is of more importance than the actual level of vision achieved and to assess quality of vision ingenuity is needed to devise ways of gaining this information in patients with communication difficulties. Initially it is essential to know whether or not there is any pre-existing ophthalmic condition such as myopia (short sight) or hypermetropia (long sight) and whether or not glasses or contact lenses are usually worn by the patient and for what activities. If a squint is present one must ask the patient or relatives whether the squint is recent or longstanding. If the squint has been present from childhood, amblyopia will have developed and diplopia is unlikely to be a problem.

Visual acuity should be measured with the patient wearing glasses appropriate to the distance being tested. If glasses are only suitable for close work and reading, they are of no use for television or walking unless they are bifocals or graduated lenses. If circumstances permit visual acuity will be tested monocularly and binocularly. If it improves when tested binocularly it is an indication that the patient is likely to have stereoscopic vision, i.e. the ability to perceive depth. An inappropriate test which is beyond the patient's ability to perform may cause confusion and frustration, which will undermine the usefulness of the test, and confidence in the examiner. This is important as visual acuity tests are usually carried out before any other ophthalmic investigations, enabling the examiner to interpret the findings and relevance of other tests.

Distance visual acuity must be measured for accuracy at a distance of 6 m which, if space does not allow, can be performed at 3 m using a mirror. Each case must be viewed individually and it may only be possible to assess the vision at a closer distance. The distance at which the test is performed is always recorded in the notes for comparison on subsequent testing.

Patients with communication difficulties may be able to perform the Sheridan Gardiner Test which was initially devised for testing children before they knew the alphabet and were able to read the Snellens Test Type. This test requires the patient to match the letter held up the examiner to a letter on a card held by the patient. The Kay Picture Test is based on similar lines and can be either used as a matching test or with the patient responding verbally.

To assess visual acuity in less able patients the Preferential Looking Test is useful. The patient is required to sit in front of a grey screen and a sequence of gratings of reducing spatial frequency are presented from behind the screen by the examiner who observes the patients' responses. The Cardiff Acuity Test is based on similar principles and can be useful for assessment of these patients. Ingenuity is required and everyday commonplace objects such as small cake decorations may be part of the armoury used by the orthoptist to assess visual acuity. If a patient is to return to driving, a corrected (i.e. wearing of appropriate glasses) visual acuity of 6/9 binocularly and a visual field extending to 120° horizontally and 20° above and 20° below the horizontal, is the minimum visual requirement (Chapter 50).

DIPLOPIA

Normal eye movement and the use of both eyes together results in a single image of the world, associated with depth perception and clarity. When there is a misalignment of the eyes or a weakness of movement, the consequences can be diplopia, loss of depth perception and associated visual confusion. Diplopia may be constant or intermittent and can be of different types or combinations of types: horizontal (images side by side), vertical (one above the other) or oblique (tilted). One of the commonest signs which demonstrates the presence of diplopia is that the patient is noted to consistently close or cover one eye, thereby eliminating the double image. Main causes of diplopia are cranial nerve palsies, mechanical restrictions of the eye muscles, or loss of control of a pre-existing muscle imbalance. There are six muscles which move each eye in different directions, as demonstrated in Figure 21.1. These muscles are supplied by the following cranial nerves:

- Medial rectus, superior rectus, inferior rectus and inferior oblique by the IIIrd cranial nerve.
- Lateral rectus VIth cranial nerve.
- Superior oblique IVth cranial nerve.

Cranial nerve palsies are most commonly caused by trauma, intercranial aneurysm, diabetes, multiple sclerosis or tumours.

Mechanical restrictions of the muscles may also cause diplopia, particularly when associated with orbital fractures or severe facial injury. In its most minor form diplopia may be transient if associated with bruising and swelling which subsides. The presence of diplopia can be recorded using various methods. One of these is the use of the Hess Chart, which provides a diagram indicating which eye muscles are affected and therefore helps in diagnosis. There are several types of Hess Chart in existence, all of which are based on the principle of dissociation, i.e. each eye receives a different image. This can be done either by using a mirror, or by presenting different coloured/shaped images to each eye. One of the methods used is the Electric Hess. A grey metal screen of approximately 1 m square, which incorporates a tangent pattern, is fixed to a wall. Small red spots are shown on the screen in different positions at regular intervals, produced by holes in the screen with red bulbs inside. The patient sits facing the screen holding a torch which projects a short green line of light, and wears red/green goggles. The eye with the red filter in front of it sees the red dots; the other eye looking through the green filter sees the green line. The patient is asked to place the green line on to each red spot in turn,

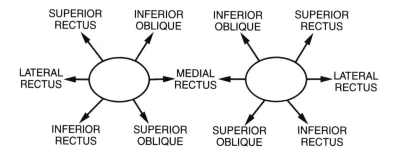

Figure 21.1 Six muscles which move the eyes in different directions.

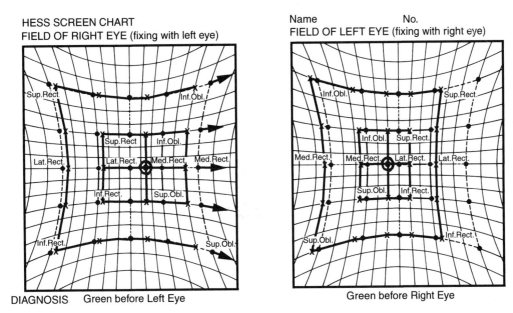

Figure 21.2 Hess screen chart of a recent onset right lateral rectus paresis. (Courtesy of Clement Clarke, Harlow, Essex, UK.)

thereby indicating to the examiner any discrepancy between the balance of each eye. All of the information is plotted on a chart.

Serial charting produces a clear picture of stability, improvement or deterioration of a condition. The example shown (in Figure 21.2) is of a recent onset right lateral rectus paresis. Another method of recording the presence and position of diplopia is by plotting the field of binocular single vision. This indicates the direction in which the patient appreciates diplopia, and the position of gaze in which this does not occur. This is done by using the Amark or Lister Perimeter. The patient is seated with the head level and immobile, and moves the eyes to follow a small white target which travels from the central area of vision towards the periphery at a slow pace, along regular meridians at 15–30° intervals. The patient indicates when diplopia occurs, and also the relative position of the two images.

Each point at which diplopia begins is recorded manually on a chart, and the final

result is an accurate representation of where diplopia occurs in the binocular field of vision. This produces a clear picture that is extremely useful to other professionals in interpreting subjective symptoms.

Figure 21.3 shows the field of binocular single vision for the same patient as before, with a right lateral rectus palsy.

The orthoptist not only diagnoses the type and area of diplopia present, but in many cases can provide relief from this symptom. This may be simply by the use of an eye occluder or eye patch covering one eye which, rather like closing one eye, can eliminate the double image. Another more useful method of treating diplopia is by the use of Fresnel prisms. These are produced by mounting multiple small prisms on to a 2 mm plastic base, which can be applied on to a spectacle lens using water. Prisms have the effect of refracting light so that its direction is changed, thereby allowing an image to fall centrally on to the retina in an eye which is out of alignment. A small prism has the same

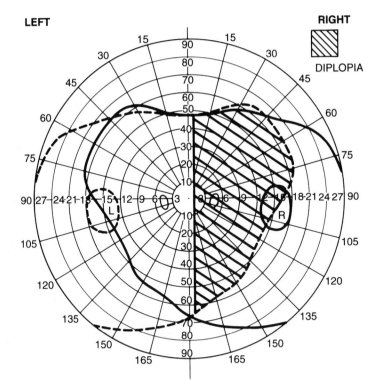

Figure 21.3 Field of binocular single vision for patient shown in Figure 21.2.

refracting power as a larger prism with the same angle at its apex, therefore multiple small prisms can take the place of a larger and thicker prism, without the weight problem.

The correct application of Fresnel prisms by the orthoptist can quickly eliminate diplopia in many patients. If the patient does not wear glasses a pair may be obtained solely for this purpose.

Figure 21.4 shows a patient with a complete VIth cranial nerve palsy and the resulting effective use of corrective lenses.

VISUAL FIELDS AND VISUAL NEGLECT

Visual fields

The normal visual field extends to 100° temporally, 60° nasally, 60° upwards and 70° downwards, allowing for slight variations depending on the individual's facial bone structure. The fields of the two eyes overlap, giving the horizontal binocular field of 120° when tested with a white target. The field will be smaller if tested with a red target as there are less cones at the periphery of the retina and red has a lower luminosity than white.

Visual field loss (Figure 21.5) is one of the most common visual symptoms in patients who have suffered a stroke or head injury but the patient usually does not complain of this symptom or of visual neglect. It is important that a diagnosis is made of the presence of either or both these conditions to ensure that the rehabilitation programme takes these difficulties into account.

The orthoptist's role in the management of field defects is largely in diagnosis and in devising ways of minimizing their effects on the patient by advising other team members

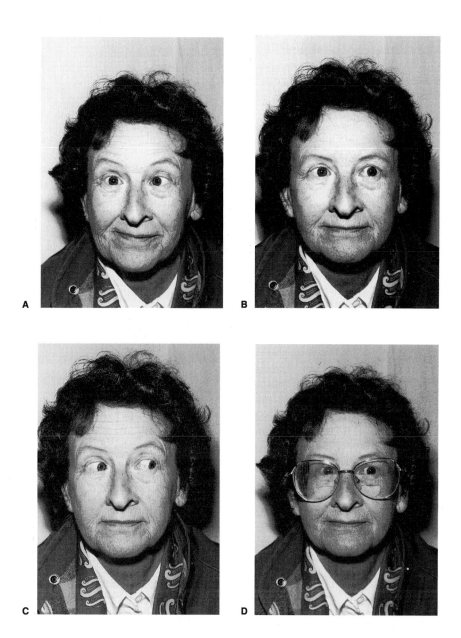

Figure 21.4 Patient with a complete VIth cranial nerve palsy: A, gaze directed to the right; B, looking straight ahead; C, looking left; D, wearing base out Fresnel prism on the right lens of her spectacles.

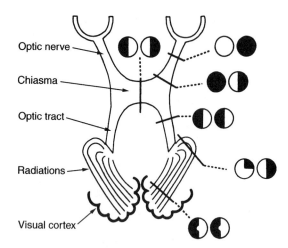

Optic nerve

Chiasma

Optic tract

Radiations

Visual cortex

Figure 21.5 Visual field loss.

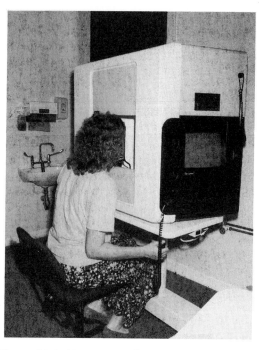

Figure 21.6 Assessment of visual field loss. (Courtesy of Zeiss Ltd, Welwyn Garden City, Hertfordshire, UK.)

of the defect and the most suitable way of dealing with the problem. Homonymous hemianopia is the most common field defect. It can be useful for carers to try specially adapted spectacles to simulate the condition to enable them to gain an insight into one of their patient's more difficult visual problems. The patient can also be helped by staff being made aware that it is reassuring for the patient to be approached from their sighted area and to speak to the patient by name as they are approached. The positioning of the patient's bed in the ward also needs consideration in cases with visual field loss. It is much easier for a patient to be able to look directly at a television, or other patients and staff, on their sighted side rather than to uncomfortably turn their head in an extreme position.

Visual fields can be assessed by confrontation or, if it is practical, formal visual fields can be recorded on equipment especially developed for the purpose (Figure 21.6). To perform the Confrontation Test of visual fields the examiner sits on the same level as the patient at a distance of 50 cm. The patient, with his/her left eye covered, fixes the examiner's left eye and the examiner closes his/her right eye. In this way the patient's

right visual field can be compared with the examiner's 'normal' field. The target is moved slowly from the periphery towards the centre from the superior, lateral, inferior and nasal positions.

This sequence is then repeated with the other eye occluded. If a patient is unable to cooperate with this test then it will be necessary to perform an adaptation which requires the aid of an assistant. The patient's attention is maintained by the examiner whilst the assistant introduces the target from the periphery in all the positions of the gaze with the examiner observing the patient's responses. Both these tests can only give an approximation of the visual fields; however, in skilled hands they can give relatively accurate results. If a patient is considering a return to driving an accurate plot of the visual fields on the appropriate equipment is essential.

There are a few ways to minimize the effect of visual field loss. The patient may be able to achieve maximum benefit of the remaining field by adopting a compensatory abnormal head posture. The patient may adopt this him/herself or the orthoptist can advise and explain the advantages, although abnormal head posture may cause undesirable changes in limb and trunk spasticity. Strategically placed mirrors can also be useful in certain circumstances. Prisms can be applied to glasses to increase the extent of the visual field.

Visual neglect

This is where a patient can see in one part of the visual field, but as soon as a second target is presented in the opposite visual field at the same time, the first target is ignored. It can remain undiagnosed until the patient is able to communicate that there is a difficulty with close work or they may bump into objects when moving around. The patient is most likely to experience difficulty with reading, losing their place and missing words out which can make the piece unintelligible. The orthoptist can help devise ways of coping with these difficulties depending on the problems experienced by each individual.

Case history 1

A 28-year-old male with severe head injury following road traffic accident. When first seen he had communication problems and a severe right convergent squint without any symptoms of diplopia. As he had no relatives to give any previous symptoms it was assumed that this was a longstanding squint. As the patient began to recover he did complain of diplopia and stated that he had no pre-existing squint. Diplopia had not been troublesome initially as the two images were widely separated. The angle of squint was too large to be overcome by Fresnel prisms so the diplopia was overcome by occlusion of alternative eyes. He will be listed for squint surgery, if it has not improved spontaneously over 6–12 months.

Case history 2

A 72-year-old female, with a diagnosis of stroke. When first seen by the orthoptist she had severe communication problems, reduced distance visual acuity and a right divergent squint. It was known that she had a pre-existing ophthalmic condition, being highly myopic, and the wearing of glasses controlled her divergent squint. Unless they are specifically asked, relatives may neglect to mention the wearing of glasses which they take for granted or consider trivial in relation to the communication difficulties.

Case history 3

A 50-year-old man was knocked from his bicycle by a van. Amongst other injuries, he suffered multiple fractures of the frontal region of the skull. Subsequent CT scan of the head showed some subarachnoid blood with contusion in the left temporoparietal region. The patient spent 3 weeks in the intensive therapy unit before being transferred to the rehabilitation ward. Once sufficiently aware, he complained of double vision, and was then seen by the orthoptist who diagnosed a complete right VIth cranial nerve palsy. Staff on the ward were made aware of the fact that he experienced horizontal diplopia when looking straight ahead and to the right, but not to the left, and he was fitted with a Fresnel prism. This gave him single vision when looking straight ahead and as he improved could be reduced in strength. The patient recovered quickly and after 4 weeks the lateral rectus paresis had completely resolved.

FURTHER READING

Fitzsimmons, R. and Fells, P. (1989) Ocular motility problems following road traffic accidents. *British Orthoptic Journal*, 40–48.

Fowler, M.S., Richardson, A.J. and Stein, J.F. (1991) Orthoptic investigation of neurological patients undergoing rehabilitation. *British Orthoptic Journal*, 2–7.

Freeman, C.F. and Ridge, N.B. (1988) Cerebrovascular accident and the orthoptist. *British Orthoptic Journal*, 8–18.

Mein, J. and Trimble, R. (1991) *Diagnosis and Management of Ocular Motility Disorders*, Blackwell Scientific Publications, Oxford.

Rossi, W., Kheyfets, S. and Reading, M.J. (1990) Fresnel prisms improve visual perception in stroke patients with homonymous hemianopia or visual neglect. *Neurology*, **40**, 1597–9.

Sankies, N. (1987) Neurological field defects. *British Orthoptic Journal*, 15–24.

USEFUL ADDRESSES

British Orthoptic Society,
Tavistock House North, Tavistock Square, London WC1H 9JP, UK.

Royal National Institute for the Blind
224 Great Portland Street, London W1N 6AA, UK.

Partially Sighted Society
Queen's Road, Doncaster DN1 2NX, UK.

22 Speech, communication and swallowing problems

P. Enderby

In the beginning was the word. The word itself, of which our works of art are fashioned, is the first art form, older than the roughest shaping of clay or stone. A word is the carving or colouring of a thought and gives to it, permanence. We do not yet know, if ever we are able to trace, how language first began, though we may deduce that words to express love were those first used, since love is the emotion, just as speech the instrument, that even in its lowest most primitive form, clearly distinguishes human beings from their humble cousins of the animal world. (Osbert Sitwell)

Speech and language are so much a part of ourselves that it is hard to distinguish one from the other. The way we relate to others, the way we express our thoughts and emotions, our angers and fears, affect the way that we see ourselves and reflect our personalities to the world. Thus, it is possible to surmise that people with communication impairments not only have difficulty in asking for what they want, and other relatively mundane aspects of daily living, but also have difficulty in reflecting their being and in being respected as a whole person. Speech and language impairment may be looked upon as one of the most fundamental difficulties, as it can strike at the very soul of the human being.

Speech and language therapy reflects the recognition that communication is an integral part of human nature not only by being involved in the surface structure of speech and articulation or of the underlying structures of language and vocabulary, but by being committed to communication in its broadest sense. Frequently we see patients who will be unable to communicate in the conventional manner, but who will benefit from therapy aimed at developing alternative methods of expression.

WHO SHOULD BE REFERRED FOR SPEECH THERAPY

As therapy extends beyond the sounds and words to their use and effectiveness, referral of persons with communication disorders for assessment by the speech and language therapist (SALT) is nearly always the most appropriate action, as it is difficult for somebody who is unfamiliar with these therapy approaches to know who will, or who will not, benefit.

Any patient who has a congenital or acquired speech or language difficulty, or who has a long-standing communication disorder, but has not received attention for this for some time, should be referred for a SALT opinion. The therapist, following

Rehabilitation of the Physically Disabled Adult. Edited by C. John Goodwill, M. Anne Chamberlain and Chris Evans. Published in 1997 by Stanley Thornes (Publishers) Ltd, Cheltenham. ISBN 0-7487-3183-0.

assessment of difficulties and retained abilities, will ascertain whether this patient would benefit from therapy. If the patient is not in a position to benefit from direct therapy either because he/she is too ill, or the situation is unstable, the therapist will arrange for an appointment at a later time and therefore patients benefit from the knowledge that at least this difficulty is not being ignored. When the therapist is unable to work directly with the patient, he/she will be able to guide the family at a time when they are greatly concerned and distressed, and do not know how to approach the patient.

WHY SHOULD YOU REFER?

The SALT is concerned with all aspects of communication and is thus involved in the following activities:

- detailed speech and language assessment;
- specific speech and language remediation;
- improving communication skills in general, and introducing non-oral means of communication where appropriate;
- advice to nursing, medical, remedial and other staff on handling specific expressive and receptive difficulties;
- advice and support to patients and relatives.

It is clear that most communicatively impaired persons may benefit by contact with the SALT, despite the fact that a large number will be unable to be rehabilitated to normal communication. Coping with disability and functioning at the highest possible level may be realistic and satisfactory from both patient's and relatives' point of view (Brown, 1981)

ASSESSMENT

Assessment of the orofacial musculature, phonology, linguistic, pragmatic and semantic abilities including those of reading and writing, will assist the therapist to plan appropriate intervention. Objective assessments are important, as a number of patients will learn to hide their socially unacceptable disorder, and it is very easy to assume or surmise inaccurate information from observation alone. Not only do assessments help to establish the degree of the defect, and the areas of retained ability, but also they can assist in the classification of the disorder, provide information required to plan treatment, and can quantify and qualify changes in abilities. This latter point is important, as subjective clinical judgement may well give a false impression with regard to progress. For example a patient with impaired articulation may be thought to be improving as people become familiar with his/her attempts to speak, and therefore can interpret the speech efforts more readily. It is imperative to ensure that the improvement is in the patient and not limited to improvement in the therapist's interpretive skills!

There are many appropriately standardized assessment procedures that detail methods of eliciting speech and language – both receptive and expressive, conversation and intelligibility.

SPEECH AND LANGUAGE DISORDERS

Four main groups of speech and language disorders are found in disabled adults:

- disorders of speech;
- disorders of language;
- disorders of fluency;
- disorders of voice.

Disorders of speech

It is important to understand the difference between the term **speech** and the term **language**. Speech may be used to express audible utterances, whereas language refers to vocabulary and grammar, or the content of those utterances which may be expressed in gesture, writing or speech. Articulation disorders are a disruption of speech, and there may be many causes of these. Damage to the structures required for speech, i.e. the tongue, the lips, the palate, the vocal cords, the lungs, etc., may affect the tone and quality. A cleft in the roof of the mouth may result in speech sounding hypernasal. A tongue badly scarred following an accident may have difficulty in moving precisely to the right place to form the different interruptions to the airflow which results in sound. Therefore, damage to a certain part of the articulatory system would affect speech in a fairly predictable fashion. (Dickson and Dickson, 1983; Enderby 1986).

Loss of neuromuscular control of the organs of articulation due to central or peripheral nerve involvement results in changes of tone, coordination or precision, resulting in speech that is commonly termed **dysarthric**. The level of the neurological lesion is strongly associated with different speech characteristics, thus analysis of the speech disorder can assist with diagnosis.

The term **anarthria** is used to describe a complete loss of speech due to impairment of neuromuscular control, and the term **dysarthria** is used to describe abnormal speech as the result of disorders of neuromuscular control affecting articulation, respiration, phonation and intonation. A knowledge of different types of dysarthria may assist in localizing the neurological damage, as the speech symptoms are frequently characteristic (Dearly, Aronson and Brown, 1975).

Disorders of language

The most commonly acquired disorder of language is dysphasia, which is a disorder of processing and formulating language. The term **aphasia** and **dysphasia** are commonly used interchangeably, although the former term strictly refers to a complete language loss. The most common cause of dysphasia is a stroke affecting the dominant hemisphere which may result in difficulty in understanding and using the vocabulary and grammatical structures required to formulate expressions. These symptoms may also be reflected in reading and writing. Although dysphasic patients frequently have receptive and expressive difficulties, there may well be a disparity between the modalities; i.e. the dysphasic person may be able to understand more than he can express, or vice versa (Darley, 1982). There are many different combinations of language symptoms, and some schools suggest there have diagnostic implications.

Disorders of fluency

The inability to express oneself fluently due to hesitations, repetitions or blocking of speech may be termed stammering or stuttering, the latter term being more frequently used in America to describe the same condition. A number of persons who stammer will develop secondary problems associated with fear of speaking, causing muscular twitching, poor eye contact, or avoidance of words and situations. Stammering is remarkably variable, and the person may go through periods when he/she has difficulty in speaking in most situations and then periods of very little difficulty in speaking (Gregory, 1979; Peters, and Guitar 1991)

Disorders of voice

Dysphonia (abnormal phonation) may be a symptom of neurological, organic or psychological disorder. Amongst the organic dysphonias are those resulting from polyps, nodules and oedema of the vocal cords. Stress, tension and vocal misuse may underlie some pathological changes of the vocal cords or cause dysphonia without any apparent organic change. Dysphonia is frequently looked upon as a cosmetic rather than an actual disability, but many patients will suffer personal and employment difficulties if this symptom is not treated (Greene, 1980; Coltan and Casper, 1990). Aphonia results from laryngectomy, which may be required following irremediable cancer or trauma to the larynx. Laryngectomy is discussed later in this chapter.

MAIN SPEECH AND LANGUAGE DISORDERS ASSOCIATED WITH COMMON DISEASES OR CONDITIONS

Learning difficulty

Those with learning disability comprise one of the largest group of persons having speech and language disability (prevalence 2.5 per 100). One of the main considerations is whether the speech and language development is in line with mental ability, or is contributing substantially to the latter. If speech and language are out of line with mental ability then therapy may substantially assist the person's functional improvement. Frequently reduced demands, limited environment and associated disabilities restrict the learning disabled person's opportunities for language development, so that treatment within realistic limits becomes possible. These clients may also suffer from phonological disorders which may be the direct result of learning difficulties, requiring therapy to improve intelligibility; or may have difficulty retaining vocabulary to express needs and wants. Simple signing systems, for example, hand signs, Makaton, or Picture Signs – Blissymbolics – can extend communication (Rhyner, 1988 Angelo and Goldstein, 1990. Therapists work closely with the relatives and carers to promote an environment which promotes and facilitates communication.

Stammering

About 1%; of the adult population are stammerers and the underlying causes of stammering are much debated. There are schools of thought which dwell upon psychological aspects, and other schools which emphasize abnormal neurological transmission. It is likely that there is more than one cause which is exacerbated by the secondary problems associated with having a speech disorder for a long period of time, such as lack of confidence and situation avoidance. Speech and language therapy occasionally resolves somebody's fluency disorder completely, but in most cases the aim is to assist the person to control the stammer using fluency techniques. In conjunction with this, it is important for the therapist to improve the person's attitude to speaking situations, to increase confidence, overcoming some of the habitual aspects of this disorder. Surprisingly it may be difficult for the person who has stammered for a long time to become accustomed to fluency if he/she has been used to being dysfluent for a long time. Frequently, children who have done poorly in therapy at school will have a different attitude to therapy when faced with motivating factors such as attracting and keeping girl/boyfriends or going for jobs.

Deafness

Approximately 200 persons per 100 000 population are severely deaf. Of these, 60% have deafness to a level which impairs speech and language. If a person is born deaf, not only speech but also vocabulary and language structure will be limited, due to restricted learning opportunities. With acquired deafness the patient will have difficulty with modulation of voice and the use of appropriate stress and pitch at an early stage, whereas articulatory precision may deteriorate later. In addition to SALT, the hearing therapists and teachers of the deaf help in the management of this disability. This may include practical advice on hearing aids, teaching lip reading and speaking skills and general advice on how to cope with such a hidden and isolating condition. A number of deaf persons will require continued assistance to ensure that the quality of speech is maintained.

Cerebral palsy

This condition is suffered by 175 per 100 000. This term is used to describe a heterogeneous group of disorders and disabilities with a variety of aetiologies that have the common elements of being developmental, neuromotor disorders that are the result of non-progressive abnormalities of the developing brain. Sixty per cent of persons with cerebral palsy will have a speech and/or language disorder. The majority will be dysarthric, but in addition there may be language disorders, due to specific problems such as dysphasia or developmental delay, memory problems or reduced intellectual function; these may be concomitant problems with the dysarthria (Hardy, 1983)

Cerebral palsied children are now attracting much more specialized educational assistance, but this has not always been the case, and there are many adults with cerebral palsy who have not had appropriate assessment and treatment. Frequently they do not get referred to SALT, as they have suffered their condition for so many years, that it is assumed that all has been done, but this is not necessarily so. Techniques and technology have developed rapidly, enabling us to help the more severely physically handicapped. Detailed assessment of the cerebral palsied person is essential to gauge the degree of mental, physical and speech disability, and thus appropriate therapy to maximize communication can be given. In some cases SALT can assist by helping the person to improve his/her speech; in other cases alternative communication via communication aids or sign systems is more appropriate.

Stroke

The prevalence of speech and/or language disorders secondary to stroke is about 150 people per 100 000. The majority of these will have a language disorder, i.e. dysphasia, which is commonly associated with lesions either in the temporal lobe or the frontal area of the dominant cerebral hemisphere. Posterior inferior lesions are suggested to cause more impairment of comprehension, whereas posterior superior lesions cause fluent expressive dysphasia and frontal lesions may give rise to non-fluent expressive dysphasia. Non-fluent dysphasia is demonstrated when the person grasps for words, repeats the same word frequently, and has a very restricted vocabulary. Fluent dysphasia is used to describe those patients who speak readily, but use jargon consisting mainly of nonsense words. Intonation may be preserved, assisting the listener to guess the speaker's intent.

Bilateral cortical damage will result in spastic dysarthria, characterized by a strained, husky, weak voice, imprecise articulation and hypernasility. The patient will commonly have problems with swallowing and dribbling, particularly in the first 2 weeks post stroke.

There is a common misconception that the main role of the therapist is to initiate and guide exercises which release, increase, develop or clarify the speech. It is important to emphasize that this is only one element of the SALT's involvement with the poststroke patient. As language is an integral part of human behaviour and relationships the approach to its remediation is necessarily eclectic. It is essential that the disorder is assessed so that all those caring for the patient are aware of the extent of the impairments and the areas of retained ability. For example, a patient who has difficulty understanding the spoken word may have greater ability in understanding what he/she reads. This knowledge will help all those involved. The shock of losing one's speech is fundamental, and can be devastating to all family members. The speech and language therapist is in a position to assist and support the family in their period of readjustment, which sometimes takes many months. A person's vocation, social life, self-esteem and personal hobbies can be destroyed by losing the power of communication; support and attention from a person with specialized knowledge may be paramount importance (Enderby and Langton-Hewer, 1985)

Other acquired neurological disease

Many people suffering from other acquired neurological diseases will have a speech disorder. The most common diseases which affect speech are: Parkinson's disease, multiple sclerosis, Friedreich's ataxia, muscular dystrophy, motor neurone disease, myasthenia gravis and Huntington's chorea, some of these are known to affect language to some extent as well. The prevalence for these acquired neurological diseases (excluding stroke) is 250 per 100 000. Of these, about half may develop a disorder of communication. The majority of patients with these disorders will have a dysarthria due to neuromuscular involvement. Additionally, many of them will have feeding and swallowing problems. The therapists work closely with relatives and carers in order to ensure communication strategies can be incorporated into everyday activities and to facilitate a supporting environment, enabling the person to try out new methods of communication

Many patients with Parkinson's disease will notice that their voice becomes quieter as the disease progresses. Others find that they have difficulty in initiating speech, or that their speaking rate increases and becomes festinant. The onset of this extrapyramidal dysarthria is insidious and the patients themselves may not notice that they are having difficulty in making themselves understood until it has become a major problem. There is some evidence that short intensive courses of speech therapy to improve self-monitoring, reestablish control over speaking rate and to improve breathing and phonation can assist the patient to re-attain some degree of clarity (Scott and Caird, 1981; Chenery, Murdoch and Ingram, 1988).

A few patients with multiple sclerosis develop dysphasia in addition to the more common dysarthria during the course of the disease. Occasionally both symptoms are temporary, and are related to an exacerbation in the condition. In other cases the symptoms persist and require attention. There may be some degree of intellectual involvement, which will affect the type of therapy appropriate. Many patients will benefit from learning compensatory methods which may assist the quality as well as the intelligibility of their speech, but a few will have difficulty retaining information; thus teaching a patient to improve the clarity of articulation would be inappropriate, and using simple communication aids, or teaching the family prompting methods, might be more realistic. Medical textbooks often cite that the dysarthria associated with multiple sclerosis is cerebellar in origin, and describe 'scanning speech'. However, more recent studies show that the most common dysarthria is associated with upper motor neurone involvement, causing spasticity to the muscles of articulation.

Nearly all patients suffering from motor neurone disease will become dysarthric during the course of their disorder. A significant number will become anarthric (Newrick and Langton-Hewer, 1984). Very few will have any intellectual impairment, and the frustrations and difficulties of coming to terms with a very distressing, progressive disease are heightened by the reduced ability to communicate effectively. The SALT's role is associated not only with ameliorating some of the bulbar symptoms, but also assisting with the management of adapting to non-vocal methods. Speech and language therapists can often understand disordered speech which others find difficult, and they frequently become the person who can most easily communicate with the patient, and have to take on the role of interpreter, as well as therapist (Yorkston, Beukelman and Bell, 1988)

The majority of patients with dysarthria will have feeding and swallowing problems. Recently, SALTs have become involved in the management of dysphagia. Certainly the techniques used to assist and improve muscular control and coordination for speech are not dissimilar to those which assist with swallowing, so this seems a natural development.

Laryngectomy

The incidence of laryngectomy is influenced by a number of different factors, including early detection of laryngeal tumour which is related to the astuteness of primary health care and general health education of the population; philosophies regarding radiotherapy as a primary intervention and surgical approaches to tumour management without total laryngectomy. Thus, the prevalence of laryngectomy varies, not only between countries but also, probably, within a country by geographical area. It has been estimated that the prevalence of laryngectomy within the UK is between 0.9 and 3 per 100 000 population (Enderby and Davies, 1989). In most cases the patient undergoes the total removal of larynx including the hyoid bone superiorly and the upper rings of the trachea inferiorly. The upper end of the trachea is brought out through the skin at the front to form a stoma. Some patients require less extensive surgery involving only a partial removal of the larynx whereas others require more extensive surgery requiring the removal of the oesophagus and larygnopharynx necessitating the transplantation of part of the colon or jejunum. There are primarily three methods of communication following laryngectomy. The most traditional way is oesophageal speech which requires the patient to develop a method of injecting the air with his tongue and cheeks into the oesophagus and then returning this air to form the sound support for speech. Many different electrolarynges have been developed and offer patients a different form of communication. Most studies show that this form of speech is not only intelligible but as acceptable as oesophageal speech. It is frequently less tiring and can be quite controllable.

The third method of vocal rehabilitation following laryngectomy is the use of vocal prostheses. These surgical speech techniques recreate the physiological situation after the larynx has been removed so that air expired from the lungs generates a vibration, albeit not of the vocal cords, and supports the articulation of speech sounds. There are different surgical techniques and different valves available (Singer, Blom and Haymaker, 1981; Perry, 1988; Parker, 1993)

All these methods of speech rehabilitation require quite a heavy commitment from a specialist speech and language therapist who not only has to teach the person how best to communicate but also support and encourage the radical changes in lifestyle, (McKenna *et al*, 1991)

Head injury

The prevalence of patients disabled following head injury is hard to establish. However, it has been suggested that 160 persons per 100 000 have a severe speech and language disorder as the result of head trauma. A number of patients will have a combination of dysarthria, dysphasia and dyspraxia. Some may have a very specific isolated disorder, but many patients following head injury, will have disorders arising from impaired concentration, cognition, memory and language. The SALT's role with the head injured patient is again as a member of the team, and input may continue for many months as improvement of communication may be slow.

PRACTICAL WAYS OF HELPING THOSE WITH COMMUNICATION DISORDERS

These guidelines will assist communication with speech- and language- impaired persons, but should be modified according to the type and severity of disorder.

A: Helping the person who has difficulty with understanding

1. Never underestimate a patient's comprehension.
2. When speaking to the speech/language impaired patient, keep in full view so that your facial movement and facial expression can be observed – do not mouth or exaggerate your facial expression.
3. Avoid long rambling conversations – they are almost always misunderstood.
4. Do not demand too much of the patient when he/she is agitated. Fatigue or emotional upset adversely affects both comprehension and expression.
5. Avoid noisy rooms. Some language-impaired patients are distractible and have difficulty in concentrating.
6. Some limited gesture may help the person to understand, but it must not be exaggerated.
7. Use repetition. If the patient has not understood a question or statement, repeat what you said but phrase it slightly differently.
8. Speech should be a little slower than normal, and if hearing is good, the voice should be clear but not raised.
9. Single words often convey less than a phrase or short sentence. Therefore it is best to talk to the patient using familiar words in short sentences pausing frequently.
10. Do not change the subject quickly.
11. The patient will understand and express himself more easily when he is in familiar surroundings talking about familiar things.
12. Allow more time for the patients to start their response. Do not assume that he/she has not understood immediately. It may take more time to assimilate what has been said.

B: Helping the patient who has difficulty with speaking

1. Communication in any way should be encouraged, for example if the person can write or do a 'thumbs-up' sign, then these should be accepted.
2. Encourage the person to use all the speech that is available to him/her and give opportunities to speak. Persons with speech difficulties often function at a lower level than they are capable of. They may well withdraw from speaking situations and inhibit their speech due to embarrassment and frustration.
3. Try to avoid asking a question of a relative about the patient when he can answer for him/herself. For example 'does he take sugar in his tea'?
4. Talking to the person on his own will often reduce embarrassment on both sides.
5. If a patient is learning to speak, he/she must 'want' to learn to speak; therefore encourage discussion which is motivating and stimulating.
6. If the patient is having difficulty in expressing him/herself, allow time. If he/she fails, supply the words for him and encourage these to be repeated.
7. If the patient uses one-word sentences, for example 'out', encourage him/her as this is meaningful, but expand the sentence for him/her by saying, 'I want to go out'.
8. Sometimes it is easier for the staff and the patient to avoid speaking, due to the obvious effort on both parts. As far as possible these occasions should never arise.
9. A dysphasic person may be at their best when the routine is familiar. Always promote some communication at regular times, for example always say, 'Good morning' 'How many sugars do you take'? etc. These questions will become familiar, encouraging an improved response.

COMMUNICATION AIDS

Some patients who have difficulty in making themselves understood may benefit from a communication aid. These may assist existing speech to be more intelligible. (e.g. an amplifier) or they may replace speech so that a person is able to communicate via the aid, (e.g. a typewriter). However, all communication aids require some degree of language ability and therefore they are mainly used by people with speech disability with some retained language. The majority of those stroke patients who have severe dysphasia are unable to use a communication aid due to the inability to recall the words that they wish to express, making it impossible to express them through any mode, be it through speech, writing or communication aid. Some aids can prompt and suggest language but there still remain a number of communicatively impaired people who cannot benefit from the technology that is presently available.

There are many communication aids available, and it is important that the patient is thoroughly assessed so that the correct equipment is selected. The SALT has to assess the language abilities, the physical abilities, eyesight, hearing and psychological factors. It is important to determine retained abilities as well as deficits, in order to determine the most suitable aid. Aids can be categorized according to the method of input. There are three groups of aids:

- direct select
- scanning
- encoding.

Direct select

This is any technique in which the desired choice is directly indicated by the user and may involve the use of any part of the body which can indicate a symbol. Whilst the easiest facility should be used, the upper body is used in preference, when possible, for example, finger, elbow, chin, fist or eyeball. If

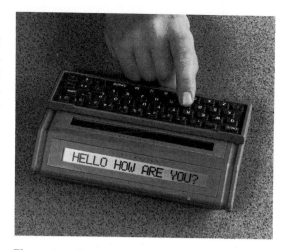

Figure 22.1 Direct select keyboard with LED display.

the patient is unable to control these then the lower body, for example foot, may be chosen. Simple appliances which might help the accuracy of indication, such as head sticks, mouth stocks, hand stick, may need to be considered. If direct selection is a possibility, then this method is preferred above the others as it requires less cognitive skills and becomes a rapid method with practice. The advantage of this method is its wide range of application. The moderately intelligible dysarthric person may use an alphabet board and point to the first letter of each word as he/she says it; or, aids using conventional keyboards such as electric typewriters and computers may be appropriate. Some aids which are specifically made for disabled persons, and which use the direct-select technique, are the Canon Communicator, which is a small, hand-held method of typing one's communication, or a Memo-writer, which has not only a print-facility, but also a light-emitting diode (LED) Figure 22.1).

Scanning

This method of indication is often chosen for those with very severe physical disability.

They tend to be relatively slow methods and are cognitively more complex than direct selection. Methods of scanning are 'any technique in which the selections are offered to the user by a person or display'. Depending on the aid, the user may respond by signalling when he/she sees the correct choice presented. The simplest scanning method is to run-through a series of 'yes–no' questions. The individual uses a prepared signal to indicate the required item.

Linear scanning involves an item-by-item scan for the individual, indicating when his chosen subject is reached. Items may be displayed on a simple communication chart, or a clock face with an indicator or scanning light. In group item scanning the letters, words or symbols are placed in rows or groups. The individual is encouraged to scan along a row, until he/she indicates when the appropriate column is reached. This column is then, in turn, scanned to reach the correct item (Figures 22.2 and 22.3).

Encoding

This technique is cognitively sophisticated, but is very useful for individuals who may wish to use a large vocabulary even though they may have limited movement. Encoding may be described as a method by which the individual makes a choice from a pattern or code of symbols which, when decoded, indicate the message. The code needs to be either memorized or set out on separate cards for reference. Morse code may be considered as such a method, where sequences of dots and dashes, when decoded, represent traditional orthography. Another simple encoding method may be to have on one card a list of commonly used phrases, with each of these being numbered. On another card there can be the numbers of the phrases. It is possible for the individual to indicate a number by an arranged method, which will then correspond to the appropriate phrase. Encoding may be combined

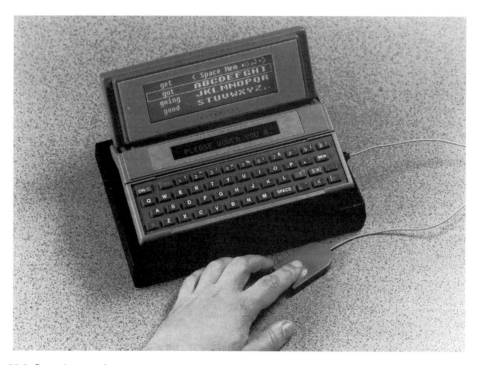

Figure 22.2 Scanning mode.

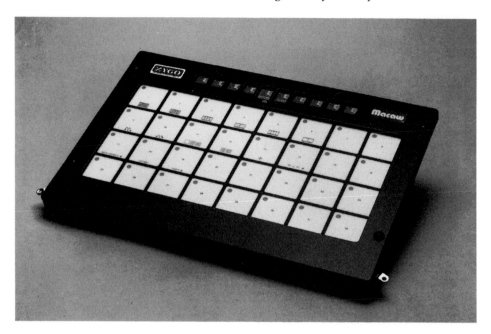

Figure 22.3 Words, symbols and pictures can be used on overlays with this aid.

with direct-selection or with scanning, in order to indicate messages.

Communication aid outputs

The outputs of aids have become more sophisticated and varied. Some communication aids allow the therapist and user to select either an LED display, printout or synthesized/digitized vocal output. Different outputs are appropriate for different users and situations and preferably maintaining flexibility is desirable.

PROMOTING SUCCESSFUL USE OF COMMUNICATION AIDS

Assessing a patient prior to a communication aid being provided is essential but complex. Not only does the therapist need to establish the linguistic and cognitive potential of the client but also physical and sensory abilities, motivation, and personal wishes of the client need to be assessed. Additionally, the therapist considers the environments in which the

patient is going to communicate, as it is essential that communication is not seen as a one-way process. For example, if the main carer has hearing or eyesight problems this may directly affect the type of equipment that is most useful in that situation.

The patient should have a total communication system, and sometimes a sophisticated technical device has to be backed up with a simple picture board or sign system which can be available to the patient for longer periods, and can be used as back-up in the event of technical problems with the aid. Continued access to the speech and language therapy department is required for any aid-user, as the interfaces may need to be adapted according to changes in the patient's condition, be it for better or worse, or if the patient's environment needs change (Musselwhite and Louis, 1982).

Considerable help is available from communication aid centres, they will:

- assess the patient;
- arrange for aids to be loaned;

- train patients and carers to use aids;
- arrange aids to be modified;
- assess whether the aid/approach should be changed when patient's needs alter.

In addition many speech therapy departments carry a stock of aids for loan. Whilst appropriate assessment is essential the therapeutic intervention to assist the person to develop effective communication skills must not be forgotten.

In all cases patients who use communication aids can be helped by the following:

- Ensure that the aid is near and accessible to the patient.
- Encourage the patient to use the aid. No communication aid can replicate the speed of speech; patience on the part of both the listener and sender is essential.
- Do not change the subject too quickly. The aid-user may be replying to one question, and if other questions are asked it is difficult to catch up.
- It is important that the communication aid is accepted and not looked upon as a toy or a joke. Some patients reject equipment that can be most useful because of the attitudes of other people around them.
- Many patients can communicate a little verbally or by facial expression. Encourage this, along with the rest of their communication, through their communication aid.

ASSISTING THE PATIENT WHO HAS SWALLOWING PROBLEMS

Many people with neuromotor speech disorders may develop problems with swallowing, which are distressing not only to the patient, but also to the relatives. Frequently dysphagia can be secondary to stroke, motor neurone disease, multiple sclerosis, and in some patients with Parkinson's disease. To help the patient eat more comfortably and safely it is important to understand what is involved in the swallowing mechanism. There are three phases to swallowing; the **oral** phase, which takes place in the mouth and is under voluntary control; the **pharyngeal** phase, which takes place in the upper part of the throat; and the **oesophageal** phase, which carries the food from the back of the throat to stomach. These last two phases are mostly under reflex control and thus we shall concern ourselves particularly with the oral phase, as it is the one over which therapists have the most influence (Groher, 1984)

SYMPTOMS CORRESPONDING TO VARIOUS NEUROMUSCULAR SWALLOWING DIFFICULTIES

Disorders affecting preparation of the bolus

The patient may have difficulty in masticating, due to weakness of the buccal musculature or restriction of tongue movement which normally distributes food between the teeth for grinding, and then retrieves the food to form the bolus. Reduced lip closure may allow food or liquid to fall from the mouth while the bolus is being prepared. Some patients have reduced oral sensitivity which would affect this preparatory phase.

Disorders affecting propulsion of the bolus.

The bolus, having been retrieved, has to be moved from the front to the back of the mouth, and this is usually done by elevation of the front of the tongue which squeezes the bolus backwards. Any restriction in the movement of the tongue will have an effect upon this propulsion. As the bolus moves posteriorly the palate is raised to seal the nose from the pharynx and prevent food from regurgitating up into the nasopharynx.

The swallow reflex

The swallow reflex is triggered by the sensory receptors in the anterior aspect of the faucial arch. Normally the timing of the reflex is such that the posterior movement of the bolus is not interrupted. Some patients do not trigger the reflex until the bolus has contacted the aryepiglotic fold, while others trigger the reflex only when the material has fallen into the pyriform sinuses. This delay in the reflex being triggered may result in slow eating or, more seriously, may give rise to aspiration.

Cricopharyngeal dysfunction

The cricopharyngeal valve is in a state of tonic contraction during rest. During swallowing, respiration is halted and the cricopharyngeus must relax as the bolus approaches. If this does not happen the patient may feel that he/she is having to force food down his/her throat and may complain of feeling an obstruction. The dysfunction of the cricopharyngeus muscle may be related to various upper motor neurone lesions, or due to fibrosis in this area.

There are many other swallowing problems which can cause distress and concern to the patient and his/her relatives. The SALT frequently works with the physiotherapist and dietician to analyse exactly the type of feeding problem that the patient is suffering, and to develop a feeding programme which will increase confidence and promote better integration of the retained facilities.

The following feeding programme should be adapted for individual patients, following appropriate assessment, but gives the basis which may assist neurologically damaged patients.

GUIDELINES TO HELP THOSE WITH SWALLOWING DISORDERS

First ensure a patient's swallowing difficulty has been assessed.

1. **Posture.** Make sure that the patient is sitting comfortably, with head upright. Support the head if this is required.
2. **Relax.** Ensure that the patient is in a calm frame of mind before eating or drinking. Stress and tension are often associated with exacerbating dysphagia.
3. **Do not talk.** Avoid speaking during the meal. It may be helpful to be silent for a couple of minutes before eating or drinking.
4. **Yawn.** Encourage the patient to yawn before eating if the throat feels tight. This may ease constriction.
5. **Feeding routine.** Encourage the patient to follow this purposeful routine:
   (a) place a small amount of food in the mouth;
   (b) close the lips tightly;
   (c) chew;
   (d) pause and hold breath;
   (e) give purposeful swallow;
   (f) pause – start routine again.
6. **Food textures.** Avoid mixing fluids and solids, e.g. minestrone soup. Also avoid any foods which are crumbly. Frequently, smooth semi-solids are easiest. Food should neither be too liquid nor too solid.
7. **Small meals.** It is advisable to have several small meals a day rather than two or three big meals.
8. **Fatigue.** The patient should stop eating if feeling tired with the effort.
9. **After the meal.** Drink a small amount of water to swill the mouth out, and cough to make sure that the throat and mouth are clear. Remain sitting for at least half an hour after eating or drinking.

CONCLUSION

Speech and language disorders are rarely restricted to the obvious defects which meet the ear. Frequently they cause misery to the patient and relatives, who may have difficulty in understanding a defect which is not visible, and which is frequently variable. The techniques available to the SALT have progressed over the past decade and our understanding, ability to analyse, and skills in remediation have grown. Therapists are now more aware of the realistic objectives which should be employed in active treatment of adult patients with chronic and acquired disorders.

REFERENCES

Angelo, D.H. and Goldstein, H. (1990) Effects of a Pragmatic Teaching Strategy for Requesting Information by Communication Board Users. *Journal of Speech and Hearing Disorders*, **55**, 231–43.

Brown, B.B. (1981) *Speech Therapy Principles and Practice*, Churchill Livingstone, Edinburgh.

Chenery, H.J., Murdoch, B.E. and Ingram. J.C. (1988) Studies in Parkinson's Diseases: perceptual speech analysis. *Australian Journal of Human Communication Disorders*, **16**(2), 17–29.

Colton, R.H. and Casper, J.K. (1990) *Understanding Voice Problems. a physiological perspective for diagnosis and treatment*, Williams and Wilkins, Baltmore, Maryland.

Darley, F. (1982) *Aphasia*, WB Saunders, Philadelphia.

Darley, F.L., Aronson, A.E. and Brown, J.R. (1975) *Motor Speech Disorders*, W.B. Saunders, Philadelphia.

Dickinson, D. and Dickson, W. (1983) *Anatomical and Physiological Bases of Speech*, Littlebrown & Co., Boston, MA.

Enderby, P. (1986), Relationships between dysarthric groups. *British Journal of Disorders of Communication*, **21**, 189–97.

Enderby, P. and Davies, P. (1989) Communication Disorders: planning a service to meet the needs. *British Journal of Disorders of Communication*, **24**, 301–31.

Enderby, P. and Langton-Hewer, R. (1985) The context and management of acquired speech and language, in *Recent Advances in Geriatric Medicine* (ed. B. Issacs), Churchill Livingstone, Edinburgh, pp. 36–54.

Gregory, H. (1979) *Controversies About Stuttering Therapy*, University Park Press, Baltimore.

Greene, M.C. (1980) *The Voice and its Disorder*, Pitman Medical, London.

Groher, M. (1984) *Dysphagia*, Butterworth, Boston, MA.

Hardy, C.J. (1983) *Cerebral Palsy*, Prentice Hall, Englewood Cliffs, NJ, pp. 200–5.

McKenna, J.P., Fornataro-Clerici, L.M., McMenamin, P.G. and Leonard, R.J. (1991) Laryngeal Cancer: diagnosis of treatment and speech rehabilitation. *American Family Physician*, **44**, 124–9.

Musselwhite, C.R. and Louis, K.W. (1982) *Communication Programming for Severely Handicapped: vocal and non-vocal strategies*, College Hill Press, San Diego, CA.

Newrick, P. and Langton-Hewer, R. (1984) Motor neurone disease: can we do better? A study of 42 patients. *British Medical Journal*, **289**, 539–42.

Parker, A.J. (1983) *Speech Rehabilitation Following Laryngectomy in the United Kingdom*. Third National Head and Neck Oncology Conference, Nottingham Conference (abstracts).

Perry, A. (1988) Surgical voice restoration following laryngectomy: the tracheoesophageal fistula technique (Singer Blom). *British Journal of Disorders of Communication*, **23**, 23–30.

Peters, T.J. and Guitar, B. (1991) *Stuttering: an integrated ppproach to its nature and treatment*, Williams and Wilkins, Baltimore.

Rhyner, P.M. (1988) Graphic symbol and speech training of young children with Down's syndrome: some preliminary findings. *Journal of Childhood Communication Disorders*, **12**(1), 25–47.

Scott, S. and Caird, A. (1981) Speech therapy for patients with Parkinson's Disease. *British Medical Journal*, **283**, 1088.

Singer, M.I., Blom E.D. and Haymaker, R.C. (1981) Voice restoration. *Annals of Otology, Rhinology and Laryngology*, **90**, 498–502.

Yorkston, K.M., Beukelman, D.R. and Bell, K.R. (1988) *Clinical Management of Dysarthric Speakers*, College Hill Press, San Diego, CA.

PART FIVE

NEUROLOGICAL DISABILITY

23 Adult cerebral palsy

E.G. Cantrell

INTRODUCTION

Many apparently insoluble problems face healthy school-leavers, so severe disability must make the future seem even more bleak for disabled teenagers. Adolescence is a time of great emotional and physical change, where the 'child' has to learn to become an independent adult. They need to break from elders who usually wish to advise, threaten their privacy, and who tend to treat the adolescent, especially if disabled, as a perpetual child. It is a time of low confidence disguised by bravado, and low status hidden in great energy.

The practical problems of learning to live independently in the community are difficult enough. With a high risk of being unable to find employment and financial security the prospects for adult life must seem depressing. There is unemployment and recession, and many of the employed adult population seem ignorant or unconcerned about such problems. The 'perfect people' in society do not give the 'imperfect' a chance, they may focus mockery on the disabled, and make close friendships difficult to make or keep. Mobility may depend on other people being free to help with transport. The worst public responses to cope with may be pity and charity, sometimes the only ways in which other people are capable of reacting. 'Childhood' status can be prolonged excessively when physical needs require daily help from other 'helpers' and their lack of sensitivity may be the main cause of handicap.

DEFINITIONS

This chapter will focus on those people, aged 16+ who have cerebral palsy (CP), defined as mixtures of:

1. Effects of brain damage from birth (or recognized in the first year of life).
2. Neurological syndromes such as hemiplegia, diplegia, tetraplegia, with or without sensory disturbances.
3. Central cognitive, perceptual or intellectual problems.
4. Disorders of movement.
5. Dysphasia and dysarthrias.

In addition there may be secondary acquired problems related to painful distorted mobility and uneven movements such as osteoarthritis, cervical myelopathy, epilepsy and social isolation.

Cerebral palsy is 'an umbrella term covering a group of non-progressive but often changing, motor impairment syndromes secondary to lesions or anomalies of the brain arising in the early stages of its development' (Mutch *et al*, 1992). Children with cerebral palsy mature and grow, but abnormal compensatory movements result in secondary musculoskeletal deformities. Adults change

Rehabilitation of the Physically Disabled Adult. Edited by C. John Goodwill, M. Anne Chamberlain and Chris Evans. Published in 1997 by Stanley Thornes (Publishers) Ltd, Cheltenham. ISBN 0-7487-3183-0.

less, but they get pain and loss of function associated with the deformities, and many have difficulty in social interaction,

The brain impairment in cerebral palsy varies in severity. It may involve a variety of motor and sensory deficits including cognitive difficulties, epilepsy and behavioural disorder, as well as the musculoskeletal deformities.

INCIDENCE, PREVALENCE AND LIFE EXPECTANCY

Cerebral palsy occurs in 1.2–2.5 per 1000 live births with a similar prevalence rate into adolescence and adulthood (Kudrjavcev *et al*, 1983; Grether, Cummins and Nelson, 1992; Bhusan, Paneth and Kiely, 1993). Information is limited, but it seems likely that people who are mildly or moderately involved can expect a normal lifespan as defined by their cultural and geographical environment. Badley, Thompson and Wood (1978) compared the relative number of people with CP with two other disabilities and impairments in an average Health District of 250 000 (Table 23.1).

In the study reported by Thomas, Bax and Smyth (1989) in areas of London and Berkshire, the diagnoses in 111 young adults (aged 18–25 years) with physical disability, were:

CP	42%
Spina bifida	17%
Others	41%

Table 23.1

Diagnoses	Total severely or very severely disabled (no.)	Age 16–44 years (no.)	Age 65+ years (no.)
Congenital disorders (CP included)	102	61	9
Stroke	427	6	316
Arthritis, back pain	1074	6	756

'Others' included seven with rheumatoid arthritis, three with multiple sclerosis and single examples of 13 other conditions.

DISABILITY AND PROGNOSIS

There are three ways of defining the disabilities which result from CP:

- **Medical model**. This views complications as intrinsic, inferred from the areas of brain damage or pathology, but ignoring reactions between the person and their part of the outside world. Medical details are important for predicting prognosis.
- **Social model**. This concentrates on the effects of a discriminating society which gives little concern to the needs of those who are impaired in any way. The disadvantages in access to buildings, transport, jobs, shops, entertainment and social grouping actually apply to all disabled people, and to us all as we get older.
- **Fusion model** (PAOM = problem/asset-oriented management). This uses a disability matrix in which the questions to be answered seek to tackle both the intrinsic (pathology) and extrinsic (society) needs of each individual. This allows sufficient information to provide a basis for life-planning.

Deteriorating brain damage, increasing epilepsy, severe depression, lack of family support are intrinsic factors which can make any person's disability worse. There are also extrinsic problems such as poor social opportunities, unemployment, isolation, poor housing, that would affect any person, disabled or not. In addition, there are important character factors to consider. Some people can rise above all the disabling pressures of uncaring society, even with deteriorating health – those people who have strong morale, never give up, remain cheerful and use every quality and skill they have, to the full. These features are called assets in analysing the personal plan for any individual. It is important that genuine choice exists so that an adult with CP can opt to use a wheelchair to save energy for other activities, or try to walk to gain their own independent form of mobility. They must be helped to find what is 'right' for them, but also know the possible results of their choice.

SPECIFIC CEREBRAL PALSY DISABILITY PROBLEMS

The common types of difficulty arising from CP pathology are either intrinsic or extrinsic:

Intrinsic problems

- **Joint contractures**. Limb-stretching routines practised daily from early childhood may help, but contractures are not always avoidable.
- **Osteoarthritis** may occur early because of distorted joints and the very hectic gait. The neck and lower limbs may be particularly affected and become painful, and so can hard-pressed ataxic or contracted hands.
- **Speech** can be incoherent or simply difficult to understand. Most young adults want to talk and be understood, and often commune with a noisy background of pop music. Distorted speech is a major disadvantage and inhibits new friendships. It can interfere with education.
- **Pain** from arthritis and contractures can affect all postures and movements.
- **Anger** is to be expected from the mismatch between aspirations and reality.
- **Fatigue** is common because more energy is needed for movement.
- **Fitness:** It is difficult to keep fit or slim.
- **Memory and perception** may be difficult and is also often better than speech will express.
- **Epilepsy** can occur and threatens independent living, mobility, safety, transport and social contacts.

Extrinsic problems

- **Isolation**. This may be from unemployment, lack of mobility or poor communication. It may result in depression and low morale. Pair-bonding is more difficult, casual acquaintances more impossible to sustain. Socializing requires more tolerance than is widely available.
- **Misunderstanding**. Adult services are not orientated towards disability present since birth, and they often do not allow the person with disability to give guidance on what they need.
- **Poverty**. Disabled people are 50% less likely to be employed than able-bodied (OPCS) and most earn less than the average for their age group if they are in work, (Chapter 52). This intensifies a condition that may need extra money for specific disability needs (e.g. transport, heating, communication aids).
- **Dependency**. Where a person cannot manage daily activities alone for 24 hours, they need help from fit carers. If this is family-based, the carers may have health problems of their own (Cantrell, Dawson and Glastonbury, 1985).
- **Guilty feelings of parents**. Transition to adulthood may be especially difficult if it involves separate existence from a family that has felt (unjustifiably) guilty.
- **Stigma**. The public often assumes that someone with funny speech and peculiar gait is intellectually limited as well.
- **Sexual rejection**. Everything conspires to make finding partners difficult.
- **Reduced education**. If a lot of time has to be spent in physical training and visiting hospitals it can seriously compromise education.
- **Transport and access**. Many people with CP cannot get on buses or trains. Few can drive.
- **Housing**. Most houses do not have good wheelchair access, or adapted equipment.

CLASSIFICATION

CP has been classified by Minear (1956) by topographical distribution and abnormalities in muscle tone, but the terminology has not been standardized. This chapters uses the terms:

- **Hemiplegia** – for unilateral distribution.
- **Diplegia** – for bilateral lower limb distribution with an ability by the person to use the hands bimanually, if abnormally.
- **Tetraplegia** – for the person with head, neck and trunk involvement.
- **Dyskinesia** – for an excess of observed unwanted, abnormal movements associated with ataxia, chorea or athetosis.
- **Spasticity** means palpable abnormal muscle tone associated with a poor movement. It is probably a heterogenous condition and that what is felt clinically is the final common effect of differing causes (Wright and Rang, 1990) (Chapter 34).

A change which can occur in adults with elements of dyskinesia is that their limbs and trunk often become more rigid with age.

AETIOLOGY

There are many disorders that may cause CP (Holm, 1982). Many people with CP, and their families and friends, still believe the main cause is birth trauma. However, prenatal causes may include genetic abnormalities, congenital malformation and *in utero* infections. Perinatal causes may be birth trauma and asphyxia but improved prenatal imaging techniques and normal Apgar scores suggest that these are not common causes. Postnatal causes may be infection and postconvulsive and vascular problems. In many cases the cause is simply not known (Nelson and Ellenberg, 1986).

As live birth weights fall in populations and survival rates increase there is a constant trend from lower to higher CP rates (Mutch *et al.* 1992). As a result of improved early care more very low birth weight infants survive, but some have severe multiple handicaps (Pape and Wigglesworth, 1979). Problems with labour occur more commonly in infants with central nervous system malformation (Biale, Brawer-Ostrovsky and Insler, 1985). Most cases of cerebral palsy with severe mental retardation are prenatal rather than perinatal in origin (Hagberg, 1979; Nelson and Ellenberg, 1981).

The timing of the damage to the central nervous system is important, as the effect on the fetus is often more dependent upon the stage of development at the time of injury than on its specific nature. The effect of rubella in the first trimester of pregnancy illustrates this phenomenon.

Hemiplegia is often associated with a lesion in the distribution of the middle cerebral artery in the hemisphere contralateral to the spasticity and it is now possible to ascertain the timing of such a lesion. Diplegia is often associated with periventricular leucomalacia and preterm birth with low weight. Tetraplegia is often associated with brain malformation. Ataxia is associated primarily with genetic factors and athetosis with hyperbulirubinaemia, not often seen in the western world today and, perinatal asphyxia.

For additional information on these subjects, the reader is referred to Aicardi (1992).

CLINICAL FEATURES

Hemiplegic cerebral palsy

This is a unilateral condition, although associated movements may be observed on the unaffected side when efforts at movement are made by the affected side. The abnormality of muscle tone is more often spastic than dyskinetic, males are affected more than females and the right side more often that the left. In order to be classified as CP the lesion must be congenital or acquired during the first 3 years of life.

If the problem is in the lower limb it is often first noticed on ambulation and the posture or movement pattern adopted is one of equinus in the ankle and equinovarus of the foot. Severity can usually be gauged by the amount the affected upper limb is used. Growth may be unequal on the two sides, the hemiplegic side being smaller. The associated problems may be epilepsy, which can be of late onset, mental retardation and behaviour. People with hemiplegic CP usually walk between the ages of 18 and 21 months (Bleck, 1987) and function as community walkers (Hoffer *et al*, 1973). People with hemiplegic CP are independent in most activities of daily living, talk, join in activities with their peers, attend mainstream schools and are employable if the associated problems of epilepsy, mental retardation and behavioural disturbance are not too severe.

Diplegic cerebral palsy

This is a bilateral condition with the lower limbs more affected than the upper limbs. The abnormality of muscle tone is usually spastic although it can be ataxic. People with spastic diplegia usually have a better prognosis if they were preterm rather than full term at birth. The problem is often first noticed on attempting weightbearing. The distribution of abnormality is often asymmetrical. The upper limbs may have flexed elbows but the manipulative skills are usually good and only fine motor problems tend to exist. Intellect is usually normal but linked proportionally to the severity of the upper limb (Beales, 1966).

The posture or movement pattern adopted in the lower limbs is one of hip flexion, internal rotation and adduction with femoral neck anteversion. A 'silent' dislocation of the hip often occurs after puberty, with a gradual increase in pain and degeneration of the cartilage leading to arthritis, so that problems become apparent much later. The knees can be flexed, extended or neutral depending

upon the movement pattern involved. The ankle is usually in equinus with pes valgus, plantarflexed talus and hindfoot equinus. The person stands with the legs internally rotated and walks, or more often runs, due to impaired coordination, on tip toes frequently with the feet inverted.

A lack of balance, trunk hypotonus and contractures will affect walking ability. The person will only walk independently if the equilibrium reactions are intact. If anterior equilibrium reactions are absent the person will require crutches and if other equilibrium reactions are absent a four-point walker or rollator (Bleck, 1987). They will usually function as household walkers. The associated problems are often visual (strabismus) and perceptual. Epilepsy is rare and intellect usually intact. The person can usually use speech for communication purposes and manage most activities of daily living. These are the people whose integration into a relatively normal adult life depends substantially upon whether they have been able to attend mainstream schools (O'Reilly, 1975), avoid spending an excessive amount of time on special treatment programmes (Goldkamp, 1984) and especially whether they and their families have come to terms with the impairments and disabilities sustained so that these have not become major handicaps.

Ataxic diplegia

Ataxic diplegia is usually congenital in origin and bilateral. The person can often stand and walk independently but lifts the feet up high at each step and has a floppy trunk. A tremor may be seen in the arms in the sitting position and there may be difficulty when reaching for objects and with writing. A staccato speech pattern is often evident. Intellect is usually intact but the person may be slow.

Tetrapleiga

Tetraplegia can show either spastic or mixed muscle tone. All four limbs are involved and the head, neck and trunk. Primitive reflexes, such as the asymmetrical and symmetrical tonic neck reflexes, are often retained and the emerging righting, equilibrium and parachute reactions are often delayed or absent. The problem is usually noticed early, how early depends on the severity. Walking is usually non-functional and sitting needs to be supported so that lying may be the person's only independent position. The bulbar muscles are often involved and mental retardation is frequently present, often associated with microcephaly. There are usually problems with feeding and care-giving and deformities may occur resulting from abnormal positions and movement.

Severity can be ranked by the ability to perform independent transfers, assisted transfers or being totally dependent on others for changes in position. Mobility will be either with an electric wheelchair or else pushed by a carer. Communication problems may range from being unable to speak but able to use non-verbal methods to not being able to communicate needs, thoughts or feelings by any method. Those with tetraplegic CP often require lifelong care (Hagberg, Edehol-Tysk and Edestrom, 1988).

Dyskinetic cerebral palsy

This usually involves all four limbs and the head, neck and trunk. There is usually a persistence of the primitive reflexes especially the asymmetrical tonic neck reflex and a predominance of either excessive extension or flexion. Imaging has proved elusive in this condition and the cause is often attributed to perinatal difficulties. The problem is often first noticed when the child changes from being floppy or hypotonic during the first year to having difficulty with executing purposeful movement. Independent walking and standing can occur but are not the norm. There is reduced trunk control and, although contractures are said to be unusual, scoliosis,

pelvic obliquity and hip dislocation occur. Pain is often present in both the spine and the limbs due to the continuous contorted movements. People with dyskinetic cerebral palsy are often thin compared to those with immobility who put on weight.

Their speech is often difficult to understand, drooling is often present. Other associated problems can be hearing loss, visual problems and grimacing. Intellect is usually intact, writing is difficult but a keyboard may be practical. Epilepsy is rare. They will require adaptive equipment and bioengineering technology available to enable them to function as independently as possible.

For additional information on development the reader is referred to Sheridan (1973) and Illingworth (1966), and for additional information on the motor development of children with cerebral palsy to Bobath and Bobath (1975).

PROGNOSIS

The prognosis for movement of at-risk infants before they are a year old is difficult and often inaccurate (Nelson and Ellenberg, 1982). This may explain why parents often say that they were not told that anything was wrong, even though they suspected a problem.

Functional ability levels

Hoffer *et al.* (1973) has classified the following useful functional ability levels:

Sitting
1   Propped sitter – upright in brace needing loose hips and a straight back.
2   Self sitter – uses hands and a wheelchair.
3   Independent sitter – needing no support.

Walking
1   Non-functional – stands and weight bears.
2   Household – kitchen/bathroom.
3   Community – out of doors.

DEVELOPMENT OF CONTRACTURES AND DEFORMITY

If the musculoskeletal system is used abnormally, problems follow. Active movement enables movements to be practised and perfected. Inability to do this often leads to deformity. Deformities in the soft tissues and bones of joints may be mobile, fixed or structural. The effect of abnormal posture on the development of joint deformity in CP has been described by Fulford and Brown (1976). Muscle contractures in CNS dysfunction is primarily due to a shortened muscle and is a response to prolonged abnormal functioning (Tabery *et al*, 1981). Structure of muscles is conditioned by its use (Lieber, 1986) or nonuse.

Contractures

Contractures may affect the spine leading to scoliosis and an impaired respiratory function. In the legs they may affect the hips leading to poor mobility and weightbearing and later to difficulty in sitting, with consequent problems with perineal and skin care. They may affect the knees producing pain, a loss of mobility and weightbearing. The feet may be involved, also making walking difficult, and possibly needing special shoes. In the arms shoulder, elbow and hand function may be affected. There is often a rapid deterioration during the growth spurt at puberty.

Place of surgery

Muscle releases, lengthening and transfers are frequently done to increase joint range of motion and hopefully prevent later problems; stability and pain control are more important priorities for adults with CP so that bony surgery is more likely to be undertaken. Orthopaedic surgeons often feel that results are more predictable in people with spasticity who display a stable EMG than in people with dyskinesia who display a variable EMG and therefore prefer not to operate on the latter. It can be difficult to distinguish between spasticity and dystonia (Gage, 1991). Skeletal maturity is usually delayed in people with CP and deformity is often increased as a result of the growth spurt at puberty, so that bony surgery is sometimes delayed until after this time.

Procedures which might be undertaken in young adults include:

1. Spinal fusion in tetraplegia if sitting and lying become difficult.
2. Remodelling of the hip joint to maintain function if the articular cartilage is relatively intact, using a femoral osteotomy and acetabular reconstruction.
3. Femoral head and neck resection for pain relief if the articular cartilage has degenerated. Heterotopic bone following surgery can be a problem.
4. Hip arthrodesis in tetraplegia to regain a sitting position.
5. Total hip arthroplasty in diplegia with painful subluxation in a person who has lost the ability to household walk. Loosening following surgery can be a problem.
6. Correction of knee flexion if the flexed knee interferes with transfer or if positioning becomes difficult in tetraplegia.
7. Supracondylar closed wedge osteotomy of the femur to correct flexion deformity in the knees of a person with diplegia who has lost mobility and is experiencing pain.
8. Triple arthrodesis of the foot in people with diplegia or hemiplegia who are experiencing difficulties with weightbearing.
9. Correction of the skeletal deformity in hallux valgus and bunion and in dorsal bunion.
10. Cosmetic surgery to the hand.

For additional information on these subjects the reader is referred to Bleck (1987).

TRAINING AND MANAGEMENT

There are a number of different 'schools' for the treatment, training or management of children with CP (Bower, 1993), and many children with CP are likely to have undergone at least one such method and more if their carers were searching for the cure. The 'schools' in most common use at the present time are:

- **Bobath** (Bobath and Bobath, 1984; Mayston, 1992) which is a neurodevelopmental treatment aimed at normalization of movement to prevent deformity.
- **Conductive education or Peto** (Hari and Tillemans, 1984; Cottam and Sutton, 1986) which is a training programme aimed at learning movement, language and functional skills.
- **Doman Delacato** (Doman *et al*, 1960, developed from the ideas of Fay, 1948) which is both a neurophysiological treatment and a training aimed at influencing: (a) the brain impairment and (b) the development of cognition.
- **Portage** (Shearer and Shearer, 1972; Jesien, 1984) which is a training programme aimed at improving general skills and cognition.
- **Vojta** (Jones, 1975; Vojta, 1984) which is a neurophysiological treatment aimed at influencing impairment so that normal skills are developed.

Many physiotherapists use an eclectic, management approach tailored to the needs of each individual person and often influenced by Phelps (1990). His ideas on diagnosis, assessment using slow-motion pictures, team approach, orthopaedic management of the peripheral musculoskeletal problems, aids, equipment and exercise are still largely in evidence today.

Table 23.2 illustrates the principal emphases of the different schools.

As yet, no single school of therapy has been proven to be more successful than any other. While this issue remains unresolved, the

Table 23.2 Differing emphases among the most widely known treatment methods in cerebral palsy

School of therapy	Theories covering the selection of goals for therapy
1. BOBATH (Bobath and Bobath, 1984)	A neurodevelopmental treatment using reflex inhibiting patterns (not static) from key points of control (head, neck, spine, shoulders and hips) to inhibit abnormal spasm, spasticity or rigidity and facilitate normal movement by initiation from the therapist guiding the movement and the child taking it over gradually
2. CONDUCTIVE EDUCATION (Hari and Tillemans, 1984)	The use of movement, language and function initiated by the child in an all-embracing day-long educational process in groups led by a conductor
3. DOMAN DELACATO (Doman *et al*, 1960; developed from, Fay, 1948)	The reprogramming of the brain by teaching motion according to phylogenetic development through evolution from the fish to the amphibian to the reptile to the mammal on all fours to the anthropoid, that is through five stages of progressive patterning movements – swim, squirm, creep, crawl and walk first passively then actively.
4. PHELPS (Phelps, 1990)	The encouragement of self-help to reach one's full potential as an adult based on a eclectic treatment approach including both orthopaedic and neurological elements individual to each child's needs in an institutional setting
5. PORTAGE (Jessien, 1984)	A home education programme comprising 580 developmentally progressive skills for children from birth to 6 years taught by a visiting teacher and practised by parents with the child
6 VOJTA (Jones, 1975)	The use of manual pressure on 'trigger zones' to elicit normal patterns of reflex motion, especially creeping and rolling

choice of whether any school of therapy is requested or which school of therapy is requested should be left to the choice of each individual child and his/her family (Bower and McLellan, 1994).

GOAL SETTING

It is suggested that the following points are important when formulating goals for people with CP:

1. There are no studies on humans or animals proving conclusively that the effects of CNS lesions have been either cured or even profoundly or permanently influenced by therapy.
2. Hubel and Weisel (1970) investigated the effects of visual deprivation on cortical development in kittens, demonstrating that there was a critical time during which sensory stimulation was important for the development of normal vision.
3. Lorenz (1970) in his studies with greylag geese demonstrated that there was a sensitive period for fixing on and following a moving figure which he called imprinting. If a gosling imprinted on a human figure during the sensitive period, it would ignore other adult geese when the time came to pair and mate.

PRIORITIES OF TREATMENT

When a child is diagnosed as cerebral palsied the first question asked by the parent is always 'Will he walk?' The second is 'When?' and the third is 'What can we do to make him walk?' (Bleck, 1987).

The priorities for adults with CP are likely to be different from those of parents for their children. This difference can be detrimental to the development of the emerging adult, especially if the emphases on the management difficulties are not adapted as time passes. Cogher, Savage and Smith (1992) have suggested that during the early years care should

be centred on the home environment and focus on the family and child. In the school years care should be centred on the school environment and focus on the school, child and family, and in adolescence and early adulthood, care should be self-centred and concentrate on life skills.

Bower and McLellan (1992) have suggested that goals of therapy should be negotiated with the child and carers and that the goals often fall into one of three categories. The first was called 'achieve a state' and it was concerned with relationships and ease of handling a child. The second was called 'establish a daily programme' and it was concerned with equipment and compliance, and the third was called 'achieve a motor skill'. Motor skills were only achieved if the child's neural mechanisms were ready (McGraw, 1989) or, to put it another way, if the child was at the appropriate developmental age and if the skills were associated with daily functional activities understood and desired by the child and not requiring increased assistance from the carers. Rang (1982) suggested that the main problems for the chronically disabled are that their difficulties never go away, the physical difficulties impede emotional development and that the problems remain a lifetime preoccupation for the entire family. He pointed out that three of the important problems faced by chronically disabled teenagers and young adults are that on reaching that stage they begin to comprehend their own future, recognize their own social insecurity and lack of interpersonal skills and so may emerge from being a protected child to being a social reject.

Maybe these are some of the reasons why Gillberg (1992) has found that people with CP have an increased rate of psychiatric problems. He suggest that the milder forms of CP display anxiety states and that the more severe forms often display autism.

Sadly, the often encountered persistence of parents and therapists in treatment and training programmes to make the child, adolescent or young adult improve basic skills, even though the 'critical periods' for attaining the particular skills are probably long past, may hinder the ability which is probably of paramount importance in later life, namely, the capacity to integrate socially in to the community.

INDEPENDENCE

Bleck (1987) has suggested that the needs for optimum independent living for adults with CP ranked in order of priority are:

1. communication
2. independence in activities of daily living
3. mobility
4. walking.

Communication can be either by verbal or non-verbal methods and a yes/no response is the basic requirement. Independence in activities of daily living is facilitated by the availability of one good hand but the important aspect is independence from parental help. Mobility can be either by self-locomotion or mechanical devices and control over just one part of the body (foot, chin, etc.) is the basic requirement. It is very important that the individual person's requirements for communication, independence and mobility are regularly reassessed and updated as their needs change. Unfortunately this is an area which is often neglected in the young adult with CP. People with CP are restricted in their movement abilities but this does not mean that they do not need to keep fit, healthy and active in the same way as other people throughout their lives. The necessary facilities for this should be made available.

EMPLOYMENT

Factors likely to favour long-term independence and employment Bleck (1987) are:

1. mainstream schooling;
2. independent mobility in the community;

3. manual dexterity;
4. habitation in provincial towns rather than large cities;
5. spasticity rather than dyskinesia and hemiplegia or diplegia rather than tetraplegia.

Factors suggesting less likelihood of independence and employment are:

1. intellectual inability;
2. severe handicap;
3. prolonged treatment programmes and special schooling;
4. over-protection, especially from the family.

For additional information on these subjects, the reader is referred to: Bleck (1987), Cogher, Savage and Smith (1992), Thomas, Bax and Smyth (1989) and Ingram *et al*, (1964).

LIFE PLANNING (PERSONAL PLAN)

If an individual with CP is to become an independent adult then every opportunity must be taken to evaluate his/her strengths (assets) and weaknesses and to look at options for the adult life. The process is difficult and complex, because cognitive, memory or perception skills may be lacking. Parents and professionals may have better understanding of what can/ cannot be done with limitations of finance, housing, social support and local services. However, the life plan the young adult follows will contain anger and frustration if they have not been involved in choices. The personal plan should not be the property of family and therapists; every effort should be made to guide the person with CP to make decisions.

Careful documentation of assets and problems can lead to better sharing of information between professions and the family. From this base it is possible to chose options and objectives.

Assets

Two people with exactly the same levels of intrinsic impairment may end up with totally different lifestyles, because one has far more assets. These are personal features (not just finance) and social factors that make some people much more capable of succeeding in coping with a competitive and unhelpful environment than others. Examples are:

1. **Humour**, the person who can laugh at all misfortune, the absurdities of the situation, or even at themselves is more likely to find their own solutions, and will also attract more help from other people than the morose defeated ones.
2. **Determination**. Some people never give up, and whatever the barriers or disabilities they face, they keep trying, they have faith in themselves that they will succeed. Many physical and social problems respond well to this positive approach.
3. **Interests**. If a person can show enthusiasm in a wide range of activities, subjects and hobbies, it gives them a wider perspective on life anyway, and can often lead to a greater choice of occupations to chose from in future. Interests also lead to social links outside the family more successfully than apathy.
4. **Stamina**. It is not always easy to know why some people keep going in spite of the physical demands of spastic limbs, pain levels and a full programme. Tiredness may of course relate to depression, lack of sleep, anaemia or poor nutrition, but endurance can also have personal and mental components that some people have more of than others.
5. **Finance** options are clearly greater if adequate finance can be found.

Even the most talented, cheerful and interested person can be worn down by repeated failure or by lack of support or animosity from family, professionals or neighbours.

DEPENDENCY, FAMILIES AND CARERS

If the needs of a disabled person are plotted on a time scale or 24-hour chart (Cantrell and Dawson, 1983), then it can be seen how much help they need each day. The example given in Figure 23.1 shows several important results:

1. The independence times are short because nowhere in the daytime did the person manage without personal help for more than 2 hours, largely because of the problem of transferring from a wheelchair to the WC, or to other chairs.
2. Rehabilitation scope. There is one particular area of difficulty (WC) which should be a target for intensive investigation and training, because if it could solved (and removed from the chart) then the person might manage for longer periods without help. This could make a difference socially and in the search for work.
3. Carers have barely any chance to be involved with other activities, other relatives or their own needs if the independence times are only 1–2 hours. It hardly gives enough time to visit shops, do another job, or take time for recreation or respite. If this chart applied for 7 days per week then the family or partners as carers could become worn out rapidly.

The family of a person with CP, when he/she is a teenager, may well be very heavily involved in supplying the needs of the individual 7 days per week. This could be 'mothering or smothering', it could be genuine concern to do for an offspring what they really could do alone, or it could represent an imposed dependency from years of exaggerated 'care' that has produced a state of passive defeat and apathy. Families should be helped to learn to live apart, if they do not they can end up in bondage to each other. If intensive training, special equipment

Name.... A. YOUNGMAN ....

Ward.... Home ....No:............Diagnosis CP(Tetra)...Date..........

Functions/can't be Done Alone	Helpers Needed	Helping Hours Time	Equipment/aids Needed
Day GETTING UP, WASH ⎫		6.0	
WC, DRESS, TRANSFERS ⎭	1	7.0	
		8.0	
		9.0	
ON/OFF WC.	1	10.0	?Retrain
		11.0	
PREPARE MEAL	1	12.0	
ON/OFF WC.	1	1.0	
		2.0	
TRANSPORT TO/FROM SHOPS	1	3.0	
		4.0	
ON/OFF WC.	1	5.0	
		6.0	
FOOD PREPARATION	1	7.0	
BATH	2	8.0	
		9.0	
Night		10.0	
TRANSFER TO BED	1	11.0	?HOIST
		12.0	
		1.0	
		2.0	
		3.0	
		4.0	
		5.0	

(Dependence (Total Time (4.25 Hours)

Figure 23.1 Twenty-four hour dependency chart.

and alternative carers can be shown to be compatible, and work perfectly well, then the person with CP can become a person with a choice of how to live. Family can then be welcome because they are not dominant and essential. This independence is an essential transition.

Residential 'homes' can equally create habits of involvement by other 'people' which make a person with CP over-dependent and remove all motivation to learn to do things by themselves.

Partnerships outside the original family, or arising within a sheltered environment (day centres, social clubs, residential centre) may seem to be a welcome chance to escape from an earlier restricted group to a 'free' life, but that does assume that the partnership is stable, the new carers capable of providing the same amount of physical and mental support, and that escape is not from over-care to isolation.

INDEPENDENCE TRAINING (REHABILITATION) OR INDEPENDENT STRAINING?

There are centres in the UK where a young person with CP can be given a chance to reduce all the dependency problems on the 24-hour chart and be pushed (or helped) to do much more alone. This process may need prolonged practice and practice training with all the remedial therapists involved (physiotherapy, occupational therapy, psychology, engineering, speech training, education). It can only happen if:

1. Needs assessment is comprehensive.
2. The customer (CP) is trying hard to be independent.
3. The unit staff practice 'planned withdrawal of assistance' (another definition of rehabilitation).
4. Funding is available for this training to be completed.
5. There are choices in housing and care in the community available.

PAOM (problem- and asset-orientated management)

Lawrence Weed (1969) was instrumental in publicizing a system of data organization which has been debated widely and used by many (POMR, problem-orientated medical records). He stressed the need for any medical practitioner to define more precisely the specific disorders presented by a patient, so that elements of the whole could be tackled separately. One difficulty with applying Weed's system to disabled people is that it concentrates on the negative side of a person; on what is wrong. As often used by medical people this may be restricted to medical comments (e.g. hypertension, poor visual acuity, hemiplegia), whereas it really should be a list that includes all disabilities, or practical outcomes of the condition (e.g. job impossible, reactive apathy, inadequate finance). Another difficulty is that the standard list does not include details of the family, or the context from which a person comes, or the people able and willing to be helpers in community life.

The Household Matrix System (Cantrell and Dawson, 1983) records both positive and negative factors for both the primary disabled person and the main helpers (Figure 23.2). It is a simple, practical scheme.

It is clear from this example that the problems of this individual could be so great as to make totally independent life and employment difficult to achieve. Because of the range of personal assets it would seem likely that intensive further training (if wanted) might allow greater development of the personal abilities and lead to some opportunities for independent living and perhaps employment. The family side of the matrix indicates that home care will probably be available for as long as it is wanted, but that A.P. Erson will be competing for limited resources with two younger children whose needs are as yet undefined.

The matrix also highlights an important

Name: A. P. Erson (age 18)

Diagnosis: Cerebral palsy (diplegia and ataxia)

	Problems	Assets
Individual	Easily fatigued	CSE 2 subjects
	Slow	Motivated to improve
	Tendency to trip	Almost ADL-independent
	Awkward gait	Intelligent
	Slurred speech	Interest in music
	Ataxic hands	Sense of humour
Family	Mother: backache	Supportive relatives
	Two younger children	Own house
	Low income	Father in regular work

Figure 23.2 The Household Matrix System: Example of problem and asset-orientated management.

medical problem in the mother, since a history of backache identifies a recurrent condition that is likely to give more trouble if she has to do regular lifting. Hence independence training, especially in mobility and the activities of daily living (ADL), and good equipment is of great importance.

If this example contained a less motivated person, totally dependent on others, with a single parent in difficult social circumstances, the whole balance of the family matrix would shift adversely.

	Problems	Assets
Individual	++	0
Family	++	0

OBJECTIVES AND PERSONAL PLAN

What should follow from a holistic review of the specific needs of the individual is a personal plan, with specific objectives that could be achieved (potentially). It is essential that the person involved is an integral part of the planning process and the choices are their own. If their plans lack insight and are thought to be unrealistic, they still may need to be considered and tried. There is no evidence that professionals are always right.

The final disability chart can be summarized in a six-space personal plan which includes an agreed programme of targets to be tried for that are a reasonable objective (Figure 23.3). Over time the plan may need to be rewritten as circumstances change, relatives move or become ill, or the individual's abilities do (or do not) develop. Occupations and housing may be very important issues that can dominate a personal plan.

Who makes the plan?

It is easy for case conferences and rehabilitation plans to be dominated by professionals. It is far better if the drawing up of a personal plan is a process of partnership with the disabled individual plus expert advice from medical, remedial and social work colleagues on possible future changes, and current resources. Lack of clear thinking or insight does not remove the right of a person to plan their own lives.

PERSONAL PLAN

Client problems	Assets	
		Objectives
Family problems	Assets	

Figure 23.3 Personal plan chart.

Medically there may be factors which will become important in avoidance of contractures, pressure sores, joint disorders, malnutrition and avoidable respiratory or cardiac complications.

Therapists may be able to offer a wide range of ideas, equipment and exercises for self-maintenance, and better mobility and communication. Psychology or counselling may be able to help with some of the complex problems of facing disability, coping with public avoidance or aggression, and adjustments to life in the community.

No outsider can produce a working plan unless the individual with CP can be involved, or make their own plans that suit their own choices. There are problems if choices are impossible or funding cannot be found to suit expectations. Family involvement, for an adult or even teenager, may need to be included with caution because the individual with CP (if capable) should be asked to outline their own lifestyle choices, even if these conflict with those of parents or siblings.

Supporters

Each adult with CP should develop a link with a group of other people to whom they may look for regular help (physical or social). Although independence is a most important factor in allowing a person to reach their maximum freedom of choice, it is essential that this does not destroy the roles of family or friendships from being maintained as supporters. To practice doing most activities alone is not the same as rejecting parents, spouses or friends – on the contrary their company and help may be more readily available because they do not have to undertake every lift, transfer, dressing session or mealtime. In a study of 100 families in Southampton (Cantrell, Dawson and Glastonbury, 1985) where mixed diagnoses resulted in significant dependency in young people (16–65), two results were very important:

1. There were very high levels of illness, tiredness, isolation and depression in main helpers; their disabilities threatened the community care of the disabled people they helped.
2. Family breakdown, and the need for alternative care arrangements, was the result in 50% of the series over 3 years, a very high rate. Carer health is vulnerable.

The study pointed to the need for regular visiting of all such families annually at least. This is now the basis for the Young Disabled

Dependency Register. It was also found in a proportion of families that home care was much more capable of surviving if periods of respite care were available, for all to recover from each other.

The Care Attendant Schemes that now exist in many parts of the UK, do allow regular care to be offered to disabled people to replace relatives who cannot cope, or give essential help where there are no relatives to help. It has meant that more people with CP can now live in the community rather than in residential centres.

Useful resources (for clients, carers or professionals)

If needs are identified that cannot be met easily within the family or by the individual, then there is an important role for information services (Chapter 55).

Enquiries may come from the CP individual, their relative, therapists, GP, care attendants or voluntary group.

Access may be by telephone, visiting demonstration centres or browsing through information systems at the public library or Citizen's Advice Bureau.

Expertise is sometimes related to experience in the form of fellow sufferers who have CP, or from organizations which specialize in 24-hour calling systems and very comprehensive databases with up-to-date information.

Equipment centres are available in many centres of the UK and allow a CP adult to spend time trying out specially designed furniture, electronic equipment or gadgets. They can also provide advice on quality, cost and where to find the money.

The Help for Health Trust, an information service in Winchester, received 8666 enquiries from professionals and disabled people in 1994, 80% from the general public. It has details of several thousand national bodies concerned with some aspect of disability, and local groups throughout Wessex. The Mental Health Foundation claim to have 10 000

groups on their lists, all involved in some voluntary or statutory work for people in need. Detailed studies in Wiltshire show large numbers of groups including self-help, playgroups and social clubs. Many groups have been criticized by disabled people as basically amateur collections of patronizing busybodies, but nearly always they are organized by people who are very keen to give their services, often highly motivated by having had to cope with a severe disability in their own families.

Special mention should be made of some types of resource group that are of particular relevance to the young disabled person, and these are described below.

Disorder-specific groups

These offer a kind of practical expertise in the form of other families who have been though the same sort of trials and tribulations. They can offer help to the disabled, support for families, encourage independence, promote better research and lobby for improved services.

Social links

It is essential to find local groups prepared to offer a place where young people can get to know each other informally, whether disabled or able-bodies. Many local clubs, sports centres and coffee bars are available to help remove the barriers of the shy and embarrassed generation, also allowing some release of energy though physical activities. PHAB is one group that sponsors special meeting places between the physically handicapped and able-bodied.

Centres for independent living

These are growing as the British response to the very political and successful American CIL movement. These groups can give enormous support to disabled people though the experience of people with similar disabilities. This promotes increased activity and self-confidence. Some have been so militant in their approach as to raise barriers, but when well led they can offer a great deal of help to young people who are trying to develop lives of their own in the community.

Sports clubs

Sports clubs exist in many places with special facilities or equipment for disabled people to use, if they wish, or times set aside for swimming, gym games, angling and many other activities. Much interest is being raised by special boats (e.g. *Lord Nelson*) and holidays or training courses for those who wish to sail.

Family replacement schemes

A number of voluntary and statutory groups offer considerable help to those families who have to give daily assistance to a young person living in the community. The whole care attendant movement has proved to be of enormous value to many people, and was inspired by the original Rugby 'Crossroads' scheme. Many other systems now exist.

Day centres

These are places where a wide range of occupations (and sometimes special training) is available. They give time out from home care, relieve relatives or carers and may give opportunities to learn special skills that may lead to open or sheltered employment.

CONCLUSION

Adult CP requires detailed planning for the maximum independence and choice of lifestyle for each person. It is complicated by the need to develop adult life-patterns from what is often a very closely knit family dependency. Details are given of some of the features of

CP, and complications that may develop, but also the factors which affect personal planning.

REFERENCES

Aicardi, J. (1992) *Diseases of the Nervous System in Childhood. Clinics in Developmental Medicine,* MacKeith Press, Blackwell Scientific, Oxford, pp. 115–18.

Badley, E.M., Thompson, R.P. and Wood, P.H. (1978). The prevalence and severity of major disabling conditions – a reappraisal of the government social survey on the handicapped and impaired in Great Britain. *International Journal of Epidemiology,* 7, 145–51.

Beales, R.K. (1966), Spastic paraplegia and diplegia: an evaluation of non-surgical and surgical factors influencing prognosis for ambulation. *Journal of Bone and Joint Surgery,* 48A, 827–46.

Bhusan, V., Paneth, N. and Kiely, J. (1993) Impact of improved survival of very low birth weight infants on recent secular trends in the prevalence of cerebral palsy. *Pediatrics,* 91, 1094–100.

Biale, Y., Brawer-Ostrovsky, J. and Insler, V. (1985) Fetal heart tracings in fetuses with congenital malformations. *Journal of Reproductive Medicine,* 30, 43–7.

Bleck, E.E. (1987) *Orthopaedic Management in Cerebral Palsy. Clinics in Developmental Medicine* 99/100, SIMP with Blackwell Scientific, London.

Bobath, B. and Bobath, K. (1975) *Motor Development in Different Types of Cerebral Palsy,* Heinemann Medical, London.

Bobath, K. and Bobath, B. (1984) The neuro-developmental treatment, in Scrutton D. (Ed) *Management of the Motor Disorders of Children with Cerebral Palsy. Clinics in Developmental Medicine,* 90, SIMP with Blackwell Scientific, London.

Bower, E. (1993), Physiotherapy for cerebral palsy – a historical review. In Ward CD (Ed) Rehabilitation of Motor Disorders. *Balliere's Clinical Neurology,* 3, 29–55.

Bower, E. and McLellan, D.L. (1992) Effect of increased exposure to physiotherapy on skill acquisition in children with cerebral palsy. *Developmental Medicine and Child Neurology,* 34, 25–39.

Bower, E. and McLellan, D.L. (1994) Assessing motor skill acquisition in 4 centres for the treatment of children with cerebral palsy. *Developmental Medicine and Child Neurology,* 36, 902–9.

Cantrell, E.G. and Dawson, J. (1983) Young disabled in the community, in *Pressure Sores* (eds J. Barbenel, C.D. Forbes and G.D.O. Lowe), Macmillan, London, pp. 103–114.

Cantrell, E.G., Dawson, J. and Glastonbury, G. (1985) *Prisoners of Handicap*, RADAR, London.

Cogher, L., Savage, E. and Smith, M. (1992) *Cerebral Palsy in the Child and Young Person*, London, Chapman and Hall Medical.

Cottom, P.J. and Sutton, A. (1986) *Conductive Education. A system for overcoming motor disorder*, Croom Helm, London.

Doman, R., Spitz, E., Zuckman, E., Delcato, C. and Doman, G. (1960) Children with severe brain injuries, results of treatment. *Journal of the Americal Medical Association*, **174**, 247–62.

Fay, T. (1948) The neurophysiological effects of therapy in cerebral palsy. *Archives of Physical Medicine and Rehabilitation*, **29**, 327–34.

Fulford, G.E. and Brown, J.K. (1976) Position as a cause of deformity in children with cerebral palsy. *Developmental Medicine and Child Neurology*, **18**, 305–14.

Gage, J. (1991) *Gait analysis in cerebral palsy. Clinics in Developmental Medicine*. MacKeith Press Blackwell Scientific, Oxford, pp. 13–14.

Gillberg, C. (1992) Developmental and neuropsychiatric disorders of childhood, in *Diseases of the Nervous System in Childhood. Clinics in Developmental Medicine* (ed. J. Aicardi), Mackeith Press Blackwell Scientific, Oxford, pp. 1357–1363.

Goldkamp, O. (1984) Treatment effectiveness in cerebral palsy. *Archives of Physical Medicine and Rehabilitation*, **65**, 232–4.

Grethar, J.K., Cummins, S.K. and Nelson, K.B. (1992) The Californian Cerebral Palsy Project. *Pediatric and Perinatal Epidemiology*, **6**, 339–51.

Hagberg, B. (1979) Epidemiological and preventative aspects of cerebral palsy and severe mental retardation in Sweden. *European Journal of Pediatrics*, **130**, 71–8.

Hagberg, B., Edehol-Tysk, K. and Edestrom, B. (1988) The basic care needs of profoundly mentally retarded children with multiple handicaps. *Developmental Medicine and Child Neurology*, **30**, 287–93.

Hari, M. and Tillemans, T. (1984) Conductive education, in *Management of the Motor Disorders of Children with Cerebral Palsy*, vol. 2 (ed. D. Scrutton), SIMP with Blackwell Scientific, Oxford, pp. 19–36.

Hoffer, M.M., Fiewell, E., Perry, R., Perry, J. and Bonnett, C. (1973) Functional ambulation in patients with myelomeningocele. *Journal of Bone and Joint Surgery*, **55A**, 137–48.

Holm, V. (1982) The causes of cerebral palsy: a contemporary perspective. *Journal of American Medical Association*, **247**, 1473– 7.

Hubel, D.H. and Weisel, T.N. (1970) The period of susceptibility to the physiological effects of unilateral eye closure in kittens. *London Journal of Physiology*, **206**, 418–36.

Illingworth, R.S. (1966) *The Development of the Infant and Young Child. Normal and abnormal*, 3rd edn, Livingstone, Edinburgh.

Ingram, T.T.S., Jameson, S., Errington, J. and Mitchell, R.G. (1964) Living with cerebral palsy, in *Clinics in Developmental Medicine*, 14, The Spastics Society Medical Education and Information Unit with Heinemann Medical, London.

Jesien, G. (1984) Home-based early intervention: a description of the Portage Model, in *Management of the Motor Disorders of Children with Cerebral Palsy. Clinics in Developmental Medicine*, vol. 3 (ed. D. Scrutton), 90 SIMP with Blackwell Scientific, London. pp. 36–49.

Jones, R.B. (1975) The Vojta method of treatment of cerebral palsy. *Physiotherapy*, **61**, 112–13.

Kudrjavcev, A., Schoeberg, B., Kurland, L.T. and Groover, R.U. (1983) Cerebral palsy – trends in incidence and changes in concurrent neonatal mortality. Rochester MN 1950–1976. *Neurology*, **33**, 1433–8.

Lieber, R.L. (1986) Skeletal muscle adaptability, I: Review of basic properties. *Developmental Medicine and Child Neurology*, **28**, 390–7.

Lorenz, K. (1970) *Studies in Animal and Human Behaviour*, vol I, Harvard University Press, Cambridge, MA.

Mayston, M. (1992) The Bobath Concept. Evolution and application, in *Movement Disorders in Children. Medicine and Sports Science*, vol. 36 (eds H. Forssberg and H. Hirschfeld). Karger, Basel, pp. 1–66.

McGraw, M. (1989) *The Neuromuscular Maturation of the Human Infant. Clinics in Developmental Medicine*. Blackwell Scientific Mackeith Press, pp. 9–13.

Minear, W.I. (1956) A classification of cerebral palsy. *Paediatrics*, **18**, 841.

Mutch, L., Alberman, E., Hagberg, B., Kodama, K. and Perat, M.V. (1992) Cerebral palsy epidemiology: where are we now and where are we going? *Developmental Medicine and Child Neurology*, **34**, 547–51.

Nelson, K.B. and Ellenberg, J.H. (1981) Apgar scores as predictors of chronic neurological disability. *Pediatrics*, **68**, 36–44.

Nelson, K.B. and Ellenberg, J.H. (1982) Children who outgrew cerebral palsy. *Pediatrics*, **69**, 529–36.

Nelson, K.B. and Ellenberg, J.H. (1986) Antecedents of cerebral palsy: I univariate analysis of risks. *New England Journal of Medicine*, **315**, 81–6.

O'Reilly, E.D. (1975) Care of the cerebral palsied: outcomes of the past and needs for the future. *Developmental Medicine and Child Neurology*, **17**, 141–9.

Pape, K. and Wigglesworth, J.S. (1979) Hemorrhage ischaemia and the perinatal brain, in *Clinics in Developmental Medicine*, SIMP with William Heinemann Medical Books, London, pp. 69–70.

Phelps, W.M. (1990) Cerebral birth injuries; their orthopaedic classification and subsequent treatment. *Clinical Orthopaedics and Related Research*, **253**, 4–12.

Rang, M. (1982) *The Easter Seal Guide to Children's Orthopaedics*, The Easter Seal Society, Ontario.

Shearer, M.S. and Shearer, D. (1972) The portage Project: a model for early education. *Exceptional Children*, **39**, 210–17.

Sheridan, M.D. (1973) *From Birth to Give Years Children's Developmental Progress*, Nfer-Nelson, Windsor, Berks, UK.

Tabery, J.C., Tardieu, C., Tardieu, G. and Tabery, C. (1981) Experimental rapid sarcomere loss with concomitant hypo-extensibility. *Muscle and Nerve*, **4**, 198–203.

Thomas, A.P., Bax, M.C.O. and Smyth, D.P.L. (1989) *The Health and Social Needs of Young Adults with Physical Disabilities*, MacKeith Press, Blackwell Scientific, Oxford.

Vojta, V. (1984) The basic elements of treatment according to Vojte, in *Management of the Motor Disorders of Children with Cerebral Palsy. Clinics in Developmental Medicine*, 90, vol. 6 (ed. D. Scrutton), SIMP with Blackwell Scientific London, pp. 75–86.

Weed, L. (1969) *Medical Records, Medication Education and Patient Care*, Case Western Reserve University.

Wright, J. and Rang, M. (1990) The spastic mouse, and the search for an animal model of spasticity in human beings. *Clinical Orthopaedics*, **253**, 12–19.

USEFUL ADDRESSES

The Help for Health Trust, Health Information Service, FREEPOST, Winchester SO22 53R. Tel: 0800 665544.

24 Epilepsy

P. Crawford and A.M. Stewart

INTRODUCTION

'Living with epilepsy', he said, 'is like playing Hamlet standing on a trap door which can open suddenly at any moment. When it does, you fall into a black hole, only to come round after a few minutes with your face smashed in and your pants wet. But unlike the theatre, this audience has seen everything. Sometimes they laugh; others are embarrassed; most, I guess, feel pretty helpless.' He looked up and smiled. 'You say that I won't have another fit if I take these tablets, but you can never be sure. I hate that bit of me that you call "epilepsy".'

Epilepsy is one of the commonest neurological diagnoses with a lifetime prevalence of 2% and an incidence of 0.6/1000. The peak ages of onset are in childhood (20/100 000) and old age (80/100 000).

Epilepsy is defined as the tendency to recurrent seizures, excluding febrile convulsions. A single seizure is not considered as 'epilepsy', but as recent studies have suggested that up to 75% of people go on to have a second seizure this definition may have to be reconsidered. A seizure results from a paroxysmal abnormal synchronous electrical discharge in the brain. It is not a 'diagnosis' itself, but is an endpoint of many diverse neurochemical, neuropathological and neurophysiological abnormalities.

Epilepsy is a clinical diagnosis based on an eyewitness description of an episode. About 10% of people given a diagnosis of 'epilepsy' do not have the disorder. One of the commonest causes of misdiagnosis is reflex anoxic seizures. These occur when someone feels faint and is kept upright, a few muscle jerks occur and a diagnosis of an 'epileptic' seizure is made. As epilepsy has such serious consequences with regards to driving, employment and schooling, it is a diagnosis which should not be made lightly. If there is doubt, it is better to await clear evidence. An electroencephalogram (EEG) does not **make** the diagnosis of epilepsy as many trivial abnormalities are often overinterpreted. An EEG helps **classify** the kind of epilepsy; localization related or generalized.

CLASSIFICATION

The International League Against Epilepsy has produced a classification of seizures, epilepsies and epileptic syndromes but it is complicated to use. Epilepsy is broadly divided into two group: the generalized epilepsies where abnormal electrical activity arises over the hemispheres synchronously (usually 3-Hz spike wave) and is often genetic in aetiology, and the partial epilepsies where the abnormal electrical activity arises in one area in the brain and spreads. It is important to differentiate between the two types, as in the primary generalized epilepsies the prog-

Rehabilitation of the Physically Disabled Adult. Edited by C. John Goodwill, M. Anne Chamberlain and Chris Evans. Published in 1997 by Stanley Thornes (Publishers) Ltd, Cheltenham. ISBN 0-7487-3183-0.

nosis is usually excellent, the syndromes have an age-specific onset, and respond best to therapy with sodium valproate and possibly lamotrigine. People with primary generalized epilepsies do not need computerized tomography (CT) or magnetic resonance imaging (MRT) scans as the syndromes are genetic in aetiology and many cease by adult life. A variety of seizure types are seen in association with the characteristic EEG abnormality.

Absence seizures begin in childhood between the ages of 5 and 8 and usually cease by adult life. They consist of a stare, often with fluttering of the eyelids and occasionally followed by short-lived automatisms.

Tonic-clonic seizures may occur as part of the childhood absence syndrome or other primary generalized syndromes.

Juvenile myoclonic epilepsy begins in adolescence and is characterized by tonic-clonic seizures and myoclonic jerks on awakening. The diagnosis of often missed, as leading questions are needed to elicit the history of myoclonic jerks. This is a very important syndrome to identify as the prognosis is excellent. The majority become seizure free with sodium valproate therapy, but over 95% relapse if treatment is stopped. These are the rare group of people with epilepsy that need treatment for life. A related syndrome is that of **tonic-clonic seizures on awakening**.

Symptomatic generalized epilepsy occurs in people who have a syndrome with brain damage from many different aetiologies together with epilepsy. A variety of seizures types occur including absence, atypical absence, myoclonic jerks, atonic and tonic attacks and tonic-clonic seizures. The EEG shows generalized spike wave activity but not at the classical 3-Hz spike wave of primary generalized epilepsy. Symptomatic generalized epilepsy comprises a variety of syndromes such as West's syndrome (infantile spasms) and the Lennox – Gastaut syndrome. It is often very difficult to treat and seems to respond best to drugs such as sodium valproate, lamotrigine and benzodiazepines. Vigabatrin has been recently shown to be useful in the treatment of infantile spasms.

As the **partial epilepsies (localization related)** arise in one area of the brain, the symptomology is related to the area of onset and the extent of spread. **Simple partial seizures** occur when consciousness is retained, for example the feelings of *déjà* or *jamais vu*, rising sensations, macropsia, abnormal smells or tastes. A **complex partial seizure** occurs if the seizure activity spreads further and consciousness is lost. If the seizure activity then spreads to the other hemisphere, a **secondary generalized tonic-clonic seizure** results.

An EEG during an episode will show the abnormal activity arising in one area of the brain. Interictal focal EEG changes may be present. Those in this group need investigation of the cause of their seizure disorder, preferably with a MRI scan. The prognosis is much poorer compared to the primary generalized epilepsies, only about 50% will enter a seizure-free remission. All anti-epileptic drugs are equally effective (or ineffective!). People with a focal onset to their seizures form the majority of so-called 'drug-resistant' patients.

AETIOLOGY

Primary generalized epilepsy is likely to be genetic in aetiology and disorders such as childhood absence seizures are probably inherited as an autosomal dominant with incomplete penetrance. As yet, the genes responsible have not been identified.

Since the advent of MRI, it has been realized that, with appropriate scanning techniques, the majority of people with partial seizures have an abnormality identified to account for their seizure disorder, such as mesial temporal sclerosis or neuronal migrational abnormalities.

Epilepsy occurs in 25% of people with

learning difficulties. The incidence is related to the severity of the handicap and the aetiological reason, for instance epilepsy, is very common in people with tuberous sclerosis. About a third of people with cerebral palsy have epilepsy. The incidence of epilepsy is higher in relatives of those with cerebral palsy and epilepsy than in the general population. There is a reduced risk of epilepsy in the relatives of those who only have cerebral palsy, showing that even after cerebral insults, genetic factors are important.

Risk factors for the development of epilepsy after severe head injury include intracranial blood clot, depressed skull fracture, severity of the injury and operative intervention. Cerebral tumours are a relatively rare cause of epilepsy. The incidence of epilepsy in the elderly now exceeds that of childhood. This is predominantly secondary to cerebrovascular and other neurodegenerative diseases.

INVESTIGATIONS

These are usually undertaken to see if there are any reasons for the development of the seizure disorder. An EEG is used to classify the seizure disorder. If it shows generalized spike wave (3 Hz) and the diagnosis of a primary generalized epilepsy is made, further investigations are not indicated.

If seizures are focal in origin, an MRI scan is the most sensitive investigation to look for underlying pathological changes, although this is not at present universally available. A CT scan will exclude any major underlying pathology, but a small low grade glioma may be missed. A change in seizure frequency or the development of neurological signs is an indication for re-scanning. Other investigations, for example basic haematology, biochemistry and an ECG, are usually performed. In elderly patients a 24-hour ECG may be indicated if cardiac arrhythmias are suspected.

TREATMENT

The aim of treatment is to suppress seizures totally with the lowest possible dose of one anti-epileptic drug. This can be achieved in about 70% of people developing epilepsy. The choice of drug is dependent on the type of seizure disorder, the use of the oral contraceptive pill or the desire to become pregnant.

In primary and symptomatic generalized epilepsy the treatment of choice is sodium valproate, unless there are absence seizures only when ethosuximide is a useful alternative. Recent studies suggest that lamotrigine is also of value.

In those with localization-related epilepsy, all the first line drugs are equally effective, they just differ in side-effects. It is therefore advisable to choose a drug with a low side-effect profile such as carbamazepine or sodium valproate. Barbiturates (phenobarbitone, mysoline) have no place in today's treatment of epilepsy. Phenytoin, although an effective drug, is difficult to use because of interactions and a saturable metabolism and therefore should be reserved for people with drug-resistant epilepsy. Lamotrigine and gabapentin, two recently introduced anti-epileptic drugs, may in the future be used as first line therapy as they both appear to have low side-effect profiles. Currently gabapentin is licensed as add-on medication in therapy-resistant patients while lamotrigine has a new patient licence. None of the anti-epileptic drugs, apart from gabapentin, need to be given more frequently than twice daily.

First line anti-epileptic drugs

Carbamazepine is one of the first line drugs for the treatment of partial seizures. It is an hepatic microsomal enzyme inducer and therefore speeds up the metabolism of other anti-epileptic drugs such as phenytoin, phenobarbitone and lamotrigine as well as inducing its own metabolism. Its main side-effect is a rash which occurs in about 10% of people. In high dosages double vision and drowsiness may occur. If this occurs after a dosage increase, it is worth waiting a week to see if symptoms resolves as induction occurs and blood levels fall. Maximum tolerated mono-therapy dosages tend to be between 800 and 1200 mg/day. If dose-related side-effects are a problem then a change to carbamazepine retard can be helpful.

Carbamazepine induces the metabolism of the oral contraceptive pill so a higher dose pill (50 μg or more of oestradiol) needs to be given. Women also need to be warned that it might not be 100% effective as contraception. Carbamazepine is at present the recom-mended anti-epileptic drug for partial sei-zures during pregnancy and a recent overview suggests that there may be slightly less risk compared to the other first line drugs. Pregnant women who receive carba-mazepine should have ultrasound screening for spina bifida and other malformations such as congenital heart disease, cleft lip, etc.

Sodium valproate is the treatment of choice for the generalized epilepsies and the other first line drug for localization-related epilep-sies. A recent American study suggested that sodium valproate was less effective against complex partial seizures than carbamazepine but other studies have failed to confirm these findings. It is the drug of choice for women on the oral contraceptive pill as they can remain on a low dose preparation. Sodium valproate is teratogenic, particularly when combined with other anti-epileptic drugs, as it slows down the metabolism of drugs such as phenytoin and carbamazepine leading to an increase in intermediary metabolites which are teratogenic. Therefore sodium valproate should only be used as monotherapy in women wishing to become pregnant and the fetus screened for spina bifida.

The main side-effects of sodium valproate are weight gain, tremor and hair loss at higher doses. The weight gain can be a problem in young women and is due to stimulation of the appetite.

Phenytoin is a difficult drug to use as it has a saturable metabolism. Small changes in dosage or interactions with other drugs can precipitate toxicity such as ataxia or an increase in seizures. The main problems encountered in clinical practice are the cos-metic side-effects such as hirsutism, acne, gum hyperplasia and coarsening of the facial features.

Phenobarbitone and mysoline have no place in today's management of epilepsy because of the high degree of sedation encountered.

Newer anti-epileptic drugs

Vigabatrin is an irreversible GABA-transami-nase inhibitor and is active against complex partial seizures. It is an effective anti-epileptic drug but is usefulness has been limited by a high incidence of psychiatric side-effects, in particular psychosis, anxiety and depression. The starting dose is 500 mg at night, increasing two weekly by 500 mg increments to a maximum of between 2 and 3 g/day.

Lamotrigine is an effective, broad-spec-trum anti-epileptic drug that appears from clinical trials to be active against both partial seizures and the generalized epilepsies. It is difficult drug to use because the dose and dosage schedule differ according to whether it is added to enzyme-inducing drugs or sodium valproate. Its main side-effect is rash, the incidence of which can be reduced by a slow dose titration. Lamotrigine appears to have a low side-effect profile but it can precipitate toxicity of background anti-epi-leptic drugs such as carbamazepine. It may become a first line anti-epileptic drug in the future due to its broad spectrum of action, low side-effect profile, lack of interactions with the oral contraceptive pill and the fact that it does not appear teratogenic in animal models, although pregnancies at the moment are few.

Gabapentin is a new add-on drug and probably the first choice to try in people who have failed to respond to a first line drug because of gabapentin's low side-effect profile and ease of use. It is active against partial seizures. It is taken up by a specific amino acid uptake system in the gut and excreted unchanged in the urine. This means that the dose needs to be reduced in people in renal failure. It does not interact with any of the other anti-epileptic drugs nor with the oral contraceptive pill. There are minor interactions with antacids and cimetidine.

The dosage titration is fast. Gabapentin can be titrated to an initial maintenance dose of 1200 mg over 2 weeks and then increase by 400 mg weekly in non-responders up to a maximum dosage, at present, of 2400 mg/day, although trials of dosages up to 4800 mg/day are currently in progress. With such a fast titration it is easy to identify responders, so if there is no benefit after 1 month's treatment, gabapentin can be withdrawn over the next 6 weeks.

Gabapentin may also become a useful first line drug for partial seizures because of its low side-effect profile, ease of use, it is not teratogenic in animal models and does not interact with the oral contraceptive pill.

Topiramate (Cilag) is the newest of the licensed anti-epileptic drugs. It is a novel anti-epileptic drug which is proving very effective in people with drug-resistant partial seizures. It appears relatively toxic compared to the other new anti-epileptic drugs, the most worrying side-effect being that of 'abnormal thinking' where the person's speech and thought processes appear very slowed. Weight loss and gastrointestinal symptoms can also cause problems.

Clobazam is a useful adjunctive therapy in people with predictable seizures. If used daily, tolerance often develops. People who have seizures which cluster or are predictable, such as perimenstrual seizures or who have preceding symptoms or prolonged auras, can benefit from intermittent therapy with clobazam.

Clonazepam is related to clobazam but has a shorter half-life and a higher side-effect profile, in particular sedation. Its usefulness is limited by the development of tolerance.

Ethosuximide is only of value in absence seizures.

Anti-epileptic drugs being clinically evaluated

Tiagabine (Novo Nordisk) is a GABA re-uptake inhibitor which appears effective in people with complex partial seizure, particularly those who have responded to vigabatrin. At present it appears to have a lower side-effect profile than vigabatrin and may provide a useful alternative.

Remacemide (Fisons) is an NMDA glutamate receptor blocker that is looking promising in clinical studies. Because of its actions on glutamate, it also has neuroprotective actions in animal models of stroke and head injury. It may also have a role in Parkinson's disease and neurodegenerative diseases where excess glutamate release may be involved.

Anti-epileptic drug level monitoring

In the majority of people this is a waste of time and money. People are their own *in vivo* drug assays. If seizure free they are receiving the correct dosage and no alterations are indicated. If seizures continue without side-effects then the dose can be increased. If dose-related side-effects occur, the dosage is too high. There is no bottom limit to the so-called therapeutic range and many people are able to tolerate plasma level in excess of the top. Anti-epileptic drug level are useful in checking compliance, a common reason for treatment failure. They can be of value for drugs such as phenytoin which have difficult kinetics and can be helpful in giving an idea of the scope for dose increments in someone with continuing seizures.

Management of drug-resistant epilepsies

If seizures have failed to respond to a first line anti-epileptic drug, various questions need to be asked.

1. Is this epilepsy?
2. Is this the best anti-epileptic drug for the seizure type?
3. Is it an adequate dosage?
4. Is the person actually taking the drug?

If someone has genuinely failed to respond, alternative therapies need to be considered. If seizures are predictable, intermittent clobazam is a useful adjunctive therapy. If not, another drug needs to be added, and the dosage increased until a response is obtained or side-effects develop. If the second drug is ineffective, then it should be stopped before another therapy is considered. If it is effective, then the first drug needs to be gradually withdrawn, as the aim of treatment is someone seizure free on monotherapy.

CONTRACEPTION

A high dose oral contraceptive pill ($>50\,\mu g$ oestradiol) needs to be given if a women is on an enzyme inducing anti-epileptic drug, such as carbamazepine, phenytoin or topiramate, and women warned that the contraceptive might not be totally effective. If adequate contraception is needed, it is better to choose an anti-epileptic drug that does not alter the metabolism of the pill, such as sodium valproate, gabapentin or lamotrigine.

PREGNANCY

All first line anti-epileptic drugs are teratogenic. The risk factors are:

1. total daily dosage;
2. polytherapy;
3. sodium valproate in combination with other anti-epileptic drugs.

The aim of treating women with epilepsy who wish to become pregnant is to obtain optimal seizure control on low dose monotherapy of the drug most appropriate for their seizure type. Women should consult for preconception counselling to reconsider the need for therapy and, if necessary, their drug therapy changed. Women need to take high dose folate supplements before and in the early stages of pregnancy. In the future, women may be advised to change therapy to either gabapentin or lamotrigine as they do not appear to be teratogenic in animal models but at the moment data relating to pregnancies is insufficient. The new drug topiramate is teratogenic in animal studies.

Anti-epileptic drug dosages may need increasing in response to an alteration in seizure pattern during pregnancy because of changes in metabolism, fluid distribution, etc. This will need reducing in the puerperium back to prepregnancy levels.

NEUROSURGERY

Neurosurgical treatment may be of benefit in people, particularly those whose seizures originate in the temporal lobes. The work-up involves neuropsychological assessments, monitoring EEG activity during at least one seizure, MRI, and the Wada test to localize speech centres and sometimes depth electrode recordings to localize the epileptic focus. In carefully selected patients up to 70% will become seizure free after temporal lobe surgery, particularly younger people of normal intelligence and who have mesial temporal sclerosis after prolonged febrile convulsions. Other surgical techniques include callosotomy and subpial resections or hemispherectomy.

SOCIAL MANAGEMENT/ REHABILITATION

Acquiring a physical disability, for whatever reason, will have an immediate impact on day-to-day living for both the individual and their family. A diagnosis of epilepsy compounds these effects. Both legislation and regulations limit people with epilepsy in the areas of employment, leisure activities and civil and criminal law. These difficulties will occur whatever the severity or origins of the epilepsy.

To enable individuals to re-take their place as actively as possible in the community it is important to provide them with the opportunity to learn more about the condition. Counselling in this particular kind of situation should include factual information as well as a listening ear.

EMPLOYMENT

There are a number of occupations which are prohibited if a patient has a diagnosis of epilepsy and there are others where the individual will initially be suspended. This suspension may be temporary or permanent. Therefore, it is imperative that the diagnosis of epilepsy is accurate. Details of the prohibited occupations can be obtained from the epilepsy associations. In addition to those jobs which are precluded, there are others where the type and severity of the seizure pattern can result in rejection. Working at heights, in exposed areas, near water or with fragile objects may be difficult. For those whose seizures occur only during sleep there should not be any risk factor. But who is going to appraise a prospective employer of this fact unless the person with epilepsy does?

SOCIAL LIFE AND LEISURE

In 1990 a survey of nearly 2000 people with epilepsy indicated that their social lives and leisure activities were their second highest problem area. Of the 1958 respondents, 71.1% reported some problems or serious problems with this aspect of their lives. Difficulties in forming relationships – a well-documented outcome of a diagnosis of epilepsy – may be prevented by enabling people with the condition to take calculated risks; to support the building of self-esteem by not over-protecting them; and also provide education about the condition thereby eliminating fear based on

ignorance. There is a known lower frequency of marriages amongst people with epilepsy which is related to the age at which epilepsy develops. Young men developing epilepsy under the age of 19 years are also more likely than women of that age group not to marry if they have epilepsy.

Discrimination within leisure activities prevents people with epilepsy from developing and retaining independence and integration. Team and individual sports events provide opportunities to feel comfortable with one's peers and grow in confidence amongst them. Swimming, riding, cycling and climbing are some of the activities people with epilepsy are often excluded from. These can however be enjoyed if some practical commonsense supervision is offered.

DRIVING

Prior to 1972 people who had been diagnosed as having epilepsy were not legally entitled to drive. Since then laws about driving after a diagnosis of epilepsy have been materially changed. Driving has become a feature of most people's lives, whether as a means of getting to work, part of a job or for leisure. With the reduction of the public transport system and more people opting to live outside of the cities, the driving licence has steadily gained importance with regard to employment.

In August 1994, changes were made so that people who have been free of seizures for 12 months or more may apply for a provisional licence or re-apply for their 'lost' licence. For those who continue to experience their seizures only during sleep, they may drive if that pattern of attacks has been established for 3 or more years. The law makes no distinction between the different causes or types of epileptic seizure nor between their infinite variations of severity, frequency or precipitating factors (*Medical Aspects of Fitness to Drive*, 1995).

Being physically disabled and having the additional disability of epilepsy will be an even greater blow to self-esteem when mobility is also threatened. The freedom to get from one place to another independently may well rely upon the ability to drive. The restriction of this accepted liberty can be a severe disadvantage.

Obtaining driving insurance, once a licence is restored, will almost certainly be a further limitation to mobility. There are some insurance companies who view each application individually. Details of these companies can be obtained from the epilepsy associations.

THE CRIMINAL LAW

This continues to view people with epilepsy as having a 'disease of the mind' despite the medical profession having determined that this is not so. In July 1991 interested organizations joined together to encourage the Government to review the sentencing procedure for someone who had committed a criminal act during an epileptic seizure there being no 'guilty intent'. The joining together was successful and the previous automatic committal to a psychiatric hospital, although still retained, became one of a number of alternative methods of disposal at the hearing of such cases.

SUMMARY

Good medical care and management by a consultant with an in-depth knowledge of epilepsy will be the quickest route to rehabilitation. Epilepsy has been written about for well over 2000 years; however, there are still medical personnel whose knowledge of the complexities of epilepsy is incomplete. Living with the condition, in the knowledge that you are being treated by someone who has both the expertise and the support of a multidisciplinary team, is essential to being rehabilitated in the fullest sense of the word.

REFERENCES

Medical Aspects of Fitness to Drive (1995) Medical Commission on Accident Prevention, London.

FURTHER READING

Chadwick, D., Orme, Appleton, Baker and Roagan (1991) *The Management of Epilepsy in General Practice*, Roby Education, Liverpool.

Crawford, P.M. (1993) Epilepsy and pregnancy, *Seizure*, **2**, 87–90.

Epilepsy and Getting a Job (1995) British Epilepsy Association, Leeds.

Epilepsy and pregnancy (1994) *Drug and Therapeutics Bulletin*, **32**, (7), 49–51.

Frequency of Problems Survey. 'Charter for Epilepsy 1990' (1990) British Epilepsy Association, Leeds.

Hopkins, A., Shorvon, S. and Cascino, G. (eds) (1995) *Epilepsy*, 2nd edn, Chapman & Hall, London.

ADDRESS OF VOLUNTARY BODIES

British Epilepsy Association
35–43 Lincoln's Inn Fields, London, WC2A 3PN Tel: 0113 243 9393; Help-line 0800 309030. The Old Postgraduate Medical Centre, Belfast City Hospital, Lisburn Road, Belfast, BT9 7AB, UK. Tel: 01232 248414.

The National Society for Epilepsy
Chalfont Centre, Chalfont St Peter, Bucks SL9 ORJ, UK. Tel: 01494 873991.

The Epilepsy Association of Scotland
48 Govan Road, Glasgow, G51 1JL, UK. Tel: 0141 427 4911.

The Irish Epilepsy Association
Brain Wave, 249 Crumlin Road, Crumlin, Dublin 12, UK. Tel: 01 557500.

USEFUL ADDRESSES

British Sports Association for the Diabled
Solecast House, 13/27 Brunswick Place, London N1 6DX, UK. Tel: 0171 490 4919.

Disabled Drivers' Motor Club
Cottingham Way, Thrapston, Northampton NN14 4PL, UK. Tel: 01832 734724.

Disabled Living Foundation
380/384 Harrow Road, London W9 2HU, UK. Tel: 0171 289 6111.

Queen Elizabeth's Foundation for the Disabled
Leatherhead, Surrey, KT 22 OBN, UK. Tel: 01372 8422204.

Riding for the Disabled
Aveunue R, National Agriculture Centre, Kenilworth, Warwickshire CV8, 2LY, UK. Tel: 01203 696510.

Appendix

RESTRICTED EMPLOYMENT AND STATUTORY BARRIERS

AIRCRAFT PILOT: applicants shall have no established medical history or clinical diagnosis of epilepsy. (Manual of Civil Aviation Medicine.)

AMBULANCE DRIVER: applicants shall have been free from any epileptic seizures and off anti-epileptic medication for 10 years or more. They must pass a medical examination. (PCV Regulations.)

ARMY: applicants rejected on the grounds of epilepsy. (Army Act 1955 – reviewed regularly.)

COAST GUARD: there are no specific epilepsy regulations but applicants require 'a high standard of fitness' and have to pass a medical.

DIVER: any history of seizures (apart from febrile convulsions) will preclude granting of a Certificate of Fitness to dive. ((Diving Operations at Work Regulations 1981) (S1 1981/399).)

FIRE BRIGADE: a history of epilepsy renders a person unsuitable for operational fire duties. (Fire Service Act 1947.) Those who have been free of seizures since age of 5 any be considered individually.

MERCHANT SEAFARER: absolute barrier for applicants with a history of seizures since age of 5. (DOT Merchant Shipping Regulations 1983.)

NAVY: medical regulations state that any seizures at any age debar entry.

POLICE: applicants currently having seizures not recruited. Those with a past history dealt with on an individual basis. Also applies to traffic wardens and drivers. (Police Regulations 1979.)

PRISON SERVICE: recent history debars applicant on the grounds of security for posts at Prison Officer Grade. Applicants to other grades of prison service considered individually.

ROYAL AIR FORCE: proven epilepsy with few exceptions is a ban to recruitment. (Air Force Acts 1955 and others.)

TEACHER: applicants for teacher training should have been seizure free from seizures for 2 years at the time of applying. (Physical and Mental Fitness to Teach of Teachers and of Entrants to Initial Teacher Training – Circular number 13/93 Department of Education.)

TRAIN DRIVER: absolute barrier if seizures have occurred after the age of 5 years. (London Regional Transport and British Rail.)

25 Motor neurone disease

R. Langton Hewer

INTRODUCTION

Motor neurone disease (MND) is one of those conditions which we all hope we shall never develop ourselves. It involves progressive weakness of the limb and bulbar muscles. The cause of the disorder is unknown and no treatment is yet available to halt its progress. The majority of patients die within 3 years of onset. That said, because of some of the variants, it is often not possible to predict outcome for an individual accurately.

A number of well-known people have suffered with MND so the disorder is better known that it was previously. In addition, there is much current research in progress and a number of drugs are being evaluated. One, Riluzole, has recently been released for use in the United Kingdom. Despite our therapeutic impotence, much can be done to reduce the distressing effects of the disorder. Informed and compassionate management can undoubtedly ease the distress and discomfort of patients and their relatives. The object of this chapter is to show how this may be achieved.

WHAT IS MOTOR NEURONE DISEASE?

In MND degeneration occurs in the motor neurones, i.e. those that control certain specific components of muscle movement. The vast majority of the remaining portions of the nervous system remain normal.

There are two main groups of motor neurones. The first group originates in the cells of the motor and pre-motor cortex and travels through the brain to terminate either in the brainstem or in the spinal cord, in close relation to the bulbar nuclei or the anterior horn cells. The second group have their origin in the brainstem or in the spinal cord and terminate on the muscle fibres. Thus four main structures are involved in MND:

1. **The anterior horns of the spinal cord.** Degeneration of these cells results in wasting and weakness of muscles. The term **progressive muscular atrophy (PMA)** is applied when muscle wasting and weakness predominate.

2. **The corticospinal tracts.** These tracts lie in the lateral columns of the spinal cord and contain the long nerve fibres which originate in the motor and pre-motor cortex of the brain. Involvement of this structure produces **upper motor neurone** signs in the limbs – weakness, spasticity and extensor plantar responses. The term **amyotrophic lateral sclerosis (ALS)** is applied when these upper motor neurone signs predominate. In practice **there is usually a combination of upper and lower motor neurone signs** (i.e. muscle wasting with exaggerated tendon reflexes and **spasticity**).

Rehabilitation of the Physically Disabled Adult. Edited by C. John Goodwill, M. Anne Chamberlain and Chris Evans. Published in 1997 by Stanley Thornes (Publishers) Ltd, Cheltenham. ISBN 0-7487-3183-0.

3. **The nuclei of the nerves to the bulbar muscles.** These nuclei are the counterparts of the anterior horn cells discussed above. For example, there may be degeneration of cells in the hypoglossal nuclei (situated in the medulla) producing wasting of the tongue. The term **bulbar palsy** is applied when wasting of bulbar muscles occurs.

4. **The corticobulbar fibres.** These fibres (counterparts of the corticospinal fibres discussed above) contain the nerve fibres of cells which originate in the motor and pre-motor cortex. Involvement occurs in the brainstem territory; for example, a spastic tongue which cannot be protruded, and an exaggerated jaw and facial jerk.

When upper motor neurone signs predominate, the term pseudobulbar palsy is applied. In practice there are usually signs of both upper and lower motor neurone involvement (e.g. a wasted but spastic tongue).

The fibres in the spinal cord subserving sensation are not usually involved. Precisely why such specific areas of the central nervous system are affected in motor neurone disease is not known. Vision, hearing, intellectual function and sphincter function usually remain intact.

The disorder is characterized clinically by progressive wasting of muscles combined with evidence of upper motor neurone abnormality. It is common to observe brisk tendon reflexes in a spinal segment which also includes wasted muscles.

HOW MANY CASES?

The disorder is usually sporadic, but in about 5% of cases it appears to be familial – with an autosomal dominant mode of inheritance. The annual incidence rate is 1–2 persons per 100 000 and the prevalence is about 6 per 100 000. Most patients are aged between 50 and 70.

EARLY SYMPTOMS

The early clinical features vary considerably, depending upon which structures in the central nervous system are affected. Common early symptoms include the following:

1. Wasting and weakness of a hand. This may produce difficulty in writing and doing up buttons.

2. A foot-drop due to weakness of dorsiflexion of one foot.

3. Weakness of the proximal limb muscles, producing difficulty with washing the hair and shaving if the arms are affected, and difficulty with mounting stairs if the legs are involved. In many instances there is spontaneous twitching of muscles (fasciculation).

4. If upper motor neurone signs predominate there may be a complaint of stiffness in the legs and inability to walk fast.

5. In about 20% of cases the first symptoms involve the bulbar muscles causing slurred speech and choking with fluids.

DIAGNOSIS

The diagnosis is made largely on clinical grounds, i.e. after carefully taking a history and examining the patient. In general, diagnosing MND is easy for a neurologist to make in about 80% of cases. In 10% there are some difficulties and in a further 10% the diagnosis may be almost impossible to make.

The diagnosis of motor neurone disease should depend on the presence of upper and lower motor neurone involvement in a single spinal segment. In addition, there is usually motor involvement of at least two limbs or one limb and the bulbar muscles. Sensory dysfunction must be absent. Conditions causing confusion may include cervical spondylotic myelopathy and syringomyelia. However, sensory loss is usual in these conditions and it can be clarified by MRI scan. If muscle wasting predominates a large number of conditions need to be considered, including diabetic amyotrophy and various types of motor peripheral neuropathy. Primary muscle disease rarely causes major confusion.

The postpolio syndrome does not cause upper motor neurone dysfunction. The differential diagnosis of progressive bulbar palsy includes myaesthenia gravis and vascular lesions involving the brainstem.

Some patients with slowly progressive neuropathies have been previously diagnosed as suffering from motor neurone disease. Motor nerve conduction studies may show multifocal motor conduction block, prolonged or absent F-waves, prolonged distal latencies and reduced motor nerve conduction velocities. Serum antibodies to GM-1 gangliosides are present in over 80% of cases, and it is a treatable condition.

PROGNOSIS

No treatment has been shown to alter the course of the disease. The majority of patients die within 3 years, but up to 30% may survive 5 years or even more. The prognosis is particularly bad in patients who show dysphagia and choking at an early stage.

WHAT SHOULD THE PATIENT BE TOLD?

The question arises as to what the patient should be told (Carey, 1986). Current practice usually involves telling the patient and their spouse the diagnosis as soon as this is reasonably certain. However, the certainty with which the diagnosis can be made will influence what and when the patient is told. There is a great deal to be said for obtaining a second opinion in most cases.

Giving bad news is difficult and it is not always done well. Often, as with telling people that they have cancer, once the diagnosis has been named then all the rest of the interview becomes a poorly remem-

bered nightmare. In general it should be given to the patient with their spouse or prime carer at the same time. If there is no family then another person such as a social worker can help by their presence, so that information can be discussed afterwards. A second interview should be offered, with a suggestion that the patient might care to bring up written notes, so that important issues are not forgotten. A 'hot line' for support should be given, with the name and address of the Motor Neurone Disease Association (MNDA), both nationally and locally.

It is not possible to predict the future in great detail at this early stage, but as time goes on more details can be given. Much sensitivity is required and it is totally unsatisfactory for these delicate matters to be dealt with by inexperienced junior staff. However, it is important that each member of the team should be aware of what has been said. It is worth telling the patient and family that the disease does not affect touch, taste, sight, smell and hearing nor, directly, bladder, bowel or sexual function. Neither is it likely to be transmitted to anyone.

COMMON PROBLEMS

The nature and range of problems experienced by MND patients and their families is very considerable, and much expertise is necessary in handling them.

Mental distress

There is ample evidence that many patients and their relatives experience distress at various stages of the disease. Distress is sometimes related to fruitless consultations and lack of advice about the disease and its course. Some patients have been resentful that they are told half-truths, learning from others because 'the neurologist would not say plainly, and my family doctor was honest enough to say that he did not know' (Carus, 1980). Particular 'crisis' points include the time at which the diagnosis is made, the point at which the patient has to give up work, the time at which a wheelchair has to be introduced, when it is no longer possible to go upstairs and when permanent admission to hospital becomes necessary. There may be worries about dying from suffocation or from gradually worsening respiratory muscle paralysis, or in some other frightening way. Many patients fear the unknown.

Bulbar problems

Dribbling, dysphagia, choking and dysarthria are particularly distressing symptoms. At any one time more than 50% of MND patients will be experiencing some or all of these problems (Newrick and Langton Hewer, 1984). The vast majority will do so eventually. These various problems can be a cause of social isolation due to the patient becoming embarrassed and friends being upset and sometimes frightened. In most instances the problems are due to a combination of both upper and lower motor neurone disturbance.

Salivary dribbling

A normal person produces about 2 litres of saliva per day. This is swallowed automatically. Salivary dribbling is a common problem in patients with MND. There are a number of different causative factors, but there is no definite evidence that volume of saliva is increased. A reduction in the frequency of automatic swallowing is probably a major factor. Dribbling tends to be associated in the public mind with mental disorder. The patient will require constant reassurance about this. Later in the disease he/she may fear that he/she may drown in his/her own saliva, but it seems unlikely that this ever occurs. The detailed management of the problem is discussed below:

1. **Oral candidiasis** (thrush) is common and should be treated.
2. **Head position.** Many patients have weakness of the neck muscles and dribbling may occur when the head falls forward. This problem can frequently be controlled by appropriate posture, including a reclining backrest and/or the provision of a collar (Figure 25.1).
3. **Stimulation of swallowing.** Automatic swallowing can sometimes be stimulated if the patient sucks sweets. Great care must be taken with this technique, especially if there is a tendency for choking to occur.
4. **Lip closure.** Weakness of the lips may make dribbling worse. Attempts to improve this can be made by, for instance, getting the patient to hold a spatula between the lips whilst he/she is otherwise relaxing, for example watching television.
5. **Cosmetic.** The patient's blouse or shirt should not be allowed to become saturated with saliva. A false shirt front or polo-neck which could be changed frequently may be helpful. 'Bibs' can appear degrading.
6. **Medication.** Atropine 0.6 mg three times a day is frequently appropriate. Many of the antidepressant drugs also have an atropine-like action. It should be remembered that pyridostigmine (Mestinon) can increase the amount of saliva.
7. **Suction.** Some patients wake up in the middle of the night with a feeling that they are choking on their own saliva. The provision of a simple portable suction apparatus in this situation can be helpful, but both the patient and carer must be properly instructed in its use.
8. **Surgery.** Various operations have been tried. The most useful operation is bilateral division of the corda tympani via the middle ear. Surgery is not required in the vast majority of cases.

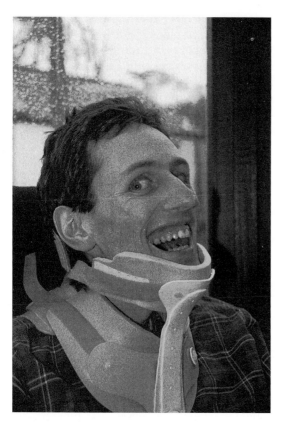

Figure 25.1 Head support in use.

Dysphagia (see also Chapter 22)

Once again several different factors contribute to swallowing problems in MND. These include weakness of the masseter muscles (producing difficulty with chewing), impaired tongue mobility (making it difficult for a bolus to be formed), palatal weakness (resulting in reduced intra-oral pressure) and weakness of the pharyngeal muscles. In addition, there may be spasm of the pharyngeal muscles.

In each case a careful evaluation of the swallowing problem should be undertaken by taking a history and watching the patient eat and drink. In appropriate cases it may be helpful to undertake video-fluoroscopy. The patient's weight will need to be monitored.

The precise advice that is given to the patient will clearly depend on the result of the assessment. In each case the mechanism of swallowing should be explained to the patient, as should an account of what has gone wrong. The patient will need to be seen at regular intervals during the course of the disease as the dysphagia, and attendant problems, may change rapidly. The following specific points need to be emphasized:

1. **Diet.** Solids are often better tolerated than fluid. Foods that crumble should be avoided. Smooth, liquidized food may be required in the later stages. It may be necessary to experiment so that the texture of the most appropriate food can be found for each patient.
2. **Ice.** Spasticity can often be reduced for a few minutes by the local application of ice. The patient can be asked to suck ice cubes for 10 minutes prior to a meal or ice can be applied to the outside of the throat.
3. **Medication.** Some clinicians find that Mestinon can be helpful, but in our experience this drug has been of doubtful use. Baclofen, in a dose of 20–60 mg a day, may reduce spasticity and can be tried. The actual swallowing of drugs needs to be carefully assessed, as some patients have great difficulty with swallowing large tablets or capsules.
4. **Head position.** It is important that the head and neck should be supported if necessary and maintained in a position which will facilitate swallowing. If the head is allowed to fall forwards, then swallowing will probably become more difficult. A collar may be helpful, just as some patients find it helpful to turn the head to one side when swallowing.
5. **Feeding.** It may be necessary to use a nasogastric tube during the later stages of the disease. The narrow-bore tubes are more acceptable than the old-fashioned wide-bore Ryles tube. Indications for a nasogastric tube include frequent

choking, repeated inhalation pneumonia, severe dehydration, severe weight loss and taking an unacceptable time to eat a meal.

In many cases, it may be preferable to establish a gastrostomy. Percutaneous endoscopic gastrostomy (PEG) has now been used for some time as a safe and highly acceptable alternative to nasogastric feeding. The tubes can be inserted under a local anaesthetic and maintained for many months without complication. Many people regard percutaneous endoscopic gastrostomy as a major advance in the management of MND. It needs to be carefully discussed with the patient before undertaking the procedure. Not all patients choose to have one.

6. **Surgery.** A number of different surgical techniques are available, but in our experience surgery is rarely required.

Cricopharyngeal myotomy is only undertaken if there is demonstrable and consistent hold-up of food at the level of the cricopharyngeus muscle. The procedure has a mortality (Loizou *et al.*, 1980) but can bring benefit, not only of improved swallowing but of choking (Leighton *et al.*, 1994). Occasionally pharyngostomy has a place.

Choking

It is necessary to remember that choking and coughing are defence mechanisms which prevent aspiration into the air passages. The symptoms can be very frightening.

Choking can occur in various situations. It most commonly occurs when the patient is drinking or eating. Occasionally it occurs at night if there is pooling of saliva at the back of the throat. This latter problem may be dealt with by the use of a sucker (see above).

Anxiety and panic will make choking worse and therefore calm reassurance is necessary at all times. It is particularly important to avoid ingesting substances that trigger choking, including crumbly food, strong curry, whisky and brandy. If a severe bout of choking occurs the carer should be prepared to apply the 'hug of life'. It should be remembered that choking is probably an uncommon cause of death (Saunders, Summers and Teller, 1981).

Dysarthria

Initially the speech may become slightly slurred, but ultimately many patients become totally unable to articulate. The first symptom is often a weak palate associated with nasal escape. Weakness of the lips may be a further important problem. In this early stage intelligibility may be improved by training and by the supply of a palatal support. Some patients can compensate for the loss of speech by writing. However, many are too weak to write, and for these a communication aid will need to be provided. Recent experience in Bristol indicates that patients require as many as five or six different aids during the course of their illness. With the help of a competent speech therapist, who is familiar with communication aids, most patients can be enabled to communicate with their families up to the time of death (Chapter 22).

Pain

A study (Newrick and Langton Hewer, 1985) has shown that pain may occur in as many as 64% of people with MND. Cramp in the limbs is common. Pain may be experienced in various sites, including the shoulders and back. The cause for this is frequently not obvious. Late in the disease, discomfort at night can be distressing, and can only be relieved by a change in position. It is particularly important that the patient is provided with a well fitting chair. If pain and/or mental distress become severe then opiates should be used. Diamorphine in a dose of 2.5 mg initially is usually acceptable and this dose can be gradually increased (it may need to be administered via a syringe driver). Cramp may be helped by the use of quinine (in an initial dose of 300 mg at night).

Poor sleeping (Table 25.1)

Poor sleeping may itself result in depression and feelings of chronic tiredness. These feelings may also be experienced by the spouse, whose sleep is liable to be disturbed, with the resultant risk of breakdown in his/her ability to cope. The management of insomnia requires careful assessment of the causes. The uncritical use of hypnotics should be avoided.

If the problem remains intractable it may be necessary to admit the patient to hospital or to a hospice for a short while in order to give the spouse some respite (see below).

Table 25.1 Factors contributing to poor sleep in motor neurone disease patients

Problem	Management
Inability to change position without help	An electric turning bed or pressure-relieving mattress may be helpful
Pain (see above) and general discomfort	It is important to make sure that the bed is as comfortable as possible. A small dose of diamorphine may be helpful
Depression and anxiety	Counselling, antidepressant drugs
Frequency of micturition	Nocturia is a common symptom in older people. Management includes fluid restriction during the previous evening

Weakness of the arms

Marked weakness of the proximal arm muscles produces difficulty with feeding, combing and washing the hair, and donning vests and shirts. Mobile arm supports, attached to the wheelchair, can help some patients. Clothes may need adapting (e.g. shirts and vests should be front opening).

Weakness of the hand muscles produces difficulty with a multitude of tasks, including writing, doing up buttons, knitting and feeding. A wrist-drop support, the use of wide-handled cutlery and velcro instead of buttons, may be indicated. Communication aids are discussed elsewhere (Chapter 22).

Weakness of the legs

Difficulty with climbing stairs, standing and walking, together with falls (which may lead to fractures), are the principal results of weakness of the leg muscles. Leg oedema is an important secondary effect. The management includes housing modifications (e.g. ensuring easy access to the toilet and to the garden) and the supply of a wheelchair (Chapter 44).

Respiratory insufficiency and breathlessness

Respiratory insufficiency occurs ultimately in most cases. This is frequently, but not always, accompanied by a sensation of breathlessness. Nocturnal breathlessness may be helped by giving the patient several pillows so that he/she sleeps in a semi-recumbent position. Chest infections require treatment. Medication can worsen respiratory insufficiency, particularly large doses of diazepam or morphine.

Some patients require assisted ventilation, particularly at night. In occasional cases a tracheostomy may be performed and artificial ventilation instituted (Norris, Smith and Denys 1985). Distressing breathlessness can be relieved by using diamorphine in a small dose (e.g. 1 mg at a time initially). This should ultimately be given regularly and the dose increased as necessary.

Nasal intermittent positive pressure ventilation, mainly at night, is the most practical form of assisted ventilation. It can be used for patients with relatively mild breathlessness and is usually applied by a nasal mask. Negative pressure ventilation by cuirass is more cumbersome to apply and requires the assistance of a fit carer. Again, it is essential to include the patient and family in all discussions about this procedure; it is easier to start ventilation than to stop it once established.

Constipation

Constipation is a frequent and distressing symptom in many patients. Contributing factors include weakness of the abdominal muscles, difficulty in maintaining a sitting position, decrease in intake of bulky foods and of fluids (in patients with dysphagia) and medication (particularly opiates and anti-cholinergic agents). Effective management involves, as always, making a careful assessment of the problem to find out precisely what has gone wrong. Simple measures include increasing fluid intake with careful use of purgatives. However, in many cases the problem remains intractable. Regular enemas may be required. Faecal impaction is common in the later stages of the disease. Manual evacuation by the spouse should be avoided if possible.

TECHNICAL AIDS AND APPLIANCES

Some of the problems encountered by MND patients can be eased considerably by the supply of effective aids and appliances. The most commonly needed pieces of equipment are listed in Table 25.2. There should be no delay in their provision; indeed, anticipation of needs is essential. The Motor Neurone Disease Association is very helpful in providing loan equipment in the UK. Similar societies are developing worldwide.

ORGANIZATION OF CARE

There has been criticism of the way in which MND is handled (Newrick and Langton Hewer, 1984). The criticisms include lack of interest by doctors, insufficient psychosocial support, and long delays in the supply of equipment such as wheelchairs which may be unsuitable when they do arrive. Patients clearly dislike attending clinics where they are seen by junior doctors who have no specific experience, or training, in the management of the disorder. The pattern is easily seen as being disorganized and uncaring.

SOMEONE 'IN CHARGE'

The management of MND should ideally be coordinated by one person. The general practitioner should clearly be involved, although he is unlikely to have much experience of the disease. An interested consultant, either in neurology or rehabilitation medicine, is also in a position to provide continuity and support, although this frequently does not happen in practice. Hospices or the Macmillan Service can offer much help (Saunders, Summers and Teller, 1981).

Newrick and Langton Hewer (1984) have suggested the concept of a key worker who would work closely with the general practitioner and hospital consultant. No proper evaluation of this suggestion has yet been undertaken. Experience in Bristol has been that a speech therapist, working closely with a hospital consultant, can provide a satisfactory level of support. This arrangement seems particularly appropriate in view of the fact that the most intractable problems involve the bulbar musculature. Such support could probably also be given by a properly trained nurse, social worker or remedial therapist.

Other forms of carer support are available. The MND Association provides quick, effective counselling and support. They also train volunteer visitors and most districts in the UK at least will have a local organization. The

Table 25.2 Aids and appliances used in motor neurone disease

Appliance	Indication	Type
Collar	Significant weakness of the neck muscles. This is particularly liable to occur when the patient is a passenger in a car. Pain in the neck and inability to look up are other indicators	Must be lightweight, washable cosmetically acceptable and comfortable, e.g. an MND collar
Wrist splint	Severe wrist and/or finger-drop with preservation of hand movement	A lightweight cosmetically acceptable splint is needed, e.g. Futuro splint
Mobile arm supports	Severe weakness of arm abductor muscles with some preservation of hand function. Some patients may be enabled to feed independently	The supports are usually attached to a wheelchair
Ankle–foot orthoses (AFO)	The tip of the shoe catches on the ground in walking. This may result in falls, with resultant fracture of long bones	The AFO is of lightweight plastic and is made for the individual
Wheelchair	1. Frequent falls 2. Inability to walk inside the house 3. Inability to walk outside, e.g. to get to the garden, pub or shops	A self-propelled chair is suitable for many people. Later an electric wheelchair may be required. If the patient needs to sit in the chair for long periods a headrest, proper seating and leg supports are essential
Environmental control with suction apparatus	Inability to use switches, e.g. TV control. Dysphagia, choking	See Chapter 49
Armchair, possibly electric	Discomfort in ordinary chair, inability to get out of ordinary chair	The chair should be comfortable, the back should recline, with proper support for the head, back and legs
Communication aid	Inability to speak intelligibly combined with inability to write	A wide variety of aids is available

main MND Association has a helpline and equipment banks. The health service has established a multidisciplinary community approach; similar responses in the forms of specialized support workers and community nurses may be models which should be followed. It is important that these various approaches are evaluated because support is not uniformly good and sound protocols with rapid response need to be universal.

Much research is being undertaken and some of it is promising. It is claimed that some prolongation of life (not as yet of statistical significance) may be achieved by the use of Riluzole which alters glutamate levels in the CNS.

SUGGESTED MODEL OF CARE

Five arbitrary stages may be recognized in the management of MND:

Early

At this point the patient will probably have little, or no, disability.

1. The diagnosis should be made correctly and effectively.
2. The patient should be told the diagnosis in general terms. The spouse should be present at this interview. They should be given as much information as seems appropriate in their particular case. They should be told that proper support will be given throughout the course of the disease, and that the general practitioner, the hospital consultant and their supporting staff will do everything possible to provide support.

    Certain positive aspects of the disease need to be emphasized. Many patients are relieved to know that they have not got multiple sclerosis and that the disorder is not usually familial. It is also worth emphasizing that the majority of patients retain their intellectual faculties until the end, and that vision, hearing and continence are usually preserved.
3. Because of the nature of the disease, it is recommended that a second consultant opinion should usually be sought at this stage. Unnecessary diagnostic doubt should be avoided if at all possible.

Stage of mild disability

At this stage the patient may need advice on employment, driving, and how to cope with work and home duties. The diagnosis will need to be further discussed.

Stage of severe disability

It is at this point that considerable support is needed. It is particularly important that the various groups of workers should liaise closely together, avoiding overlap and underlap. A key worker, if available, becomes particularly important at this stage. **It is absolutely essential that the patient and spouse should be able to get immediate advice and help if a crisis arises.**

Specific needs include the following:

1. Intermittent admission to hospital or hospice. This may be needed in order to give the spouse a regular break or if an emergency occurs (e.g. if the patient develops pneumonia, or if the spouse becomes unwell). As the terminal stages of the disease approach, more frequent admissions to hospital may be required.

    It is particularly important that the ward staff should be properly trained in the management of the bulbar problems itemized above. They should be as expert as the spouse, otherwise the spouse may refuse to allow the patient to go into hospital to receive such care, however much the carer needs a rest. Sometimes other ways of supporting them may be necessary.
2. The effective provision of equipment and the undertaking of housing adaptations.

    Equipment such as walking aids, commodes and wheelchairs should be supplied as soon as possible after the need is demonstrated. It is necessary to anticipate the patient's needs. Whilst it is also important to avoid suggesting equipment which is not yet required (e.g. the premature provision of a wheelchair may upset the patient unnecessarily), delays in supply are unacceptable. Similarly, housing adaptations, for example to provide proper access to the toilet or a stair rail to enable the patient to get upstairs, should be provided quickly. (Pentland, Rainey and MacNeill, 1985)

    A range of equipment may be required including a wheelchair, a proper chair to sit in, a collar, a proper bed and various types of communication aid.
3. Complications should be avoided if possible. If they do occur they must be dealt with efficiently. They include limb fractures, fungal infections of the mouth, pressure sores, severe dependent oedema, uncontrolled pain, contractures and breakdown in the health of the spouse.

Terminal stage

The objective is to help the patient live and to die with dignity, with the minimum of pain and distress. Many patients prefer to remain at home for as long as possible. The policy of gradually increasing the amount of time spent in hospital or hospice has been found to be satisfactory for many patients. Indeed, some patients still regard themselves as 'living at home' even when they only have a single home visit once a fortnight.

The principles of care at this stage have been discussed by Saunders, Summers and Teller (1981), and include unhurried and sympathetic handling by staff, and the use of appropriate analgesic drugs (particularly diamorphine).

After death

A major objective of management is to prevent the relatives from feeling guilty that they have failed to do everything possible. An interview with the one of the senior doctors shortly after the patient's death may be helpful. Additionally, the key worker or social worker may remain in contact with the relatives for a few weeks, or even longer in some cases.

CONCLUSIONS

It will be seen from the above discussion that MND presents a large number of complex problems. The efficient handling of the disease requires considerable knowledge, expertise, patience and sympathy. The present evidence appears to be that many patients with MND could be handled better. Because of the rarity of the disease it is suggested that management should ideally be centred on departments who have proven expertise. However, other organizations may well have an important role to play, and the lead being taken by the hospice movement is helpful and important. It is suggested that there should be a key worker who would work closely with the consultant and medical staff in charge and the general practitioner. Other medical and paramedical staff are also involved and the speech therapist has a particularly important role in managing the distressing problems of dysphagia, choking, dribbling and dysarthria.

As has already been pointed out, much research is being undertaken and there is the promise of real therapeutic advance. It is claimed that some prolongation of life may be achieved with Riluzole which alters the level of glutamate in the central nervous system. This drug has recently been released for use in the United Kingdom.

MND presents a challenge to all those involved – doctors, nurses, therapists and social workers. We need to monitor our quality of care and strive to improve the service we offer to our patients.

ACKNOWLEDGEMENTS

I gratefully acknowledge the help given by Dr. P.M. Enderby in the preparation of this chapter.

REFERENCES

Carey, J.S. (1986) Motor neurone disease – a challenge to medical ethics. *Journal of the Royal Society of Medicine*, **79**, 216–20.

Carus, R. (1980) Motor Neurone disease: a demeaning illness. *British Medical Journal*, **280**, 455–6.

Leighton, S.E.J., Burton, M.J., Lund, W.C. and Cochrane, G.M. (1994) Swallowing in motor neurone disease. *Journal of the Royal Society of Medicine*, **87**, 801–5.

Loizou, L.A., Small, M. and Dalton, G.A. (1980) Cricopharyngeal myotomy in motor neurone disease. *Journal of Neurology, Neurosurgery and Psychiatry*, **43**, 42–5.

Newrick, P.G. and Langton Hewer, R. (1984) Motor neurone disease: can we do better? A study of 42 patients. *British Medical Journal*, **289**, 539–42.

Newrick, P.G. and Langton Hewer, R. (1985) Pain in motor neurone disease. *Journal of Neurology, Neurosurgery and Psychiatry*, **48**, 838–40.

Norris, F.H., Smith, F.A. and Denys, E.H. (1985) Motor neurone disease: towards better care. *British Medical Journal*, **291**, 259–62.

Pentland, B., Rainey, M.E. and MacNeill, R. (1985) Wheelchair provision for patients with motor neurone disease. *Health Bulletin (Edinburgh)*, **43**, 72–5.

Saunders, C., Summers, D.H. and Teller, N. (1981) *Hospice – the living idea*, Edward Arnold, London.

USEFUL ADDRESSES

Motor Neurone Disease Association,
PO Box 246, Northampton, NN1 2PR (Publishes much useful information for patients and professionals.) (Tel: 01604 250505. Helpline: 0345 626262.)

There are many local branches and many carry equipment banks and have trained visitors.

26 Multiple sclerosis

M. Roberts

INTRODUCTION

Multiple sclerosis (MS) is a disease of unknown cause characterized clinically by relapse and remission and pathologically by patches of demyelination of different ages in separate parts of the central nervous system. It may progress and lead to severe disability, but the rate of progression is not, for an individual, predictable.

Until recently there was little evidence that treatment influences the natural history. Nevertheless, most accounts of the illness concentrate on the attempt to do so and do not give prominence to the management of symptoms (Matthews *et al*, 1991, Rudick and Goodkin, 1992). Much, however, can be done and fortunately there are now fuller accounts of symptom management and rehabilitation (Barnes, 1993, British Society of Rehabilitation Medicine, 1993).

Patients and relatives want information and a description of the disease is presented below. A brief account of attempts to treat relapse and influence the natural history follows. The management of common symptoms is then discussed. MS presents challenges and frustrations precisely because of its disseminated character. Although different symptoms are described separately, it is the combination in an individual that is relevant. For example, vision, intellect, upper limb strength, sensation and coordination must be assessed when considering intermittent self-catheterization. The final section is a short account of the social context of MS in terms of handicap, implications for other family members and sources of support, followed by a personal account by a patient suffering from the disease.

BACKGROUND INFORMATION

Pathology and pathogenesis

The axons of myelinated nerves in the CNS are surrounded by sheaths derived from oligodendrocytes. It is these sheathes, especially in the optic nerve, brainstem, spinal cord and periventricular region, which when damaged lead to slowed nerve conduction. Acute lesions show inflammatory infiltration with T and B lymphocytes, macrophages and oligodendrocytes loss. Chronic lesions show dense processes and loss of myelin and oligodendrocytes.

The breakdown of the blood–brain barrier and the entry of T cells into the cerebrospinal fluid seem central to the process. That perivascular inflammation is also seen in the retina, which has no myelinated axons, suggests it is primarily an endothelial cell abnormality that triggers this penetration. Magnetic resonance imaging (MRI) is more sensitive than Computer tomography (CT) scanning or clinical examination at detecting

Rehabilitation of the Physically Disabled Adult. Edited by C. John Goodwill, M. Anne Chamberlain and Chris Evans. Published in 1997 by Stanley Thornes (Publishers) Ltd, Cheltenham. ISBN 0-7487-3183-0.

lesions which appear more frequently than clinical episodes. Blood–brain barrier breakdown, as shown by gadolinium DTPA enhancement, appears to precede other MRI evidence of new lesions.

The cause, or causes, remain obscure. The geographical prevalence variation and studies on migrants led to a research emphasis on environmental causes but the discovery of HLA associations rekindled interest in the genetic contribution. In 10–15% of cases more than one family member is affected. A population study in British Columbia has shown the risk for siblings of an affected person is 4%, for parents 3% and for offspring 2.5%. The concordance rate for monozygotic twins is at least 26%.

Epidemiology

There have been many studies of prevalence of MS but fewer studies of incidence. These, and the problem of case definition, have been critically reviewed (Sadovnick and Ebers, 1993). The prevalence rises in both hemispheres with distance from the equator. Within the mainland UK the prevalence appears to rise from 99/100 000 in Southampton in the south to 155/100 000 in North East Scotland. Controversy remains about whether a gradient exists and there are problems with case definition (Robertson and Compston, 1995). In New Zealand the prevalence is 24/100 000 in the north whereas the prevalence is 69/100 000 in the south. There are however exceptions to this generalization, of which the prevalence in Sicily of 44/100 000 and in Malta of 4/100 000 is a good example.

A very complex situation exists in South Africa where in black southern Africans the disease is very rare and recent white immigrants have a higher incidence than white African born English speakers in whom the disease is more common than in white African born Afrikaans speakers (Dean, Bhighee and Bill, 1994).

Better case detection is probably the reason that more recent epidemiological studies tend to show higher prevalence rates. Incidence rates show complex temporal trends and in North East Scotland appear to have risen from 5.3 to 7.5 between 1959 and 1980. Assuming a prevalence of 100/100 000 and an incidence of 5/100 000 per annum, a general practitioner with 2 000 patients may expect to have two with established MS and see a new case every 10 years.

Both prevalence and incidence studies show that the disease is more common in females and the ratio of females to males is between 1.9 and 3.1. The disease is rare in childhood. The incidence is maximum around the age of 30, slightly later in men, remains high in the fourth decade with a mean age of onset at 32–34. Between 5 and 10% will have an age of onset over 50, more often with a progressive course. The age-specific prevalence rates often show a peak in the late forties. These age patterns have implications for services. In an MS population, about a quarter will be aged 60 or over as will half of the more seriously disabled. There is thus little sense in arbitrary age limits to service provision.

Diagnosis

The diagnosis may be made on clinical evidence of lesions separate in time and location within the CNS supplemented by investigations. Visual evoked potentials (VEPs) and MRI scanning may provide evidence of lesions which may not be clinically apparent. Oligoclonal bands may be shown in the CSF but not serum and suggest intrathecal inflammation. Investigations help to exclude conditions which may closely mimic MS, such as structural abnormalities, inflammatory and inherited diseases (Compston, 1993). The early clinical and epidemiological literature has a confusing array of diagnostic terms, but the Poser Committee criteria are much more clearly defined (Mathews *et al*, 1991).

The significance of symptoms at the onset may not be correctly appreciated and an initial psychiatric diagnosis is not uncommon. The diagnosis is often made over a period of time and this contributes to the difficulty in conveying this to the patient and relatives in a timely, appropriate and sensitive manner or with good communication between neurologist and general practitioner. In Southampton, 9% had found out inadvertently and 38% were dissatisfied with the manner in which it was conveyed. The period of diagnosis is a crucial one in which future attitudes to available services can be shaped.

Onset, relapse and remission

Onset symptoms, sometimes multiple, are commonly limb weakness, pain and loss of vision due to retrobulbar neuritis, paraesthesiae or numbness and vertigo, double vision, ataxia and dysarthria. Bladder and sexual symptoms may be present at the onset as may paroxysmal symptoms described below. Given the disseminated nature of the disease it is not surprising that a huge variety of onset symptoms have been described and occasionally intellectual deterioration will be the predominant feature. Not all patients with isolated symptoms attributed to demyelination go on to develop MS but the proportion in those with optic neuritis approaches 75% within 15 years, at least in the UK. Some with a clinically isolated episode of demyelination have multiple MRI abnormalities at the onset and a high proportion of these go on to develop MS. However, this finding is not in itself sufficient to diagnose MS – some will have acute disseminated encephalomyelitis.

A relapse (sometimes referred to as a bout, episode, attack or exacerbation) is the occurrence of new or worsening symptoms of neurological dysfunction lasting for more than 24 hours and often lasting for several weeks. A remission is simply a definite improvement in these and, for clinical trial purposes, is often required to last 1 month to be considered significant. Although it is known that the administration of gamma-interferon increases relapse rate, it is not known what usually precipitates relapses and this may be multifactorial. In a prospective study the relapse rate during periods exposed to viral infections was 0.64 per annum compared with 0.23 per annum in periods not exposed.

There are case reports of trauma (including surgery) being associated with onset or relapse and this is sometimes a matter of legal dispute. Sibley *et al* (1991) did not confirm this association. Overall, there was a negative correlation between trauma and exacerbation rate, and certainly there is no evidence that trauma is a common precipitant of relapse. There is much speculation and some evidence about the role of 'stressful life events' in the exacerbation or onset of MS. There are major methodological difficulties but in a careful study Grant *et al*, (1989) found a positive association. Other than to avoid needless exposure to viral infections the literature does not translate into simple advice to patients – there are seldom choices about trauma or life events.

There may be an opportunity for more informed choice about pregnancy. The relapse rate during pregnancy appears to be lower but there is an increased rate in the post-partum period (Hutchinson, 1993). From retrospective studies there is no evidence that pregnancy affects long-term disability, and in one study pregnancy decreased the risk of a progressive course (Runmarker and Anderson, 1995). Each patient needs careful evaluation and advice and it can be anticipated that extra support will be required postpartum.

Assessment/rating scales

The rating scales described by Kurtzke Rudick and Goodkin, 1992, chap. 3 should be understood by anyone wishing to read further about MS but are largely research oriented and less relevant to clinical management. An initial 0–10 'Disability Status Scale' (DSS) was later, to increase sensitivity, subdivided into an 'Expanded Disability Status Scale' (EDSS).

Rating requires a neurological examination to place the impairments found in eight subscales – the 'functional systems'. In essence the point on the lower part of EDSS is determined by the number and grade in different functional systems rated at examination. In the mid part of the scale it is heavily weighted by locomotor function and in the upper part by upper limb function and independence in activities of daily living. The scale is confusing in terms of the ICIDH impairment, disability and handicap model and has been heavily criticized. There are concerns about interobserver agreement and although in a clinical trial it may be reasonable to suggest that differences of up to 1.0 may be due to interobserver variation, this cannot be adequate to guide individual management. A person rated 6.0 should be able to walk 100 metres with one stick whereas someone rated 7.0 should in essence be restricted to a wheelchair. This is an enormous transition into which much rehabilitation input will be required. The scale is ordinal and in cross-sectional population studies there is a bimodel distribution with relatively few in EDSS 4.0–5.0.

There have been other attempts at neurological scales and of standardized ratings of disability and handicap in MS. The Incapacity Status Scale and Environmental Status Scale are however not widely used and in the author's experience are unwieldy and inadequately defined. Ease of communication is a cogent reason why rating scales not specific to MS, such as the Barthel Index or Functional Incapacity Measure, should be used. Clearly it is important to use descriptors of function as no impairment scale will describe the common and complex interaction of different impairments, for example motor weakness, ataxia, sensory loss and visual impairment, or the ability to walk.

Prevalence of disability, prognosis and disease type

Those planning health services will be interested in cross-sectional studies of MS populations. The literature and the methodological problems have been well reviewed (Goodkin, 1992).

In UK studies approximately 25–30% of people with MS are wheelchair users (EDSS 7.0 or over) and similar proportions have been found in studies in Canada (28%) and Australia (23–25%).

Individuals with MS are more concerned with their own prognosis. The extremes are a fulminant rapidly fatal course and 'silent' MS in which typical lesions may be found incidentally at post mortem in those dying of other causes. Can anything useful be said? Some (perhaps 15% and a higher proportion in those with later age of onset) have a disease which is progressive from the onset without any obvious tendency to relapse and remit. Some are relapsing and remitting and others develop progression after relapsing and remitting disease. Progression is not inevitable and without strict operational definitions there is some arbitrariness in such classifications. In one study adherence to disease type was not strong at 2-year follow-up. A proportion, between 25 and 40%, are said to have a benign course (sometimes defined as EDSS of 3 or less at 10 years), but with more prolonged follow-up this proportion drops. This description is framed in terms of impairment and even those people who turn out to have 'benign' disease may have irrevocably altered lives as will be discussed below.

In an important series of studies (Weinshenker *et al*, 1991) one in three had reached DSS 6 (walking with one stick) by 10 years. Certain clinical features are associated with a worse prognosis although studies are inconsistent. Weinshenker *et al* (1991), who used more detailed statistical analysis than most studies, found that males, and those with older age of onset, insidious motor deficit, impaired balance or ataxia had a shorter time to DSS 6. Those with optic neuritis had a longer time. Disease that was progressive from the onset was associated with poor outcome. However, even with such sophisticated modelling, this does not provide clinically useful risk estimates for individuals and in most studies present disability, as measured by DSS, is the strongest predictor.

It is not certain that serial MRI scanning will prove to be more useful. There is little evidence of correlation between MRI lesion load in the brain or spinal cord and global measures of disability in cross-sectional studies. However there is some evidence that lesion load in serial scans and the appearance of new lesions may be associated with prognosis. Thus those with benign disease had fewer new or enlarging lesions and less enhancement as compared with those with relapsing and remitting disease of more recent onset (Kidd *et al*, 1994). The number of brain lesions at presentation, the number of new lesions and the disability at follow-up were correlated in a study of people with clinically isolated lesions (Morrisey *et al* 1993). However, there appears to be a lower rate of appearance of new lesions in those with primary rather than secondarily progressive disease and it may be that the pathological process is different.

The prognosis in terms of life expectancy has probably increased with modern management of complications. In essence, although the average life expectancy is not greatly reduced overall (perhaps by 6–7 years), those who have acquired significant physical disability have a higher mortality. Suicide is a significant cause of death, over seven times that in an age-matched population, and is more common in those with less severe disability.

TREATMENT OF RELAPSE AND THE DISEASE PROCESS

Of relapse

Relapses may be treated with intravenous methyl prednisolone (Griffiths and Newman 1994). A possible regime might be 500 mg or 1 gm on three consecutive days, with or without an alternate-day steroid tail. This has been shown to reduce the blood–brain barrier abnormalities as shown by gadolinium-DTPA enhancement on MRI scans. Other mechanisms of action might be resolution of oedema, immunosuppression, inhibition of demyelination or a direct effect on nerve conduction. The effect is to decrease the duration of a relapse but not to influence the outcome of that relapse. Thus it would be reasonable to use steroids only when a relapse causes significant symptoms. However, in a trial of treatment of isolated optic neuritis (a common presentation of MS), those treated with intravenous methyl prednisolone and a short steroid tail showed a lower rate of development of multiple sclerosis over the subsequent 2 years as compared with those treated with placebo or oral prednisolone alone (Wray, 1995). Further studies are needed to see if the relapse rate is influenced.

There is no established role for long-term treatment with oral steroids but all clinicians will be familiar with some patients who will bitterly complain if an attempt is made to wean them off the drug. Anaphylaxis to intravenous methyl prednisolone has been described, so it should be given in circumstances where resuscitation is possible. If high dose oral steroids were as effective as intravenous methyl prednisolone in the treatment of relapse they would be more convenient. However, the relative effectiveness has not been fully established.

Aimed at influencing natural history

Randomized controlled trials of treatment in MS have been conducted in the face of major difficulties. MS tends to relapse and remit unpredictably, progresses often slowly and variably, and the relapse rate may decrease with time. The Kurtzke EDSS, as discussed above, has rather crude intervals yet there are concerns about interobserver variability. With the introduction of MRI scanning into clinical trial outcome measurement there is now much greater optimism that treatment effects can be detected relatively rapidly. In a study of 'independent ambulatory' patients between 18 and 50, with relapsing and remitting disease and at least two documented relapses in the previous 2 years, interferon beta-1-b subcutaneously on alternate days in a dose of 8.0×10^6 IU reduced exacerbation rate by 34% compared to placebo. The mean lesion area measured by MRI increased over 3 years by 17% in the placebo group as compared to 6% decrease in the 8×10^6 IU treatment group (Hughes, 1994; IFNB MS Study Group and University of British Colombia MS/MRI Study Group, 1995). The disability as measured by the Kurtzke EDSS, however, did not differ between the two groups. Although one interpretation is that neither treatment nor placebo group changed much in terms of disability over the trial period, the relationship between MRI appearances and disability is an area of active research. Final proof is lacking but it seems logical that agents which decrease the rate of acquisition of MRI-detectable lesions will on average decrease the accumulation of impairments. However, some patients develop disability without new MRI activity and it may be that progressive axonal loss in pre-existing lesions is the mechanism (Kidd *et al* 1996).

Other trials, of interferons and other agents such as copolymer-1 and monoclonal antibodies such as Campath 1, are in progress. In particular, interferon beta trials are needed in those with more severe disability and with progressive disease. Rudick and Goodkin (1992) is an excellent summary of clinical trials (and their tribulations) to that date. Even if agents are found which will at least slow the rate of accumulation of new lesions this leaves a large cohort in which damage has already been done.

SYMPTOM MANAGEMENT

Locomotor impairment

The ability to walk may deteriorate with pyramidal weakness and spasticity, proprioceptive loss, ataxia, decreasing vision and vertigo. Secondary mechanical problems such as arthritis and low back pain may occur. A careful programme of stretching, gait training and exercise under the supervision of a physiotherapist is vital; for example, even a minor worsening of achilles tendon shortening can seriously impede gait. Walking aids are described in Chapter 48. Often poor grip and upper limb ataxia make them less effective.

Many who can only walk short distances restrict their range of activities because of reluctance to acquire a wheelchair for occasional outdoor use. It may take gentle suggestions of use on trips away or on holiday or careful explanation that provision of a chair will not decrease walking ability – the 'if you don't use it, you lose it' fear – before a chair will be accepted. In those who walk little or not at all, a physiotherapist can help maintain the ability to transfer and, in conjunction with an occupational therapist, give advice to relatives on assisted transfers. Orthoses, most commonly ankle–foot orthoses, can be helpful in walking and providing stability of weightbearing in transfers (Chapters 44 and 47).

Ataxia

The person with ataxia who has inadequate social support may give the appearance of self-neglect with long nails, poor dentition, cigarette burnt clothing and scalds from over-hot drinks. Weight loss may be present due to the inability to prepare adequate meals or unwillingness to accept the need to be fed. Unfortunately, except in the context of steroid treatment of a relapse, drug treatment has little to offer, although the use of isoniazid, clonazepam or sodium valproate has been suggested. Stereotactic thalamotomy, where there is severe intention tremor, can only apply to the very few. Weighted bands on the wrists, with the intention of damping tremor, may be tried but equipment to compensate for poor upper limb function, for example electric toothbrushes, plate guards, adapted cutlery, keyboard guards and hands-free telephones are likely to be more successful (Chapter 41). A Neater Eater may help in feeding as may the use of straws in drinking. A wheeled walking frame may allow walking to continue but prolong exposure to risk of falling. Those with powered wheelchairs may need reassessment of controls.

Spasticity

The management of spasticity is considered elsewhere (Chapter 34). Attention to detail is required. Painful stimuli may exacerbate spasticity. Therefore, footwear, the need for chiropody, seating and pressure area care, management of pain syndromes, constipation and bladder management should be reviewed. Many patients would benefit from a regular stretching programme and the only feasible way this can be delivered in the UK is for relatives and professional carers to incorporate such regimes into daily care. This may improve symptoms and ease of handling in transfers, personal care and dressing.

Drug therapy with baclofen or dantrolene has a role, especially in the control of positive symptoms such as spasms. Phenol or botulinum injections are also useful, particularly where adductor spasticity interferes with perineal hygiene. In more severe cases techniques such as intrathecal baclofen infusion may be used. Lumbar intrathecal phenol may be used if spasms are severe and bladder function and sensation is lost. It has however

been suggested that care must be taken with this technique and that there is in place an adequate pressure-relieving programme (British Society of Rehabilitation Medicine, 1993).

Bladder disturbance

Bladder function may be disturbed by lesions as distant as in the frontal lobes, the pontine micturition centre and the length of the spinal cord. It is not therefore surprising that bladder symptoms often occur in MS. The most common symptoms are 'irritative' (urgency, frequency, urge incontinence) and difficulty in initiating voiding. Irritative symptoms and incomplete urine may exacerbate frequency. Upper tract damage is uncommon (Chapter 35).

In the Southampton epidemiological study, 61% had urgency and a further 10% had indwelling catheters or had urinary diversions. Hesitancy was experienced by 20%. Overall 33% were incontinent more than once per fortnight and this was as common in males as females. Although clearly related to disability; 14% of the mildly affected also had incontinence and 11% had never discussed the incontinence outside the family. Other studies of those with bladder symptoms (i.e. not population based) have found urgency in 24–86%, frequency in 17–65%, urge incontinence in 34–72% and hesitancy in 25–49% (Betts, D'Mellow and Fowler, 1993).

The commonest abnormality found in those who undergo cystometry is detrusor hyperreflexia (52–78%). In 18–66% there is loss of the coordination in voiding between detrusor contractions and the external striated urethral sphincter – 'detrusor-sphincter dyssynergia'. In Betts, D'Mellow and Fowler's (1993) study, 85% had urgency, 82% frequency, 63% urge incontinence, 43% poor or interrupted stream, and 34% had a sensation of incomplete emptying. Ninety-five per cent had pyramidal signs and the degree correlated with severity of urinary symptoms. Postmicturition residuals of over 100 ml were present in 63% and although 83% of those who had the sensation of incomplete emptying had significant residuals, only 47% of those with high residuals had the sensation of incomplete emptying. Detrusor hyperreflexia, which correlated well with the symptoms of urgency, frequency and urge incontinence, was found in 91% of those in whom urodynamics were carried out.

In the majority of people symptoms can be improved by careful use of medication to control detrusor hyperreflexia, for example tricyclic antidepressants, flavoxate or oxybutynin, or, in those with high postmicturition residual urines, clean intermittent catheterization by self or other.

Thus, in those with significant bladder symptoms, diabetes and infection should be excluded and then a postmicturition residual measured by ultrasound. A rectal examination, though in itself insufficient to exclude outflow obstruction, should be done – MS does not protect against prostatic hypertrophy and cancer. It there is no significant residual the author uses oxybutynin for urgency except where depression is also present. Residual urine should be checked when treatment is established.

If there is a significant residual, referral to a continence nurse advisor should be made for teaching self-catheterization. If urgency persists technique and frequency of catheterization is checked, infection again excluded and oxybutynin may be added. In those intolerant of oral oxybutynin, intravesical oxybutynin has been tried but this is not at present a licensed indication in the UK. Urodynamics will inform decisions about treatment but it is impractical to request this in every case and urinary symptoms may fluctuate. For some, when skin care becomes a problem, when it is not possible for a carer to be available for transfers or when intermittent catheterization is difficult because of obesity, immobility or adductor spasticity, urinary catheters continue to be necessary. Blocking and bypassing require management by an appro-

priately small balloon, exclusion of stones or debris and are sometimes helped by suprapubic catheter. Urinary diversion should seldom be required.

It should be emphasized that time and careful tactful questioning may be required to elucidate how important bladder symptoms are to the person and their carer, especially where there is poor recall. Many will say they have some urgency and no incontinence when what is nearer to the truth is that they avoid ever being far from a lavatory or that continence is only maintained with the help and ready availability of a carer day and night. It is only when a minor further loss of dexterity or mobility happens or a carer becomes less able to assist in transfers that the true extent of bladder symptoms emerge.

Bowel disturbance

This has been less extensively studied. Constipation, sometimes related to analgesics, antidepressants and oxybutynin, is common. Urgency and faecal incontinence may occur and this may have a profound effect on an individual's morale and willingness to go out. In a postal survey of MS society members in the USA, (Hinds, Eidelman and Wald, 1990) constipation was present in 43%. Faecal incontinence, the involuntary passage of stool at least once in the previous 3 months, was found in 51%. A quarter of those with little locomotor impairment and 40% of those without bladder disturbance nevertheless had faecal incontinence. In a uroneurology clinic study 20% had current faecal incontinence, (Chia, Fowler and Kamm, 1995). In contrast in Southampton, only 4% had regular faecal incontinence but 21% had never been faecally incontinent (Roberts, 1991). Although the prevalence of bowel disturbance is less clearly defined than is the case with urinary symptoms, the practical message is the same – that symptoms should be sought by careful and tactful inquiry. Constipation usually responds to dietary change and faecal softeners but stronger laxatives should be used with caution and may precipitate incontinence. Manual evacuation and enemas may be required to avoid impaction with overflow. Urgency may respond to anticholinergics.

Sexual difficulties

These are very common in both males and females and may result from a wide variety of causes (Dupont, 1993). Sexual difficulties may, for example, occur when a role changes from being a spouse to being a carer even if 'function' is unchanged. In Southampton 61% of females reported an effect on their sex lives for a wide variety of reasons, including sensory loss, spasticity, incontinence and fatigue. Seventy-two per cent of males felt MS had affected their sex lives, with 51% reporting erectile impotence. Those with erectile problems may be helped by intracavernosal injection of alprostadil or papaverine. Referral to specialist clinics should be made after a careful assessment of the nature of a relationship has been made. Erectile impotence may be only one factor in a more complex change in a relationship. This appreciation should not be taken as the excuse not to enquire. Only half of the males with erectile impotence in Southampton recalled ever having discussed the subject yet the majority felt the matter was of current concern.

Communication disorders and dysphagia

Dysphasia may occur in MS but dysarthria is much more common. Communication difficulties, present in perhaps 4% (Benkelman, Kraft and Freal, 1985), have not been extensively studied. Referral to a speech therapist may be helpful with advice about posture and techniques to increase intelligibility such as advice on speech rate, intonation and breath control. Advice about communication aids can also be given, sometimes with referral to a Communication Aids Centre when the use of keyboards in the more common aids is made problematical by weakness, ataxia, poor vision or sensory loss. Cognitive function should be assessed, otherwise expensive errors in provision will be made (Chapter 22).

Speech therapists have a major role in assessing dysphagia. Although the prevalence is not known, there are suggestions from studies of swallowing speed that impaired swallowing is common, and bulbar involvement can contribute to the respiratory complications sometimes observed (Howard *et al*, 1992). Swallowing should not be assessed independently of feeding position and seating. Careful instruction of carers by a dietician or speech therapist may be required. In those in whom it is a lengthy daily chore to try and get adequate food intake, who have chest infections due to aspiration and in whom weight loss leads to pressure area problems, percutaneous endoscopic gastrostomy may be recommended either as an adjunct to or substitute for oral feeding.

Vision

This may be impaired both by optic neuritis (with scotomata, altered colour vision and, much less commonly, severe visual loss which may be bilateral) and by a variety of eye movement disorders (McDonald and Barnes, 1992). Relapse can be treated by steroids. Referral for low vision aids may be appropriate as may be a home occupational therapy review of hazards in the home (Chapter 20).

Pain and paroxysmal syndromes

These are considered together but pain is much more common, affecting about a half of patients. Pain is often the discomfort from poor sitting posture, inadequate wheelchair seating or leg spasms, but in addition there are specific pain syndromes. Persistent dysaesthesiae, especially in the lower limbs, may be present. Lhermitte's sign, a symptom provoked by neck flexion of an unpleasant 'electric' sensation passing down the spine to the lower limbs and sometimes the arms, is usually adapted to by the avoidance of flexion. There are a number of stereotypical motor or sensory symptoms, some of which are painful, which occur in brief frequent episodes which may be triggered. The most widely known is trigeminal neuralgia which affects at least 1% of those with MS. Treatment is as with the idiopathic condition.

Less well known paroxysmal symptoms are paroxysmal dysarthria and ataxia, tonic seizures and paroxysms of paraesthesiae, pain or itching. The importance of recognizing such symptoms is that they respond readily to treatment with carbamazepine. Movement disorders have been reviewed (Tranchant, 1995).

Cognitive problems

Cognitive impairment is extremely common and a large number of studies have demonstrated detectable abnormalities on standardized psychometric assessments (Rao, 1990, 1995). The study populations are often clinic based and the prevalence of cognitive impairment is in the range of 50–60% but much lower if clinical assessment rather than detailed testing is used. A population based cross-sectional study has also confirmed these findings (McIntosh-Michaelis *et al*, 1991). Intellectual change is not confined to those with major physical disability and occasionally it may be the presenting feature. There is evidence that neither disease type or duration is strongly predictive of the presence of cognitive impairment. (Beatty, *et al*, 1990). Detectable abnormalities have been found in those who present with a clinically isolated lesion yet have MRI evidence of multiple lesions. There are correlations between MRI lesions load and cognitive impairment and it may be that the notion of a clinically silent lesion should be revised. Memory is commonly impaired and this may be present without awareness or insight. Problems with

shifting set, formation of concepts and perseveration may occur with preservation of language. There is some evidence of correlation between specific lesions in the frontal lobes and performance on tests of abstract reasoning such as the Wisconsin Card Sorting Test. It is important to detect cognitive impairment for several reasons. Firstly, some patients and relatives value information and counselling about such changes and strategies adapt to them. The risk without such counselling is that changes may be misinterpreted as personality attributes or the patient and the family believe they have an additional illness such as Alzheimer's. Secondly, rehabilitation goals must be tempered by a person's ability to learn and recall new information. Thirdly, where cognitive impairment is present the compliance with, and need for, potentially sedative medication should be reviewed. There is evidence that clinical assessment is inaccurate and insensitive and the availability of a clinical psychologist, who may also be involved in more general counselling, is essential. The need for a standard screening instrument is clear. Although the utility of Folstein's MMSE has been explored in a number of articles, it is relatively insensitive. The 'core battery' suggested by Peyser *et al* (1990) is impractical in ordinary clinical work. There has however been insufficient work on how abnormalities on psychometric tests are related to changes in function and social engagement. How important intellectual change may be to quality of life is shown in a study (Rao *et al*, 1991) in which those with cognitive impairment were less likely to engage in social activities, routine household tasks, and to be employed, but reported more sexual dysfunction.

Mood disorders

'The association of euphoria with multiple sclerosis has proved ineradicably memorable among those who see and know little of the disease...' (Matthews *et al*, 1991). Accounts of mental changes in MS often give undue prominence to euphoria, which means a sustained elevation of mood or an inappropriate sense of well-being, and the subject is discussed by Rabins in Rao (1990). In the former sense euphoria is present in probably under 10%, and in the latter sense is correlated with more extensive brain lesions and global cognitive decline but it should be emphasized that the subject, surprisingly, has not been extensively studied.

Depression is far more common, occurring in about 40–50% of patients. In some the symptom is part of a bipolar affective disorder. There is a debate as to whether depression is related to structural brain lesions or is reactive in nature or some interaction of the two. Minden and Schiffer (1990) suggested that this debate is the 'vexing question for clinical research in this field'. Perhaps more important is the question of what treatments are effective and there are surprisingly few clinical trials to guide treatment. In the absence of evidence, the approach must be adopted that depression should be treated as one would with depression without MS. In some the diagnosis is all too clear but in others careful evaluation of the symptoms of tiredness or memory impairment need to be made. Non-verbal cues to depression, such as lack of care in appearance, poverty of facial expression and poor eye contact, may be altered by the disease in the absence of depression. Screening instruments for depression, such as the BDI (Back Depression Inventory) and HAD (Hospital Anxiety and Depression) scales, and for mood disorder, such as the GHQ (General Health Questionnaire), have been widely used. Minden and Schiffer (1990) recommend the use of the BDI, although this itself was developed as a 'quantitative measure of the intensity of depression'.

Paroxysms of easily provoked laughter or crying, 'pathological emotionalism', may show a gratifying response to antidepressants and fluoxetine has been found to be effective in a number of reports.

Fatigue

Fatigue can be defined as a sensation of tiredness or lack of energy disproportionate to the effort required for a task or for the degree of disability. It is a very common symptom and is often puzzling to patients and their relatives. It requires careful explanation as to why function may vary from day to day if fluctuations are not to be interpreted as psychologically based. Particular difficulty may be caused at work especially if the diagnosis is not known by colleagues. It is difficult to evaluate in clinical trials but amantadine has been found to be modestly effective in several trials (Cohen and Fisher, 1989). There is no precise relationship of the sensation of fatigue to exertion, but some will find it helpful to adjust their daily patterns to provide adequate periods of rest. The symptom of fatigue should prompt a review of medication and an enquiry into whether sleep is being lost due to bladder symptoms, leg spasms or depression. MS does not protect against other conditions; for example, anaemia or hypothyroidism. In some, what is being described is a transient worsening of symptoms occurring after exercise or a hot bath (Uhthoff's phenomenon).

General

People with MS are not exempt from other illnesses and it should always be borne in mind that deterioration may not be due to MS, especially where there is a history of falls. A fractured femur or a subdural haematoma needs surgery not steroids. If more severe disability is present physical examination may be difficult at home or in a clinic without a variable height examination couch or hoist. Breast self-examination is impossible with ataxia or a quadriparesis and general examination during an admission should be thorough not cursory. Advice on diet should not be restricted to consideration of decreasing fat intake to under 20 g a day or linoleic acid and N-3 fatty acid supplementation for which there is evidence of efficacy. Energetic attempts to avoid the development of obesity should be made, as this may have disastrous consequences on ease of handling in transfers.

SOCIAL CONTEXT AND SOURCES OF SUPPORT

Impact of MS

There is no fixed relationship between the impairments that someone may have and the resultant handicaps and indeed just being diagnosed may have very significant consequences.

> *Life and health insurance at once become more expensive or unobtainable and house purchase may be adversely affected. Job applications must either be falsified or carry the risk of automatic rejection. Immigration may be barred. Fiance(e)s or spouses may depart. Child adoption is usually no longer possible.* (Matthews *et al*, 1991, p. 222).

In Southampton, although the impact on employment was more with worsening disability, 31% of those with EDSS 4.5 or less had altered or lost employment because of MS with consequent alteration to standard of living. Referral to employment services, for example in the UK the Disability Employment Advisor, may be helpful with grants to enable continued access to work.

The impact on social life may be severe and only 3% of those with EDSS 7.0 or over went out daily, compared to 81% of those with EDSS 4.5 and below. This is partly related to environmental barriers, the cost of transport and loss of ability to drive or transfer into cars and poor availability of accessible toilets. For many, more severely affected, contact with

other people will become restricted to relatives and professional carers.

Sources of support

As will be discussed below, most support in practice comes from relatives and often a single individual, the spouse. The medical supervision and review in the UK remains largely with general practitioners, as there are insufficient neurologists. Those with mild or more severe disability are less likely to be attending than those with moderate (EDSS 5.0–6.5) disability, but this pattern is likely to change rapidly with the introduction of treatments like beta interferon.

Voluntary organizations such as the Multiple Sclerosis Society play a vital role in funding basic research, but also produce information both for patients and their families and professional carers. They can support individuals with counselling and advice, both by telephone and in person, and may be able to fund items of equipment and support holidays. Not all will use this resource as some people cope, at least initially, by denial.

Relatives and carers

> *When one member of the family has MS, the whole family will be affected.* (Burnfield, 1985, p. 66)

Parents may face the prospect of ageing whilst caring for an increasingly dependent child with MS. However, given the median age of onset, it is spouses who most often share the worry of the uncertain prognosis and the economic impact of being unable to work or having to give up work to look after someone with MS. In the Southampton prevalence study, 305/411 people with MS were interviewed and of these 25 were in residential care and 88 were living at home regularly dependent on a carer for help in ADL. The carer was aged 60 or over in 36% of cases and in 90% of cases was a spouse. With a prevalence of 100 000 this would suggest that a population of 250 000 would have 70 carers of people with MS. MS is said to have a particularly destructive effect on families, with a high rate of divorce. Marriages, however, may survive despite considerable problems. These include the physical burden of helping those who are dependent, the role change from spouse to carer, the gradual shrinking of social contacts outside the immediate family, and the altered interaction that happens when cognitive impairment is present. It is vital that everything possible is done to support carers. This may mean adequate recognition of the needs and contribution of carers, tuition in transfer techniques, optimal bladder management to decrease the number of transfers and night disturbance and the provision of respite care. Although research may have over-emphasized the psychological rather than the practical needs of carers, depression and anxiety are not uncommon. In the Southampton study 27% of carers were borderline or cases of depression as measured by the HAD as compared with 8% of relatives where there was no regular dependency in ADL. The interests of the patients and the carer may conflict, most commonly when respite away from home is poorly tolerated by the patient. Flexible 'respite at home' should be available but seldom is.

LIVING WITH MULTIPLE SCLEROSIS AND A FAMILY

Contributed by Mary Smith

I was 14 when I had my first episode of MS, weakness in the left side of the body. My father (a doctor), the neurologist, and the GP felt I was too young to be told that it was probably MS and after 3 months when I was 'better' I was told that though it might return 'and if it did we'll deal with it then', that I should carry on with life as normal.

During the next 20 or so years I followed that advice. I had the occasional problem caused by 'my illness'; not being able to run fast, sleep problems, and at one time I had steroid injections, and though I paid attention to these incidents I was not too concerned as they seemed rare and relatively minor. I also married and had four sons, and I practised as an antenatal teacher, was a parent governor at the children's school, trained to become a counsellor and practised as an officiant for non-religious weddings and funerals. My life seemed to be taking a predictable path as my forties approached and I was beginning to look forward to the future and consider what I would do now my children were growing up. I had it in mind to develop various of my part-time activities in order to earn a second income for some of the extras in life.

It was about 9 years ago that my brother went blind in one eye and it was found he had MS. It was then that I was asked if I had realized that this was what 'my illness' was. Somehow I had not, but I was still not too concerned for myself as it had not caused me much pain or trouble so far. I did not rush to read any books on the subject, I suppose I was trying to keep it at a distance.

My attitude has, however, changed considerably over the last 5 years. As the MS has gradually taken over my body my laid-back approach based on an assumption of the predictability of life has been seriously reviewed. Although it is my body that is affected by the illness every other area of my life is affected; my feelings about myself, my assumptions, plans for the future, my roles as wife, mother, and even daughter, sister and friend as well as my situation in relation to strangers as I sit in my wheelchair. Instead of taking life for granted I feel I am living at the 'sharp end' having to consider and weigh up the whats and whys of things; there is a strange exultant feeling of being in this position. I, in my forties, am having to contemplate my mortality, a situation usually reserved for older people; it is both challenging and awesome.

My physical condition has worsened over the last 5 years. It is now 15 months since I have been catheterized. I have numb hands and legs, strong and painful leg spasms and need a wheelchair. In physical terms I am disabled, I need help with dressing, showering and getting in and out of bed. I cannot do many of the jobs around the house, including cooking, that I used to do but I am not affected mentally.

The challenge comes from living with the many very painful, sad and difficult aspects of the situation. These will vary from one individual to another as the symptoms and lifestyles vary, but anger, frustration, fear and a sense of loss (of the old lifestyle, the old 'me', etc.) must be felt by all sufferers. Each individual will take up the challenge, or not, in their own way gaining support from where and from whom they can. At times, though, one can feel very alone even when surrounded by people. As new symptoms appear, perhaps a new area of numbness or blurring of vision, gradually one recognizes that more adjusting has to be done and it has to be explained to the doctor/carer/husband/mother/sister/or child as appropriate.

There is, however, also the awesome aspect; I have found it an unexpected opportunity to learn and develop. It is a rare opportunity to be able to look at oneself again, take stock and readjust one's view. If the latter sounds 'virtuous in adversity', then I can only say, I have one life and I want to make the best of it for myself and also for the many people whose support and love make it possible for me to feel this way. One of the most moving experiences has been the generosity of spirit and feeling that has come from such a wide range of people, from those closest to me to some who hardly know me.

In practical terms the physical limitations and uncertainty of living with MS have produced a massive rearrangement of the running of family life as well as creating all sorts of emotional adjustments for us all. Suddenly, over the last 6 months since I have been largely in a wheelchair, going out in the car has become complicated and anything more adventurous a major operation. In terms of wider family activities, like planning holidays, we cannot do many of the things we used to do and at home there has been an enormous shift in how things are done and who does what. In both areas of life we have had to find other ways of operating and enjoying ourselves, an enormous adjustment for us all. The handing over of many of my motherly and homemaking responsibilities to others, mainly my husband, has been a sad loss for me and not an entirely welcome change for him, who is also in full-time employment. The effect on our relationship is complex almost beyond imagining.

In order not to become isolated from the family as I cannot be as practically involved as I used to be, I try to keep an administrative role as well as a caring one. I try also to keep the family informed of what is happening to me emotionally and health-wise. This is not always gladly received but overall it seems to allow the children (aged 17, 15, 12 and 9) to have an honest and realistic view of what is happening and it also keeps them in touch with me. Reconciling the needs and demands of the family with my health needs is a constant preoccupation of mine.

As a relatively private person I have found the involvement in my life of so many individuals, professionals or otherwise, a considerable intrusion. My body and its functions out of necessity seems a constant cause for discussion whether it is with health professionals or relatives, and I am now having to share many of the previously most automatic and straightforward functions of my life (dressing and shopping for example) with other people. Although I welcome the helpers' knowledge and expertise or just their support (and it is given out of necessity), it is not easy for someone who is used to doing the caring to be cared for. I am often told 'it is up to you' presumably so I can still feel some sense of being in control but my lack of experience and knowledge about this condition and situation makes me wonder whether I want to or can make the best decisions, though I grant in the end it should be 'up to me'. The trouble is I have lost so many of my areas of control not through my choosing that it is hard to take up new ones.

When I first had a carer come to our home to help me to shower and dress not surprisingly I did not find it an easy situation, after all the last person to care for me so intimately was my mother some 40 years ago. I have found, however, so long as the carer was not near my mother's age that her professionalism and reliability has become a reassurance making my disabilities seem surmountable or at least liveable with. A tactful, sensitive and professional carer who gives no hint of judgement or criticism and who respects my routines helps build my confidence and also takes the pressure off others in the house, giving me some independent activity away from them. I have come to welcome her visits.

The medical support where I live has proved to be reliable and consistent, whether it is from the community or the rehabilitation unit. I have become acquainted with the individuals involved and they with me so there is a comfort in the feeling of familiarity whether they are from the unit or people I contact from home. I feel very reassured that there is always someone at the end of a phone or even prepared to visit when an unforeseen drama occurs, this is also a reassurance for my husband.

A big problem lies in the large number of people that are involved with me, each one with their own particular area of interest – the GP, district and continence nurses, community physiotherapist, social worker, informal carer, home carers, and occupational therapist from the community, and doctor, consultants (rehabilitation and urologist), nurses, physiotherapists and occupational therapists from the rehabilitation unit on the medical side alone. At home the situation also involves a large number of people from close to wider family and friends, to the wheelchair providers, the window cleaner, the grocer and the milkman, etc., all of whom take an interest. I appreciate their interest and enjoy to talk, but I do feel, I am at the fulcrum of a large amount of concern, at times it feels life a weighty responsibility.

With so many people helping me and willing it, it is hard not to take on myself the responsibility for 'getting better' from this incurable condition...perhaps if I practised the physiotherapy more?...rested more?... tried one of the alternative remedies (homeopathy, special diet etc.)?... Because of the variable nature of the condition there are few answers to the serious questions one asks (or dares not to ask); it is accepting this situation that is so hard for all involved. A key worker who could help me sort out some of the practical priorities, sifting family versus health decisions, would perhaps lighten my sense of responsibility.

I am helped emotionally by a psychotherapist and an art therapist who allow me to express my feelings without my having to protect them from those feelings or worry about their reactions (as I do with other people). They are there solely for me and **I set the agenda**, a rare and welcome bit of privacy and control.

My sense of dependency is based on physical reality, it has an unmistakeable childlike quality as I have to be cared for in many ways like a child does. What saves me from feeling like a child is my sense that those around me value me as an individual with experience of life, ideas, and views, etc. That I feel I still have something worthwhile to offer my family and others despite my physical condition and uncertain future is the key factor which keeps me from being overwhelmed by what is happening to me.

From Henry Smith, aged 15

My mum's illness has affected me in the same way as my brothers, like her not being able to make my packed lunch or take me to school.

It also affects me differently to my brothers and dad. I sorely miss my mum cheering on the sidelines in football games and watching me being captain of the cricket team. Before, when she was more able, she came to the primary school matches which I probably took for granted.

From Jonathan Smith, aged 12

My mother has MS and it has a big effect on me and the rest of the family. I am a chorister and when I joined my mother came quite often but now she hardly ever comes. I also have to be taken home by my best friend's mother every evening and we are always having total strangers (who are actually helpers for mum) wandering in and out of our home. The thing I really used to get annoyed about was when my friends at school used to say when they forgot something 'my mother forgot to pack it'. I was annoyed at this because I wished that my mother could pack my things and I got annoyed when I remembered that this could never happen.

CONCLUSION

Pessimism about what can be done when confronted with a sometimes progressive disease helps no one. Information can be given and some symptoms can be treated. Aids and adaptations can be provided and sources of financial and practical support can be explored. This requires input from a multidisciplinary team and may be aided by voluntary organizations. At the time of writing there are grounds for cautious optimism that a treatment that will influence the natural history is in sight.

REFERENCES

Barnes, M.P. (1993) Multiple Sclerosis, in *Neurological Rehabilitation* (eds R.G. Greenwood *et al.*), Churchill Livingstone, London, pp. 485–504.

Beatty, W.W., Goodkin, D.E., Hertsgaard, D. *et al.* (1990) Clinical and demographic predictors of cognitive impairment in multiple sclerosis. *Archives of Neurology*, **47**, 305–308.

Benkelman, D.R., Kraft, G.H. and Freal, J. (1985) Expressive communicative disorders in persons with multiple sclerosis. *Archives of Physical Medicine and Rehabilitation*, **66**, 675–679.

Betts, C.D., D'Mellow, M.T. and Fowler, C.J. (1993) Urinary symptoms and urological features of bladder dysfunction in multiple sclerosis. *Journal of Neurology, Neurosurgery and Psychiatry*, **56**, 245–250.

British Society of Rehabilitation Medicine (1993) *Multiple Sclerosis*, A working Party Report of the British Society of Rehabilitation Medicine.

Burnfield, A. (1985) *Multiple Sclerosis: a personal exploration*, Souvenir Press, London.

Chia, R.A., Fowler, C.J. and Kamm, M.A. (1995) Prevalence of bowel dysfunction in patients with multiple sclerosis and bladder dysfunction. Journal of *Neurology* **242**, 105–108.

Cohen, R.A. and Fisher, M. (1989) Amantadine treatment of fatigue associated with multiple sclerosis. *Archives of Neurology*, **46**, 676–680.

Compston, D.A.S. (1993) The diagnosis of multiple sclerosis. *Proceedings of the Royal College of Physicians of Edinburgh*, **23**, 433–445.

Dean, G. Bhighee, A.I.G, and Bill, P.L.A. (1994) Multiple sclerosis in black South Africans and Zimbabweans, Journal of *Neurology and Psychiatry*, **57**, 1064–1069.

Dupont, S. (1993) Multiple sclerosis and sexual functioning – a review. *Clinical Rehabilitation*, **9**, 135–141.

Goodkin, D.E. (1992) The natural history of multiple sclerosis in *Treatment of Multiple Sclerosis* (eds R.A. Rudick and D.E. Goodkin), Springer Verlag, London, pp. 17–45.

Grant, I., Brown, G.W., Harris, T. *et al.* (1989) Severely threatening events and marked life difficulties preceding onset or exacerbation of multiple sclerosis. *Journal of Neurology, Neurosurgery and Psychiatry*, **52**, 8–13.

Griffiths, T. and Newman, P.K. (1994) Steroids in multiple sclerosis. *Journal of clinical pharmacology Therapeutics*, **19(4)**, 219–222.

Hinds, J.P., Eidelman, B.H. and Wald, A. (1990) Prevalence of bowel dysfunction in multiple sclerosis – a population survey. *Gastroenterology*, **98**, 1538–1542.

Howard, R.S., Wiles. C.M., Hirsch, N P *et al.* (1992) Respiratory involvement in multiple sclerosis. *Brain*, **115**, 479–494.

Hughes, R.A.C. (1994) Immunotherapy for multiple sclerosis. *Journal of Neurology, Neurosurgery and Psychiatry*, **57**, 3–6.

Hutchinson, M. (1993) Pregnancy in multiple sclerosis. *Journal of Neurology, Neurosurgery and Psychiatry*, **56**, 1043–1045.

The INFB MS Study Group and University of British Columbia MS/MRI Study Group (1995) Interferon beta 1-6 in the treatment of MS. *Neurology*, **45**, 1277–1285.

Kidd, D., Thompson, A.J., Kendall, B.E. *et al.* (1994) Benign form of multiple sclerosis: MRI evidence for less frequent and less inflammatory disease activity. *Journal of Neurology, Neurosurgery and Psychiatry*, **57**, 1070–1072.

Kidd, D., Thorpe, J.W., Kendall, B.E. *et al.* (1996) MRI dynamics of brain and spinal cord in progressive multiple sclerosis. *Journal of Neurology, Neurosurgery and Psychiatry*, **60**, 15–19.

Matthews, W.B., Compston, A., Allen, I.V. *et al.* (edn) (1994) in *McAlpine's Multiple sclerosis*, 2nd edn, Churchill Livingstone, Edinburgh.

McDonald, W.I., and Barnes, D. (1992) The ocular manifestations of multiple sclerosis, I and II. *Journal of Neurology, Neurosurgery and Psychiatry*, **55**, 747–752, 863–868.

McIntosh-Michaelis, S.A., Roberts, M.H.J., Wilkinson, S.M. *et al.* (1991) The prevalence of cognitive impairment in a community survey of multiple sclerosis. *British journal of Clinical Psychology*, **30**, 333–348.

Minden, S.L. and Schiffer, R.B. (1990) Affective disorders in multiple sclerosis. Review and recommendations for clinical research. *Archives of Neurology*, **47**, 98–104.

Morrisey, S.P., Miller, D.H., Kendal, B.E. *et al.* (1993) The significance of brain magnetic resonance imaging abnormalities at presentation with clinically isolated syndromes suggestive of multiple sclerosis. A five year follow up study. *Brain*, **116**, 135–146.

Peyser, J.M., Rao, S.M., La Rocca, N.G. *et al.* (1990) Guidelines for neuropsychological research in multiple sclerosis. *Archives of Neurology*, **47**, 94–97.

Rao, S.A. (ed.) (1990) *Neurobehavioural Aspects of Multiple Sclerosis*, Oxford University Press, New York.

Rao, S.M. (1995) Neuropsychology of multiple sclerosis. *Current Opinion in Neurology*, **8**, 216–220.

Rao, S.M., Leo, G.J., Ellington, L. *et al.* (1991) Cognitive dysfunction in multiple sclerosis, II. Impact on employment and social functioning. *Neurology*, **41**, 692–696.

Roberts, M.H.W. (1991) The Southampton MS Study: disablement in a commonly survey of multiple sclerosis, University of Southampton. DM Thesis.

Roberts, N. and Compston, A. (1995) Surveying multiple sclerosis in the United Kingdom. *Journal of Neurology, Neurosurgery and Psychiatry*, **58**, 2–6.

Rudick, R.A. and Goodkin, D.E. (eds) 1992) *Treatment of multiple sclerosis* Springer-Verlag, London.

Runmarker, B. and Anderson, O. (1995) Pregnancy is associated with a lower risk of onset and a better prognosis in multiple sclerosis. *Brain*, **118**, (Pt 1), 252–261.

Sadovnick, A.D. and Ebers, G.C. (1993) Epidemiology of multiple sclerosis: a critical overview. *Canadian Journal of Neurological Sciences*, **20**, 17–29.

Sibley, W.A., Bamford, C.R., Clark, K. *et al.* (1991) A prospective study of physical trauma and multiple sclerosis. *Journal of Neurology, Neurosurgery and Psychiatry*, **54**, 584–589.

Tranchant, C., Bhatia, K.P. and Marsden, C.D. (1995) Movement disorders in multiple sclerosis. *Movement Disorders*, **10**, 418–423.

Weinshenker, B.E., Rice, G.P.A., Noseworthy, J.H. *et al.* (1991) The natural history of multiple sclerosis: a geographically based study. 4. Applications to planning and the interpretation of clinical therapeutic trials. *Brain*, **114**, 1057–1067.

Wray, S.H. (1995) Optic neuritis: guidelines. *Current Opinion in Neurology*, **8**, 72–76.

A BOOK FOR PATIENTS AND RELATIVES

Burnfield, A. (1985) *Multiple Sclerosis: a personal exploration*, Souvenir Press, London.

USEFUL ADDRESSES

International Federation of Multiple Sclerosis Societies
10 Heddon Street, London W1R 7LJ, UK. Tel: 0171 734 9120.

Internet: this is a condition on which there is a wealth of information available on the Internet.

The Multiple Sclerosis Society of Great Britain and Northern Ireland
25 Effie Road, Fulham, London SW6 1EE, UK. Tel: 0171 736 6267.

27 Rarer neurological conditions

P.E.M. Smith

MUSCLE DISEASES

Hereditary myopathies

The hereditary myopathies comprise the muscular dystrophies, hereditary dystrophic myotonias and various inherited metabolic disorders of muscle including those caused by disorders of mitochondrial function.

Muscular dystrophies

The understanding of the muscular dystrophies has been revolutionized by the identification of the genetic and molecular basis for several of these conditions. Furthermore, genetic markers have allowed a precise diagnosis to be established for many neuromuscular disorders; those with similar phenotypes can now readily be distinguished. The muscular dystrophies are classified according to their inheritance pattern: X-linked recessive, autosomal dominant, autosomal recessive or 'congenital'.

X-linked muscular dystrophies The commonest X-linked recessive muscular dystrophies, traditionally known as Duchenne and Becker muscular dystrophies, are considered together as 'dystrophinopathies' since their molecular basis is a disorder of the protein, dystrophin. Emerin, the defective gene product in Emery–Dreifuss syndrome, another X-linked dystrophy, has also been identified (Nagano et al., 1996).

Duchenne muscular dystrophy

The disease is one of the most interesting and at the same time most sad, of all those with which we have to deal: interesting on account of its peculiar features and mysterious nature; sad on account of our powerlessness to influence its course, except in a very slight degree. It is a disease of early life and early growth. Manifesting itself commonly at the transition from infancy to childhood, it develops with the child's development, grows with his growth so that every increase in stature means an increase in weakness, and each year takes him a step further on the road to a helpless infirmity, and in most cases an early and inevitable death. (Gowers, 1879).

Gowers' poignant description of Duchenne muscular dystrophy remains as relevant and accurate over a century after his writing.

Typically, a boy with previous mild delay in motor milestones presents aged 3–5 years with declining ability to climb stairs, a waddling gait and paradoxically large calves. The decline in mobility is remorseless to wheelchair confinement aged 9–12 years. Contractures around the hips and ankles lead to toe-walking and further limit function. Death at 17–20 years results from ventilatory failure from progressive respiratory muscle weakness, compounded by scoliosis. The typical extent of skeletal muscle wasting is illustrated in Figure 27.1.

Rehabilitation of the Physically Disabled Adult. Edited by C. John Goodwill, M. Anne Chamberlain and Chris Evans. Published in 1997 by Stanley Thornes (Publishers) Ltd, Cheltenham. ISBN 0-7487-3183-0.

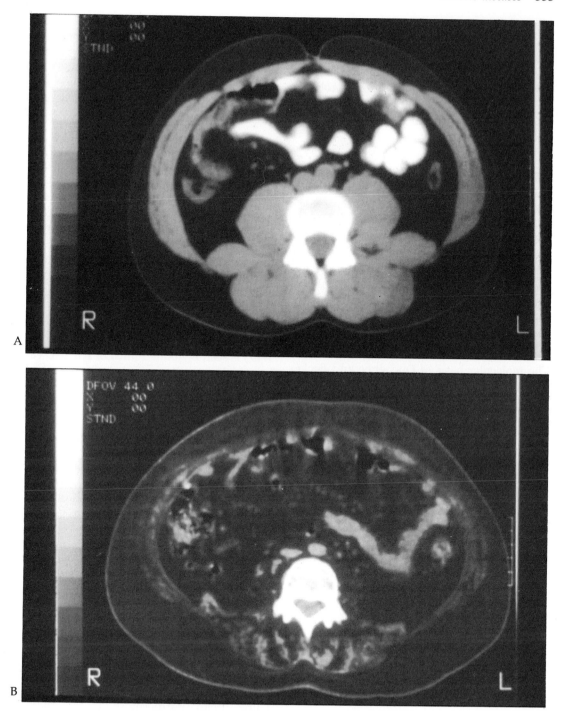

Figure 27.1 CT scans at the level of the L4 vertebral body in (A) a healthy 18-year-old male and (B) in 18-year-old with Duchenne muscular dystrophy. The Duchenne patient's psoas and paraspinal musculature show marked wasting and fatty replacement.

Although predominantly a skeletal muscle disorder, cardiomyopathy is also common and electrocardiogram changes may even be seen in non-manifesting female carriers. The presence of dystrophin in the brain probably accounts for the marginally but consistently lower than average intelligence scores in boys with dystrophinopathy.

Becker muscular dystrophy   This presents with similar progressive muscle weakness, but more variably, and is milder and of later onset. Where there is no known family history, Becker muscular dystrophy can mimic other myopathies; erroneous genetic advice may be given. Calf hypertrophy and toe-walking in a boy with muscle weakness should alert the physician to a dystrophino-pathy.

Genetics of Duchenne and Becker dystrophies
The molecular basis of Duchenne and Becker dystrophies is a deletion at Xp21, the gene coding for the muscle membrane protein, dystrophin. This was the first major disease gene to be identified by positional cloning (Monaco and Kunkel, 1988). Duchenne and Becker dystrophy differ pathologically only in that dystrophin is absent from Duchenne muscle whereas in Becker, dystrophin is abnormal or present in reduced amounts. The spectrum of clinical phenotype in Becker dystrophy reflects the varying expression of the abnormal, though partially functioning, dystrophin (Comi *et al.* 1994). The conditions can be considered together as 'Xp21 myopa-thies' or 'dystrophinopathies'. The X-linked recessive disorders, for practical purposes, occur only in males, but manifesting female carriers of the Xp21 deletion do occur rarely and present diagnostic problems unless there is a clear family history.

Emery–Dreifuss syndrome   This is a similar X-linked condition characterized by progressive skeletal muscle weakness complicated by early contractures particularly of the Achilles tendons, elbow flexors and spine, and a cardiac conduction defect or other evidence of a cardiomyopathy (Yates, 1991). The cardiac involvement is of particular impor-tance as even non-manifesting female carriers of the gene may be at risk of sudden death.

Autosomal dominant muscular dystro-phies   The commonest autosomal dominant dystrophy is facioscapulohumeral muscular dystrophy (FSHMD), characterized, as its name implies, by a curious distribution of skeletal muscle involvement. The combination of scapular winging (Figure 27.2) and facial weakness is characteristic. A wide spectrum of clinical severity is seen, ranging from only minimal facial involvement and normal life expectancy, to wheelchair-bound childhood cases with ventilatory failure. An exudative retinopathy (Fitzsimons, Gurwin and Bird, 1987) is seen in about a third of FSHMD cases for which early diagnosis is important since it may be amenable to photocoagulative treat-ment to prevent retinal detachment. Although most FSHMD families show linkage to 4q35, the molecular basis and gene product for the disease are unknown. Mitochondrial disor-ders and spinal muscular atrophies may occasionally present with the FSHMD pheno-type causing diagnostic confusion. Other autosomal dominant dystrophies are the self-explanatory scapuloperoneal, oculophar-yngeal and distal muscular dystrophies.

Autosomal recessive muscular dystrophies
Limb Girdle Muscular Dystrophy (LGMD) is the diagnosis traditionally ascribed to an autosomal recessive progressive muscular wasting and weakness often beginning in childhood. Increasingly, the condition is recog-nized as heterogeneous having at least seven different genetic varieties (Mastaglia and Laing, 1996). Furthermore, LGMD may be mimicked by certain spinal muscular atrophies, congenital myopathies and metabolic disor-ders. Cases of Becker dystrophy previously

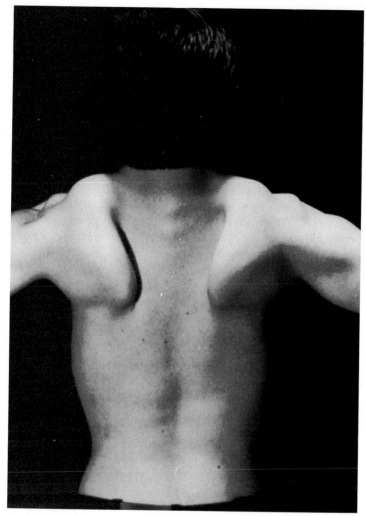

Figure 27.2 Scapular winging in facioscapulohumeral muscular dystrophy.

diagnosed as LGMD, for example, have led to important changes in genetic advice.

Many childhood-onset muscular dystrophies, clinically similar to Duchenne muscular dystrophy but autosomal recessive, have mutations of dystophin-associated proteins (α-, β-, or γ-sarcoglycans) and are known as 'sarcoglycanopathies' (Kakulas, 1996).

'Congenital' muscular dystrophies (CMD) This is a heterogeneous group of genetically determined disorders characterized by severe dystrophic muscle wasting dating from infancy. Conditions in this group include Fukuyama CMD, and the 'classical' form of CMD (Arahata, Ishii and Hayashi, 1995).

Investigations in muscular dystrophy The serum creatine kinase (CK) is almost invariably elevated in muscular dystrophy and often grossly so in the early stages of Duchenne dystrophy while the patient is still ambulant. Electromyography shows myopathic changes, its main role being the distinction of dystrophy from spinal muscular atrophy and the exclusion of myotonia. Muscle biopsy is necessary for a definite diagnosis of muscular dystrophy. Typically this shows variation in muscle fibre size, central nuclei, and fatty and fibrotic replacement of muscle. The muscle pathology of FSHMD is occasionally surprising in showing prominent inflammation as well as dystrophic changes (Fitzsimmons, 1994). More importantly, in the dystrophinopathies, diagnostic changes in dystrophin immunocytochemistry are found.

Management of muscular dystrophy Despite exciting advances in the understanding of the genetics of muscular dystrophy, there is still no specific treatment. Preliminary results using myoblast transfer in Duchenne muscular dystrophy have yet to have any practical impact, although experience with gene therapy in other diseases suggests that engineered myoblasts will eventually benefit patients (Karpati *et al*, 1993). Surprisingly, corticosteroid treatment may help in dystrophinopathy (Mendell *et al*, 1989) but predictable side-effects will prevent its widespread use. Several general management strategies must be considered in muscular dystrophy.

Diet and weight optimization Weight control is frequently necessary in patients with muscular dystrophy. Not only do obese patients add extra loads to already weak skeletal muscles, but also they risk a deleterious effect on their ventilatory function (Sharp, 1985). Nevertheless, many patients with Duchenne and other muscular dystrophies become overweight through a combination of inactivity, reduced energy turnover in wasted muscle and a misguided desire to improve muscle bulk by overeating. Weight loss through dieting has been shown to be safe and effective in muscular dystrophy (Edwards *et al*, 1984). Target weights for people who have lost muscle bulk are

correspondingly lower than that of persons of similar height but with normal muscle mass; at his optimal weight, a boy with muscular dystrophy will, at first glance, appear too thin.

Physiotherapy and training The main aims of physiotherapy in muscular dystrophy are to build morale, maintain posture and prevent contractures. Where contractures are an early feature, for example in Emery-Dreifuss syndrome, physiotherapy is of particular importance. Vigorous muscle training programmes in muscular dystrophy must be viewed with caution, however, since the development and progression of muscle weakness in these conditions is partly driven by mechanical factors (Brouwer *et al*, 1992). Deep breathing exercises, assisted coughing and forced expiration manoeuvres can improve symptoms and perhaps temporarily preserve the vital capacity in children with Duchenne dystrophy (Smith *et al*, 1987). The role of respiratory muscle training remains controversial and short-term studies have shown no benefit (Smith *et al*, 1988). Again, vigorous training may be inappropriate and even hazardous in advanced respiratory muscle weakness.

Role of surgery In FHSMD, scapulothoracic arthrodesis may improve arm function (Bunch and Siegel, 1993). In LGMD and FHSMD ankle–foot orthoses may improve gait, and later, mobile arm supports may be needed (Chapter 47). Referral to a mobility centre for advice on driving or other outdoor mobility chairs is often useful (Chapter 50).

Assisted ventilation The role of assisted ventilation in muscular dystrophy remains an area of controversy.

Management of scoliosis Scoliosis develops in up to 80% of children with Duchenne muscular dystrophy, markedly worsening the ventilatory deficit. Spinal orthoses or moulded wheelchair inserts may delay, but cannot prevent, the spinal curve progression. Spinal bracing may actually reduce the vital capacity by 20% (Noble-Jamieson *et al*, 1986); patients with very low vital capacities, especially during chest infections, should not wear orthotic jackets. Surgical techniques in segmental spinal instrumentation have proved an important advance in limiting scoliosis, improving morale and quality of life. This surgical option is now readily offered to selected teenagers with progressive myopathic scoliosis.

Genetic advice A definite diagnosis of a genetic condition may have little advantage to the affected individual but allows information to be disseminated to 'at–risk' family members who can use this knowledge to plan their own families. A prompt diagnosis and proper communication of the genetic implications to other family members will help to prevent the tragedy too often seen of a second or even third affected sibling with Duchenne dystrophy.

Hereditary myotonias

The hereditary myotonias comprise several conditions whose common clinical feature is myotonia, a failure of a contracted muscle to relax voluntarily. Included are the hereditary dystrophic myotonias (myotonic dystrophy and proximal myotonic myopathy), and also myotonias caused by channelopathies including disorders of chloride (formerly myotonia congenita) and sodium transport (e.g. paramyotonia congenita) (Lehmann-Horn and Rudel, 1995).

Myotonic dystrophy

This autosomal dominant condition is probably the most easily diagnosed muscle condition. Despite its name, it is now re-classified as an hereditary dystrophic myotonia, distinct from the muscular dystrophies. It is clearly a systemic condition with manifestations outside the musculoskeletal system. There is a predominantly distal pattern of muscle wasting, weakness and myotonia, with facial and sternomastoid muscle weakness. In addition, almost all patients show subcapsular cataracts. Men show frontal balding and hypogonadism and there is often sleep apnoea and daytime somnolence (Harper, 1979). Electrocardiographic abnormalities are common and the risk of sudden death relatively high (Editorial, 1992).

Myotonic dystrophy is caused by an unstable expansion of triplet repeats (CTG) in the myotonin protein kinase gene on the long arm of chromosome 19 (Buxton *et al*, 1992). With each generation, the repeat number increases with worsening clinical state, a phenomenon known as **anticipation**. Particularly severe childhood disease can result when a moderately severely affected mother (rather than the father) passes on the expanded gene. Other affected family members may be so mildly affected that their condition passes unnoticed. Specific treatment measures in myotonic dystrophy include attention to the possibility of heart block and sleep apnoea; cataract treatment and androgen replacement may be necessary. Particular caution with surgery is necessary as ventilator weaning problems following general anaesthesia occasionally occur. Genetic advice together with examination of family members is very important. The condition is often subclinical but, owing to anticipation, severe disease may still occur in the offspring of seemingly unaffected relatives.

Congenital myopathies

Central core disease and nemaline myopathy are examples of a rare group of disorders of unknown cause and inheritance, named from their muscle biopsy appearance and classified as congenital myopathies. Clinically the onset is in childhood with slowly progressive muscle weakness but often normal life expectancy. There may be skeletal abnormalities such as kyphoscoliosis, pes cavus and high arched palate. Nemaline myopathy is important as a cause of diaphragm weakness presenting with potentially treatable ventilatory failure.

Metabolic myopathies

Examples of these rare autosomally recessive enzyme deficiency conditions are McArdle's disease and phosphofructokinase deficiency. Typically, they present in childhood or early adult life with muscle pain and cramps on exertion. They can be readily diagnosed on muscle biopsy but treatment is limited to simple advice and glucose supplements. A rare but important metabolic myopathy is acid maltase deficiency (adult Pompe's disease), as this can cause life-threatening diaphragm weakness at a time when the patient is still ambulant.

Mitochondrial diseases

Characteristically, mitochondrial disease presents as a myopathy affecting the limbs and eye muscles leading to ptosis and progressive failure of eye movement (Schapira and Di Mauro, 1994). However, the clinical spectrum is extremely broad, encompassing myopathy, central nervous system, ocular and cardiac disorders. Even the myopathy can, within a family, range between a fatal infantile myopathy to a barely noticeable adult myopathy. Patients with all types of mitochondrial disorder may also show short stature, deafness, diabetes mellitus, basal ganglia calcification and elevated fasting venous lactate. The pathological hallmark of mitochondrial disease is the ragged red fibre, subsarcolemmal mitochondrial aggregates demonstrated by Gomori trichrome or NADH dehydrogenase. Electron microscopy confirms the abnormal mitochondrial morphology (Figure 27.3).

The Kearns–Sayre syndrome (KSS) comprises progressive external ophthalmoplegia with retinitis pigmentosa and sometimes heart block, elevated cerebrospinal fluid protein and cerebellar signs. The clinical features of other mitochondrial disorders are summarized in their acronyms: Myoclonic Epilepsy with Ragged Red Fibres (MERRF) and Mitochondrial Encephalopathy with Lactic Acidosis and Stroke-like episodes (MELAS).

Treatment is largely symptomatic. Meaningful genetic advice is very difficult owing to the range of phenotypes. Furthermore the mitochondrial genetic abnormality does not always match the clinical presentation nor does the size of the mitochondrial gene deletion match the degree of disordered biochemistry. An interesting feature of some of the mitochondrial disorders is maternal inheritance. The fertilizing sperm contains only nuclear material and so the mother's ovum is the embryo's sole source of cytoplasm and hence of mitochondrial DNA.

Non-hereditary myopathies

There is a wide range of acquired myopathy. This review focuses upon disorders most amenable to treatment. Although not primarily myopathies, chronic fatigue syndrome and stiff man syndrome are also considered here.

Inflammatory myopathies

The inflammatory myopathies comprise the major group of treatable myopathies (Dakalas, 1991): polymyositis, dermatomyositis and inclusion body myositis.

Polymyositis This is a sporadic immune-mediated condition of unknown cause. It affects predominantly females presenting with symmetrical proximal muscle weakness, sometimes with pain and tenderness, and is occasionally strikingly focal in nature. The

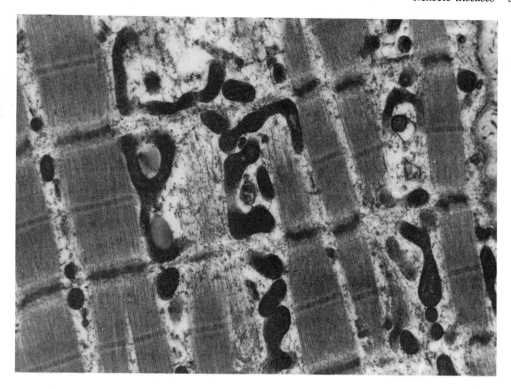

Figure 27.3 Abnormal muscle mitochondrial morphology on electron microscopy in mitochondrial disease. Quadriceps biopsy ($\times$ 10 000).

serum creatine kinase (CK) and the erythrocyte sedimentation rate (ESR) are usually, though not invariably, elevated. Electromyography may show abundant brief low amplitude polyphasic potentials and the muscle biopsy shows perivascular infiltration with muscle ischaemia.

Treatment is with immunosuppression, usually with daily prednisolone 40–60 mg initially, perhaps together with azathioprine 2.5 mg kg day, switching to alternate-day prednisolone when there is clear clinical improvement. Cyclosporin, pulsed cyclophosphamide or high dose intravenous immunoglobulin may be necessary if the response to steroids is inadequate. An important element in monitoring treatment progress in inflammatory myopathy is the use of muscle strength measurements (Wiles, Kami

and Nicklin, 1990). The encouragement of mobility (especially in the elderly) and intensive physiotherapy aimed at preventing contractures is essential. A high protein diet is advisable. Attention to the safety of swallowing and the adequacy of ventilation may be necessary in severe cases.

Dermatomyositis Although pathologically distinct from polymyositis, the clinical presentation is similar although with a rash over the extensor surfaces and trunk in 90% of cases. Surprisingly, therefore, a rash is not essential for the diagnosis. Its immunopathology is unique, being a complement-mediated intramuscular microangiopathy. In about 15% there is an underlying malignancy and some basic screening investigations are required with this in mind. The treatment is as for polymyositis.

Inclusion body myositis This is the commonest myopathy presenting in men over 50 years. The onset is insidious and painless with a curious distribution of weakness affecting especially the quadriceps and forearm flexors, particularly flexor digitorum profundus (Garlepp and Mastaglia, 1996). Dysphagia occurs in a third of cases. There is no skin involvement. Serum CK is usually normal but muscle biopsy shows rimmed vacuoles and amyloid-containing filamentous inclusions in muscle. It seems likely that the condition is primarily degenerative with a secondary inflammatory response and this probably explains why the amount of inflammation on biopsy is variable and the response to immunosuppression is poor.

Myopathy of systemic disease

Since muscle comprises 40% of body weight, it is not surprising that many systemic disorders are associated with myopathy. The cachexia associated with malignant disease is the best known example. Various endocrine disorders, for example hyper- or hypothyroidism, Cushing's disease or osteomalacia, can be accompanied by reversible muscle weakness as the major symptom. Certain drugs, including alcohol and certain cholesterol-lowering agents, are known to cause a painful necrotizing myopathy (Argov and Mastaglia, 1994).

Miscellaneous muscle-related disorders

Chronic fatigue syndrome Muscle fatigue is a feature of many disorders but in the chronic fatigue syndrome, the patient's life becomes dominated by abnormally persistent or recurrent fatigue for which no consistent physical basis can be determined. The complex interplay between physical and psychological factors seen in this condition does not fit well with traditional medical teaching of a clear divide between 'organic' and 'non-organic' disease. Symptoms are no less distressing or disabling for having no discernible cause and the frustrations of such patients are understandable. The clinical features differ between patients and vary within the individual. Usually there is no identifiable cause although the symptoms often first appear with a viral infection. The major symptoms are of exhaustion, fatigue and muscle aching, exacerbated by exertion and partially relieved by rest. Additional factors, often the non-specific effect of illness, colour the presenting symptoms. Thus, prolonged bed rest may provoke symptoms of postural hypotension. Anxiety, hyperventilation (breathlessness, light headedness and tingling of the fingers and face), negative feelings and depression (impaired sleep (Morriss *et al*, 1993) and appetite, negative thoughts and crying) often are superimposed, provoking a vicious cycle of symptoms. An over-caring partner or over-involved family may adversely influence illness behaviour. Behan (1996) reviews the definition and investigation and gives as clear diagnostic criteria as is possible at present.

Neurological investigations and tests of muscle physiology are normal (Gibson *et al*, 1993) and repeated investigations are unnecessary. The condition is often self-limiting but the treatment strategy should include an explicit acceptance of the patient's symptoms, a clear explanation and appropriate reassurance. The reversible aspects of the condition (hyperventilation, postural hypotension, too little or too much sleep) must be emphasized; a routine of sleep and meals is important and a sensible graded exercise programme should be encouraged. Psychosocial factors and the role of the partner can be addressed. The use of antidepressant agents is often surprisingly helpful, probably as much through treating sleep disorder and muscle pain as any effect on depression (Wessely, 1991). The worst outcomes are in the those who view the condition as having an entirely physical basis and who advocate complete rest (Lawrie and Pelosi, 1994).

Stiff man syndrome This is a rare auto-immune central nervous system (CNS) disorder which may give diagnostic confusion with muscle disease. Despite its name it is commoner in females than males. It is characterized by a gradual onset progressive symmetrical increase in axial muscle tone with a painful startle response to noise or emotion.

The mechanism of muscle stiffness is presumed to be an impairment of the CNS inhibitory neurotransmitter gamma-aminobutyric acid (GABA). Antibodies to glutamic acid decarboxylase are found in 60% (Editorial, 1991) and an autoimmune aetiology is also implied by an increased incidence of insulin-dependent diabetes, cerebrospinal oligoclonal bands and response to plasma exchange (Harding *et al*, 1989).

NEUROMUSCULAR JUNCTION DISORDERS

Non-hereditary neuromuscular junction disorders

Myasthenia gravis

This is an acquired immune-mediated disorder in which circulating autoantibodies damage the muscle's motor end plates, impairing neuromuscular transmission. It is most commonly seen in young adult females who present with ocular and bulbar symptoms giving fatiguable ptosis, diplopia, dysarthria and dysphagia. There may be facial, neck and limb weakness but no sensory signs or reflex change. The symptoms worsen after muscle use and towards the end of the day.

Myasthenia is confirmed by the identification of circulating antibody to acetylcholine receptors, present in 90% of cases. A transient response to intravenous edrophonium (Tensilon) is usual (Figure 27.4). Enhancement of the quantity of acetylcholine at the neuromuscular junction can be achieved using

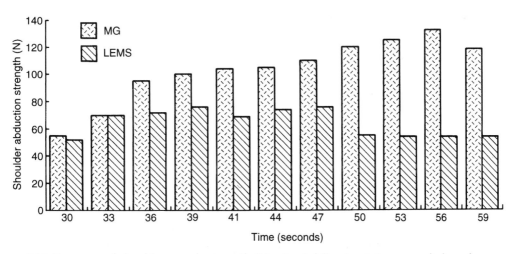

Figure 27.4 Response of shoulder muscle strength (Newtons) following intravenous bolus of edrophonium chloride (Tensilon) 10 mg in myasthenia gravis (MG) and Lamber–Eaton Myasthenic Syndrome (LEMS).

acetylcholinesterase inhibitors (e.g. pyridostigmine). Often, immunosuppression using steroids, azathioprine or even plasma exchange is necessary. Myasthenia gravis is associated with hyperplasia and sometimes even tumour of the thymus gland. Thymectomy is indicated for any myasthenic patient with thymoma and also for patients with antibody-positive generalized myasthenia presenting aged less than about 50 years.

Myasthenic syndromes

The best-known example is Lambert–Eaton myasthenic syndrome (O'Neill, Murray and Newson Davis, 1988). This is also an antibody-mediated neuromuscular junction disorder usually, in adults, associated with an underlying small cell carcinoma of the bronchus. Antibodies to the voltage-gated calcium channels on the tumour cell surface cross-react with the calcium channels on the motor nerve terminals, impairing acetylcholine release. It is distinguished clinically from myasthenia by the predominant limb involvement (though ptosis is usual), autonomic involvement including dry mouth and temporary enhancement of diminished reflexes and strength following a sustained voluntary contraction. There is a partial Tensilon response (Figure 27.4). Treatment is first to remove any underlying malignancy and, if still necessary, to enhance acetylcholine release using oral 3 : 4 diaminopyridine (McEvoy *et al*, 1989).

Hereditary neuromuscular junction disorders

Congenital myasthenia

This is a rare group of inherited non-immune disorders presenting in early childhood with ptosis, ophthalmoplegia, feeding difficulties and apnoeic episodes.

PERIPHERAL NEUROPATHY

The term 'peripheral neuropathy' covers disorders ranging from mononeuropathy and radiculopathy to widespread polyneuropathy and has been reviewed in detail (Dyck and Thomas, 1993). Here the advances in the understanding of the genetically determined neuropathies and the more treatable acquired forms, is addressed.

Hereditary neuropathies

The nosology of the hereditary peripheral neuropathies has changed with increasing knowledge of their genetics. For example, the clinical syndrome formerly known as Charcot–Marie–Tooth disease is now recognized to comprise several distinct disorders, the main three being hereditary motor and sensory neuropathy types I and II and distal spinal muscular atrophy.

Hereditary motor and sensory neuropathy (HMSN)

HMSN types I and II are autosomal dominant conditions with similar clinical presentations, distinguished by their neurophysiological characteristics. In each case the onset is usually before the age of 10 years, with initially distal wasting and weakness, particularly of the legs. Deep tendon reflexes are lost and there is altered distal sensation particularly to light touch, vibration and position sense. Pes cavus and scoliosis occasionally occur. Although equally prevalent in the two sexes, HMSN may be more severe in males.

HMSN type I is distinguished from type II by slowed motor (Harding and Thomas, 1980) and sensory nerve conduction and by evidence of nerve biopsy demyelination and remyelination, with 'onion bulb' formation. The molecular basis for the HMSNs has been clarified recently, considerable genetic heterogeneity existing even within the known clinical subgroups. Seventy per cent of HMSN type I are associated with a tandem DNA duplication of the 17p 11.2–12 gene (HMSN-1A) encoding peripheral nerve myelin protein PMP22. Most of the remainder map to chromosome 1 (HMSN-1B) and to the X chromosome (HMSN-X).

Treatment is symptomatic but again with emphasis upon genetic advice to other family members.

Hereditary liability to pressure palsies

This is a related though milder condition due to a deletion of the PMP22 gene. The patient presents, usually as an adult, with pressure palsies for example ulnar or common peroneal, which slowly, often incompletely, resolve. Nerve conduction studies show slowed conduction in asymptomatic nerves. The treatment priority is to protect vulnerable superficial nerves from further trauma, for example by wearing foam elbow or knee supports to aid healing of these nerves.

Non-hereditary neuropathies

The availability of treatment for several groups of neuropathy in recent years has given new purpose to the detailed investigation of peripheral neuropathy. Whilst it has long been recognized that vasculitic inflammatory neuropathy improves with immunosuppressive treatment, other treatable inflammatory neuropathies have recently been distinguished.

Chronic inflammatory demyelinating polyradiculoneuropathy

This condition presents with motor and sensory symptoms, gradually progressive over at least 2 months. The arms may be more involved than the legs. The reflexes are diminished or absent. Nerve conduction studies show evidence of demyelination and nerve biopsy may show active demyelination with an inflammatory cell infiltrate. Some patients have an IgG monoclonal gammopathy. The condition usually responds to high dose steroids or to intravenous pooled gamma globulin infusions, although about half of cases subsequently relapse and require repeated treatments.

Chronic demyelinating peripheral neuropathy

These disorders also offer potential for immunosuppressive treatment. The usually elderly patient presents with progressive, predominantly sensory, limb symptoms, sometimes with severe sensory ataxia. Nerve biopsy shows demyelination without inflammation. Most cases show an associated 'benign' monoclonal gammopathy, usually IgM and half show antibodies to myelin-associated glycoprotein (MAG). Often the condition is mild and specific treatment unnecessary but steroids or intravenous immunoglobulin can produce a limited response in progressive cases. Those without anti-MAG antibodies respond best to treatment (Glass and Cornblath, 1994).

Multifocal motor neuropathy

Multifocal motor neuropathy with conduction block, as defined electrophysiologically, is important since it can mimic motor neurone disease yet is readily treatable with immunosuppression. It presents with patchy, asymmetrical wasting, weakness and fasciculations, often most marked in the upper limbs (Krarup *et al*, 1990). The reflexes are preserved but, unlike motor neurone disease, not brisk. Circulating anti-ganglioside antibodies are occasionally seen.

ANTERIOR HORN CELL DISORDERS

The anterior horn cells are the motor neurones in the anterior horn grey matter of the spinal cord; they are sometimes referred to as the lower motor neurones.

Hereditary anterior horn cell disorders

Autosomal recessive spinal muscular atrophy

Several inherited conditions, known as the spinal muscular atrophies (SMA) are associated with depletion or degeneration of the anterior horn cell neurones. SMA is one of the commonest autosomal recessive conditions in Europe. Clinically, it can cause diagnostic confusion with muscular dystrophy although it is distinguished by the presence of fasciculations and early loss of deep tendon reflexes. The traditional division of the SMAs into the severe 'acute' infant-onset form (Werdnig–Hoffmann disease), the milder 'subacute' juvenile-onset form (Kugelberg–Welander disease) and the 'chronic' adult-onset form has been blurred by the knowledge that all these conditions map to the same gene, 5q12–14 (Gillam *et al.*, 1990). Most cases of Werdnig–Hoffmann disease are homozygous for the genetic abnormality and show a high probability of parental consanguinity whereas Kugelberg–Welander disease indicates genetic heterozygosity.

X-linked bulbo-spinal neuronopathy

The importance of this rare variant of SMA is that it can mimic motor neurone disease although with a much more benign course and with little effect on longevity. Typically, adult males present with weakness and wasting of bulbar and facial musculature, proximal limb weakness, cramps, tremor and gynaecomastia. The diagnosis can be confirmed by detecting an abnormal trinucleotide repeat (CAG) in the androgen receptor gene.

Distal spinal muscular atrophy

This disorder represents 10% of the SMAs. It can mimic the Charcot–Marie–Tooth phenotype although is distinguished by the normal sensation and sensory nerve action potentials and by only minor slowing of peripheral motor conduction velocity.

Monomelic spinal muscular atrophy

This is a rare adult-onset condition in which wasting of an arm or leg occurs, almost always in men, apparently from anterior horn cell disease. It may run a very benign course and so its distinction from motor neurone disease is essential.

Non-hereditary anterior horn cell disorders

Motor neurone disease

Motor neurone disease is considered in detail elsewhere.

Post-poliomyelitis syndrome

The late development of new muscular weakness and atrophy in patients with previous paralytic poliomyelitis led to speculation that post-polio syndrome was a re-awakening of the disease. More likely, however, the disorder represents the effect of normal ageing on a depleted population of anterior horn cells, combined with the increased vulnerability of neurones previously partially damaged and supplying expanded motor units. In addition, there may be secondary myopathic changes in muscles already weakened by excessive demands. There is no evidence for viral persistence and no evidence that previous poliomyelitis predisposes to sporadic motor neurone disease. It has been comprehensively reviewed by Gawne and Halstead (1995).

Guillain–Barré syndrome

The Guillain–Barré syndrome (GBS) is the commonest cause of acute onset lower motor neurone weakness in adults. The onset is with progressive motor and sensory symptoms over less than 4 weeks and complete recovery is usual. An inflammatory autoimmune reaction against myelin gangliosides appears to damage the peripheral nerves and proximal nerve roots. Often, a preceding infection (e.g.

Campylobacter jejuni) or vaccination is reported. The cerebrospinal fluid protein is typically raised but without excess inflammatory cells. Nerve conduction studies may suggest patchy peripheral demyelination. A variant of GBS, known as acute motor axonal neuropathy and comprising 20% of cases, has a more rapid onset, a higher proportion of preceding *C. jejuni* infection, more frequent GM1 ganglioside antibodies and a generally worse prognosis (Gregson *et al*, 1991).

The Miller Fisher syndrome of acute ophthalmoplegia, ataxia and areflexia without limb weakness is considered a GBS variant; its diagnosis is assisted by its close association with the specific antibody to GQ1b ganglioside (Willison *et al*, 1993).

Careful monitoring and supportive treatment may be life-saving in GBS. Vital capacity must be monitored closely and elective ventilation instituted as necessary. Cardiac monitoring is advisable in the early stages as acute autonomic neuropathy can provoke cardiac arrhythmias. Plasma exchange and intravenous immunoglobulin are each of proven benefit in GBS (Van der Meche and Schmitz 1992), whereas, perhaps surprisingly, steroids are of no help. Prevention of deep venous thrombosis is very important. Acutely inflamed nerves may be unusually vulnerable to pressure palsies and foam elbow supports may be appropriate early in the illness. Depression, common in severely affected patients, may require medication.

Although the overall prognosis for complete recovery is good, fatalities and long-term disability still occur. Factors suggesting a poor prognosis are increasing age, a preceding *C. jejuni* infection, evidence of axonal damage, rapid onset of weakness and the need for assisted ventilation. Winer *et al* (1985) reported 51 out of 71 patients had some difficulty with walking 1 year after onset of the illness. Rees (1995) discussing recent management of the condition noted a mortality of 5% but 80% of the patients made a full recovery. A further recent review is by

McKhann (1990). Roper and Alani (1995) discussed 49 patients who had recurrence of the condition, although this is relatively uncommon.

Physiotherapy can help to prevent chest infections and contractures and aid mobility. As strength gradually improves resisted exercises are started to restore muscle strength, the patient is mobilized on a tilt table, and only slowly brought to the upright position, otherwise postural hypotension may occur, due partly to voluntary muscle weakness and partly to autonomic dysfunction. Persistent flaccid drop-foot requires ankle–foot orthoses (Chapter 47).

Even when the patient has survived the acute stage of the illness there may still be need for prolonged physiotherapy and sometimes the use of orthoses, walking aids or car modifications (Chapters 47, 48 and 50). The residual disability may require changes in lifestyle, work and social activities. Even with good recovery and no relapse, fatigue may persist for at least 12–18 months.

ATAXIAS

Hereditary ataxias

The inherited ataxias were reclassified on clinical grounds in the 1980s (Harding, 1983). Improved knowledge of their genetics has allowed an increasingly rational classification.

Recessively inherited ataxias

Friedreich's ataxia This is the major cause of childhood-onset ataxia. It is autosomal recessive, mapping to chromosome 9. The child presents at a mean age of 10 years with cerebellar ataxia, accompanied variously by dysarthria, pyramidal weakness, absent or reduced reflexes, extensor plantar responses and impaired position sense. About half develop symptoms of cardiomyopathy; all show absent or reduced amplitude sensory nerve potentials. A few develop deafness, optic atrophy or diabetes (Ackroyd, Finnegan and Green, 1984).

Spastic ataxia of childhood   This condition can be distinguished from Friedreich's ataxia by the retained reflexes, normal sensory nerve conduction and absence of cardiomyopathy

Autosomal dominant late-onset cerebellar ataxias (ADCA)

The classification of this varied group of disorders (Harding, 1993) is evolving from descriptive to genetic as knowledge of their genetic substrates advances. For example, the clinically defined ADCA type I includes at least four genetic mutations now known as spinocerebellar ataxia (SCA) types 1–4. A genetic classification also brings unexpected problems. SCA3 and Machado–Joseph disease, for example, previously were considered as separate disorders but both map to the same unstable triplet repeat sequence (CAG) on chromosome 14q. The same mutation has also been identified in a family with little ataxia but with parkinsonism, peripheral neuropathy and dystonia (Guinti, Sweeney and Harding, 1995). The clinical phenotypes of the major autosomal dominant ataxias are considered here.

ADCA type I (spinocerebellar atrophy) This presents aged 20–50 with gait disturbance, dysarthria and, almost invariably, truncal ataxia, hyperreflexia and nystagmus. As the disorder progresses, limb ataxia and dysarthria predominate and the nystagmus lessens. The four genetic varieties are clinically indistinguishable.

Olivopontocerebellar atrophy   This is a descriptive term covering the remainder of the ADCA type I phenotype whose genetic loci are undefined. The onset is aged 20–60 years with ataxic gait and dysarthria, diminished reflexes, eye movement disorder and often extrapyramidal features (akinetic-rigid syndrome). Its genetic heterogeneity is emphasized by the variability of associated features, including optic atrophy, supranuclear gaze palsy, dementia and akinetic-rigid syndrome; sometimes these even occur in otherwise unaffected relatives (Bundy, 1992).

ADCA type 2 and ADCA type 3   These terms respectively refer to ADCA with pigmentary macular dystrophy (Enevoldson, Sanders and Harding, 1994) and a pure cerebellar syndrome.

Machado–Joseph disease   This condition has, until recently (see above), been considered a discrete entity characterized by progressive ataxia, pyramidal and extrapyramidal signs and sometimes staring eyes, facial and tongue fasciculations, and peripheral muscle wasting.

Dentatorubropallidoluysian atrophy   This is another triplet repeat disorder (chromosome 12p) and presenting with myoclonic epilepsy, ataxia, chorea and dementia.

Non-hereditary ataxias

Damage to the cerebellum and its central connections in the brainstem can result from many causes, although is most commonly seen with vascular lesions or demyelination.

MOVEMENT DISORDERS

Hereditary movement disorders

Dystonias

Despite apparently normal central and peripheral motor function, patients with dystonia exhibit repeated involuntary, often bizarre, posturing and movements when attempting to use a muscle group. Until surprisingly recently many of the dystonias were considered to have a strong psychological component. Despite real advances in the understanding of the genetics and treatment of dystonia, the condition remains one of the enigmas of neurology. Although there appears to be a common genetic aetiology, the dystonias show a bimodal age of onset, the more severe generalized condition occurring only in children and the less severe focal dystonias predominantly in adults.

Idiopathic torsion dystonia This childhood-onset condition, formerly known as dystonia musculorum deformans, begins with abnormal posturing in the legs and feet. In severe cases, it spreads to involve the whole body and results in major disability.

Focal dystonia This is the cause of most adult-onset dystonias, involving either the cranial musculature or occurring in association with certain occupations. Cranial dystonia comprises spasmodic torticollis (jerky movements of the head to one side), blepharospasm (repetitive or sustained forcible eye closure), oromandibular and laryngeal dystonia, any or all of which can occur in a patient. The full house of cranial dystonia is known as Bruegel's syndrome after Pieter Bruegel the Elder's *The Yawner* (1577), a portrait of a gaping man with apparent blepharospasm (Marsden, 1976). Occupational dystonias, or 'craft palsies', include writer's cramp (involuntary limb movements on attempting to write) and various conditions associated with occupational repetitive movements best recognized in musicians. Occasionally a focal dystonia in a limb follows an episode of trauma; involuntary repetitive movements are well recognized in amputation stumps.

Genetics of dystonia All idiopathic dystonias appear to be autosomal dominantly inherited, mapping to chromosome 9q32–34 (Gasser, Farn and Breakfield, 1992). The abnormal gene shows a penetrance of only 40%. A widely variable clinical presentation is often seen even within single families, unexplained by environmental factors (Fletcher, Harding and Marsden, 1991). This variability makes it difficult to give clear genetic advice to affected families.

Treatment of dystonia A correct diagnosis of idiopathic dystonia is clearly imperative and investigations to exclude rare but more treatable conditions, such as Wilson's disease, must be considered. Until the mid-1980s, dystonia was largely untreatable. Partial response to anticholinergic agents in high doses can be obtained, but with troublesome side-effects.

The recognition that a subgroup of generalized dystonia, characterized by diurnal variation of symptoms (Segawa *et al*, 1976), dramatically responds to L-dopa, led to some miraculous cures. Since this disorder is clinically indistinguishable from idiopathic torsion dystonia, it is now considered imperative to give a trial of L-dopa to all patients presenting with generalized dystonia (Nygaard, Marsden and Duvoisin, 1988).

The major breakthrough in dystonia treatment has been the therapeutic use of botulinum toxin (Jancovic and Brin, 1991), which is now the treatment of first choice. Injections of the toxin derived from Clostridium botulinum into affected muscles can bring about significant improvement in focal dystonia, sustained for about 3 months before repeat injection becomes necessary. Despite the injection of the most potent known biological toxin, surprisingly few problems are encountered and there appear to be no major long-term sequelae to repeated injections.

Surgery to ablate the motor nerve supply to affected muscles is still under investigation but might be considered for severe cases resistant to botulinum toxin.

Huntington's disease

Clinical features Huntington's disease (HD) is a slowly progressive autosomal dominant neurodegenerative disorder of adult onset. The first symptoms appear at a mean age of between 35 and 44 years typically with involuntary non-stereotyped jerky movements (chorea) together with gradually progressive cognitive decline and personality change; death occurs prematurely after about 15 years from onset (Harper 1991). In the more severe juvenile-onset form (5–10% of cases), there may be severe behavioural disorder or frank psychosis: rigidity is more likely than chorea and there may be epilepsy or cerebellar signs. CT brain scan shows cerebral atrophy, particularly of the caudate nucleus heads (Figure 27.5). The investigation of patients with chorea has been enormously

facilitated by the availability of a diagnostic genetic blood test for HD; the diagnosis can now be confidently made even without a family history.

Genetics HD is caused by an unstable trinucleotide repeat (CAG) at the gene locus 4p16.3 (Huntington's Disease Collaborative Research Group, 1993). The repeat length correlates with the clinical features, the more expanded repeats (usually from the father) being associated with earlier age of onset and more severe disease (Kremer *et al*, 1994).

Treatment As with many genetic disorders, the priority of treatment in HD is the provision

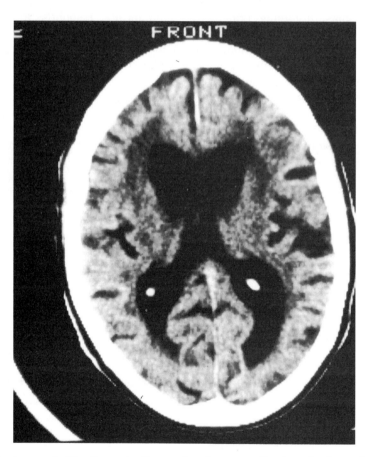

Figure 27.5 CT brain scan in Huntington's disease showing generalized cerebral atrophy and characteristic atrophy of the caudate heads.

of accurate genetic advice to other family members who have yet to plan their families. The persistence of Huntington's disease in the population is largely the consequence of its late presentation; most patients have finished their families and may well be grandparents at the time of their diagnosis. The temptation by the patient to suppress knowledge of the disease can only compound the family's difficulties. Important ethical principles must be applied to asymptomatic predictive testing for HD and an extended protocol of counselling should be followed.

The mental changes of HD are unresponsive to medication although the possibility of additional depression must be considered as in any dementia. The chorea can be very troublesome but so can the side-effects of therapeutic attempts to suppress it. If treatment is necessary, tetrabenazine or haloperidol, alone or in combination, are the preferred choices although sedation, lethargy, inattention or depression can occur. Sometimes, stopping such treatments gives surprising benefit.

REFERENCES

Ackroyd, R.S., Finnegan, J.A. and Green, S.H. (1984). Friedrech's ataxia, a clinical review with neurophysiological and echocardiographic findings. *Archives of Disease in Childhood*, **89**, 217–21.

Arahata, K., Ishii, H. and Hayashi, Y.K. (1995) Congenital muscular dystrophies. *Current Opinion in Neurology*, **8**, 385–90.

Argov, Z. and Mastaglia, F.L. (1994) Drug induced neuromuscular disorders in man, in *Disorders of Voluntary Muscle*, 6th edn (eds J.N. Walton, G. Karpati and D. Hilton-Jones), Churchill Livingstone, Edinburgh, pp. 898–1029.

Behan, W.M.H. (1996) Chronic fatigue syndrome – diagnosis and treatment. *Rheumatology in Practice*, **3**, 12–16.

Brouwer, O.F., Padberg, G.W., van der Ploeg, R.J.O., Ruyes, C.J.M. and Brand, R. (1992). The influence of handedness on the distribution of muscular weakness of the arm in facioscapulohumeral muscular dystrophy. *Brain*, **115**, 1587–98.

Bunch, W.H. and Siegel, I.M. (1993) Scapulothoracic arthrodesis in facioscapulohumeral muscular dystrophy. Review of seventeen procedures with three to twenty one year follow-up *Journal of Bone and Joint Surgery, American Volume*, **75**, 372–6.

Bundy, S. (1992) Genetics and Neurology 2nd edn, Churchill Livingstone, Edinburgh.

Buxton, J., Shelbourne, P., Davies, J. *et al* (1992) Detection of an unstable fragment of DNA specific to individuals with myotonic dystrophy. *Nature*, **355**, 547–8.

Comi, G.P., Prelle, A., Bresolin, N. *et al.* (1994) Clinical variability in Becker muscular dystrophy. Genetic, biochemical and immunohistochemical correlates. *Brain*, **117**, 1–14.

Dalakas, M.C., (1991) Polymyositis, Dermatomyositis and inclusion body myositis. *New England Journal of Medicine*, **325**, 1487–98.

Dyck, P.J. and Thomas, P.K. (1993), *Peripheral Neuropathies*, WB Saunders, Philadelphia.

Editorial (1991) Of stiff men and sweet mice: GAD and diabetes. *Lancet*, **338**, 1428–9.

Editorial (1992) The heart in myotonic dystrophy *Lancet*, **339**, 528–9.

Edwards, R.H.T., Round, J.M., Jackson, M.J., Griffiths, R.D. and Lilburn, M.F. (1984) Weight reduction in boys with muscular dystrophy. *Developmental Medicine and Child Neurology*, **26**, 384–90.

Enevoldson, T.P., Sanders, M.D. and Harding, A.E. (1994) Autosomal dominant cerebellar ataxia with pigmentary macular dystrophy: a clinical and genetic study of eight families. *Brain*, **117**, 445–60.

Fitzsimons, R.B. (1994) Facioscapulohumeral dystrophy: the role of inflammation (editorial). *Lancet*, **344**, 902–3.

Fitzsimons, R.B., Gurwin, E.B. and Bird, A.C. (1987) Retinal vascular abnormalities in facioscapulohumeral muscular dystrophy. *Brain*, **110**, 631–48.

Fletcher, N.A., Harding, A.E. and Marsden, C.D. (1991) Intrafamilial correlation in idiopathic torsion dystonia. *Movement Disorders*, **6**, 310–14.

Garlepp, M.J. and Mastaglia, F.L. (1996) Inclusion body myositis (editorial). *Journal of Neurology, Neurosurgery and Psychiatry*, **60**, 251–5.

Gasser, T., Fahn, S. and Breakfield, X.O. (1992) The autosomal dominant dystonias. *Brain Pathology*, **2**, 297–308.

Gawne, A.C. and Halstead, L.S. (1995) Post-polio syndrome: pathophysiology and clinical management. *Critical Reviews in Physical and Rehabilitation Medicine*, **7**, 147–88.

Gibson, H., Carroll, N., Clague, J.E. and Edwards,

R.H.T. (1993) Exercise performance and fatigu-ability in patients with chronic fatigue syn-drome. *Journal of Neurology, Neurosurgery and Psychiatry*, **56**, 993–8.

Gillam, T.C., Brzustowicz, L.M., Castilla, L.H. *et al.* (1990) Genetic homogeneity between acute and chronic forms of spinal muscular atrophy. *Nature*, **345**, 823–5.

Glass, J.D. and Cornblath, D.R. (1994) Chronic inflammatory demyelinating polyneuropathy and paraproteinemic neuropathies. *Current Opinion in Neurology*, **7**, 393–7.

Gowers, W.R. (1879) *Pseudo-hypertrophic Muscular Paralysis – a clinical lecture*, J & A Churchill, London.

Gregson, N.A., Jones, D., Thomas, P.K. and Will-ison, H.J. (1991) Acute motor neuropathy with antibody to GM1 ganglioside. *Neurology*, **238**, 447–541.

Guinti, P., Sweeney, M.G. and Harding, A.E. (1995) Detection of the Machado–Joseph disease/spinocerebellar ataxia three trinucleo-tide repeat expansion in families with auto-somal dominant motor disorders, including the Drew family of Walworth. *Brain*, **118**, 1077–85.

Harding, A.E. (1983) Classification of the heredi-tary ataxias and paraplegias. *Lancet*, **i**, 151–5.

Harding, A.E. (1993) Clinical features and classifi-cation of inherited ataxias. *Advances in Neu-rology*, **61**, 1–14.

Harding, A.E. and Thomas, P.K. (1980) The clin-ical features of motor and sensory neuropathies types I and II. *Brain*, **103**, 2599–280.

Harding, A.E., Thompson, P.D., Kocen, R.S., Bathcelor, J.R., Davey, N. and Marsden, C.D. (1989) Plasma exchange and immunosuppres-sion in the stiff man syndrome. *Lancet*, **ii**, 91–5.

Harper, P.S. (1979) Myotonic dystrophy in *Major Problems in Neurology*, vol 9, W.B. Saunders, Philadelphia, pp. 321–344.

Harper, P.S. (ed.) (1991) The natural history of Huntington's disease, *Huntington's disease*, W.B. Saunders, London, pp. 127–139.

Huntington's Disease Collaborative Research Group *Major problems in neurosurgery* vol 11, (1993) A novel gene containing a trinucleo-tide repeat that is expanded and unstable on Huntington's Disease chromosomes. *Cell*, **72**, 971–83.

Jankovic, J. and Brin, M.F. (1991), Therapeutic uses of botulinum toxin. *New England Journal of Medicine*, **324**, 1186–94.

Kakulas, B.A. (1996) The differential diagnosis of the human dystrophinopathies and related dis-orders. *Current Opinion in Neurology*, **9**, 380–8.

Karpati, G., Ajdukovic, D., Arnold, D. *et al.* (1993) Myoblast transfer in Duchenne muscular dys-trophy. *Annals of Neurology*, **34**, 8–17.

Krarup, C., Stewart, J.D., Sumner, A.J., Pestronk, A. and Lipton, S.A. (1990) A syndrome of asymmetric limb weakness with motor conduc-tion block. *Neurology*, **40**, 118–27.

Kremer, H.P.H., Goldberg, Y.P., Andrew, S.E. *et al.* (1994) Worldwide study of the Huntington's disease mutation: the sensitivity and specificity of repeated CAG sequences. *New England Journal of Medicine*, **330**, 1401–6.

Lawrie, S.M. and Pelosi, A.J. (1994) Chronic fatigue syndrome: prevalence and outcome (editorial). *British Medical Journal*, **308**, 732–3.

Lehmann-Horn, F. and Rudel, R. (1995) Heredi-tary nondystrophic myotonias and periodic paralyses. *Current Opinion in Neurology* **8**, 402–10.

McEvoy, K.M., Windebank, A.J. Daubent and Low, P.A. (1989) 3,4-diaminopyridine in the treatment of Lambert–Eaton myasthenic syn-drome. *New England Journal of Medicine*, **321**, 1567–71.

McKhann, G.M. (1990) Guillain Barré Syndrome: clinical and therapeutic observations. *Annals of Neurology*, **27**, (Suppl.), 13–16.

Marsden, C.D. (1976) Blepharospasm-oromandib-ular dystonia syndrome (Brueghel's syndrome). A variant of adult-onset torsion dystonia? *Journal of Neurology, Neurosurgory and Psy-chiatry*, **39**, 120–9.

Mastaglia, F.L. and Laing, N.G. (1996) Investiga-tion of muscle disease. *Journal of Neurology, Neurosurgery and Psychiatry*, **60**, 256–274.

Mendell, J.R., Moxley, R.T., Griggs, R.C. *et al.* (1989) Randomised double blind six month trial of prednisolone in Duchenne's muscular dystrophy. *New England Journal of Medicine*, **320**, 1592–7.

Monaco, A.P. and Kunkel, L.M. (1988) Cloning of the Duchenne/Becker muscular dystrophy locus, *Advances in Human Genetics* (eds H. Harris and K. Hirschhom), Plenum Press, New York pp. 61–98.

Morriss, R., Sharpe, M., Sharpley, A.L., Cowen, P.J., Hawton, K.K. and Morris, J. (1993) Abnormalities of sleep in patients with chronic fatigue syndrome. *British Medical Journal*, **306**, 1161–3.

Nagano, A., Koga, R., Ogawa, M. *et al.* (1996) Emerin deficiency at the nuclear membrane in patients with Emery-Dreifuss muscular dys-trophy. *Nature Genetics*, **12**, 254–9.

Noble-Jamieson, C.M., Heckmatt, J.Z., Dubowitz, V. and Silvemman, M. (1986) Effects of posture

28 Paraplegia and tetraplegia

W.S. El Masry

IMPAIRMENT, DISABILITY AND COMPLICATIONS

Impairment of cervical cord functions results in tetraplegia or paralysis in the upper and lower limbs. When the lesion is below the cervical spinal cord the upper limbs are spared and paraplegia or paralysis of the lower limbs will occur. Impairment of the spinal cord or cauda equina functions result also in impairment of functions in most body systems. In turn, each system malfunction causes a number of disabilities and potential complications. The cumulative effects of system malfunctions cause a wide range of disabilities and remain the source of many potential complications for the rest of the patient's life.

The terms paraplegia and tetraplegia are therefore hardly descriptive of the effects of neural dysfunction, as they do not encompass the multisystem impairment. Furthermore, the non-medical effects of the paralysis (psychosocial, financial, psychosexual,) usually extend beyond the paralysed individual. The partner, family members, relatives and friends, employer, community and society in general, are also affected.

Paraplegia and tetraplegia are either spastic or flaccid. This depends on the location of the lesion in the spinal cord/cauda equina and on the integrity of the vascular supply below the level of the lesion. A patient with a complete cauda equina lesion, or a patient who becomes paralysed following surgery on the aorta, is likely to have flaccid paralysis, while a patient with multiple sclerosis or a supra-lumbar traumatic lesion is likely to have spastic paralysis. Paraplegia and tetraplegia can be complete or partial, depending on the density of the lesion and the sparing of ascending and descending tracts in the spinal cord or nerve roots in the cauda equina.

DIAGNOSIS

The clinician should be able, from the history, clinical signs and investigations, to identify surgically or medically treatable pathologies, for example benign tumours (meningioma or neurofibroma), infection, epidural haemorrhage, acute disc protrusion and vitamin B_{12} deficiency, following the treatment of which the patient may improve. CT and MRI scanning have made this possible with greater ease than a few years ago. These two investigations are complementary as the CT scan will demonstrate the bone but not the soft tissue or the spinal cord, while MRI scanning will demonstrate the spinal cord and the soft tissue better than the bony element. A bone scan is also valuable in the detection of early infection and metastasis.

An accurate diagnosis whenever possible will also be helpful in determining the extent

Rehabilitation of the Physically Disabled Adult. Edited by C. John Goodwill, M. Anne Chamberlain and Chris Evans. Published in 1997 by Stanley Thornes (Publishers) Ltd, Cheltenham. ISBN 0-7487-3183-0.

of the impairment and disability as well as the course of the pathology and the disability. Paraplegia and tetraplegia are occasional complications of systemic diseases, such as rheumatoid arthritis, systemic lupus erythematosus, polyarteritis nodosa, sarcoidosis or Behçet's syndrome. Although acute polyneuritis (Guillain–Barré syndrome), paralytic polyneuritis, amyotrophic lateral sclerosis (motor neurone disease) and poliomyelitis can cause paraplegia and tetraplegia, in these conditions the bladder, bowels and autonomic functions are rarely impaired. A thorough neurological examination of these patients is unlikely to reveal a sensory level. A bulbar palsy on the other hand is likely to increase the disability with added requirements from the rehabilitation team. The relevance of a diagnosis is also necessary to determine the course of the disease (reversible, permanent or progressive) in order to counsel the patient and his/her carers and to acquire their cooperation with the planning and implementation of the rehabilitation process. Recovery of spinal cord function is rare following acute or subacute onset paralysis from transverse myelitis, spinal cord infarction, dissecting aortic aneurysm, epidural abscess and metastasis to the spine from carcinoma, leukaemia and reticulosis, but partial paralysis from pyogenic or tuberculous spinal disease may recover with prompt treatment. Although in general the course of multiple sclerosis is progressive, patients usually have remission followed by relapses. Progressive paralysis usually occurs with hereditary spastic paraplegia, syringomyelia, arachnoiditis, Friedreich's ataxia, amyotrophic lateral sclerosis and radiation myelopathy.

In traumatic paraplegia and tetraplegia the course of the paralysis varies depending on the density of the initial damage to the neural tissue and on the subsequent quality of treatment. What must be emphasized is whether the condition that has caused the paralysis will improve, deteriorate or become static. A dynamic and flexible rehabilitation infrastructure is required in order to minimize the impact of the disability on the patient and on the partner both in the short and in the long term.

NEUROLOGICAL ASSESSMENT

A detailed neurological assessment to determine the level of the lesion and the density of the lesion is important. In general, the higher the level of the lesion of the spinal cord the greater is the degree of disability. The patient with complete somatosensory loss is likely to be more at risk of certain complications like pressure sores than a patient who has some sparing of sensation. It is also important to determine whether the paralysis is spastic or flaccid, as the bodily functions may behave differently and require different treatment. The bladder of a patient with a spastic paraplegia below the level of T 10, for example, is likely to automatically empty itself, while a patient with a complete flaccid paralysis above the level of T10 is likely to require some form of bladder drainage on a permanent basis. Regular and frequent neurological assessments following discharge are important for the early detection and treatment of further neurological deterioration. For example, the incidence of post-traumatic syringomyelia following spinal injury is about 4.5%. Without early detection and treatment of this condition, a paraplegic patient can deteriorate and develop tetraplegia.

MULTISYSTEM IMPAIRMENT

The spinal cord is involved with the innervation of almost every system of the body; the interruption of its function usually results in paralysis associated with a multisystem impairment of functions. Examples of how the multisystem impairment of functions results in various disabilities and potential

Table 28.1 Examples of impairment, disability and potential complications caused by spinal paralysis

System impairment	Disability	Potential complications
Musculoskeletal	Paralysis Restricted mobility Limitation of independence Diminished ability of self-protection	Contractures of muscles, spasticity, pressure sores, osteoporosis, fractures of long bones, heterotrophic calcification
	Difficulty in fitting shoes	Oedema of lower limbs
	Sensation of fainting and weakness	Postural hypotension, pulmonary oedema, bradycardia, cardiac arrest, deep venous thrombosis, pulmonary embolism
	Fainting	Postural hypotension
Autonomic	Severe disabling headaches	Autonomic hyperreflexia
Urinary	Incontinence of urine	Skin sores, urinary tract infections, urinary tract calculi, renal failure, urethral strictures, diverticula, fistula
	Social embarrassment	Excess spasticity
Gastrointestinal	Incontinence of faeces and flatus	Constipation, haemorrhoids, anal fissure
Respiratory	Difficulty of breathing, weakness Inability to cough and expectorate	Upper respiratory tract infections, bronchopneumonia, respiratory failure
Sexuality and fertility	Alteration of mechanics of sexual activity Loss of pleasure Alteration of body image Male infertility	Autonomic hyperreflexia, anxiety, depression, disharmony

complications are demonstrated in Table 28.1.

Unfortunately, the behaviour of a pathological spinal cord is dynamic, labile and unstable (El Masry and Jaffray, 1992). This is usually reflected in the way the various systems of the body behave at various times. For example, during the stage of spinal shock the bladder wall is flaccid. Following return of reflex activity, the bladder wall contracts reflexly and empties some urine spontaneously. The return of this reflex activity is however slow and incremental. It may, therefore, take weeks or months before automatic voiding with low residual urine is achieved. The level of reflex activity in the spinal cord remains labile throughout the patient's life and can be a source of further disability and complications. For example, a patient who develops an ingrowing toenail or any other pathology below the level of the lesion is likely to develop excess spasticity. This is likely to interfere further with activities of daily living and may be the cause of complications such as contractures of muscles, pressure sores or long bone fractures. When the spasticity involves the pelvic floor muscles, urinary retention, infections and autonomic dysreflexia may occur. It is, therefore, common to have a cascade of complications after spinal injury arising from

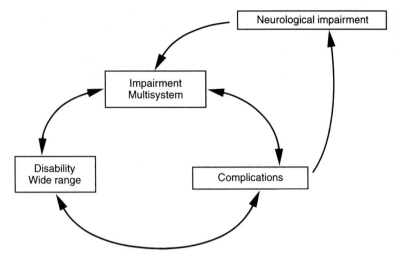

Figure 28.1 Interactions occurring in patient with spinal paralysis.

one system of the body and spreading to other systems causing further disability and complications.

A pathological spinal cord is physiologically unstable (El Masry, 1993) and vulnerable to complications outside its own vicinity. For example, infections, pyrexia, hypoxia and hypotension can cause neurological deterioration in a patient with multiple sclerosis or spinal cord injury. This may cause further disability and complications. A vicious circle of further impairment, disability and complications can therefore easily occur in the individual with spinal paralysis (Figure 28.1).

MANAGEMENT

The management of the tetraplegic and paraplegic patient requires planning by various members of a multidisciplinary team from the very early stages of paralysis. The clinician will establish a diagnosis and, whenever possible, treat the cause of the paralysis. Together with the physiotherapist, the occupational therapist and the nurse, the level and the degree of the neurological impairment and disability should be assessed taking into consideration the patient's age,

personal circumstances, prognosis, needs and potentials. Both the acute medical treatment and the rehabilitation process should, whenever possible, be commenced simultaneously from the onset of paralysis. The management of patients with paraplegia and tetraplegia should ensure the following:

- Maintenance of good general health of the patient.
- The choice of a suitable treatment for each of the systems impaired, including the paralysis, should be tailored to the individual patient.
- It is paramount that established complications are diagnosed and treated as soon as they occur in order to prevent further impairment and disability.
- It is essential that the programme of physical, psychological and social rehabilitation is comprehensive and well coordinated. This should include the provision of the necessary equipment, education, training and appropriate support to the individual and partner/carer. It is important to establish an environment which allows individual personal growth and development (Schalock and Kiernan, 1990).

• Management must ensure that the patient suffers no further iatrogenic disability from complications that could have been prevented and that abilities are maximized within the limitation of the neurological impairment and disability. A partnership between the patient and the team is essential to achieve these goals. An education programme using simple lay terms and, whenever possible, pictures and diagrams about bodily functions, the impairment sustained and the methods of management is almost always rewarding to patients and clinicians alike. This usually results in better cooperation from the patient and facilities the often arduous rehabilitation process.

Fact finding about the patient

This process should commence at a very early stage and usually extends over the first few weeks of paralysis. Information is gathered from the patient, his/her partner, relatives and friends. The collection of information is usually done formally by the clinician. However, informal information gathering by any member of the team should be encouraged. The marital status of the patient, employment, accommodation, hobbies, education and financial status are important factors that can influence the outcome of treatment and rehabilitation. A visit by a member of the team to the patient's home is very useful. Often advice is required on home alterations to facilitate access and mobility as well as to ensure health and safety. Assessment of the community resources and liaison with the community services from an early stage has many advantages. It reduces the anxieties and concerns of the patient and the family members, enhances their motivation, reduces hospitalization time and often reduces the frequency of re-hospitalization post-discharge.

Psychological assessment

A formal psychological assessment is not always necessary. A psychologist should, however, be available for assessment of cognitive functions, attention, orientation and learning when necessary. Impairment of any of these functions is likely to influence the planning of management, the rehabilitation process, the goals to be achieved and the subsequent support the patient will require. The trauma these patients sustain is both psychological and physical. The combination of sensory deprivation, paralysis and loss of control over bodily functions is both frightening and degrading. Not knowing what the future holds and the perception of loss of control over one's life is unsettling and disturbing.

One of the main advantages of treating paraplegic and tetraplegic patients together in relatively large numbers is the peer support that the patient and the relatives obtain from other patients and their relatives. This support from an early stage helps minimize anxiety, increase confidence and enhance the necessary motivation the patient and family usually require to battle through the often arduous and periodically frustrating rehabilitation process. Attention to the patient mix is, however, important in order to avoid inappropriate expectations and/or unnecessary depression and frustration. For example, patients with non-deteriorating paralysis such as transverse myelitis, benign tumours or spinal injuries usually mix well because they have similar expectations of outcome. Patients with deteriorating conditions such as motor neurone disease, metastasis to the spine or chronic myelopathies do not mix well with patients whose conditions are stable. Both groups of patients tend to compare progress and outcome to everybody's disadvantage. The two groups can be treated in the same institution but in different wards. Despite the appropriate patient mix, each patient ought to be encouraged to use his/her own strategy for coping. Anger, denial, over-assertiveness, blame and depressive moods should not be regarded as abnormal reactions following spinal cord paralysis. Transference of anger to medical and paramedical staff is not unusual. Psychological support should be made available to staff as well as patients when required.

General health

The general health of the patient is almost always at risk because of complications related to the multisystem impairment. Poor general health can also cause complications in patients with paraplegia and tetraplegia. Untreated anaemia, diabetes or a protein-deficient diet are likely to result in further weakness of the non-paralysed muscles as well as impairment of motivation and neglect of self-care. This can increase the risk of pressure sores, urinary infections and contractures of paralysed muscles. Hypertension, anaemia or diabetes are common coexisting conditions in the higher age group of patients with non-traumatic paralysis and require special medical attention. There may be undue sensitivity to drugs used in hypertension.

Depending on the cause of paralysis and general health, the patient may require a period of bedrest. During the period of bedrest, the patient requires regular turning. This is beneficial for the prevention of pressure sores and also for postural drainage of the bronchi. Passive movements, with appropriate positioning of the paralysed limbs, helps prevent contractures of muscles and limitation of range of movement in the joints. Patients without instability of the spinal column would benefit from a period of lying prone, with the ankles kept at a right angle, avoiding plantarflexion. This helps to stretch the knees and hips and avoid the development of contractures of hip and knee flexors.

Following traumatic spinal injuries, deep venous thrombosis and pulmonary embolism (El Masry and Silver, 1981) may necessitate the administration of prophylactic oral anticoagulant therapy (warfarin) during the period of bedrest. This is advisable in acute and subacute tetraplegia and paraplegia. Close monitoring of the level of anticoagulation is essential since patients are also at risk of developing gastrointestinal bleeding from stress ulcers (El Masry, Cochrane and Silver, 1982) as well as haemothorax (Gopalakrishnan and El Masry, 1986). If the paralysis is due to an epidural haemorrhage, anticoagulation is not advisable. If paralysis is associated with paralytic ileus as in the early stages of traumatic spinal injury, subcutaneous heparin is commenced until the bowel sounds return, when oral anticoagulants should be commenced. Once the International Normalization Ratio (INR) is in the therapeutic range subcutaneous heparin may be discontinued.

Early mobilization of patients with traumatic paralysis above the level of T6 during the stage of spinal shock is likely to result in postural hypotension, reduced vital capacity and possible neurological deterioration (El Masry and Jaffray, 1992). Pyrexia in a paraplegic or tetraplegic patient is often a clinical challenge, as the patient is unable to feel pain and direct the clinician to its origin. The commonest causes of pyrexia are urinary or chest infections. It is advisable to secure an intravenous line for hydration as delays may cause difficulties in finding a vein if autonomic hyperreflexia occurs. Pain and the conventional clinical signs are often unreliable in these patients. The spasticity may be increased in the initial stages but when the patient becomes very ill, spasticity may become greatly diminished. A patient who is pyrexial and who complains of pain in the tip of the shoulder may have an intra-abdominal pathology such as a perforated ulcer (Walsh, Nuseibah and El Masry, 1973).

Impairment of respiratory function

Impaired breathing is probably one of the commonest causes of morbidity and mortality in patients will paraplegia and tetraplegia. Bergofsky (1964) reported that in normal subjects expansion of the rib cage appears to be responsible for 60% of the tidal volume and descent of the diaphragm accomplishes the remaining 40%. Tetraplegic patients have impairment of rib cage expansion due to the paralysis of the intercostal muscles and the rib cage moves paradoxically (Moulton and Silver, 1970). Patients with paralysis of the abdominal muscles have weakness of forced expiration. The patient's ability to cough, expectorate and clear their bronchi is impaired. Retention of secretions and poor alveolar ventilation can result in chest infections, bronchopneumonia and respiratory failure. Prophylactic antibiotics are not advisable for the prevention of these complications unless there is a pre-existing chest problem. Deep breathing exercises, postural drainage of the lungs, vibration and percussion of the chest wall and assisted coughing reduce these complications significantly. A mini-tracheotomy inserted under local anaesthesia may further facilitate the suction of secretions (Gupta *et al.*, 1989). Patient-triggered intermittent positive pressure breathing (IPPB) to assist the patient during inspiration can be used prophylactically to improve ventilation and perfusion. It should, however, be avoided in patients with bronchospasm, asthma, pneumothorax, haemothorax or paralytic ileus.

Patients with good motor power in the deltoid and elbow flexors are able, with training, to assist their cough and clear their respiratory tubes by self-assisted coughing. This is achieved by triggering a spasm in the abdominal muscles and enhancing the abdominal pressure by pushing both wrists under the diaphragm. Patients with spinal cord pathology above the level of C4 are likely to have paralysis of one or both diaphragm. Training of the accessory muscles of respiration is, therefore, essential. When both phrenic nerve functions are impaired a tracheostomy and ventilation will be required. The patient with a lower motor neurone lesion of the phrenic nerve is likely to require ventilation for life. A portable ventilator fitted to the wheelchair will enable the patient to retain mobility. Some patients with a previously healthy respiratory system are able to maintain ventilation with hemidiaphragm paralysis. When the spinal cord lesion is above the level of the anterior horn cells of the phrenic nerves (C3 to C5), electrophrenic nerve respiration can be achieved by implanting electrodes on the phrenic nerves (Glenn and Phelps, 1985). The patient achieves ventilator independence for substantial periods of time during the day.

Impairment of the autonomic nervous system

The autonomic nervous system outflow which traverses all regions of the spinal cord is impaired in all patients with spinal cord lesions. The activity of the autonomic nervous system, however, is also dependent on the afferent nervous system. Activation of viscera, skin and muscle receptors also influences the efferent outflow in the spinal man (Mathias and Frankel, 1988). In general, there are three factors that govern the effects of the autonomic impairment in paralysed patients. The level of the lesion, the speed at which the lesion develops and the completeness of the damage to the spinal cord at the site of the lesion. Lesions in the cervical spine or above the 5th thoracic spinal cord segment will affect the autonomic supply to the heart. Sudden complete cord lesions are usually followed by a period of autonomic areflexia before the reflex activity of the autonomic system returns. Lesions that spare longitudinal tracts often result in relatively less autonomic dysfunction. Acute onset complete lesions above the level of T5 result in an overall reduction in sympathetic nervous activity which is reflected in low plasma noradrenaline and adrenaline levels (Mathias *et al.*, 1979). In the stage of spinal shock, the patient usually has low blood pressure and bradycardia. The hypotension does not as a rule warrant corrective measures; however, even a minor degree of bleeding or dehydration or indeed a degree of head-up tilt may substantially lower the blood pressure further. On the other hand, restraint is recommended in attempting to correct the hypotension with excess intravenous fluid since the failure of the autonomic reflexes to respond to hypervolaemia is likely to result in pulmonary oedema and congestive heart failure. Reflex bradycardia during tracheal suction in recently injured tetraplegic patients (Frankel, Mathias and Spalding, 1975), hypothermia (Pledger, 1962) and hypoxia could lead to cardiac arrest. Atropine 0.3 mg IV should be at hand and administered intravenously if the pulse rate falls below 40 per minute.

Peripheral vasodilatation may predispose to increased vascular permeability, venous stasis, subcutaneous oedema and skin breakdown. This is further aggravated by the loss of the pumping action of the paralysed muscles, especially during the stage of spinal shock and when the paralysis is flaccid. Long-term gravitational oedema can be minimized by treatment of the patient in recumbency until the reflexes return by gradual tilting up of the patient in bed prior to mobilization, frequent elevation of the legs during the initial stages of mobilization and the use of elastic stockings. Postural hypotension occurs due to the impairment of baroreceptor reflexes following transection of descending sympathetic pathways. This occurs during the initial stages of mobilization with complete lesion of the spinal cord. The treatment is similar to that of gravitational oedema. In addition, the use of an abdominal binder usually helps. The symptoms diminish with frequent tilt (Guttman, 1976). Tilting the wheelchair back-wards helps to elevate the blood pressure and reduces the feeling of faintness. Oral ephedrine 15 mg may be administered about an hour prior to mobilization when postural hypotension has not resolved within a period of 2–3 weeks. The injudicious use of ephedrine should be avoided as this could contribute to excess activity in the bladder outlet and urinary retention.

Thermogenesis is impaired as the patient is unable to shiver in a cold environment below the level of the lesion. This, together with peripheral vasodilatation caused by the sympathetic inactivity, may lower the core temperature substantially. A persistent bradycardia may provide a vital clue to hypothermia. This may be missed if oral temperature is recorded (Pledger, 1962). The temperature should, therefore, be monitored with a low reading rectal thermometer.

Autonomic dysreflexia affects patients with complete tetraplegia and paraplegia, usually above the level of T5. It occurs due to the activation of afferent pathways from organs supplied by the sympathetic and parasympathetic nervous system. This results in an uncoordinated autonomic discharge which causes constriction of blood vessels, high blood pressure, bradycardia and cold limbs. This condition can occur suddenly in a previously asymptomatic patient. The patient complains of a throbbing headache, sweats profusely, becomes vasoconstricted below the level of the lesion and has a striking vasodilatation in the face and neck. The commonest causes are acute retention of urine, an acute viscus dilatation, during electro-ejaculation and vibro-ejaculation. When urinary retention is the cause, often the high blood pressure can be seen to come down to normality during catheter drainage of the bladder. If it occurs while lying down, the patient should be sat up as soon as possible and the pulse and blood pressure should be monitored. Glyceryl trinitrate 0.3 mg sublingually as an adjuvant treatment will usually reduce the blood pressure by acting directly on the blood vessels. Reserpine 2–5 mg intramuscularly may be of benefit in persistent cases to prevent the actions of monoamine neural transmitters and some of the associated peptides which are released from the sympathetic nerve endings (Lundberg *et al.*, 1985). A milder and more chronic form with symptoms of headaches and perspiration occurs with chronic constipation and chronic pathology in the abdomen or pelvis (anal fissure, thrombosed haemorrhoids, detrusor sphincter dyssynergia). Lignocaine suppositories should be used prior to manual evacuation of the bowels when these symptoms occur with bowel evacuation. Rarely, procedures such as rhizotomy, hypogastric neurotomy, cordotomy or subarachnoid block with alcohol or phenol are required. These are likely to cause further denervation to the bladder and bowels, retention of urine and constipation.

Impairment of urinary bladder functions

The urinary bladder functions both as a reservoir and a pump. Neurogenic impairment of the bladder usually results in loss of control over both functions. Both retention of urine and incontinence can occur simultaneously. When the paralysis is flaccid (cauda equina lesions or in the stage of spinal areflexia), retention of urine with overflow incontinence can occur. Drainage is, therefore, necessary. Following the stage of spinal areflexia, reflex contraction of the detrusor muscles occurs gradually. Effective voiding with an automatic bladder (residual less than 100 ml) is achieved over periods of weeks or months following the return of the tendon reflexes. Some patients with an automatic bladder develop detrusor sphincter dyssynergia with simultaneous contraction of the detrusor and the muscles of the bladder outlet. This may cause poor emptying and/or high vesical pressure, and may predispose to urine infections and upper urinary tract dilatation. The eventual aim of bladder management is to have a bladder with low residual urine (below 100 ml), free from infections and a healthy upper urinary tract. The containment of urinary incontinence is also important since incontinence can result in maceration of the skin and the development of sores.

Overdistension of the bladder can delay the onset of reflex contractions and diminish subsequent bladder contractility (Hinman, 1976). Bladder expression by applying suprapubic pressure has been advocated, but it is associated with a high incidence of upper tract dilatation (Smith, Cock and Rhind, 1972). Drainage with 4–6-hourly intermittent catheterization using a 14-gauge catheter (Guttman and Frankel, 1966) has dramatically reduced the incidence of urethritis, urethral strictures, urethral diverticula, urethral fistula and epidydimo-orchitis, which occur with indwelling urinary catheters. With intermittent catheterization the majority of the patients can be discharged from spinal injury centres catheter free and with sterile urine (Ott and Rossier, 1971). To avoid overdistension of the bladder, restriction of fluid intake may be required. Alternatively, more frequent (4-hourly) catheterization is commenced and the frequency diminished according to the residual urine. The residual volume should not exceed 500 ml. Intermittent catheterization is discontinued when the residual urine is consistently below 100 ml on three consecutive catheterizations. An ambulant patient with good hand functions can be taught to do clean self-intermittent catheterization with good results (Lapides, Diokno and Silber, 1972). This can be continued in the patient's own home if necessary. A local anaesthetic (2% lignocaine) instilled in the urethra may be required if urethral sensation is spared. Suprapubic catheter drainage (Grundy *et al.*, 1983) is an alternative method of management. This is particularly convenient in the female tetraplegic patient with poor hand function. Suprapubic catheterization reduces the incidence of urethral complications. In a recumbent patient, however, drainage is against gravity.

Hypercalciuria and hyperphosphaturia, together with oliguria, during the period of immobilization can lead to stone formation (Burr, 1978), especially in the presence of a foreign body in the bladder. Teflon-and silicone-coated indwelling urethral catheters are an improvement on the old rubber catheter; however, they should only be used as a last resort. Indwelling urethral catheter care is paramount if urethral and bladder complications are to be minimized. The catheter should be changed every 3–4 weeks. The mechanical washout of the bladder with normal saline is recommended once or twice a week. Antibiotics should only be used if the patient is pyrexial or if the urine grows proteus or klebsiella organisms. A fluid intake of about 3 litres a day is much more beneficial to the patient. Frequent clamping of the suprapubic or urethral indwelling catheter for up to 4 hours or a volume of 400 ml from an early stage during the day also helps preserve the reservoir function of the bladder. The pharmacological management of lower urinary tract dysfunction (Wein, 1987) is beyond the scope of this chapter.

In general, the drugs used are those which promote or inhibit detrusor contractions and those which increase or inhibit bladder outlet resistance. They are used either individually or in combination to improve continence or drainage. Most of these pharmacological agents have side-effects and require monitoring. A trial of these medications is however, worthwhile prior to considering surgery. Simple procedures to promote voiding include suprapubic tapping, applying pressure with both fists on the lower abdomen while leaning forward or stimulating bladder contraction by inserting a gloved finger in the anal canal. Anterior sacral root stimulation by placing the anterior root of S2, S3 and S4 within electrodes connected to a subcutaneous receiver placed in the chest wall and activated by a hand-held transmitter is an alternative way to promote voiding (Brindley et al., 1986). The motor neurones of the sacral roots must not be damaged for the procedure to succeed. Section of the posterior root of S2 and S3 helps abolish hyperreflexia during stimulation. The procedure involves a major operation. It results, however, in diminution of residual urine, increase in the capacity of the bladder, reduces urine infections and improves continence (Cardozo et al., 1984). Bladder outlet surgery in the male patient with an automatic bladder is considered when there is failure of voiding or upper urinary tract dilatation. A demonstrable obstruction by a transrectal ultrasound or cystourethrometrography (urodynamics) is usually seen. The value of endoscopic sphincterotomy (internal membranous urethrotomy) in facilitating bladder emptying (Gibbon, 1974) and reducing the peak of high pressure in the urethral pressure profile (Abel et al., 1975) is well established. There is, however, a risk of postoperative impotence. Endoscopic bladder neck incision or resection may be necessary when the patient fails to void following a sphincterotomy. Concomitant bladder neck incision or resection with a sphincterotomy is carried out when outflow resistance is required to be at a minimum, e.g. in upper tract dilatation with ureteric reflux. Bladder neck surgery usually results in further incontinence and retrograde ejaculation. The patient will require an incontinence appliance consisting of a penile sheath attached to a leg bag. The excess spasticity and sweating of which the patient may complain during micturition often resolves within 3–4 weeks after bladder outlet surgery.

Tetraplegic and paraplegic patients are potentially incontinent. With good bladder training, many patients manage to remain continent with regular toileting every 3–4 hours. Incontinence can be contained in the male patient with the use of an incontinence appliance attached to a leg bag. It is advisable to incise the ring of the penile sheath opposite

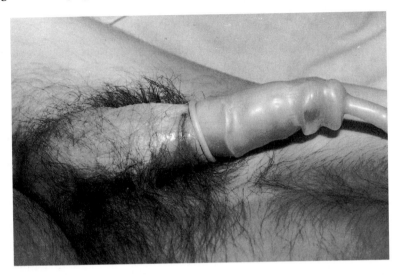

Figure 28.2 Penile sheath.

the urethral surface of the penis, in order to prevent pressure sores on the penile skin (Figure 28.2) and obstruction of urine outflow. Augmentation cystoplasty and clam cystoplasty (Mundy and Stephenson, 1985) convert a high pressure, small volume bladder to a low pressure, high volume bladder. Periurethral Teflon injection (Schulman *et al.*, 1984) and artificial urinary sphincters (Scott, Bradley and Timm, 1974) promote continence by increasing outflow resistance. Endoscopic bladder neck suspension (Stamey, 1973) can prevent incontinence in female patients provided the intravesical pressures are not too high.

Paraplegic and tetraplegic patients are at risk of developing urinary complications for the rest of their lives. Urinary infections, renal and vesical calculi, hydronephrosis and ureteric reflux can develop unnoticed by the patient who is sensory compromised. Urethral complications also develop in the presence of an indwelling urethral catheter. Lifelong careful, regular and frequent clinical assessment of the urinary tract is, therefore, essential (England and Low, 1985). This should include a history, physical examina-

tion and neurological assessment, urine culture and sensitivity, haemoglobin, urea and electrolytes estimation and an intravenous urogram or an ultrasound scan of the urinary tract on an annual or bi-annual basis. An isotope scan may be required if there is doubt about the renal function. Urodynamic studies should be carried out if there is upper tract dilatation, recurrent urinary tract infections, increasing difficulty with voiding, acute excess spasticity or sweating during micturition. Paraplegic and tetraplegic patients on indwelling catheters require a yearly cystoscopy as they are at a high risk of developing urinary calculi and carcinoma of the bladder, usually of the squamous type (El Masry and Fellow 1981).

Impairment of bowel function

Paraplegic and tetraplegic patients have loss of sensation of bowel fullness, tend to constipate and are incontinent of faeces and flatus. Spurious diarrhoea is not uncommon when bowel care is neglected. Constipation is one of the commonest causes of acute excess spasticity. An adequate fibrous diet and a rigorous bowel regime are required from the very initial stages of paralysis. It should be explained to the patient that a high fibre diet without increased fluid intake can result in further constipation. The patient should be encouraged to empty the bowels at a fixed suitable time and a fixed interval, preferably 24–48 hours. Patients usually require oral laxatives, suppositories and digital manual evacuation. Sennokot tablets can be taken (12 hours) and glycerine suppositories (inserted half an hour) prior to digital manual evacuation of the bowels. Most paraplegic patients are able to care for their bowels themselves. A tetraplegic patient is likely to require assistance from a carer.

Occasionally oral lactulose and enemas are required to keep the bowels clear. With a regular bowel regime, the majority of paraplegic and tetraplegic patients can achieve containment of their incontinence and avoid constipation.

Impairment of sensory functions

Sensory deprivation in patients with paraplegia and tetraplegia can cause disorientation, anxiety and loss of confidence, especially in the early stages following paralysis. Sensory impairment with paralysis causes difficulties with sitting balance and increases the risk of skin sores. Hyperpathia, phantom pain, allodynia and dysaesthesia can occur in a small number of patients with traumatic or vascular paralysis. Medical complications usually exaggerate these conditions. The impairment or loss of sensation can present diagnostic difficulties to the clinician, since the patient is unable to complain or localize pain, especially in acute abdominal and pelvic pathologies. Shoulder tip pain due to irritation of the diaphragm can be the only sign of peritonitis in a patient whose general condition is poor. Fractures of long bones can go unnoticed by the patient for many days. The patient may notice, however, an increased level of spasticity and a bruise or swelling

without pain. The anaesthetic skin of paraplegic and tetraplegic patients is vulnerable to asymptomatic burns, superficial friction sores and pressure sores.

Pressure sores (tissue viability)

Pressure sores occur mainly over bony prominences. Pressure, however, from tight garments or tightly fitted appliances can also cause pressure sores in areas of skin with no underlying bony prominences. The risk of pressure sores in paraplegic and tetraplegic patients is high. This is due to the concomitant impairment of the mobility (Berlowitz and Wilking, 1989), sensation and vasomotor control. The risk is highest in the stage of spinal shock. Other risk factors include a systolic blood pressure below 100 mmHg (Gosnell, 1973), flaccidity with muscle atrophy (Mawson *et al.*, 1988) and hypoalbuminaemia (Pinchcofsky-Devin and Kaminski, 1986).

Infection, pyrexia, dehydration and hypoxia are all added factors in the acutely ill patient. Despite all these factors pressure sores are preventable, except occasionally in the terminally ill patient. Pressure sores will result in added disability from complications such as excess spasticity and contractures which further limit the patient's mobility, independence and employment. Pressure sores can also be a cause of morbidity such as anaemia, bacteraemia, septicaemia, osteomyelitis and septic arthritis. Multiple recurrences can cause amyloidosis. Pressure sores cause prolonged hospitalization (Hibbs, 1990) and add unnecessary cost. It is estimated that the National Health Service spends, on average, 755 million pounds for the treatment of pressure sores annually (West and Priestley, 1994). Following healing, the residual scar is likely to be permanently vulnerable to recurrences, especially if it adheres to underlying tissue such as bone. This is not to mention that the sight and the smell of the sore is likely to affect not only the patient but also the partner or carer and possibly the family members.

Prevention of pressure sores requires an education programme. The patient and carer should be made aware of the risk factors, the methods of prevention and the effects of pressure sores on health, disability and environment. The patient should be provided with an adequate mattress and adequate seating (cushion and wheelchair) so that pressure is well distributed and not localized over the bony prominences. Both the patient and the carer should be trained in the methods of prevention, such as turning in bed every 3–4 hours, lifting from the wheelchair or rocking from side to side or bending forward every 10–15 minutes and inspecting the skin daily. A paraplegic patient can inspect his/her skin independently using a mirror. The patient and carer should be made aware of the premonitory signs of pressure sore development. Erythema which takes longer than 10 minutes to fade, a fixed erythema that does not fade, induration of the skin and subcutaneous tissues, require immediate pressure relief until the skin looks and feels healthy again. This may take up to 3 weeks, following which remobilization ought to be gradual and the skin closely monitored, It must be highlighted that the breakdown of the skin may be the last stage in the development of a pressure sore.

The management of an established pressure sore requires a thorough investigation of how and why it happened. The following should be investigated:

- The nutritional state and the general health of the patient.
- His/her habits (drinking and smoking).
- The assessment of seating (if the pressure sore is over the seating area).
- The assessment of the mattress (if the pressure sore is over the shoulder blades, spinous processes, iliac crest or sacrum).
- The patient's habits and techniques of pressure relief.

- The ability of the patient to transfer into and from a wheelchair without applying shearing forces to the skin and subcutaneous tissues during transfer.
- A neurological examination may highlight further deterioration and weakness in the upper limbs.
- Assessment of the psychosocial circumstances surrounding the development of the pressure sore may be necessary if self-neglect or neglect by the carer is suspected.
- The state of bladder and bowel incontinence as well as the degree of perspiration also need to be assessed since excess moisture can lead to maceration of the epidermis and introduction of infection.

The core management of an established pressure sore consists of the following:

- Complete relief of pressure.
- Thorough, regular and frequent cleaning either by surgical debridement or by using topical agents.
- Attention to the nutritional state of the patient.
- Protein depletion that will lead to decreased perfusion and impaired immune response should be rectified.
- The deficiency of zinc (which stabilizes membrane structure and function) impairs healing (Liszewski, 1981); may require local application of zinc preparation.
- Vitamin C is recommended since it has been shown to be important in healing pressure sores in spinal cord injury patients (Hunter and Rajan, 1971) and is necessary for protein hydroxylation.
- Adequate hydration is important for cellular metabolism and nutrition delivery (Bogie, Nuseibeh and Bader, 1992).

Once the pressure sore is clean and the general health of the patient has improved, a choice of management is available. Conservative management (nursing care) may be all that is required for a small superficial sore. Depending on the weight of the patient and the presence or absence of concomitant sores, the patient may require nursing on a special bed or mattress, i.e. the low air loss bed, the fluidized silicone bed, the Roho mattress or the Pegasus mattress. Systemic antibiotics are not recommended unless there is pyrexia or evidence of septicaemia. Weekly or bi-weekly culture and sensitivity from the pressure sore is likely to be useful in the event of the patient becoming pyrexial or septicaemic. The healing could be expedited by the application of a split-skin graft. If more aggressive treatment is contemplated, primary excision and direct closure should, in the author's opinion, be considered first, especially when there is sensory loss and potential recurrence (Nuseibeh and El Masry, 1979).

With primary excision and direct closure there is minimal disturbance to the vascular anatomy of the area. Future recurrences can therefore be dealt with easily. A large sore may require the application of a split-skin graft until it reaches a manageable size for primary excision and direct closure. Excision of the underlying bony prominence, for example the greater trochanter underlying a sore, will facilitate surgical closure and is mandatory when the bone is infected. Closure of a pressure sore defect by using a full-thickness skin flap or a myocutaneous rotation flap is a third option and may achieve faster healing. Recurrence of sores within these flaps are, however, slower to heal and more difficult to manage than following primary excision and direct closure. A latissimus dorsi musculocutaneous flap should be avoided in patients who are able to use this muscle for sitting balance. Following surgery (except split-skin graft) one or two suction drains are often left in the wound for about 10 days and sometimes longer. This is a longer period than is usually necessary: however, prolonged oozing related to loss of vasomotor control in paraplegic and tetraplegic patients usually occurs. Antibiotics with good bone penetration, such as flucloxacilin, are usually

administered for about 2 weeks postoperatively. The patient is gradually mobilized after 3 weeks of postoperative bedrest (relief of pressure).

Impairment of sexual function

The sexuality of the paraplegic and tetraplegic man and woman is impaired in many ways; the paralysis is only one factor. The patient with spinal paralysis may suffer an impairment of body image and low self-esteem, compounded by fear of rejection and loss of control of bodily functions, especially bladder and bowel functions. The restricted mobility may further limit the opportunities of meeting a sexual partner. Restricted mobility and spasticity may cause embarrassment during sexual activity. Sensory deprivation from the genital areas below the level of the lesion affects gratification and consequently possibly sexual drive. Culture and religious beliefs, personal views and previous experience may all influence sexuality.

Concerns about sexuality are usually experienced at a relatively early stage by the great majority of patients. These concerns may not be easily expressed verbally. The role of the clinician is to learn about these concerns from the patient in a sensitive manner, at an early stage and counsel the patient when he or she is ready. Group teaching, in lay terms, of the physiology of sexuality, followed by an open discussion, will often ease the burden of the shy patient. The importance of adhering to a rigorous bowel regime to avoid faecal incontinence and to empty the bladder before embarking on sexual activity in order to prevent urinary incontinence and autonomic dysreflexia ought to be highlighted to the patient. Indwelling catheters need not be removed and can be taped to the abdomen of the female patient or backwards to the dorsal surface of the penis in the male patient. Lubrication of the catheter will avoid friction. Libido usually remains strong in the male patient. It may, however, be reduced in the female because of psychodynamic factors. Male patients with suprasacral spinal cord injuries are unlikely to achieve psychogenic erections, with visual, auditory or olfactory stimuli, recall or perception. Intercourse can, however, be achieved with reflex erection. Male patients with lower motor neurone lesions of the sacral area may have impaired psychogenic erections but no reflex erections. Women whose lesions are at T9 and above have reflex lubrication and those with lesions below T12 may have psychogenic lubrication. Lubricants, such as KY jelly, may further ease penetration, especially in the presence of excess spasticity. Orgasm remotely similar to what the patient used to experience before the paralysis is absent. Indeed, discomfort from autonomic dysreflexia or excess spasticity may occur, especially if the patient is constipated or has a full bladder. However, many patients (men and women) state that following the paralysis they derive more pleasure from the erogenous areas above the level of the lesion.

In the male, erections can be further enhanced with external aids, intracavernosal injections of vasoactive drugs, penile implants or stimulation of the anterior sacral root of S2. External devices (Erectaid and Correctaid) depend on passive expansion of the penis by an external cuff or a vacuum (Witherington, 1989). Erection is maintained by a band around the base of the penis. The patient should be made aware that pressure sores can develop. Intracavernosal injections of vasoactive drugs are gaining in popularity (Wyndaele *et al.*, 1986; Sidi *et al.*, 1987; Stackl, Hasun and Marberger, 1990). They all produce smooth muscle relaxation. Papaverine is a non-specific smooth muscle relaxant. Phentolamine produces vascular dilatation through a relatively transient but potent alpha-adrenergic blockade. Prostoglandin El has a potent relaxant action on the corpus-cavernosus muscles, a dilating effect on arteries, smooth muscle relaxation and an adrenergic receptor inhibition effect. Papaverine and phentolamine have also been used in combination. Titration of the dose is required for the individual patient. The commonest complications are pain in a patient with sensory sparing, ecchymosis and priapism (an erection lasting longer that 6 hours) and fibrosis. When priapism occurs, syphoning of the penis, the injection of an antidote (metaraminol for papaverine and phenylephrine for prostaglandin El) should be used in this order. Occasionally a shunt operation is required, An implant in the corpora cavernosa (semi-regid or inflatable) should be used with caution in the sensory impaired patient. Semi-rigid implants have been known to extrude through sexual intercourse. Sacral anterior root stimulation to S2 provides the patient with control over the duration of erection and offers the advantage over intracavernosal injections by including the corpus spongiosum of the penis.

Fertility

Amenorrhoea usually occurs during the initial stages of paralysis and can last for up to 9 months and sometimes longer. Many female patients may be fertile later. During pregnancy, urinary tract infection, constipation and deep venous thrombosis can occur. Lower limb oedema usually occurs and requires elastic stockings. Fetal movement and uterine contractions are appreciated when the lesion is below T12. Women with T6 lesions and above may develop autonomic hyperreflexia and a close liaison between the obstetrician and the clinician looking after the patient is important.

The fertility of the male patient is compromised on many accounts. Ejaculation occurs rarely in patients with complete upper motor neurone lesions. The sperm quality is poor in the majority of patients (Lissenmyer and Perkash, 1991). Urinary tract infections and prostatitis would lower the sperm cell count and motility. Epididymitis and chronic inflammation due to reflux of urine in the ejaculatory duct play an important role in lowering the sperm quality (Ohl *et al.*, 1989). Histological and hormonal testicular changes in spinal cord patients, including atrophy of the seminiferous tubules (Perkash *et al.*, 1985), further impair spermatogenesis and maturation of sperm. The scrotal temperature in paraplegic men in wheelchairs averages about 0.9°C higher than in normal sitting men and may contribute to the impairment (Brindley, 1982). It is, therefore, essential to minimize urinary tract complications and avoid tight clothing as a first step towards solving the problem of infertility in male paraplegic and tetraplegic patients. Methods of obtaining semen in these patients include electro-ejaculation with a transrectal electrode (Perkash *et al.*, 1985), vibro-ejaculation (Francois, Jouannet and Maury, 1983), injection of intrathecal neostigmine (Guttman and Walsh, 1971) or subcutaneous physostigmine (Chappelle *et al.*, 1983). The patient should be warned of the risk of autonomic hyperre-flexia occurring with all these methods. The sperm can be directly aspirated from the vas deferens. Alternatively, the vas deferens can be cannulated and connected to a reservoir implanted subcutaneously above the inguinal ligament. Semen can be aspirated subsequently from the reservoir and used for direct insemination (Brindley, Scott and Hendry 1986). Hypogastric plexus stimulation with implanted electrodes (Brindley, Saverwein and Hendry, 1989) produces semen on volition but is unsuitable in patients with intact pelvic sensation. The treatment of the able-bodied female partner of the paraplegic or the tetraplegic man may also be necessary. The methods of *in vivo* and *in vitro* fertilization are beyond the scope of this chapter. It is paramount that adequate counselling to the couple be provided in order not to give unrealistic expectations which, if unfulfilled, may cause psychological problems and disharmony.

Impairment of lower limb function and mobility

Paralysis of the lower limbs results in inability to stand unsupported in the upright position, inability to walk without arm support and limitation of sexual activity. Excess spasticity, contractures of muscles and heterotrophic calcification will further increase these limitations. However high the level of the injury, the patient can be helped in the upright position with bracing of the hips, knees and ankles in the Oswestry Standing Frame (Figure 28.3) or any similar device. This is psychologically beneficial and helps reduce osteoporosis and spasticity. When the lesion is above T12 (with no motor power in the hip flexors) the patient is capable of walking with

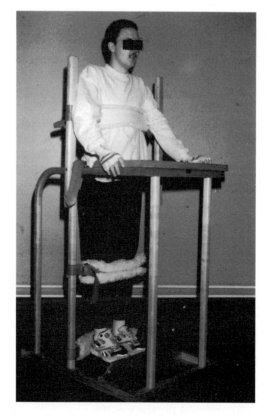

Figure 28.3 Oswestry Standing Frame.

a swing-through gait using crutches. This requires good upper limb function. With training, patients can cover reasonable distances speedily. Patients can also achieve a four-point gait by using their abdominal muscles and gravity while pushing down on the crutches to lift the foot off the ground. This is, however, more time and energy consuming. Knee, ankle and foot orthoses or the newer orthosis like the HGO (hip guidance orthosis) or the RGO (reciprocating gait orthosis) are likely to reduce the energy cost of walking and improve the gait. A hybrid system of orthosis and functional electrical stimulation is likely to improve the gait further (Chapter 47). Many patients eventually prefer to use a wheelchair for mobility.

Patients with sparing of the hip flexors are usually able to walk with knee–ankle–foot orthoses. Many patients still prefer the wheelchair in the long term. When the knee extensors are spared, ankle–foot orthoses will be required. If the position sense is impaired the patient may still require arm support during ambulation.

Wheelchair-dependent patients have problems with loss of sensory input from the periphery and loss of motor ability to realign the point of gravity. Sitting balance is therefore affected. Over a period of time and with training, the patient learns to compensate for the sensory loss by using vision and sensory input from above the level of the lesion. The patient will also learn to use the head and upper limbs to alter the point of gravity and maintain balance. In the initial stages of training mirrors will facilitate the process and will further help in making the patient aware of the limits within which movement is safe. A paraplegic patient in good health will be able to use a self-propelling wheelchair. The wheelchair should be comfortable, light, durable and ergonomically sound. Good posture and seating in the wheelchair is paramount to avoid spasticity, contractures of muscles and pressure sores.

Tetraplegic patients in good health can also use self-propelled wheelchairs when there is good motor power in the biceps brachii. Patients with weak or absent biceps muscles will depend on an electric wheelchair. The patient should be involved in the choice of the appropriate control (lever stick, head control, chin control or puff and suck) to ensure comfort and ease of use. The wheelchair should be regarded as the lifeline for the paraplegic and tetraplegic patient and most patients will require a spare wheelchair and a spare cushion. Seating assessment of the patient is paramount in order to provide an appropriate wheelchair and cushion.

Most paraplegic and tetraplegic patients without impairment of cognitive functions are able to drive vehicles with hand controls and automatic gears provided the deltoid and biceps muscles are functioning. The patient may require a forearm splint to stabilize the wrist. Special vehicles are available to enable the patient with a higher lesion to drive (Chapter 50).

Impairment of upper limb functions

Activities of daily living, personal care and hygiene depend to a great extent on the integrity of the upper limb and hand function. Paraplegic patients in good health are usually independent in almost all activities of daily living, personal care and hygiene. Tetraplegic patients with paralysed hands but with good power in the elbow flexors and wrist extensor should be able to feed provided the food is cut up, brush their teeth, wash their face and the upper part of their bodies, comb their hair, as well as dress and undress independently or with minimal help and propel their wheelchair. A strap around the palm of the hand with a pocket in which a spoon or a toothbrush or a hairbrush or a sponge can be inserted or attached will facilitate many of these activities (Figure 28.4). Although fine finger movements are absent, a tetraplegic patient may be able to pick up objects (the size of an apple) using a tenodesis grip. By

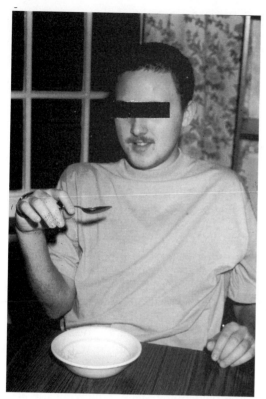

Figure 28.4 Adaptive device in use for facilitating use of the hand.

extending the wrist, the fingers flex and a hold is achieved on a reasonable size and weight object. The fingers should not be allowed to go into fixed flexion or extension deformity. This can be prevented from an early stage by passive movement to the fingers and by maintaining them in a slightly flexed position during the night using a boxing glove bandage (Figure 28.5). The patient with paralysis of wrist extensors may benefit from a forearm splint to give stability to the wrist and enable the patient to feed or brush his/her teeth.

Those who have paralysis of the triceps muscle find great difficulty in transferring, they can, however, lift their bodies and transfer, though with difficulty, by locking their elbows in extension. The functions of the upper limbs of tetraplegic patients can be improved by surgery (Moberg, 1978). Tendon transfer from the extensor radialis longus to the flexor digitorum profundus is likely to improve the tenodesis grip. This should not be contemplated when the course of the paralysis is progressive or improving. Such operations are usually deferred for a

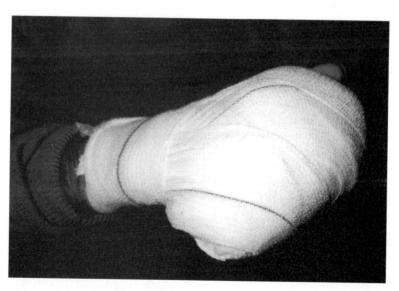

Figure 28.5 Boxing glove bandage protection.

year after paralysis. The motor power in the wrist extensor should be at least grade 4 or 5. A key grip is useful in enabling the patient to pick up small objects (a sheet of paper or a sandwich) between the thumb and index finger. The key grip can also be surgically enhanced with arthrodesis of the thumb. Paralysis of the triceps will also cause difficulty in orientating the hand in space. A tendon transfer between the deltoid muscle and the insertion of the triceps aponeurosis can help the patient orient the hand in space.

Spinal cord damage above the level of the phrenic nerves requires use of ventilation, and long term there is the possibility of phrenic nerve pacing (Chapter 17).

Spasms and spasticity

Spasms in the lower limbs are useful to patients with spinal injuries. They can be used for standing transfers, triggering reflex micturition or an erection. They also improve the venous return from the lower limbs.

In general, patients with incomplete cord lesions are usually more spastic than patients with complete cord lesions. The level of spasticity is also higher in cervical and upper dorsal injuries than in the lower lesions. Acute excess spasticity is both a nuisance and a danger to the patient. It is usually a symptom of some pathology below the level of the lesion of which the patient may not be aware due to the loss/impairment of sensation. A thorough examination of the patient in order to diagnose and cure the underlying pathology is therefore essential (El Masry, 1984). Whenever possible antispasticity medication should only be used on a temporary basis until such pathology is diagnosed and treated:

- Bladder irritation from fluid retention, infection or calculi.
- Loaded bowel, thrombosed haemorrhoids, and fissure.
- Pressure sores or ingrowing toenails.

- Pressure from tight clothing or orthoses, undetected by patient.
- Joint contractures
- Poor positioning.

Skeletal system

Bone metabolism is impaired in patients with spinal cord injuries. Osteoporosis is not an uncommon finding in patients with spinal paralysis, exposing them to an added risk of developing long bone fractures with minimal trauma. Biering-Sorensen, Bohr and Schaadt (1990) showed a significant decline of bone mineral content in the neck and shaft of the femur and in the tibia, and fractures of the tibia, fibula or femur are not uncommon. Heterotrophic calcification is rarely seen in patients with medical spinal paralysis. The incidence in traumatic cord injuries varies between centres. The hips, knees and elbow are in that order the commonest site affected. In the acute stage, the area is red, hot and swollen and can mimic an underlying abscess in the developing stage. Following the acute stage it can mimic deep vein thrombosis in the lower limbs. Radiographic appearances are usually delayed; however, the condition can be detected from a very early stage with an ultrasound scan (Pullicino *et al*, 1993). Bedrest and diphosphonates, initially for 6 months or longer, will often limit the pathology. Surgery is not advisable, if necessary it should be delayed.

FOLLOW-UP

A regular follow-up system should be made available to the individual with spinal paralysis in order to ensure good general health and maintenance of a good state of rehabilitation. The patient should have a full assessment of the multisystem impairment (both clinically and with the appropriate investigations), the equipment that is frequently used and upon which the patient relies, the quality of self-care or that provided by carers and the psychosocial circumstances that influence the quality of life of the patient. The members of the multidisciplinary team should also contribute to the follow-up assessment in order to provide a full comprehensive and relevant assessment. The aim of the follow-up should be to ensure prevention of avoidable complications and the early diagnosis and treatment of established complications. This is especially necessary as these patients have impairment or loss of sensation below the level of their lesion.

Many years after spinal injury the cord damage may progress due to development of a syrinx and neurosurgical advice should be obtained.

EMPLOYMENT

Provided there is no impairment of cognitive functions, healthy paraplegic and tetraplegic individuals who have undergone a comprehensive rehabilitation programme assisted by new technology can enjoy a reasonable quality of life. Many individuals with non-progressive paraplegia and tetraplegia work and contribute to society. Liaison and advocacy with employers from an early stage is likely to facilitate re-employment of many individuals. The person with spinal paralysis may require retraining. The computer has made it possible for many tetraplegic individuals to work. Life is likely to remain a challenge for these patients; however, with some modest help from a willing team of professionals, most difficulties can be surmounted.

LIFE EXPECTANCY

This will depend mainly on the pathology that has caused the paralysis, the health of the patient, his/her age, the quality of personal care provided, as well as the quality and expertise of the team who provide the follow-up. It is not uncommon now to find patients with traumatic paraplegia and tetraplegia sustained at a young age alive and well 40 years after their injury.

REFERENCES

Abel,, B.J., Ross, C.I., Gibbon, N.O.K. and Jameson, R.M. (1975) Urethral pressure measurement after division of the external sphincter. *Paraplegia*, **13**, 37–41.

Bergofsky, E.H. (1964) Mechanism for respiratory insufficiency after cervical cord injury. *Annals of Internal Medicine*, **61**, 435–447.

Bergstrom, E.M.K. and Rose, L.S. (1992) Physical rehabilitation, principles and outcome, in *Handbook of Clinical Neurology*, vol. (ed. H.L. Frankel), Elsevier Science, Oxford, pp. 457–478.

Berlowitz, D.R. and Wilking, S.V.B. (1989) Risk factors for pressure sores. A comparison of cross sectional and cohort derived data. *Journal of the American Geriatric Society*, **37**, 1043–1050.

Biering-Sorensen, F, Bohr, H.H. and Schaadt, O.P. (1990) Longitudinal study of bone mineral content in the lumbar spine, the forearm and lower extremities after spinal cord injury. *European Journal of Clinical Investigation*, **20**, 330–335.

Bogie, K.M., Nuseibeh, I. and Bader, D.L. (1992) New concepts in the prevention of pressure sores, in *Handbook of Clinical Neurology*, vol. 61 (ed. H.L. Frankel), Elsevier Science, Oxford, pp. 347–366.

Brindley, G.S. (1982) Deep scrotal temperature and the effect on it of clothing, air temperature, activity, posture and paraplegia. *British Journal of Urology*, **54**, 46–55.

Brindley, G.S., Polkey, C.E., Rushton, D.N. and Cardozo, L. (1986) Sacral anterior root stimulation for bladder control in paraplegics: the first 50 cases. *Journal of Neurology and Psychiatry*, **49**, 1104–1114.

Brindley, G.S., Saverwein, D. and Hendry W.F. (1989) Hypogastric plexus stimulation for obtaining semen from paraplegic men. *British Journal of Urology*, **64**, 72–77.

Brindley, G.S., Scott, G.I. and Hendry, W.F. (1986) Vas cannulation with implanted sperm reservoirs for azoospermia or ejaculatory failure. *British Journal of Urology*, **58**, 721–723.

Burr, R.G. (1978) A relationship between the composition of urine and that of urinary tract calculi in spinal patients. *Paraplegia*, **16**, 59–64.

Cardozo, L., Krishnan, K.R., Polkey, C.E., Rushton, D.L. and Brindley, G.S. (1984) Urodynamic observations on patients with sacral anterior root stimulators. *Paraplegia*, **22**, 201–209.

Chapelle, P.A., Blanquart, F., Puech, A.J. and Held, J.P. (1983) Treatment of anejaculation in the total paraplegic by subcutaneous injection of physostigmine. *Paraplegia*, **21**, 30.

El Masry, W.S. (1984) in *Clinical Management of Spasticity in Patients with Spinal Cord Injury, Paraplegia and Tetraplegia*. (eds Milan, Rossier and Ghedini), pp. 29, 289–298.

El Masry, W.S. (1993) Physiological instability of the spinal cord following injury. *Paraplegia*, **31**, 273–275.

El Masry, W.S., Cochrane, P. and Silver, J.R. (1982) Gastrointestinal bleeding in patients with acute spinal injuries. *Injury*, **14**, 162–167.

El Masry, W.S. and Fellow, G.J. (1981) Bladder cancer after spinal cord injury. *Paraplegia*, **19**, 265–270.

El Masry, W.S. and Jaffray, D. (1992) Recent development in the management of injuries of the cervical spine, in *Handbook of Neurology*, vol. 61 (ed. M.L. Frankel), Elsevier Science, Oxford, pp. 55–75.

El Masry, W.S. and Silver, J.R. (1981) Prophylactic anticoagulant therapy in patients with spinal cord injury. *Paraplegia*, **19**, 334–42.

England, E.J. and Low, A.I. (1985) Long term management and prevention of urinary tract disease, in *Lifetime Care of the Paraplegic Patient*, (ed G.M. Bedbrook), Churchill Livingstone, Edinburgh, pp. 94–108.

Francois, N., Jouannet, P. and Maury, M. (1983) Les aspects genito sexuels de la paraplegie chez le homme. *Journal of Urology*, **89**, 159–164.

Frankel, H.L., Mathias, C.J. and Spalding, J.M.D. (1975) Mechanisms of reflex cardiac arrest in tetraplegic patients. *Lancet*, **ii**, 1183–1185.

Gibbon, N.O.K. (1974) Neurogenic bladder in spinal cord injury. Management of patients in Liverpool, England. *Urological Clinics of North America*, **1**, 147–154.

Glenn, W.W.L. and Phelps, M.L. (1985) Diaphragm pacing by electrical stimulation of the phrenic nerves. *Neurosurgery*, **17**, 974–984.

Gopalakrishnan, K.C. and El Masry, W.S. (1986) Fracture of the sternum associated with spinal injury. *Journal of Bone and Joint Surgery*, **68** [Br], 178–182.

Gosnell, D.J. (1973) An assessment tool to identify pressure sores *Nursing Research*, **22**, 55–59.

Grundy, D.J., Fellows, G.J., Nuseibeh, I., Gillette, A.P. and Silver, J.R. (1983) A comparison of fine bore suprapubic and intermittent urethral catheterisation regime after spinal cord injury. *Paraplegia*, **21**, 227–232.

Gupta, A., McClelland, M.R., Evans, A. and El Masry, W.S. (1989) Mini-tracheotomy in the early respiratory management of patients with spinal injuries. *Paraplegia*, **27**, 269–277.

Guttman, L. (1976) Spinal Cord Injuries, Comprehensive Management and Research, 2nd edn, Blackwell Scientific Publications, Oxford.

Guttman, L. and Frankel, H.L. (1966) The value of intermittent catheterisation in the early management of traumatic paraplegia and tetraplegia. *Paraplegia*, **4**, 63–83.

Guttman, L. and Walsh, J.J. (1971) Prostigmine assessment test of fertility in spinal men. *Paraplegia*, **9**, 39–51.

Hibbs, P. (1990) The economics of pressure sore prevention, *Pressure Sores – clinical practice and scientific approach* (ed. D.L. Bader), McMillan Press, London, pp. 35–42.

Hinman, F. (1976) Post operative distention of the bladder. *Surgery, Gynaecology and Obstetrics*, **142**, 901–902.

Hunter, T. and Rajan, K.T. (1971) The role of ascorbic acid in the pathogenesis and treatment of pressure sores. *Paraplegia*, **8**, 211–215.

Lapides, J., Diokno, A.C. and Silber, S.J. (1972) Clean self intermittent catheterisation in the treatment of urinary tract disease. *Journal of Urology*, **107**, 458–461.

Lissenmyer, T.A. and Perkash, I. (1991) Infertility in men with spinal cord injury. *Archives of Physical Medicine and Rehabilitation*, **72**, 747–754.

Liszewski, R.F. (1981) The effects of zinc on wound healing: a collective review. *Journal of the American Medical Association*, **81**, 79–81.

Lundberg, J.M., Saria, A., Franco-Cereceda, A. and Theodossan-Norheim, E. (1985) Mechanisms underlying changes in the content of neuropeptide Y in cardiovascular nerves and adrenal gland induced by sympatholytic drugs. *Acta Physiologica Scandanavia*, **124**, 603–611.

Mathias, C.J., Christenssen, N.J., Frankel, H.L. and Spalding, N.M.K. (1979) Cardiovascular control in recently injured tetraplegics in spinal shock. *Quarterly Journal of Medicine (New series)*, **48**, 273–279.

Mathias, C.J. and Frankel, H.L. (1988) Cardiovascular control in spinal men. *Annual Reviews of Physiology*, **50**, 577–592.

Mawson, A.R., Biundo, J.J., Neville, P., Linares, H.A., Winchester, Y. and Lopez, A. (1988) Risk factors of early occurring pressure ulcers following spinal cord injury. *American Journal of Physical Rehabilitation*, **67**, 123–127.

Moberg, E. (1978) *The Upper Limb in Tetraplegia. A New Approach to Surgical Rehabilitation*, Georg Thieme Publishers, Struttgart.

Moulton, A. and Silver, J.R. (1970) Chest measurements in patients with traumatic injuries of the cervical spine. *Clinical Science*, **39**, 407–422.

Mundy, A.R. and Stephenson, T.P. (1985), 'Clam' ileocystoplasty for the treatment of refactory urge incontinence. *Journal of Urology*, **57**, 641–646.

Nuseibeh, I. and El Masry, W.S. (1979) The surgical treatment of pressure sores in spinal injuries. *Paraplegia*, **17**, 409–413.

Ohl, D.A., Bennett, C.J., McCabe, M., Menge, A.C. and McGuire, E.J. (1989) Predictors of success in electro-ejaculation of spinal cord injured men. *Journal of Urology*, **142**, 1483–1486.

Ott, R. and Rossier, A.B. (1971) L'interêt du sondage intermittent dans la rééducation vesicale des lesions medullaires traumatiques aigues. *Urologia Internationalis*, **27**, 51–65.

Perkash, I., Martin, D.E., Warner, H., Blank, M.S. and Collins, D.C. (1985) Reproductive biology of paraplegics. Results of semen collection, testicular biopsy and serum hormone evaluation. *Journal of Urology*, **134**, 284–288.

Pinchofsky-Devin, G.D. and Kaminski, M.V. (1986) Correlation of pressure sores and nutritional status. *Journal of the American Geriatric Society*, **34**, 435–440.

Pledger, H.G. (1962) Disorders of temperature regulation in acute traumatic paraplegia. *Journal of Bone and Joint Surgery*, **44B**, 110–113.

Pullicino, V.N.C., McClelland, M., Badwan, D.A.H., McCall, I.M., Pringle, R.G. and El Masry, W. (1993) Sonographic diagnosis of heterotopic bone formation in spinal injury patients *Paraplegia*, **31**, 40–50.

Schulman, C.C., Simon, J., Wespes, E. and Germeau, F. (1984) Endoscopic injections of teflon to treat urinary incontinence in women. *British Medical Journal*, **288**, 192.

Scott, F.B., Bradley, W.E. and Timm, G.W. (1974) Treatment of urinary incontinence by an implantable prosthetic urinary sphincter. *Journal of Urology*, **112**, 75–80.

Shalock, R.L. and Kierman, W.E. (1990), *Habilitation Planning for Adults with Disabilities*, Springer-Verlag, Berlin, p. 41.

Sidi, A.A., Cameron, J.S., Dijksta, D.D., Reinburg, Y. and Lange, P.H. (1987) Vasoactive intracavernous pharmacotherapy for the treatment of erectile impotence in men with spinal cord injury. *Journal of Urology*, **138**, 539–542.

Smith, P.H., Cock, J.B. and Rhind, J.R. (1972), Manual expression of the bladder following spinal cord injury. *Paraplegia*, **9**, 213–21.

Stackl, W., Hasun, R. and Marberger, M. (1990) The use of prostoglandin El for diagnosis and treatment of erectile dysfunction. *Journal of Urology*, **8**, 84–86.

Stamey, T.A. (1973) Endoscopic suspension of the vesical neck for urinary incontinence. *Surgery, Gynaecology and Obstetrics*, **136**, 547–554.

Walsh, J.J., Nuseibeh, I. and El Masry, W.S. (1973) Perforated peptic ulcers in paraplegia. *Paraplegia*, **2**, 310–313.

Wein, A.J. (1987) Lower urinary tract function and pharmacological management of lower urinary tract dysfunction. *Urological Clinics of North America*, **14**, 273–296.

West, P. and Priestley, J. (1994) Money under the mattress. *Health Service Journal*, 20–22.

Witherington, R. (1989) Constriction device for management of erectile impotence. *Journal of Urology*, **141**, 320–322.

Wyndaele, J.J., De Meyer, J.M., De Sy, W.A. and Claessens, H. (1986) Intracavernosal injection of vasoactive drugs. An alternative for treating impotence in spinal cord injury patients. *Paraplegia*, **24**, 271–275.

FURTHER READING

Bedbrook, G.M. (1981) *Care and Management of Spinal Cord Injury*, Springer, Berlin.

Bedbrook, G.M. (1985) *Lifetime Care of the Paraplegic Patient*, Churchill Livingstone, Edinburgh.

Guttmann, L. (1976) *Spinal Cord Injuries: comprehensive management and research*, Blackwell, Scientific Publications, Oxford.

Life After Spinal Cord Injury, (1991) The Midlands Centre for Spinal Injuries, Oswestry SY10 7AG, UK.

Ozer, M.N. (1988) *The Management of Persons with Spinal Cord Injury*, Demos Publications, New York.

Paraplegia, The Journal of the International Medical Society of Paraplegia.

Trieschmann, R.B. (1988) *Spinal Cord Injuries: psychological, social and vocational rehabilitation*, 2nd edn, Demos Publications, New York.

Whiteneck, G. (1992) *Ageing with Spinal Cord Injury*, Demos Publications, New York.

Whiteneck, G., Charlifue, S.W., Gerhart, K.A., Lammertse, D.P., Manley, S., Menter R.R., Seedroff, K.R. (1989) *The Management of High Quadriplegia*, Demos Publications, New York.

USEFUL ADDRESS

Spinal Injuries Association
76 St James Lane, London N10 3DF, UK. Tel. 0181 444 2121. Counselling Line: 0181 8834296.

29 *Head injury: early rehabilitation*

C.D. Evans and G.A. Morgan

INTRODUCTION

Over the last two or three decades, much accurate information about the incidence and prevalence of traumatic brain injury (TBI) has been accumulated. It is now recognized as a problem, but even so, rehabilitation after traumatic brain injury still does not attract the funding or the attention it needs. TBI is more prevalent than spinal injury, yet for this condition there are clear routes for long-term management and specialized units available. For traumatic brain injury, there is no comparable comprehensive provision widely available. This has been emphasized in a recent report by the Welsh Affairs Committee (1995).

Aims of management of TBI

A modern ambulance service staffed by paramedics allows the opportunity to prevent the 'second injury'. The rapid transfer to accident and emergency centres, the development of specialist intensive treatment units and improved access to neurosurgical units, have helped to reduce the consequences of TBI. A district general hospital with 800 beds serving a population of 400 000 treats 1500 brain injuries each year. This figure represents patients between 16 and 65. There are almost as many again if children under 16 and adults over 65 are included. About 25% will be severe or very severe with Glasgow Coma

Scores of 8 or less and the mortality in this group is relatively high.. These figures are confirmed by the results from the National Traumatic Brain Injury Survey (1996).

In the UK most head injuries, mild or severe, are initially managed in district general hospitals with no neurosurgical services on site. Such hospitals must have access to computerized axial tomography and surgical staff who can perform craniotomies to evacuate life-threatening intracranial haematoma.

The main initial objectives in early management are:

- Maintenance of oxygenation.
- Maintenance of adequate cerebral circulation.
- Maintenance of a normal intracranial pressure and adequate cerebral perfusion.
- Diagnosis and management of intracranial pathology.
- Treatment of other injuries, particularly of chest or abdomen.

Ideally, patients with disability sufficiently severe to stop them going home directly from the intensive treatment unit (ITU) should go through a unit designed to deal with the recovery of brain-injured patients. Most district hospitals are too small to sustain such for TBI patients only, but if the facility undertakes management of younger patients with stroke or subarachnoid haemorrhage there are suffi-

Rehabilitation of the Physically Disabled Adult. Edited by C. John Goodwill, M. Anne Chamberlain and Chris Evans. Published in 1997 by Stanley Thornes (Publishers) Ltd, Cheltenham. ISBN 0-7487-3183-0.

cient numbers. It is unsatisfactory to lodge patients either on medical or surgical wards, as with few exceptions they are not catered for or well managed there. Untoward behaviour often leads to inappropriate sedation. There is not usually enough therapy time available to prevent physical deterioration.

Patients should not reach rehabilitation facilities cachectic, and undernourished, or with flexion contractures and pressure sores. On all wards which deal with TBI there must be policies prepared and enough staff to prevent such happenings. Percutaneous endoscopic gastrostomy and minimal sedation are important techniques by which a good quality of survival can be achieved. Staff should be trained to cope with aggression.

EPIDEMIOLOGY

Krause *et al* (1984) looked at the incidence of brain injury and serious impairment in San Diego, California. Bryden (1989) focused on the incidence in North West Scotland. Tennant (1995) looked at figures from the North of England and compared them with data from the rest of the world in an attempt to get complete statistics. The difficulty is that most of the groups used slightly different criteria in measuring the incidence and prevalence.

Peak incidence in the late teens and early twenties is noted in all studies, with a secondary, smaller peak in the elderly population. In the earlier peak, males predominate, but males and females are approximately equal in the elderly group. Road accidents were the biggest cause in the younger group, falls were more significant in the elderly group.

In 1990 the Department of Health commissioned the National Traumatic Brain Injury Study. The purpose of this was to assess methods of rehabilitation, and to attempt to establish links between services – volumes, types of therapy – and outcomes. It would, if possible, identify good practice and look at issues of cost effectiveness, and would make recommendations concerning purchasing strategies. Twelve centres were designated to take part, each being given a grant of between £50 000 and £200 000 per year, depending upon the nature of the service development for which they were responsible. The University of Warwick was given the responsibility for conducting the evaluation. One of the remits held by Cornwall was to search for all people whose head injuries were severe enough to get them to the accident and emergency departments of district general hospitals. The study was set up to cover patients between the ages of 16 and 65, but during the study useful information about the rest of the population was obtained.

Two other areas of research were incorporated into the study. The first was to follow-up 10% of all the people classified as having a mild head injury to see how many of these were still suffering from symptoms at the end of 6 months. In addition, there has been constant monitoring of the management of those who sustained severe brain injury. This ran parallel with a programme funded by the Nuffield Provincial Hospitals Trust which looked at patients known to the rehabilitation services in Cornwall who had sustained TBI in the last 11 years. It has measured the outcomes of TBI not just for the patient, but also for their family and other carers (Sansom, 1995).

DEFINITIONS

Most of these definitions are from the working party of the British Society of Rehabilitation Medicine. They produced a working document in 1988 (McLellan, 1988).

Traumatic brain injury

'Brain injury caused by trauma to the head or which may follow lack of oxygen or low blood pressure. This definition includes collapse during anaesthesia or after cardiac arrest.'

Unconsciousness

In earlier studies the definition of end of unconsciousness by Plum and Posner (1972) was 'when communication returns to better than "yes" or "no" allowing for local impedimenta (e.g. tracheostomy, jaw injury)'.

More recently unconsciousness is defined as when 'the level of consciousness scores 9 or less on the Glasgow Coma Score (GCS)'. The GCS has become accepted as the standard measurement and is in use throughout the world.

Post-traumatic amnesia

'When continuous day to day memory is re-established'. This is different from the first remembered event or 'island' and it implies the ability to acquire and retain new information. It is difficult to apply universally because some sequelae of head injury may mean that memory never returns to what it was before, but it would not be likely that post-traumatic amnesia (PTA) was an indefinite event.

Measuring the duration of unconsciousness and PTA is complicated by more recent approaches in ITUs where ventilation with paralysis is part of standard management. In this case unconsciousness may be considered as induced by treatment and can only be established as truly being present after the anaesthetic agents have been withdrawn. In practice most people remain unconscious for significant periods after withdrawal of sedation (e.g. more than 24 hours). It may then be reasonable to assume that the unconsciousness is due to the head injury rather than sedation. Similarly, sometimes where unconsciousness lasts for hours or only one or two days, the influence of alcohol or drugs may still be present. In the elderly group, the possibility of dementia preceding the fall needs to be considered.

Mild brain injury

'An injury causing unconsciousness of 15 minutes or less or post-traumatic amnesia for less than 6 hours.' This group is largely ignored as most get better, yet recent figures from the Warwick study suggest a significant number have problems after 6 months and some help for this group to prevent unnecessary loss of work should be available.

Moderate brain injury

'An injury causing unconsciousness for more than 15 minutes, less than 6 hours or a post-traumatic amnesia of between 6 and 24 hours.'

Severe brain injury

'An injury causing unconsciousness for more than 6 hours, but less than 2 days or a post-traumatic amnesia for more than 24 hours, but less than a week.'

Very severe brain injury

'An injury causing unconsciousness of more than 48 hours or a post-traumatic amnesia of more than 7 days'.

One further category of 'disastrous brain injury' can be identified where unconsciousness has been present for more than 4 weeks. The reason for this suggestion is described later.

Persistent vegetative state (PVS)

'A profound form of brain damage where the patient although having a sleep–awake pattern responds only in a reflex way and shows no evidence of meaningful response to the environment' (K. Andrews, 1994, personal communication). There are at the time of writing four patients in Cornwall with PVS. One of these is from a road accident, the other three from non-traumatic causes. Each district will be likely to have some patients in PVS. A clear purchasing policy for this care is needed, identifying potential providers. Exact borderlines of PVS are sometimes difficult to determine leading to clinical and legal problems, but a recent British Medical Association (1995) publication helps. It requires that a patient must have been unconscious for more than 6 months for the diagnosis to be made in cases of unconsciousness other than traumatic brain injury. The diagnosis of PVS in those with TBI can only be made soundly after 12 months' unconsciousness (Chapter 10).

LIFE EXPECTANCY

One of the most frequently asked questions after head injury is about the future. Life expectancy may be measured in two ways: duration and quality.

Duration

It seems very doubtful if patients with mild, moderate or even severe traumatic brain injury will have any reduction of length of life. The question is frequently raised in the courts by lawyers who have to decide the size of settlements (quantum) where there is a culpable party. The evidence that there is a life-shortening effect of such head injury is very poor. In such cases, reference can to be made to Government Actuarial Tables for the normal life expectancy, then considering whether there are any other factors which might decrease it. Reduction of life expectancy is usually from pre-existing illness such as hypertension or diabetes, or through habits such as smoking or excessive drinking. The exception is when epilepsy complicates the injury. Corkin, Sullivan and Carr (1984) studied those who survived penetrating injuries in World War II. They showed that patients with a head injury complicated by epilepsy died sooner than those with a head injury without epilepsy. The latter group's life expectancy was the same as the control group who had a peripheral nerve injury.

The same question is also asked about very severely brain injured patients, but there are too few survivors living long enough to yield enough data. World War II patients would have had limited acute services at that time

and to survive at all implies considerable toughness!

For patients in persistent vegetative state there has been work which suggests life expectancy is shortened (Levin *et al*, 1991: K. Andrews, 1994, personal communication). It might be, however, that given enough resources any such patient can survive, so the life expectancy reflects the quality of care as well. Whether it is feasible or desirable to keep a patient alive at all costs is a lively issue, at present unresolved.

Quality

Physical problems arising as a consequence, such as hemiparesis or spasticity, may persist despite expert rehabilitation. If the residua are confined to physical problems, it is probably less stressful for all concerned than where there are problems of memory, concentration or altered personality. Brooks (1992) has described the psychosocial consequences clearly, and Sansom (1995) has demonstrated the predictable paradox that the more severely disabled a patient is as a consequence of TBI, the victim perceives the stress less, and the relatives and carers perceive it more. Outcomes will be considered later in the chapter.

OUTCOMES

Irrespective of the variety of sequelae in TBI, it may be possible to agree some mutually acceptable goals. For example, in the Chessington series (Evans, 1989). Outcomes were recorded (*inter alia*) for employability and net earnings at review about 5 years after the head injury. Figure 29.1 shows that very few people who had been observed to be unconscious for more than 4 weeks were back in employment (though one was) and very few people who has been unconscious for less than 4 weeks were unemployable. Figure 29.2 shows the net earnings at 1982 values for the same group of patients. It is possible to put some financial figures to these results, although they are

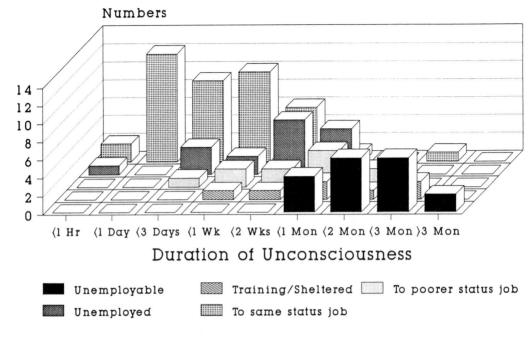

Figure 29.1 Traumatic brain injury: employment status at 5 years.

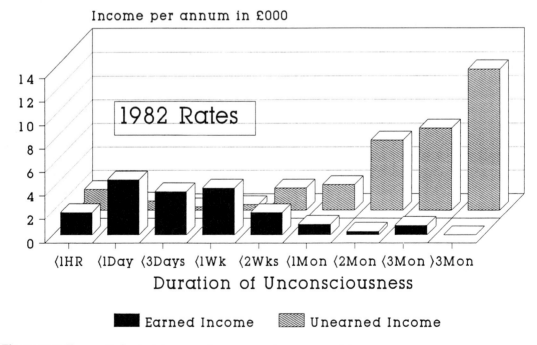

Figure 29.2 Traumatic brain injury survivors: earned vs unearned income.

derived from a series in which the young subjects were both highly motivated and intensively treated. Although they were all either severely or very severely injured, they were all in skilled employment at the time trauma occurred, unlike most civilian populations currently treated. Indeed, it is interesting to compare this group with the current series from Cornwall. In the latter there is a significant group of people who had what would have been described as a mild traumatic brain injury in the Chessington series, and so excluded, where there is a significant morbidity after 6 months.

The outcome of rehabilitation can be measured by whether the patient can return to work at the same job, or one of equivalent status, life in the same house, be independent, and sustain normal relationships with family and friends. Any restriction in any of these factors represents the residual disability, and is the measure by which the severity of the original injury has not been matched by rehabilitation. Brooks (1992) has measured these factors, and so have Wilson (1991, 1994) and Sansom (1995). The standards are now clearer than when the first report was written. Some years ago it was thought that physical recovery was the yardstick of improvement, but as more experience has been gained the impact of altered personality and behaviour have become perceived as the more disabling features of TBI. It is not that the physical aspects are unimportant, simply that all the problems after head injury need to be managed as a whole.

The use of MRI and SPECT scans, which give clearer pictures about the cerebral blood flow, may help in recording the effects of diffuse axonal damage which may be sustained in what appears at first sight to be a relatively mildly brain injured person.

EARLY MANAGEMENT

The rehabilitation ward in an acute hospital will liaise closely with the surgical wards and ITU. Ideally, the patient with brain injury should transfer as soon as medically stable to the rehabilitation ward and there should be as few changes of environment or staff during this critical time as possible.

As experienced multidisciplinary team must assess the patients. They will set short- and long-term goals, decide the management and treatment and monitor progress. They should support the family and other carers with information and help. Each patient should have a daily programme set out which should include designated rest periods. The whole rehabilitation team should review long-term goals and short-term aims of treatment at least once a week. This review should be formal and the plans discussed with the patient and his/her carers. The length of stay will depend on the operational policy of the unit and the locally available facilities to refer on to.

COGNITIVE REHABILITATION

The term cognitive rehabilitation covers any intervention, strategy or technique that enables patients and their families to come to terms with, manage or reduce acquired cognitive deficits. Several approaches to cognitive rehabilitation have been described (Miller, 1984). Modifying the environment, functional adaptations and encouraging the maximum use of retained skills may be suitable strategies to avoid problems (Wilson, 1987)

Active rehabilitation is very demanding on the patient. It is even more difficult when there are cognitive deficits. All those who are involved with the patient with brain injury must understand cognitive dysfunction and how it alters what the patient can understand, comply with and tolerate.

MODIFICATION OF BEHAVIOUR

Brain injury may cause changes in behaviour. These may cause failure to return to work and to pre-injury levels of social activity. They lead to progressively severe stress in members of the patient's family (Sansom, 1995). The disability team must try to understand and overcome these at all stages in the patient's recovery. Simple guidelines for the earliest stages have been described.

Behavioural problems may not be due only to the injury. They may be part of the patient's premorbid personality, the pattern of brain injury sustained and the cumulative effects of the patient's experiences during the process of recovery. It is most important, even in these early stages, to advise patients and their families about managing such problems; patterns may otherwise develop which place the patient beyond the reach of help from therapists, family or friends later.

The patient's previous personality is the cornerstone upon which recovery is built and the goals set must be appropriate for the patient's known attributes and interests. Assessing behaviour and setting reasonable goals requires skill and experience. It is essential that in setting goals they are agreed by the patient's relatives and family. It should go without saying that goals should be agreed by the patient, but the caveat 'where possible' must be added. Normally goal setting with patients will reflect their ability to participate. Difficulties and any controversial issues should be discussed at the team meetings; it is impossible to discuss behaviour comprehensively or to modify it except where there is a working consensus.

Where severe disturbances of behaviour occur that are not due to psychiatric disease, a formal behaviour programme should be begun. This will usually be in a specialized unit under the supervision of a clinical psychologist who has been trained in the techniques of behaviour modification. It is difficult to set up on an ordinary rehabilitation unit because of the many uncontrolled outside influences. Persisting severe behavioural disorders are discussed later in the chapter and in Chapter 30.

STAFFING FOR INPATIENT REHABILITATION TEAM

The attention span of patients with brain injury is often severely reduced. This means that they may not benefit from prolonged sessions of therapy, but require shorter intensive sessions with frequent periods of rest. Such a pattern of treatment needs more staff than for disabilities in which treatment can be managed in groups. Without adequate staffing levels, the brain-injured patient is likely to be subjected to fruitless and tiring spells of activity, alternating with prolonged periods of inactivity during which the patient becomes bored. Adequate staffing levels and tight and responsive timetabling make effective treatment possible and will help to prevent complications. Furthermore, it needs to be realized by purchasers that it will take more time to supervise a patient doing an activity such as feeding, than to take over and do it.

The following recommendations relating to the various professional staff are only guidelines; there is inadequate evidence upon which to establish the best ratios between numbers of staff and patients. In all units accepting responsibility for brain injury rehabilitation, all the following professions must be represented. The numbers of staff required to undertake these designated functions will depend upon the size of the unit, the operational policy and the physical aspects of the accommodation provided for patients, staff and rehabilitative services. The nature of the service provided to the patient is what matters rather than the professional designation of the staff member who provides it.

Nursing

Nurses are the only staff present at all times. During the evenings, throughout the night, at every meal and at weekends they will continue to develop patients' independence, concentration, social skills and behaviour. Their input needs to integrate with and complement the work of the other team members. All members of the team need an awareness of the role of the other team members. Training in physical and psychiatric rehabilitation and counselling is not given in most general nurse training courses at present; it needs to be introduced. Due to the time-consuming nature of their duties and the frequent combination of behavioural disturbance with physical dependency, the staffing ratio will normally require at least one full-time equivalent (FTE) nurse per bed in the rehabilitation ward or unit. Skill mix needs careful thought.

Clinical psychology

Clinical psychologists have two major roles. First, they assess cognitive impairments and, second, they undertake analysis of disturbed behaviour, and construct the appropriate treatment strategies. They may produce cognitive remediation programmes. In some units they may support and counsel staff. Some assessment may overlap with other professions, especially occupational therapists. It will depend upon the structure and experience of other staff. A brief outline of commonly used assessments is given in the Appendix.

Occupational therapy

Occupational therapists play a crucial role in brain injury rehabilitation, developing independence skills and planning activities that encourage initiation, planning, sequencing, concentration and social skills. They are also the team members most experienced in home assessment and identifying need for adaptations and equipment to be provided in the patient's home before discharge from hospital. Their assessment of the patient's workplace may help define goals for resettlement. One occupational therapist to five brain-injured inpatients is the minimum acceptable.

Speech therapy

Many brain-injured patients have disorders of communication and of swallowing. This needs assessment and treatment under the direction of a speech therapist. The level of support required in a unit will fluctuate according to the needs of patients present; therefore staff may sometimes be shared between in-patient and out-patient teams. Experience in the prescription and use of communication aids is an essential prerequisite of speech therapists working with brain injury. Videofluoroscopy should be available at this stage (Chapter 22)

Physiotherapy

Guidance from physiotherapists is required in positioning and handling the patient to help mobilize optimal function and to prevent contractures and deformity. Their assessment is essential in establishing appropriate means of assistance for balance and walking and in selecting and supervising appropriate movement and fitness programmes. A staffing level of one experienced specialized therapist to six brain-injured patients is the minimum.

Medical staff

Rehabilitation teams treating brain-injured patients should ideally be led by a consultant experienced in head injury rehabilitation, who has had clinical neurological experience. The speciality of the consultant is less important than the expertise and commitment to brain injury rehabilitation. Many will be drawn from the ranks of rehabilitation (disability) medicine, neurology or organic psychiatry. The consultant should be supported by junior staff in training. He or she should ensure that a written operational policy for brain injury rehabilitation is available and is followed.

Social work

Social difficulties are frequently experienced by the families of brain-injured people and professional help is often needed in assessment, counselling and advice on benefits and community support. The social worker allocated to a person in hospital should ideally keep in contact with the family after the patient returns home and needs to understand the nature of the effects of brain injury on the patient and family, so that they may be able to provide monitoring and support during the long recovery period. The staff required will depend upon the availability of effective local community social services for physically disabled people.

Art therapy

Many rehabilitation units now employ an art therapist. They can use different media to help explore moods, and help the rest of the team to understand some of the feelings and thoughts of patients with brain damage. One therapist for 16 patients seems appropriate. Art work, as opposed to art therapy, can be developed for groups and can be undertaken by volunteers under the supervision of the therapist (Chapter 43).

Orthoptics

Many patients with brain injury have problems with visual fields or with ocular imbalance. Conventional bedside testing is not precise enough to reveal all the problems and routine use of an orthoptist uncovers easily remediable defects. For example, the use of Fresnel prisms and temporary occlusions may give great help with balance problems, and can be identified by the orthoptists, working with the speech therapist if the patient's communication is impaired. The service can be given on a sessional basis (Chapter 21).

STAFFING IMPLICATIONS FOR A HEALTH DISTRICT

A health authority with a population of 250 000 is likely to generate 45 moderately and 20 severely brain-injured patients per annum. Assuming a mean length of stay in hospital of 2 months (which is probably an underestimate), approximately 10 beds will be occupied in the district general hospital at any one time by patients recovering from brain injury. This implies that for brain-injured inpatients alone the inpatient staffing requirements will be 10 FTE nurses, 2 FTE occupational therapists, 1.5 FTE physiotherapists, 0.5 FTE clinical psychologist, 0.5 FTE speech therapist and 0.5 FTE social worker. Medical staff will be required at consultant and junior level.

PHYSICAL ENVIRONMENT

Sufficient single room accommodation should be available so that any brain-injured patient who requires it can get it. It is often necessary to nurse patients soon after brain injury on mattresses on the floor. In these early stages the family must have easy access and not feel excluded or crowded. Close contact needs to be made between relatives and staff, so adequate facilities for private interviewing must be available. The standard facilities for remedial therapy include a gymnasium, hydrotherapy pool and light and heavy workshops, which must be within easy access for patients, relatives and ward staff. There also needs to be seminar rooms and quiet rooms available.

DESIGNATED BRAIN INJURY UNITS

Opinions differ about whether it is desirable for brain-injured patients to undertake rehabilitation alongside those with other disorders such as stroke. For most activities, brain-injured patients require individual treatment rather than treatment in large groups. Small

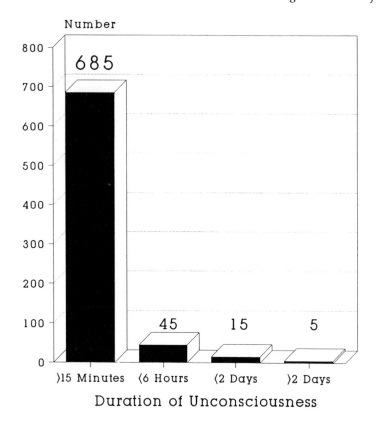

Figure 29.3 Traumatic brain injury: estimated incidence per 250 000.

group work (e.g. five or six) seems necessary for teaching some skills. Difficulties may arise if the brain-injured patient's behaviour is importunate. However, this is usually containable if there are enough staff and family available to supervise and distract. In a district hospital there may be fewer than 10 brain-injured patients having inpatient rehabilitation at a time. They can be located with other younger acutely disabled adults in a rehabilitation ward if the ward's programmes are flexible and the staffing levels and facilities are generous enough. It is not so easy to mix acutely injured patients with those with static or deteriorating disabilities such as multiple sclerosis.

Clinical research and evaluation of the service provided should be a primary require-

ment of such units which should have formal links with appropriate academic departments of a medical school. In areas of the country where the population is very dispersed, community-based models of a rehabilitation service for brain injury should be formally evaluated (Chapter 31).

It is also our experience that social workers allocated to patients with complex disability due to brain injury often do not have adequate knowledge or experience of the problems. A teacher or educational psychologist with specific experience in brain injury rehabilitation may be helpful in the rehabilitation of adolescent patients. They can link with school authorities, have expertise in group activities, and familiarity with local educational and training courses.

This general lack of specific experience and expertise would be remedied by the widespread introduction of special brain injury units, but could also be improved by the more efficient deployment and training of current staff, under the chairmanship of a properly trained consultant in disability medicine with specified responsibilities for head injury rehabilitation, as recommended for each health district by the Royal College of Physicians' Disability Committee (Royal College of Physicians), 1986).

THE MANAGEMENT OF LATER STAGES OF RECOVERY AND RESETTLEMENT AFTER SEVERE BRAIN INJURY

Discharge from hospital

With the introduction of the National Health Services and Community Care Act 1993 people are to be encouraged and helped to live in the community if they wish. A comprehensive assessment of need should be undertaken and recommendations made to meet the identified needs.

A small minority of patients, particularly those with dissociative or aggressive features, may be unable to return full time to the community and will require long-term psychiatric shared care or permanent care. Behavioural disorders often coexist with physical disability, so the resources used must be able to cope with the needs of patients with more than one handicap. It may be helpful to incorporate some professional skills of the learning disability teams into the management of behavioural difficulties. Their idea of group homes with good professional support should be explored, especially by those health authorities that at present have no identifiable resources. Such a facility could also provide short-term inpatient reassessment or breaks for the patient and the family (shared care) living in the community.

By default some health purchasers buy in specialized nursing care for managing behavioural problems and PVS from the private sector. This may be unsatisfactory as the care is often a long distance from the patient's home and family. It is also expensive.

Sometimes residential as opposed to nursing care is inevitable for a younger person, i.e. under 65. This may reflect inadequate living options in the community, difficulties with funding community care or that there are unacceptable risks for the individual. It may reflect the patient's preference. These patients should not be placed in a unit where the other residents are elderly, even if a single room has been nominally registered for this purpose.

It is essential that a patient's discharge home, or to another institution if appropriate, is carefully staged. All arrangements for the physical and psychological needs of the patient and family must be identified and arrangements made to meet them before discharge occurs. These preparations will be based on consultation with the patient and the patient's family. The members of the hospital disability team and those in the community team should liaise during this process. Where community rehabilitation or head injury teams exist, they should be used.

The strategy of rehabilitation that is to continue after discharge should be specified in writing and available to the patient, the patient's family and the general practitioner at the time of discharge. The names and contact numbers of the community teams responsible for monitoring progress or dealing with problems should be specified in writing in the medical records and be provided in writing for the patient, their relatives and the GP.

Organization of treatment after discharge from hospital

It is now known that recovery may be prolonged so that regular support and input may be required for many years after the injury. Stress increases progressively in many patients' relatives over the first 5 years (Sansom, 1995). In view of the complex nature of post brain injury patients, there is a need for a defined process of follow-up after discharge from hospital.

This should have the following functions:

- Ensure that recommendations made before discharge from the unit have been established.
- Evaluate and review the efficacy of rehabilitation measures employed.
- Formulate and coordinate any future rehabilitative procedures.
- Provide a facility for the assessment of patients not previously seen by the team who have developed post brain injury problems and to provide a crisis intervention advisory structure.

The Warwick study has found out that one of the most difficult but important areas of post acute rehabilitation is to define goals for individuals and families, and then to monitor and assess the achievement of these goals. Since rehabilitation services, like almost all services in the overstretched UK Health Service, are in short supply, there will always be a problem of allocating volumes of care. This problem is compounded if the outcomes for individual patients are not systematically and regularly assessed; patients and families who could benefit can be deprived of services because they are being devoted to those who may be experiencing little improvement. It has also become clear that post acute follow-up must cross not only the boundaries between different therapeutic professions within the Health Service, but also the boundaries between health and social services, education and employment services.

Outpatient management

In many areas this is the only reliable follow-up system available to all patients. It has an overview and can be the focus for the

management regardless of any other individual input. The outpatient clinic must have a core team consisting of medical staff, psychologist and social worker who work in cooperation with the other members of the designated brain injury team (nurses, remedial therapists and teachers). Patients already known to the team at an earlier stage would be seen for review by the member(s) of this team most appropriate to their needs at the time of discharge. The core team would review all cases at the end of the clinic session and formulate the next stage in the management plan, coordinating input from the other staff in the team and ensuring coordination with community health, employment and social services (Evans and Skidmore, 1998).

Referrals should only be accepted with the knowledge of the general practitioner. Newly referred patients would be seen in the first instance by the medical staff unless specific referral had been made for psychological or social work advice. A checklist system for clerking new patients helps to avoid problems being missed, as junior medical staff who do the clerking change frequently. It helps ensure documentation of the nature of brain injury morbidity for research purposes and also clinical management.

Case management

Case managers are extensively used in the USA. They take the general view of the rehabilitation programmers for many groups of patients, particularly those with TBI. They are supported in the USA by insurance companies who wish to make it as easy as possible to provide rehabilitation early as this has been shown to reduce long-term morbidity (and costs). In the UK the concept of case managers was started in a London teaching hospital where liaison has to be made with many local authority, social service departments and community services. Ideally a case manager is introduced to the patient and the family while the patient is in the ITU and they follow the patient through the hospital system out into the community. Contact should be kept for as long as it is helpful. There will be an element of advocacy in the job as they are responsible to the patient. The rehabilitation of the brain-injured individual requires the skill of many different health professionals and other agencies, and it is not yet proven that employing case managers is the most effective method of patients accessing services. Others, such as the use of a community head injury team or specialized, educated senior occupational therapists available to their colleagues in social services in defined areas have proven to be effective alternative means of delivering treatment (Hughes *et al*, 1995)

Key workers

The key worker concept was discussed above. Recent legislation has introduced the additional idea of an officially designated advocate for disabled people, a role that could overlap that the key worker and could be incorporated into the role of some community key workers. It can be difficult for the key worker to be a proper advocate for the patient if the role conflicts with the policies of their employing agency.

Voluntary organizations

Information about voluntary organizations such as Headway and carers associations should be given to the patient and their family when possible. Headway provides considerable support to patients' families as well as literature, and an increasing number of Headway Houses where stimulating day activities take place.

Return to work

When return to work seems attainable, liaison should be made with the employer. This is especially important if there are still some remaining cognitive or behavioural disorders likely to impair effectiveness. Occupational therapy departments need resources to initiate work practice and develop tolerance to the requirements of employment, notably stamina, noise tolerance, tolerance of interruption, communication and sequencing of activities. They also need to be the link with future employers.

The help of the Disability Employment Adviser (DEA) or the local Placement and Counselling Team (PACT) can be sought if there are problems of workplace adaptation in relation to resuming work. The Employment Service can also advise about a staged return to work in which the patient starts with light part-time duties and increases gradually to the level at which full duties are undertaken. This is particularly appropriate for head-injured patients and should be adopted wherever possible. Therapeutic earnings is a benefit that is often useful. Advice can also be given on other local alternative routes to re-employment (e.g. Link into Learning) (Chapter 51).

PLANNING FOR THE FUTURE

The Royal College of Physicians' report of 1986 has not yet been implemented in most health districts. The committee recommended that a brain injury rehabilitation service should be available in each health district. The service should identify needs of brain-injured survivors using nationally agreed outcome criteria and provide for them, drawing up a written operational policy for brain injury rehabilitation. Links with employment, social services, housing, education and voluntary organizations should be developed and formalized. The setting up of such a service should be a priority of newly designated consultants in rehabilitation medicine supported by written, widely available policy statements on TBI services by purchasing authorities. The sustained pressure by the public. aided by such policy statements and by clinical evidence of the effectiveness of interventions, should, hopefully, result in the establishment of specific services.

REFERENCES

British Medical Association (1995) *Advanced Statement About Medical Treatment*, (produced in association with the Law Society), BMJ Publishing Group, London.

Brooks, N. (1992) Psychosocial assessment after traumatic brain injury. *Scandinavian Journal of Rehabilitation Medicine Supplement*, **26**, 125–131.

Bryden, J. (1989) How many head injured? The epidemiology of post head injury disability, in *Models of Brain Injury Rehabilitation* (ed R.L. Wood and Eames), Chapman & Hall, London, pp. 17–27.

Corkin, S., Sullivan, E.V. and Carr, A. (1984) Prognostic factors for life expectancy after penetrating head injury. *Archives of Neurology*, **41**, 975–977.

Evans, C.D. (1989) Long-term follow-up, in *Models of Brain Injury Rehabilitation* (ed. R.L. Wood and P. Eames), Chapman & Hall, London, pp. 59–72.

Evans, C.D. and Skidmore, B. (1989) Rehabilitation in the community, in *Models of Brain Injury Rehabilitation* (ed. R.L.Wood and P. Eames), Chapman & Hall, London.

Hughes, D., Ward, E., Warnock, H. *et al.* (1995) An urban community service: head injury – using occupational therapy to meet the challenge of community reintegration, in *Traumatic Brain Injury Rehabilitation* (eds A. Chamberlain, Neumann and A. Tennant), Chapman & Hall, London, pp. 66–83.

Krause, J.F., Black, M.A., Hessol, N. *et al.* (1984) The incidence of acute brain injury and serious impairment in a defined population. *American Journal of Epidemiology*, **119**, 186-201.

Levin, H.S., Saydjari, C., Eisenberg, H.M. *et al.* (1991) Vegetative state after closed head injury. *Archives of Neurology*, **48**, 580–585.

McLellan, D.L. (1988) *The Management of Traumatic Brain Injury*. A working party report of the Medical Disability Society, published by the Development Trust for the Young Disabled on behalf of the Medical Disability Society, Royal College of Physicians, London. (Further edition in preparation).

Miller, E. (1984) *Recovery and Management of Neuropsychological Impairments*, John Wiley, Chichester.

National Traumatic Brain Injury Survey (1996) Health Services Research Unit, Warwick Business School, The University of Warwick, Coventry (in preparation).

Plum, F. and Posner, B. (1972) *Diagnosis of Stupor and Coma* 2nd edn, Davis, Philadelphia.

Royal College of Physicians (2986) Physical disability in 1986 and beyond. *Journal of the Royal College of Physcians, London*, **20**, 3–37.

Sansom, M. (1995) Quality of Life for Survivors of Head Injury. PhD thesis, Exeter University (in preparation).

Tennant, A. (1995) The epidemiology of head injury, in *Traumatic Brain Injury Rehabilitation* (eds A. Chamberlain, V. Neumann and A. Tennant), Chapman & Hall, London, pp. 12–24.

Welsh Affairs Committee (1995) *Severe Head Injuries: rehabilitation*, HMSO, London.

Wilson, B.A. (1987) *Rehabilitation of Memory*, Guilford Press, New York.

Wilson, B.A. (1991) Long-term prognosis of patients with severe memory disorders. *Neuropsychological Rehabilitation*, **1**, 117–134.

Wilson, B.A. (1994) Life after brain injury: long term outcome of 101 people seen for rehabilitation 5–12 years earlier, in *Treatment issues and long term outcomes* Proceedings of the 18th Annual Brain Impairment Conference, Hobart, Australia, 1994. Academic, Bowen Hills, Queensland pp. 1–6.

FURTHER READING

Chamberlain, A., Neumann, V. and Tennant A. (eds) (1995) *Traumatic Brain Injury Rehabilitation*, Chapman & Hall, London.

Crawford, J.K., Parker, D.M. and McKinkey, W.W. (eds) (1992) *A Handbook of Neuropsychological Assessment*, Lawrence Erlbaum Associates, Hove, Sussex.

Lezak, M.D. (1995) *Neuropsychological Assessment*, Oxford University Press, New York.

Appendix: psychometric tests

C. Green

In order to provide an accurate report of the presence of a given disorder, the degree to which this disorder may affect psychological functioning, and its likely course, the clinical neuropsychologist must employ a wide range of assessment measures.

Of the numerous psychometric instruments available, there are a number which tend to be used more frequently than others when assessing the head-injured patient. These include tests of individual cognitive functions such as memory and intellect, and also test batteries that contain measures of a range of skills.

A brief description of some of these tests is given below, along with their structure and their application in neuropsychological examination.

1. The Luria Nebraska Neuropsychological Battery (LNNB)

Developed by the Russian psychologist A.R. Luria and revised by researchers at the University of Nebraska. This instrument consists of 269 items designed to test a broad range of functions and is divided into the following 11 clinical scales:

- motor
- rhythm
- tactile
- visual
- receptive speech
- expressive speech
- writing
- reading
- arithmetic
- memory
- intellectual processes (intelligence).

Based on performance and a combination of items from these scales, three further summary scales can be examined:

- Pathognomic – which indicates the presence brain dysfunction.
- Left hemisphere – which measures right hand performance.
- Right hemisphere – which measures left hand performance.

The main purpose of the LNNB is to determine the nature and extent of both general and specific cognitive deficits (including the lateralization and localization of focal brain impairments) by comparing test performance against an individually calculated cut-off score based on age and level of education.

2. The Screening Test for the Luria Nebraska Neuropsychological Battery (ST–LNNB)

This very short screening test, consisting of 15 items from the LNNB, is used to predict probable performance on the full length battery. As such, the test is limited only to an indication of either 'normal' or 'abnormal'

Rehabilitation of the Physically Disabled Adult. Edited by C. John Goodwill, M. Anne Chamberlain and Chris Evans. Published in 1997 by Stanley Thornes (Publishers) Ltd, Cheltenham. ISBN 0-7487-3183-0.

performance if the full test battery were to be administered. It cannot, therefore, be employed as a separate test for diagnosing neuropsychological problems.

However, the advantage of the ST–LNNB lies primarily in its simplicity and ease of administration. It can be completed and scored, on average, within 20 minutes (the full LNNB requires a minimum of 2–3 hours), and it does not require complex interpretation in order to provide an explicit numerical result.

Thus, the ST–LNNB provides a simple means by which a patient's general psychometric requirements can be identified prior to highly intensive studies which may, upon completion, prove inappropriate.

3. Stroop Neuropsychological Screening Test (SNST)

The SNST is based on the work of J.R. Stroop who, in the mid 1930s, discovered an interference effect in the ability of individuals to switch between conflicting verbal responses modes.

The interference effect is based on the observation that the reading of colour names such as **red** or **green** requires less time than actual naming of colours themselves.

Later research indicated that this interference effect was a reliable diagnostic measure in the discrimination of brain-damaged patients from normal control subjects, with varying but stable levels of performance noted amongst various patient subgroups.

The test itself consists of a two-stage procedure. First, a list of colour names, **blue, green, red** and **tan**, printed in non-matching colours (e.g. the word **red** is printed in **blue, green** or **tan** and so on) is presented to the subject. The subject must then read aloud the words that they read.

Next the subject is presented with another similar list of colour names. This time, however, they are instructed to call out the colour of the ink that the words are printed in. Interference occurs, then, because of the natural tendency to read the word as well as identify the colour that the word is printed in.

4. The Wechsler Adult Intelligence Scale – Revised (WAIS-R)

First developed during the late 1930s by psychologist David Wechsler, the WAIS and the later revised version the WAIS-R contains 11 subtests grouped in 2 main categories. The first of these is a verbal scale containing six subtests, and the second a performance (non-verbal) scale comprising the remaining five subtests. This division allows for the calculation of both verbal and performance IQ scores as well as an overall IQ.

Subtest Components	Description
Verbal Scale	
Information	Questions covering a wide range of general knowledge.
Digit Span	Digit sequences of increasing length presented orally. After presentation the subject is required to repeat the sequence.
Vocabulary	Words of increasing difficulty are presented to the subject who must then define them.
Arithmetic	The subject is asked to solve a number of simple calculations without the use of pen and paper.
Comprehension	The subject is asked to answer questions concerning behaviour under certain specified circumstances, the meaning of certain proverbs and why certain practices are followed.

Similarities   These questions require that the subject explains the similarity between certain specified items.

Performance Scale

Picture Completion   Subjects are asked to identify the missing components of a series of line drawings

Picture Arrangement   Subjects are asked to arrange sequences of cards displaying cartoon characters performing an action so that they depict a sensible story.

Block Design   Subjects are required to complete designs of increasing complexity from coloured blocks.

Object Assembly   Subjects are provided with the pieces of a puzzle and asked to assemble them in the correct order.

Digit Symbol   Symbols paired with digits are presented to subjects who must the pair the appropriate symbol with the correct digit.

The WAIS-R, then, provides not only information on a patient's global intellectual abilities but also, through careful evaluation of the individual scales, information on most aspects of cognitive functioning. A patient's scores can then be compared with normative data to distinguish areas of deficit, while appraisals of, for example, likely vocational or educational competency, can also be made in order to design appropriate treatment strategies.

5. Wechsler Memory Scale – Revised (WMS–R)

Also developed by David Wechsler, the WMS-R provides a reliable means of mea-suring a number of different aspects of memory function in a single battery. The instrument itself contains 13 subtests and provides three major composite scores upon completion: the General Memory score (which is further subdivided into a Verbal Memory and Visual Memory), an Attention/Concen-tration score, and a Delayed Recall score.

Subtest Components	Description
Information and Orientation	The subject is asked a series of simple questions concerning biographical data, orientation, etc.
Mental Control	This subtest is designed to draw upon over learned information that most unimpaired subjects can answer without difficulty, e.g. recitation of the letters of the alphabet.
Figural Memory	This subtest involves the presentation of abstract designs to the subjects who must then, after their removal, identify them from within a larger set of designs.
Logical Memory I	The subject is asked to listen to and then recall two short stories.
Visual Paired Associates I	This subtest requires the subject to learn and recall colour associations with abstract line drawings.
Verbal Paired Associates I	Subjects are required to learn and recall a series of word pairs.
Visual Reproduction I	The subject is asked to draw from memory simple geometric shapes, each of which is presented for a period of 10 seconds.

Digit Span — The subject is asked to recall sequences of digits both forwards and backwards.

Visual Memory Span — Similar to the Digit Span subtest, the subject is required to touch a series of coloured squares in a predetermined order. The task is then repeated in reverse order.

Logical Memory II — This is a delayed recall of subtest Logical Memory I and is undertaken 30 minutes after the first presentation.

Visual Paired Associates II — Once again a delayed recall subtest based on Visual Paired Associates I.

Verbal Paired Associates II — Delayed recall trial of Verbal Paired Associates I.

Visual Reproduction II — Delayed recall trial of Visual Reproduction I.

Although not designed to elucidate problems in all facets of memory, the WMS-R does, however, provide the neuropsychologist with an immediately useful and reasonably accurate measure of global memory function. Such information can then be put to use in the design and implementation of rehabilitation programmes and the monitoring of therapeutic interventions.

6. The Rivermead Behavioural Memory Test (RBMT)

The RBMT, unlike the WMS-R, attempts to assess memory function as it applies to everyday life rather than relying on measures of the performance of a patient in the learning and recall experimental material.

The test is also quite short, comparatively easy to administer and relatively undemanding. Therefore, it has the additional advantage of being particularly effective with patients whose comprehension is poor or whose level of attention and concentration is circumscribed.

The test consists of the following subtests, some which require the immediate recall of information, and some which require delayed recall:

Subtest Components	Description
Remembering A Name	The subject is shown a photograph and asked to remember the name of the person in it.
Remembering A Hidden Belonging	An item belonging to the subject is borrowed and hidden. The subject is then instructed to ask for the item at the termination of the test.
Remembering An Appointment	An alarm is set for a predetermined number of minutes and the subject requested to ask a particular question upon its going off.
Picture Recognition	Line drawings of common objects are presented to the subject who is asked to name them and remember them for later recall.
Immediate Prose Recall	The subject is asked to listen to a short story and then repeat the story in as much detail as possible.
Test Pictures	The subject is asked to identify the line drawings presented earlier from a larger group of drawings.
Face Recognition	The subject is shown five pictures of faces and asked to remember them for later recall.

Remembering A Short Route	The subject is shown a simple route within the testing environment and asked to immediately repeat it and remember it for later recall.
Remembering To Deliver A Message	As part of the Remembering A Short Route exercise, the subject is required to pick up and deliver an envelope marked 'Message'.
Face Recognition (Delayed)	The subject is required to identify the five pictures presented earlier from a larger group of pictures.
Orientation	The subject is asked a number of orientation questions such as 'What day of the week is it?' and 'What city are we in?'.
Date	The subject is asked what the date is.
Remembering An Appointment (Delayed)	Upon the ringing of the alarm set earlier, the subject is required to ask the question they were supplied with.
Delayed Prose Recall	The subject is asked to recall the story read to them earlier.
Delayed Recall Of Route	The subject is requested to retrace the original route.
Remembering To Deliver A Message	The subject is observed to see if they recall the action required with the envelope marked 'Message'.
Remembering A Name	The subject is asked to recall the name of the person in the photograph presented at the beginning of the session.
Remembering A Belonging	Upon completion of the test the subject is required to spontaneously ask for the belonging borrowed from them at the commencement of the session.

7. The Speed and Capacity Of Language Processing Test (SCOLP)

One of the main neuropsychological symptoms following head injury is a general reduction in the speed at which patients process information. Very often, although able to perform many cognitive tasks, the head-injured patient's rate of performance is profoundly impaired.

In order to assess the degree to which this general reduction in the speed of cognitive processing occurs, the SCOLP utilizes two subsets. The first of these is the Speed of Comprehension Test which allows the actual rate of information processing to be recorded. The subject is asked to read a series of statements and identify false or bizarre items from within the set within a given time limit.

Next, in order to provide a framework for the interpretation of the first subtest, the second Spot The Word subtest requires the subject to identify pseudo words from within a series of word pairs.

Finally, when the score from the second subtest is subtracted from the score from the first subtest, a discrepancy value is derived through which the level of disturbance can be assessed.

PSYCHOMETRIC TESTS: REFERENCES

Luria Nebraska Neuropsychological Battery (LNNB) – 1984. Published by: Western Psychological Services, 12031 Wilshire Boulevard, Los Angeles, CA 90025–1251, USA.

Rivermead Behavioural Memory Test (RBMT) – 1985. Published by: Thames Valley Test Company, 7–9 The Green, Flempton, Bury St Edmunds, Suffolk IP28 6EL, UK.

Screening Test For Luria Nebraska Neuropsychological Battery (ST–LNNB) – 1987. Published by: Western Psychological Services, 12031 Wilshire Boulevard, Los Angeles, CA 90025–1251, USA.

Speed And Capacity Of Language Processing Test (SCOLP) – 1992. Published by: Thames Valley Test Company, 7–9 The Green, Flempton, Bury St Edmunds, Suffolk IP28 6EL, UK.

Stroop Neuropsychological Screening Test (SNST) – 1989. Published by: Psychological Assessment Resources Inc., PO Box 998, Odessa, Florida 33556, USA.

Wechsler Adult Intelligence Scale – Revised (WAIS-R) – 1981 Published by: The Psychological Corporation, 24–28 Oval Road, London NWI 7DX, UK.

Wechsler Memory Scale – Revised (WMS-R) – 1987. Published by: The Psychological Corporation, 24–28 Oval Road, London NW1 7DX, UK.

PSYCHOMETRIC TESTS: FURTHER READING

Evans, J.J., Wilson, B.A. and Emslie, H. *Selecting, Administering and Interpreting Cognitive Tests: guidelines for clinicians and therapists.* Published by: Thames Valley Test Company, 7–9 The Green, Flempton, Bury St Edmunds, Suffolk IP28 6EL, UK.

30 Head injury: behavioural modification

P. Eames

INTRODUCTION

Since the first edition of this book there has been an exponential increase in publications dealing with the problems of traumatic brain injury (TBI) and its rehabilitation. Two major journals devoted to these topics first appeared in 1986 (*Journal of Head Trauma Rehabilitation*) and 1987 (*Brain Injury*). In the 10 years from 1980 there was a 20-fold increase in the number of specialized units devoted to TBI rehabilitation in the USA; lesser but still significant increases occurred in many other countries, not only in the English-speaking world but also throughout Europe. The mid to late 1980s saw the establishment of the International Association for the Study of Traumatic Brain Injury (IASTBI) and the European Brain Injury Society (EBIS), as well as the appearance in this country of the British Society for Rehabilitation Medicine as a development from the Medical Disability Society, which in 1988 had published guidelines for the management and rehabilitation of head injury. International conferences examining the needs, methods and outcomes of rehabilitation have increased in number and quality, calling increasingly upon researchers in the basic neurosciences to bring their knowledge and understanding to the close attention of clinical rehabilitation workers.

Throughout the same period, families' associations have sprung up around the world, following the lead of Headway in this country, and have increased their scope to include the provision of day centres for therapeutic social activities (Headway Houses) and an active role in lobbying for the needs of head injury survivors and their families. This latter has involved increasing collaboration with professionals, both in the clinical arena and in joint meetings and conferences.

At the beginning of this era, there was a general **belief** among professionals working in TBI rehabilitation that their efforts were worthwhile, but there was a lack of **evidence** to support the belief. A major success of the past decade has been the completion and publication of an increasing number of studies examining this question. For various reasons, this has not been easy. Ethical and practical considerations make it difficult to conduct adequately controlled comparative trials; single or double blind studies are simply impossible. Comparisons with published follow-up studies of groups of patients who have been exposed to no kind of rehabilitation have been made, but tend to be confounded by technical, social and economic developments over time. Three main approaches have been used and thought valid, namely single-case

Rehabilitation of the Physically Disabled Adult. Edited by C. John Goodwill, M. Anne Chamberlain and Chris Evans. Published in 1997 by Stanley Thornes (Publishers) Ltd, Cheltenham. ISBN 0-7487-3183-0.

methods, multiple baseline group studies and group studies using subjects as their own controls (generally applied to rehabilitation initiatives undertaken a year or more after injury). (See further reading.)

Such studies have demonstrated unequivocally that prolonged intensive rehabilitation leads to greatly improved outcome for a significant proportion of individuals with severe TBI. This means not only functional improvements that enhance quality of life, but also large savings in the costs of long-term care and in the proportion who return to work (or, in the words of one neurosurgeon with a special interest in TBI, who 'pay their taxes'). Improved outcomes have been reported even for individuals with post-traumatic behaviour disorders severe enough to have prevented their acceptance in standard rehabilitation settings.

In the UK, the development of specific TBI rehabilitation facilities has been led by the private sector; this is not surprising, given the constriction and inhibition of new developments in the National Health Service (NHS) from the latter half of the 1970s. It began in 1980 with the opening of the Kemsley Unit at St Andrew's Hospital in Northampton, which aimed to provide global rehabilitation for those whose behaviour was too disturbed or difficult for them to be contained by standard rehabilitation settings. The process continued with the opening of the Brain Injury Unit at Ticehurst House, the further development of behavioural techniques at Grafton Manor and the establishment of Scotcare in Scotland. This latter demonstrated the possibility of stimulating the NHS into new activity, since not long after its inception the first steps were taken towards extending and re-capitalizing TBI rehabilitation facilities in Scotland. In the meantime, a trickle of new 'Regional Brain Damage Units' began to appear in England, to provide for the needs of those with severe behavioural disorders, though they were largely aimed at people with developmental and degenerative brain disorders as well as those with adult-acquired injuries. As had been predicted, this inappropriate mixture led to progressive exclusion of the head injured, the most difficult but potentially most rewarding group. The National Traumatic Brain Injury Survey (Chapter 29) has been a welcome, if belated, Department of Health initiative.

PRINCIPLES AND PRACTICES OF EFFECTIVE TBI REHABILITATION

'Models' and expertise

Apart from a brief period during and after World War II, when head injury rehabilitation was pioneered in the setting of an Oxford college, the problems of brain injury have usually been dealt with in general rehabilitation units, where they formed a relatively small proportion of the work. This has meant that medical and paramedical professionals had diluted experience in this field. It has also influenced the general character of the rehabilitation afforded those with brain injuries, such that efforts have been directed mainly at physical disabilities, and ideas of what might constitute sufficient treatment have been based on the expected outcomes and norms of duration appropriate to other kinds of disabilities. Only with the rise of 'categorical' brain injury rehabilitation units has there been the opportunity to develop specific expertise through concentrated experience. With this has come an appreciation of the differences, both in the nature of even the physical disorders and in effective treatment techniques.

It is a truism that there can be no expertise without experience. A particular problem, therefore, is that the incidence of severe brain injuries is too low to justify specialist rehabilitation units for populations of the size of the average health district (about 250 000). Such units would best serve populations of about one and a half million, since the numbers would then warrant some fifty places (residential and day) and use the services of a sufficient number of professionals to allow the intra- and inter-disciplinary interactions that foster the development and evaluation of optimal procedures and techniques. For continuity of long-term management, such a unit would need to work closely with smaller local (i.e. district) teams and liaise with and educate the various statutory and voluntary services necessary for community resettlement once intensive rehabilitation is completed. It is sometimes suggested that decentralized 'community rehabilitation' is an alternative model for a brain injury service, but it is worth noting that the successful examples of that approach also have central specialist units for the initial intensive part of the rehabilitation; the outreach teams then have particularly close, sustaining relationships with the central units.

The principal feature of an optimal model of brain injury rehabilitation appears likely to be coherent organization of all aspects of service, both centralized intensive and longer-term community. It must also provide for the minority of patients whose behaviour is too difficult to control without specialized skills.

Understanding

The key to the success of the developments in the field has been the clear realization that particular forms of brain injury, most typically traumatic, hypoxic, encephalitic and those resulting from subarachnoid haemorrhage, produce a combination of localized **and** diffuse damage, thus affecting in varying degrees **all** of the functions of the brain. The straight answer to the question 'What does the brain do?' is 'Everything'! Outcome research has shown that the most disabling dysfunctions are those that affect social behaviour and cognition, rather than physical abilities; they are responsible for most of the limitations on personal independence and on employability. It has thus become clear that

these areas must be tackled with vigour in TBI rehabilitation. Indeed, the recognition of their primacy has led to the notion that rehabilitation after TBI needs to be **primarily** 'neuro-behavioural'.

A further insight clearly apparent from published outcome studies is that much more can be achieved by rehabilitation than was previously assumed by many and still believed by some. Professional expectations play a large part in determining what is achieved, so that it is essential, if best outcomes are to be reached, that all those working in the field become familiar with the brain injury rehabilitation literature. If they are not, their expectations are likely to remain based on old, erroneous assumptions that place unnecessary limits on their work. This applies particularly to those who work also with stroke: it is increasingly apparent that what may be accepted as a 'good' outcome from neurological disabilities caused by stroke is likely to be much less than can routinely be achieved after traumatic brain injury; but unless the rehabilitation professionals are able to experience the differences at first hand, their expectations will not increase and efforts will be likely to cease prematurely.

The achievement of social independence and acceptance depends also on the expectations and reactions of the community at large. For this reason, it is necessary to recognize that cosmetic factors play a large part in determining the way others behave towards the survivor. Even a marked squint from, say, a residual third nerve palsy adversely affects social reintegration, so that it is always worth giving serious consideration to surgical correction, whether or not this is likely to improve vision. It is not enough to achieve independent mobility if continuing therapy might be able to improve the quality and appearance of gait, simply because a 'funny walk' tends to elicit public attitudes of distancing and rejection towards patent disability. Similarly, distorted or impoverished interpersonal social skills are alienating and therefore merit special attention and retraining.

Concepts of behaviour and behavioural disorder

Academic psychology has tended to use the term **behaviour** in a very broad way, to include anything that can be observed about an individual. In ordinary parlance, which usually includes the usage of professional and family teams working with people with head injury, however, it implies conduct or social behaviour, particularly interpersonal. It is helpful to bring this to mind, especially when studying the clinical literature: studies of **neurobehavioural disorders** often turn out to be about memory or executive functioning, whilst studies of social behaviour are still relatively sparse. There is much evidence to suggest that human social behaviour is normally acquired through conditioned, as opposed to cognitive learning, the evolutionary advantage of this being that the individual is automatically biased towards conditioned behaviours, which therefore tend to appear spontaneously and to require positive effort to over-ride. As a consequence, retraining or relearning of appropriate social behavioural patterns after brain injury is likely to be achieved more reliably through the use of techniques of behaviour modification or therapy than with counselling or traditional psychotherapies – or indeed simple exhortation!

There is also much evidence to indicate that many aspects of appropriate social behaviour depend on specific brain mechanisms. One example, recognized only in the past two decades, is the fundamental importance to interpersonal interactions of the non-dominant hemisphere areas homologous with the dominant hemisphere language areas; these are responsible for the decoding and encoding of non-verbal (pragmatic and gestural) aspects of communication. Another example

is the frontal mechanisms necessary for the inhibition of previous responses, disturbance of which underlies perseverative behaviours. Many post-traumatic disorders of social behaviour result **directly** from injury to brain mechanisms (Eames, 1990). Others may stem from the individual's emotional reactions to injury and disability, but examination of the most common forms of disorder suggests that this is a considerably less important cause of difficulties.

There is a natural tendency to equate behavioural disorder with disturbances that are actively upsetting to others, particularly aggression and disinhibition of social or sexual behaviours. It is vital to recognize that relative **absences** of behaviour, like drivelessness, lack of motivation or impaired self-awareness, are equally important to the acceptance and reintegration of the individual into family and society. In addition to these broad categories of active and passive disorders, there are behavioural disturbances that comprise clusters of abnormalities that approximate to psychiatric 'syndromes' like paranoid psychosis, manic or depressive illness or even gross hysterical states.

Duration

One of the advantages enjoyed by units specializing in the treatment and rehabilitation of individuals with very severe post-traumatic behaviour disorders has been the fact that it was already recognized that such disorders, from whatever cause, can be dealt with successfully only incrementally and therefore slowly. As a result, all aspects of rehabilitation were able to continue for much longer periods of time than were standard. By this means it has become apparent that recovery from brain injury and responsiveness to rehabilitation both continue for a very long time, so that the best results come from persistent work over at least many months and often longer. This understanding was possible only as a result of the development of specialized units, because duration of rehabilitation had previously been determined largely by the needs of those with other kinds of disorders.

Setting

One of the important implications of this need for lengthy treatment is that 'patients' are likely to spend long periods of time in the rehabilitation unit. It is therefore essential to take deliberate steps to avoid the problems of institutionalization. Most of these result from the unconscious attitudes of both treaters and treated, activated by environmental cues. Hospitals are for the sick: the sick expect to be looked after and hospital staff expect to look after them. The central idea of rehabilitation, on the other hand, is to learn new skills and relearn old ones, in order to move away from passivity and dependence and towards independence and a full life. It is all too easy to ignore the powerful tendency of signals of sickness and dependency (which include hospital furniture, fittings and procedures) to inhibit the very active efforts required of those engaging in rehabilitation. The fewer the institutional signals in the setting, both physical and social, the less is the risk of institutionalization. Hence the aim must be to create a setting that is as close to ordinary 'real life' as possible. Amongst other things, this means that there should be no room for professional uniforms and badges. Since rehabilitation is basically re-educative and centred on the idea of learning, the ideal model would appear to be an educational one in which the rehabilitation unit is structured like a college of further education. It is also important to try to separate areas for basic living, relaxation and leisure from those where work, including therapy, is undertaken.

Teamwork

The range of expertise needed for adequate brain injury rehabilitation is very broad: no one person can or should expect to possess all of the necessary knowledge or skills. At the same time, the aims of rehabilitation concern what might be called 'person functions', activities like working, enjoying oneself, developing social networks, pursuing new interests and hobbies, and so on. This means that there is an over-riding need to integrate therapies directed at specific deficits (e.g. in locomotion, language, cognition, social skills or behavioural control) so that they serve these wider aims. In part this means that professionals with different sets of skills have to learn to work closely with each other, focusing on real-life activities rather than isolated areas of deficit.

Strategies for rehabilitation

Brain first

The majority of post-traumatic disorders of behaviour and even of emotional state, as well as disorders of function, result directly from injury to areas and systems of the brain. For some of them, drug treatments are available, capable of producing greater or lesser helpful effects. Since such treatments are aimed at correcting underlying organic abnormalities, and because drug treatments generally work quite quickly (if at all), whereas other interventions achieve more gradual improvements and are, of course, labour intensive and time consuming, it is logical to try to deploy the former at the outset, in order to try to raise the starting level for the latter.

Although it is becoming apparent that some drug and nutrient treatments delivered at the roadside or at least within the first few hours after injury may have important preventive effects on ultimate outcome, and the provision of adequate nutrition and repletion of neurotransmitter stores may accelerate early recovery, many of the disorders most likely to respond to drug treatments have the characteristic of a somewhat delayed appearance. These include epilepsy and migraine, of course, but also less well known (but more common and disturbing) episodic disorders like episodic dyscontrol and temporo-limbic mood disorders, as well as extrapyramidal disorders including abulia, that can be the cause of late deterioration. Specific treatments of some of these are discussed under 'The treatment and management of disorders of social behaviour' below.

Easily overlooked is the fact that other drug treatments, used for incidental disorders (e.g. prochlorperazine for vertigo or nausea) or for the non-specific quelling of aggressive or agitated behaviour (typically haloperidol or phenothiazines), often have adverse effects on the injured brain that may retard or impede natural recovery and responsiveness to rehabilitation therapies. Thus regular critical review of all drug treatments is an important element in the optimization of conditions for best outcome.

'Functional', not discipline-led

The traditional focus of rehabilitation efforts has been on impairments, so that they have been structured by delivering different kinds of therapies in separate settings at separate times. Typically the patient would have a programme of attendances at the departments of physiotherapy, occupational therapy and so on, for work on basic functional skills. An alternative strategy that has been rapidly gaining ground is to make disabilities and handicaps the focus of attention, having therapists with different kinds of skills working with the same individual in specific real-life contexts, like the bathroom, the dining room, the supermarket or the public gymnasium. This approach has the logic of ecological validity; in practice many therapists have found it more satisfying and more effective. It is not easy to initiate, because it is such a distinct departure from traditional methods, but it has sufficient promise to be likely to become the standard rehabilitation practice of the future.

Assessment

The object of assessment is to identify strengths and disabilities in order to direct therapeutic efforts in the most appropriate directions. It also allows an attempt at prognosis and the setting of general aims for resettlement. Given the complexity of the handicaps engendered by TBI and the absolute need for a wide range of professional skills to attempt to solve them, it is essential that assessment is at least multidisciplinary (where different specialists make assessments of the various areas of disturbed functioning) and preferably interdisciplinary (where specialists work together in assessing the individual's disabilities and handicaps in real-life settings). Unfortunately, though understandably, there is a plethora of assessment instruments for most areas of functioning, the most universal and best standardized being for formal neuropsychological performance. This reflects partly the difficulty involved in devising reliable and valid scoring systems and partly the ad hoc way in which brain injury rehabilitation has developed, with individual units often having made their own scales simply because there were no recognized ones. The situation is rather better when it comes to the assessment of outcome, at least in terms of disability, but there are still competing approaches (Hall, 1994).

There are two rather different ways of proceeding beyond initial assessment. The commoner method involves the setting of goals, levels of achievement to be reached that will be reassessed at the next reassessment. The other is to recognize the aims and identify the current barriers, then work on reducing the latter and reassess the amount and rate of progress towards the former.

Resettlement or community reintegration

The conditions necessary for reintegration in the community depend on a number of factors, not least the severity of the person's ultimate disabilities and the amount of family and community support available. Optimal reintegration will mean independent accommodation and employment and satisfying social networks, but the details must depend on the person's own preferences wherever possible. When the degree of disability makes any of these aims impossible, more restricted aims have to be pursued. Examples are supported lodgings or the provision of professional carers at home, supported employment or sheltered work, a case manager to try to stimulate social and leisure activities, or attendance at day centres (ideally a Headway House).

Three main principles are relevant to the pursuit of optimal resettlement. The first is that each of the main aims will require close liaison and cooperation between the rehabilitation team and the competent authorities in the community (housing departments, disability employment advisers and work assessment centres, home care, home aid and social service departments and their network of day and support facilities, and any relevant voluntary organizations, especially Headway). This is not easy, but is considerably enhanced by funnelling through one focal site (e.g. the rehabilitation unit) and one key individual. Such organization fosters familiarity with the range of typical resettlement problems on the part of the community workers as well as oiling the wheels of communication through regular personal contacts.

The second principle is more difficult but even more important to the quality of ultimate outcome. It is that the wheres and hows of reintegration should not be decided too early in rehabilitation, since the most appropriate solutions will be those that most closely match the injured person's **ultimate** needs. The earlier decisions are made and pursued, the more likely it will be that they underestimate the final possible level of independence. Some survivors will simply leave such arrangements behind them, but

many will be effectively imprisoned by placements or supports that make life easier, but are not really necessary.

The third principle emerges from practical experience. It is essential to tackle the two main objectives, namely accommodation and work, one at a time. It is probably not so important which way round this is done, but to attempt to settle the person into new accommodation (especially if this is relatively independent) and into a job at the same time is almost certain to overwhelm his or her resources of adaptation and coping.

Fiscal restrictions on the availability of social services resources mean that the level of sophistication that can be achieved in resettlement plans (and in long-term care plans, too) is likely to be greatly enhanced if the person's injury is subject to compensation through the Courts. This is particularly unfortunate because it applies to only about 1 in 10 of severe brain injuries (Chapter 11).

Work

The statutory services for work assessment and training have changed over the past few years, such that there appear to be fewer options for the disabled person wishing to return to employment, but who are restricted from their previous areas of work. For those who have a post to go back to, the provisions of supported employment can be very helpful, but they are almost impossible to invoke for a person seeking a post. Despite this, there remain opportunities, many of them through various forms of further education. These matters are dealt with in Chapter 52.

Driving

Many survivors are extremely keen to return to driving. Physical restrictions are rarely prohibitive, apart from substantial visual field defects or persistent diplopia and, of course, epilepsy. The most important limitations are really those imposed by cognitive disorders (attention and speed of processing and reaction) and frontal lobe deficits of impulse control and judgement. These can be difficult to quantify and clinicians are often uncomfortable about making definite recommendations. The new edition of *Medical Aspects of Fitness to Drive* is clear and helpful (Taylor 1995). In difficult problems it is often helpful to refer the person to a mobility centre such as Banstead Place, (or nearest member of Forum) for formal assessment (Chapter 50).

Long-term care

Despite the most intensive and lengthy rehabilitation efforts, some survivors will never be able to reach personal or domestic independence, but will continue to have supervisory or active care needs for the rest of their lives. There is a tendency to expect that such needs will be met by relatives. This is rarely reasonable or just and it undoubtedly increases morbidity, especially emotional, in the families, both from the direct effects of the burden of caring and, more importantly, from the distress for all concerned that is generated by the gross distortions of the family roles and relationships (see also 'The family' below). Family care in the family home, with or without outside professional help, may be quite appropriate for older married (or stably cohabiting) survivors, but with younger people the stress on the spouse of the changes in the injured person ('he's not the man I married') almost inevitably leads sooner or later to breakdown and termination of the relationship. For young single adults or even late adolescents, injury tends to thrust them back into a child-like relationship with their parents, fostering dependency and over-protectiveness on the respective sides. Apart from tending to limit the achievement of potential independence, this leaves the young person unprepared and untrained for survival later on, when the parents are no longer there or able to cope. Despite the practical difficulties, therefore, the aim should always be to set the injured person up in a setting that most closely approximates the way he or she would have been living had the injury not occurred, providing whatever support may be necessary to achieve that, and of course to foster the development of new social networks.

For some survivors there will be a permanent need for nursing care or at least for constant supervision. Most will be relatively young. Long-term residential care settings that already exist are almost all designed for either the dementing elderly or the developmentally mentally handicapped, whose needs and behavioural characteristics are quite different. Some residential settings specifically created for the young brain injured are beginning to become established, and it seems likely that this area will grow over the next few years, but at the moment such facilities are in short supply. For the time being, therefore, the best quality of life for such individuals is likely to be achieved through the provision of adequate care and support in their own accommodation, with the services of a case manager experienced in the problems of acquired brain injury to maximize the chances of community involvement and stimulating social activities.

Continuing support

In a field that is actively growing and expanding, it is difficult to envisage the services and resources that may become available, even over the next few years. It is therefore desirable that regular contact be maintained with all survivors living in the community, so that they may have access to new developments. To some extent this is achieved through contact with Headway, but regular if infrequent review in a head injury follow-up clinic should be continued, probably indefinitely, but certainly until a stable niche has been established.

The family

To have a close relative with all the sequelae and problems caused by severe brain injury is a bruising and stressful experience. The initial shock and drama, often compounded by a growing awareness of the dearth of appropriate services and resources, gradually give way to the more persistent stresses of altered, often maladaptive behaviour patterns, the problem of trying to mourn for the loss of the old person and at the same time coming to terms with the new, and the knowledge that there will be need for support and care long after the family are no longer there to provide them. All this adds up to a terrible burden. Not surprisingly, there is great variation in the strain produced by these stresses and in the degree to which family members cope; such evidence as there is suggests that those who cope best are those who have coped best with life stresses in the past.

At the same time, a combination of frustration at limited resources and professional expertise, feelings of helplessness in the face of complex and mysterious disabilities and behaviours, and often irrational ideas and feelings of guilt about how and why the injury occurred, may lead to hypercritical or even aggressive attitudes towards treating staff, or to restrictively protective attitudes to the survivor that can all too easily inhibit recovery and progress in rehabilitation. Problems of these kinds are specifically exacerbated by too early discharge 'to the care of the family' (in reality determined by a desire to empty the bed) and by unavailability of appropriate rehabilitation resources. They seem to be especially likely when the injured person is young and has only recently 'flown the nest', or was just on the threshold of doing so. It is thus an important consideration to establish the nature of the pre-injury relationships and practicalities and, as suggested above, to aim for discharge and resettlement to the same kind of setting and social order that obtained or was developing at the time of the injury.

From an early stage, families and survivors should be encouraged to make contact with the nearest Headway group. Many families initially reject this idea, because they cling to a hope and belief that their injured member will quickly be restored to normality and cannot accept that Headway is relevant to them. But Headway is naturally aware of this and makes every attempt to make itself available whenever the family decides it might after all be helpful.

Needs of the team

The rehabilitation of TBI survivors is by no means easy, partly because of the complexity of their problems, both physical and psychological, but largely because of their proneness to difficult, frightening and sometimes dangerous behaviour. On the other hand, many staff, both trained and untrained, find them very rewarding to work with. Experience in independent-sector units indicates that staff are either irredeemably 'bitten by the bug' of brain injury, or decide to move on to other things, in either case quite quickly. This is an advantage in such units, but may pose problems in statutory services, especially if they are sited in larger establishments and staffed by rotation from large departments.

In both cases, there is a need for the leaders of the team and for team members themselves to be aware of the stresses and of the need to establish systems for practical and emotional support. This is all the more important in units that specifically deal with the more severe disorders of behaviour, where fear in the face of threat is a desirable characteristic, but can be overwhelming if behaviour management policies are unclear or peer support is not openly available.

An essential element in the working of the team, both for its cohesion and stability and for its heuristic and creative functions, is easy communication and the sharing of ideas. A useful practical organization is centred on a weekly team meeting at which all patients and their management are discussed, but which delegates the tasks of designing and implementing data collection, specific treatment programmes and so on, to smaller groups who report back to the full team meeting.

Open-mindedness

Physicians and therapists working with TBI recognize that the physical and functional problems they encounter are not only more complex than those that follow the more common disorders dealt with in neurological rehabilitation, but also demand different treatment approaches. This is apparent also in the TBI literature. Part of the reason for this is that TBI always produces multiple interacting deficits, the cognitive, emotional and behavioural aspects interfering with and tending to undermine the effectiveness of methods that are usually adequate when only the physical or functional deficit has to be addressed. But even the physical disorders affecting mobility and speech are often neurologically more complex that those seen, for example, in stroke. There is still much to be learned about the most appropriate methods of treatment and problems will ultimately be solved only by further experiment and research. Since the established bodies of knowledge do not provide complete answers, there is an over-riding need for creativity, which demands an open mind and a willingness to explore new approaches.

Research

This complexity also means that those who work in the field have an obligation to approach their work in ways and with procedures that will lead to increased knowledge and understanding. In other words, all rehabilitation personnel must be prepared to make careful observations and measurements in the course of their work, so that effective research can be accomplished. Over the past decade, broad-based research has shown that intensive rehabilitation in TBI is effective. What is needed now is more fine-grained research to establish which methods and which elements of the overall rehabilitation effort are valuable in themselves. This is a job for all members of the rehabilitation team. The establishment some years ago of an MSc course in Rehabilitation Research at the University of Southampton, aimed specifically at therapists, has been a valuable step in facilitating this aim.

The importance of developing and employing valid and reliable measures of outcome is not limited to the assessment of the effectiveness of specific aspects of treatment. New understandings of the processes that lead to secondary damage to the brain following primary insults are raising the possibility of a range of very acute treatments that may have powerful effects on later outcome. Unless satisfactory outcome measures exist and are sufficiently widely recognized and agreed, the kinds of large-scale collaborative studies of these early interventions that will establish or falsify them can never be done effectively.

THE TREATMENT AND MANAGEMENT OF DISORDERS OF SOCIAL BEHAVIOUR

Principles and practices of behaviour modification

Disorders of behaviour that are noticeable but relatively mild are the rule after brain injuries of any degree of severity. Many of them will show the same gradual, slow improvement seen with cognitive disorders and will not justify the kinds of treatment approaches needed for more severely disruptive ones. These require great effort, forbearance and diligence from all concerned, including relatives, but also demand that some degree of control be exercised over the individual's environment, with some consequent temporary loss of autonomy and personal rights.

There is a group of post-traumatic brain disorders, however, that tend to appear after some delay and that stem directly from brain dysfunction. They will often respond well to quite simple pharmacological treatments, without the need for more complex therapies. These are mainly episodic disorders of mood or aggression, most commonly the episodic dyscontrol syndrome and temporo-limbic mood disorder, but also include passive behavioural deficits (see next section).

It is logical to try the effects of drug treatment first, since it may obviate the need for lengthier, more difficult approaches. In some instances it may well be that a combined approach is the most effective. The behavioural problem can be unwittingly exacerbated by inappropriate reinforcement during the acute hospital stay or at home. This is increasingly likely to happen the longer the time since injury before treatment is begun, because conditioned learning is incremental and depends, amongst other things, on the number and frequency of reinforced events. Individuals differ in their susceptibility to conditioning by positive social reinforcement; they differ also in personality, not only in terms of style but in robustness. It is therefore possible to come across some whose abnormal behaviour can be completely controlled with appropriate medication alone, whereas others have developed an additional learned element in the behaviour, which will require unlearning or deconditioning if the inappropriate behaviour is to be eliminated. If the disordered behaviour is infrequent or mild, the solution (usually spontaneously discovered by the individual) may simply be to develop a new range of social contacts for whom the behaviour is neither new nor unacceptable. (Unpredictable moodiness or an explosive temper may be intolerable to those who have known a person without it, but quite within the normal range for those who have not.)

The same disorders may also underlie the more severe behavioural problems that disrupt standard rehabilitation attempts. They may contribute to these simply because of severity. It is distressing to find that patients are sometimes discharged from hospital or rehabilitation unit to the care of their families, regardless of whether or not they were living there at the time of their injury, explicitly because of behaviour that is too difficult to cope with in the hospital or unit. Not surprisingly families are exposed to enormous stress; often they can cope only by appeasement, which inevitably adds further inappropriate positive reinforcement of the aberrant behaviours. These are the patients most likely to be referred ultimately to units specializing in the management and treatment of behaviour disorders.

The essence of **behaviour modification**, nowadays sometimes known by the unwieldy and potentially misleading title of 'the experimental analysis of behaviour', is to take control of the environment and ensure, as far as possible, that positive reinforcements, whether tangible or social, are presented **only** when behaviour is appropriate and **never** in the presence of inappropriate behaviours. This sounds easier than it is. In order to ensure as consistent application of the rule as possible, all staff interacting with the person (including, for example, domestic staff) have to understand and be practised in the approach, and anyone who might deliver stray or inappropriate reinforcement must be as far as possible excluded from contact. Before treatment can begin, it is essential to survey, identify, classify and measure the behaviours the individual exhibits, so that clear targets can be declared for positive reinforcement and for 'time out from positive reinforcement' (i.e. the avoidance of any reinforcement, even social attention to the person). It is also necessary to explore the individual's responses to potential reinforcers (e.g. not everyone likes strawberries; some TBI patients have difficulty perceiving and interpreting the non-verbal signals of social approval and warmth), both immediate and 'back-up' (i.e. treats and privileges that may be linked to periods of consistently appropriate conduct), so that any treatment programme has the maximum chance of effectiveness. Moreover, meticulous, consistent recording of target behaviours must continue throughout treatment, so that changes can be identified and methods adjusted whenever necessary.

At the same time, it is implicit that difficult and dangerous behaviours must be contained effectively and safely (for the individual, fellow patients and the treaters) and must be managed with confidence.

These demands cannot be expected to be met in hospital wards or standard rehabilitation units. They can be met only in settings deliberately designed to meet them. Outcome studies from such settings have demonstrated that in a significant majority the disorders of conduct can be effectively treated and rehabilitation can become effective enough to produce radical improvements in the resettlement options, improvements that are stable on extensive follow-up (Cope, 1995). Early work in this field, first in the Kemsley Unit and then in the USA, was based on the structure of the Token Economy, where the immediate reinforcement of appropriate behaviours is by a combination of social reinforcement and the awarding of some kind of token or point, 'earnings' being exchangeable for a variety of 'back-up' privileges or commodities. Whilst this approach has the benefit of focusing the attention of staff on the need for social reinforcement, it has its critics on the grounds that delivering the tokens or points can be demeaning and may create an unhealthy division of power between treater and treated. It is in fact very difficult for staff to maintain the necessary vigilance to ensure maximum consistency of the use of social reinforcement, but if staffing stability can be achieved (which basically requires that the unit be independent so that outside managers cannot arbitrarily move staff to and from other areas), it is possible to reach a high level of efficiency without the tangible cue of the token or points recording sheet.

It is essential to the proper understanding of the workings of reinforcement to recognize that it operates willy-nilly, in other words whether or not those providing the reinforcement are aware of their actions. It is therefore all too easy to reinforce inappropriate behaviours with attention, appeasement or attempts at 'calming'. The vast research findings from the field of conditioned learning show that the increase of frequency of behaviours that emerge from any cause (i.e. stimulated or spontaneous) when they are regularly followed by positive reinforcement, and their decrease when followed by no reinforcement or by aversive consequences, represent a law of nature. It is the recognition of this law, coupled with the conscious attempt to control one's own responses to 'emergent behaviours', that constitutes the basis of the 'behavioural approach'. At the same time, it is essential to provide an environment that is generally stimulating and rewarding (i.e. reinforcing). The notion of 'time out' is crucial to the successful management and changing of social behaviour, but is easily misunderstood, largely because the expression has been purloined for a number of other uses. In behavioural terms, it stands for 'time out from positive reinforcement' and simply means the temporary avoidance and elimination of any source of positive reinforcement in the face of any behaviour one wishes to diminish. (In practice, therefore, this means any socially inappropriate behaviour.) Ideally this is achieved by withholding social reinforcement (which in its simplest form means any personal attention) for a brief period immediately following ('contingent upon') the inappropriate behaviour: this can conveniently be referred to as 'time out on the spot' (or TOOTS, for ease of communication). In group settings, it can be difficult to achieve this, since fellow patients or residents are prone to respond socially to others' maladaptive behaviours. In such circumstances, it is often necessary to remove the individual from the situation ('situational time out'), but it is important for staff to recognize that this must be done in a 'TOOTS-ful' manner, without any verbal or non-verbal interaction, since the objective is purely time out from positive reinforcement and most definitely **not** punishment or retribution. Even more difficult, but equally important, is the management of situations in which the individual's inappropriate behaviour is actively dangerous: it is simply not possible just to avoid responding to an attack on another person; moreover, such directed aggression is alarming to all concerned and it is absolutely essential that a predetermined course of action be agreed, so that everyone knows precisely what is to be done in such circumstances. It is in such situations that the use of a 'time out room' can be particularly valuable. This is a room devoid of interest and reinforcement, to which the individual is conducted, rapidly but 'TOOTS-fully', so that the risks of stray reinforcement and to others' safety are minimized. Needless to say, in order to achieve the desired aim (time out from contingent positive reinforcement) it is vital that the period of time spent in the room be brief, in practice between 2 and 5 minutes, and that immediate positive reinforcement of appropriate behaviour be provided as soon as possible.

Some specific problems of treatment, management and rehabilitation

Motivation

This is a word easy to say but hard to define, because it expresses a 'final common path' influenced by an exceedingly wide range of brain mechanisms and functions. These include basic areas like the intensity and accuracy of perception, the efficiency of attention and memory mechanisms and the capacity for self-awareness (usually the last function to recover after even moderate injury). In practice, however, there are four main areas of function that contribute to motivation and are often disturbed by injury.

The first is **drive**. This is an individual characteristic that varies widely in the general population, but when it is disturbed, the change in the person is readily recognized by relatives and friends; when drive disorder is severe, it is very obvious because of low arousal (lethargy and a tendency to fall asleep easily when inactive) and fatiguability. It is most clearly associated with brainstem injury. To some extent it can be offset by the provision of an interesting, stimulating environment. There are some case studies that show a good response to systematic positive reinforcement of increased activity. In some cases, sustained improvement has been achieved through regular specific vestibular stimulation, probably because collateral inputs from sensory systems to the brainstem arousal mechanisms are most rich in this modality. At the upper end of the continuum of severity, simple physical fitness is an important factor and can be enhanced through regular structured fitness training programmes.

The second involves the extrapyramidal (meso-cingulate) mechanisms underlying initiation and initiative (which can be seen as the initiation of behaviours, as distinct from actions). Disorder of these functions is referred to as **abulia** and results from deficits in one of the dopaminergic systems. It is distinguishable from drive disorder by the paucity of spontaneous movement and facial expressiveness (the 'butter sculpture' appearance) and often by the presence of more or less subtle extrapyramidal motor disorders (from activated rigidity to Parkinsonian signs). Moreover, whereas drive and arousal can be temporarily increased by sustained environmental stimulation and exhortation, the abulic state is typically 'broken through' by sudden bursts of novel and significant stimuli, though only briefly (perhaps because novelty never lasts for long). It is typical of the disorder that it appears after a delay, sometimes as long as several months, after the injury, though the more obvious the hypoxic element in the injury, the earlier it tends to be seen. Abulia often responds to treatment with dopaminergic drugs (bromocriptine, pergolide, and sometimes amantadine), sometimes dramatically. Clinical experience has shown that a period of just a few months at high dosage (e.g. 40 or 50 mg b.d. of bromocriptine) leads to improvements that are maintained when the drug is withdrawn. In contrast, neither encouragement nor systematic reinforcement changes the general pattern of behaviour.

A somewhat different disorder results from direct damage to the target system of the meso-cingulate projections, namely the cingulate gyrus and other parts of the medial surfaces of the frontal lobes. It is probably best described as **anergia** or **aspontaneity** and represents one of the frontal lobe syndromes, the others being described below. Some workers in the USA have reported useful effects from stimulants like methylphenidate, but experience here has been disappointing. There have been some case reports of improvement from systematic positive reinforcement of active behaviours, but at best the long-term outlook is poor.

The third major source of motivation disorders is an **absence or reduction of hedonic responsiveness**. Sometimes this reflects pre-existing psychopathic or hysterical personality disorder, but it is also an intrinsic feature of brain-injury-induced hysteria (see below). Since behaviour modification depends upon reinforcement learning, and hedonic responsiveness is the 'cement' for operant learning, behaviour modification is unavailing in such disorders (indeed it often exacerbates the behaviour disorders), so that

alternative forms of management have to be adopted.

Finally, motivation for rehabilitation and resettlement is often undermined by the individual's personal emotional reaction to the fact of having been injured and to the losses of ability and independence that have resulted. Many studies have established that there is a high incidence of **depression** in brain injury survivors, but depressive illness is by no means common and the use of antidepressant drugs is only occasionally helpful. On the other hand, supportive approaches and sometimes (when the person's cognitive state allows) more formal psychotherapies appear to be the best way of helping people through what is often a phase of recovery. Certainly a generally behavioural approach, in other words the careful deployment of positive reinforcements, is an appropriate way to deal with the motivational consequences of these all too understandable states of depression of mood.

Aggression

The most powerful element in the effective management of aggressive behaviour is to have staff who know how to manage it and, probably more important, **know** that they know. Unfortunately this element is often missing in the settings in which the problem arises (orthopaedic or medical wards, or general rehabilitation units). Indeed, it is one of the disadvantages of such settings that the broad mix of types of clinical problems makes it difficult for staff to acquire concentrated experience with disturbed behaviour. Informal enquiries of such staff invariably show that they regard aggressive behaviour as the most difficult behaviour to cope with; those with experience in settings specifically geared to head injury work, on the other hand, tend to consider it the easiest. Part of the problem is that effective techniques have to be learned practically, which requires frequent practice. It would be reasonable to assume that acute psychiatric units would be adept at this problem. In general, however, they tend to be very reluctant to take in patients with 'organic' disorders; in any case, many such patients have continuing medical or surgical needs and most have rehabilitation needs which cannot be met in psychiatric hospitals, so that transfer is not desirable. If all head-injured patients admitted to a hospital are managed in just one ward or subward, there is at least an opportunity for staff, suitably supported by appropriately experienced psychologists and medical personnel, gradually to acquire the necessary experience, skill and confidence. Most aggression occurs during the post-traumatic confusional period. When an aggressive patient is mobile, and hence wandering and interfering with other patients, there can be terrible stresses on the nursing staff, who usually have acutely ill people to tend and to worry about. In those circumstances it can be particularly helpful to engage the services of agency 'specials' with psychiatric experience, who can 'shadow' the disturbed patient and shepherd him or her away from dangers and towards more productive activities (including work with the rehabilitation therapists, of course).

Inevitably, in the acute setting, there are calls for pharmacological treatment of disturbed and aggressive behaviour. Though there is an impressive literature demonstrating that neuroleptics and benzodiazepines retard neurological recovery from trauma, and may even limit the ultimate outcome, it appears to be entirely unknown to most of the doctors, junior and senior, who usually have to deal with these calls. By far the commonest course of action is to use haloperidol or chlorpromazine, which solve the problems only in doses that also disable the person from any chance of responding to therapists. They are also epileptogenic which is of considerable importance, given the very marked deleterious effect on long-term outcome of severe head injury when post-

traumatic epilepsy supervenes. Drugs that have been shown to be both useful and safe in the acute stage include carbamazepine (400–600 mg b.d.) (which is also the anticonvulsant most recommended for epilepsy or its prophylaxis, for example in the Medical Disability Society guidelines on the management of head injury), propranolol (80–240 mg b.d.), chlormethiazole (but only for up to a week, to avoid dependence) and perhaps buspirone (10–15 mg t.d.s.).

'Hysteria'

A proportion of patients who suffer very diffuse brain injury (any form of sustained hypoxia, hypoglycaemia and sometimes encephalitis) develop disorders of behaviour that are characterized by active manipulativeness and dissociative disorders. Attempts at intensive rehabilitation with such people are usually extremely frustrating, since their response tends to be avoidant and resistive. The more direct a request or command, the more likely the person will respond adversely. This also affects attempts at cognitive and other assessments, since testing inevitably revolves largely around direct questions or requests; often much more information about the cognitive and functional state can be gleaned by observing the natural responses and production of information in 'ordinary' social or practical circumstances. (As an example, one such patient appeared on formal or 'bedside' testing to have no memory function at all, but in the pub he took half a dozen orders to the bar, delivered them to the right people, and returned the correct change.) A less obvious feature is seen when behavioural methods are tried: these individuals turn out to be nonreinforcible, perhaps as a result of the loss of hedonic responsiveness, so that their behaviour is not modified by experience. Indeed, the use of praise as reinforcement can be counter-productive, since it also gives information about what the praiser would like the person to do and thus the opportunity of doing the opposite – an opportunity that is often taken. Sometimes this can even result in dangerous escalation of the behaviour disorder, to the extent of severe self-inflicted injury (and in one case death through refusal of nutriments).

Those in whom this pattern is recognized should not be managed in any kind of explicit token economy setting. The most workable strategy appears to be to set up daily circumstances in such a way that appropriate responses are natural and are 'requested' only by the situation or circumstances, rather than directly. This requires much ingenuity and patience, especially with those whose behaviours are frankly bizarre or degraded. Nevertheless in most cases useful progress can be made towards an overall behavioural state that allows them to be acceptable in a variety of care settings. Long-term follow-up, as yet rather sketchy, suggests that some, at least, may show a marked spontaneous improvement some time between 3 and 6 years after injury, provided they are in relatively civilized settings in the meantime.

Post-traumatic psychosis

Psychosis during the acute phase, usually during post-traumatic confusion though often outlasting it, is usually self-limiting; often the leading features are hallucinations; if the manifestations are controlled with antipsychotic drugs, they can be discontinued after a short while without risking recurrence. Because the injured brain is so susceptible to the adverse effects of the classical neuroleptics, it is important to choose 'atypical' agents like sulpiride or risperidone, which produce a low incidence of extrapyramidal disorders and no anticholinergic effects to exacerbate cognitive deficits, and are less likely to be epileptogenic.

The outlook is much less good when psychotic illness appears after a latent period, which may be weeks, months or even years. In these cases the most prominent features are likely to be paranoid (ideas of reference and delusions), sometimes accompanied by auditory or tactile hallucinations and occasionally by fractured thinking or perceptual distortions. The same preference for atypical antipsychotic drugs obtains, but it has to be said that neither these nor phenothiazines are often very effective. Indeed, the development of such an illness usually indicates a rough and stormy path over the years, with quite a high risk of ultimate suicide.

The position with regard to hypomanic or severe depressive illnesses is rather different. Both lithium and carbamazepine can be effective in the prevention of recurrences; haloperidol or pimozide (for hypomania) and antidepressants usually work well, though all do carry the risk of precipitating post-traumatic epilepsy, and so should never be used lightly.

The nature of these disorders is often in some doubt. There is good evidence that the incidence of both major affective and schizophreniform illnesses is increased after severe head injury, but clearly some cases are coincidental. It seems likely that the best indicator of true post-traumatic disorders is that they are somewhat atypical in their phenomenology.

'Frontal lobe syndrome'

This name usually implies the syndrome that results from injury to the orbital part of the frontal lobe or lobes. It comprises social disinhibition, lack of judgement and realism, and a tendency to childishness and egocentricity. It is often said to involve 'loss of insight', though sensitive questioning usually shows that the individual is aware of his or her inappropriate behaviour, but quickly loses sight of the awareness when not reminded. (The anergic syndrome of medial frontal injury was discussed above under 'Motivation'; the dysexecutive syndrome of lateral frontal dysfunction appears later under 'Dys-executive disorders'. In each case it has to be remembered that dysfunction can result as easily – and much less visibly in imaging studies – from damage to the connections of the frontal areas as from local cortical lesions.)

No pharmacological treatments are available. If the behavioural pattern presents very early on and is not too marked, then considerable spontaneous recovery can be expected. On the other hand, if the features persist at a high level for several months, it is unlikely that they will become really tolerable (by family or by society at large) even in the long run. Both social disinhibition (which is likely to extend to sexual approach behaviour, since most victims are young and therefore have sexual matters much on their minds) and 'silliness' can pose great strains. It is possible to change such patterns, but this requires a very highly structured behaviour modification programme likely to be beyond the scope of any but the most formally organized setting. Consequently such patients and their families usually demand continuing support and crisis intervention, and some-times 'protective intervention' with the arms of the Law, often with worry and frustration all round.

Dysexecutive disorders

These probably represent the most complex and difficult aspect of frontal lobe dysfunc-tion, both to recognize and to explain to others, not least in the medicolegal arena, because often enough the victim may appear to be quite normal. The essence of the deficits is in the planning, organization and execution of complex tasks – how complex depends on the severity of the deficit. Perhaps the best definition is the one given by one patient's wife (he was a family doctor, still managing to practise with her constant help and super-vision): 'He shows a curious mismatch between knowing and doing'. At its worst, the person may be able to give a clear and accurate description of how to make a pot of tea, but in practice gets everything wrong. Over the past few years, neuropsychologists have been devising helpful 'ecological' testing procedures and also retraining programmes for these deficits; they can be successful, but demand a great deal of time, effort and persistence.

FUTURE DIRECTIONS

Long-term follow-up research (techniques, expectation of life, risk of epilepsy, etc.)

Whilst there is now abundant evidence of the value of prolonged, intensive rehabilitation for overall outcomes, much less is known about which techniques and elements of the rehabilitation process are most effective and efficient. This is the area of research that most needs to be developed.

At the same time, there is a lack of knowledge about long-term outcomes. The data available on expectation of life are long since out of date, since they inevitably relate to injuries sustained 30 or more years ago, when acute treatments and even nursing management were much less sophisticated than they are now. Similarly, the available data on the risks of late post-traumatic epilepsy (including the question of the value of prophylactic treatments) were gathered on cohorts injured before the CT era, so that identification of possible risk factors was a much coarser business. There will be an ever-continuing need for long-term follow-up studies of consecutive head injuries in unse-lected series from real populations. It is difficult to see how this can be achieved without some kind of ongoing register, either regional or national.

Organization of services (use of statutory services – liaison)

There are also few data on which to base conclusions about the most effective **systems** of care and rehabilitation. The Department of Health's 'initiative' of recent years appears to have been designed in such a way as to obscure rather than illuminate this question. A principal difficulty is the fact that quite large populations are needed to yield sufficient numbers to allow the acquisition of real experience and expertise. In the present style of organization of the NHS, this need easily overwhelms the willingness of Trusts to cooperate and collaborate. A second important requirement is to recognize that different areas of the UK have different patterns of population density and therefore may best be served by different kinds of service organizations. Large-scale population studies focusing on directly comparable definitions of outcome seem likely to be the only realistic way forward.

Moreover, means must be found to establish good liaison between the various statutory community services at 'ground level' through funnelled communication.

Range of facilities

Currently those with principally physical deficits (the minority, unfortunately) are reasonably will served. Those with mainly cognitive or behavioural deficits, however, may be the most recoverable, yet they are scarcely served at all and they tend to mix poorly with people with physical disability. Indeed none of these groups seems to identify readily with the others. This presupposes the need in any service organizational structure for a range of kinds of facilities that differ in environmental and staff characteristics.

REFERENCES

Cope, D.N. (1995) *Brain Injury*, **9**(7).

Eames, P. (1990) Organic bases of behaviour disorders in traumatic brain injury, in *Neurobehavioural Sequelae of Traumatic Brain Injury* (ed. R.L. Wood), Taylor & Francis, London, pp. 133–149.

Hall, K.M. and Cope D.N. (1995) The benefit of rehabilitation in traumatic brain injury: a literative review. *Journal of Head Trauma Rehabilitation*, **10**, 1–13.

Taylor, J.F. (ed.) (1995) *Medical Aspects of Fitness to Drive: a guide for medical practitioners*, 5th edn, Medical Commission on Accident prevention, London.

FURTHER READING

Classification and treatment of behaviour disorders

Journal of Head Trauma Rehabilitation, 1988, **3**(12).

Behaviour modification

Eames, P. (1988) Some aspects of the management of difficult behaviour, in *Perspectives in Psychiatry* (eds P. Hall and P.D. Stonier), John Wiley, Chichester, pp. 41–58.

Kazdin, A.E. (1981) The token economy, in *Applications of Conditioning Theory* (ed. G. Davey), Methuen, London.

Wood, R.L. and Eames, P. (1981) Application of behaviour modification in the rehabilitation of traumatically brain-injured patients, in *Applications of Conditioning Theory* (ed. G. Davey), Methuen, London.

31 Head injury: community rehabilitation

A. Tyerman

INTRODUCTION

Whilst recovery and adaptation after head injury may continue over several years, those with the more severe injuries will be faced with some permanent disability which may be physical, sensory, cognitive, emotional and/or behavioural. This complex array of disability has a marked impact on the person and their life. As the majority are under 25 years at the time of injury, many will live with the effects of their injuries for half a century. They are often enjoying new-found personal and financial independence, developing new roles and relationships and living a full leisure and social life, all of which may be threatened by the effects of head injury. Those injured at an older age may be more settled in their lives but tend to have greater responsibilities, both at work and at home, thereby presenting an even greater challenge to rehabilitation and recovery.

This chapter will review the occupational, social and family impact of head injury in adults, outline recent initiatives in community and vocational rehabilitation, and then describe the development of a specialist head injury service within a community health setting. The chapter will focus on those with more severe head injury (i.e. those unconscious more than 6 hours and/ or with a post-traumatic amnesia (PTA) of at least 24 hours) for whom long-term effects and rehabilitation needs are often extensive.

COMMUNITY OUTCOME

The long-term effects of head injury can be far-reaching, impacting on the person, their family and friends, their employers and work colleagues. Whilst those with minor head injuries will generally resume their former lifestyle, those with more severe injuries will face restrictions in their independence, work, leisure, social and family life. These restrictions are shared by members of the family who may experience great stress in caring for and supporting the person with the injury, often amidst marked changes in family relationships, roles and functioning.

Independence

Many with severe head injury experience some loss of independence. Assistance in personal and domestic care will be needed for those with severe physical disability and guidance and supervision for those with marked cognitive or personality changes. For example, in a 3–10-year rehabilitation follow-up study of 100 persons with very severe injuries in Australia, 53% were judged as able

Rehabilitation of the Physically Disabled Adult. Edited by C. John Goodwill, M. Anne Chamberlain and Chris Evans. Published in 1997 by Stanley Thornes (Publishers) Ltd, Cheltenham. ISBN 0-7487-3183-0.

to live independently (with emotional support if required), 29% as independent only with support services and/or in sheltered accommodation, and 18% as fully dependent on the family or institution (Tate *et al.*, 1989). Others may be independent in activities of daily living, but be unable to travel independently, or need help from the family in making decisions, in managing their financial affairs or be unable to return to previous employment.

Occupation

Return to education, training or work represents a major challenge after head injury. Without specialist advice, many with mild or moderate injuries return to work too soon and struggle with postconcussional symptoms such as poor memory and concentration, irritability, headaches and fatigue. After severe injuries slow speed, poor memory, limited concentration and fatigue render many uncompetitive. Others face more specific restrictions: physical disability restricts manual work; visual deficits may preclude driving; poor executive skills may exclude more managerial positions; poor behavioural control is unlikely to be tolerated in the workplace; whilst those with emotional vulnerabilities may not feel able to cope with pressure or responsibility.

Occupational outcome after severe head injury is very poor. For example, of 134 persons mainly with very severe injuries in Glasgow, only 29% were employed at 2–7 years (Brooks *et al.*, 1987). Whilst few of this group had received much rehabilitation, outcome from rehabilitation centres in the UK is equally disappointing. For example, of 44 persons admitted to the Wolfson Medical Rehabilitation Centre, only 36% were in full-time employment at 2 years, mainly working at a reduced level (Weddell, Oddy and Jenkins 1980). By 7 years, four had progressed from working in a reduced capacity to jobs comparable to pre-injury, but no-one unem-

ployed at 2 years had since found employment (Oddy *et al.*, 1985).

Whilst some persons with head injury may be fortunate to be able to attend the rising number of Headway Houses, offering specialist day care, many others are left in a vacuum without the daily structure that would otherwise serve as the foundation for personal, family and social adaptation.

Leisure and social life

Many with severe head injury also face restrictions in their leisure: activities such as sport, cycling and walking may be precluded by physical disability or impeded by inability to drive; less physical pursuits (such as art, photography, model-making) may be less rewarding due to loss of dexterity; activities such as chess or bridge may be limited by poor memory, concentration and reasoning, with reading also affected by visual/perceptual deficits. Unable to pursue former activities, the person with a head injury often lacks the imagination or initiative to explore alternatives.

The restrictions upon leisure are often paralleled by social isolation. The injured person may feel less inclined to pursue an active social life due to lack of confidence, low mood, intolerance to noise or difficulty in contributing to conversations. Friends often struggle to cope with changes in the injured person: their irritability and aggression; the impoverished content of their conversation; and their impulsivity, disinhibition and lack of refinement in social skills. As such, many friends gradually fall by the wayside. This includes boyfriends and girlfriends, leading in addition to considerable sexual frustration.

An overall indication of social outcome is provided by the rehabilitation follow-up in Australia reported by Tate *et al.*, (1989): 24% were rated as 'good'; 43% 'substantially limited' and 33% 'poor', the life of the latter group being described as 'impoverished in the extreme'. Similarly, in a 2-year rehabilitation follow-up in the UK, persons with very severe injuries reported fewer interests and hobbies, fewer friends, less social and sexual activity and a more lonely life than those with less severe injury (Weddell, Oddy and Jenkins, 1980). At 7 years the dearth of leisure and social activities remained, with half the group having very limited contact with friends and 60% with no boyfriend or girlfriend (Oddy *et al.*, 1985). Many therefore remain dependent upon partners, parents and siblings for their leisure and social life.

Marital relationships

The maintenance of an intimate relationship after head injury is uniquely difficult: physical disability may disrupt pursuit of shared activities; cognitive impairment may limit conversation and companionship; personality changes may alter the dynamics of the relationship, whilst behavioural difficulties may cause embarrassment socially and tension within the relationship. Spouses may also find the behaviour of their partner incompatible with that of a sexual partner. They may also be struggling to cope with the competing needs of work, home, partner and children. As such, whilst the injured person may feel closer to their partner, the spouse may feel trapped in a relationship they no longer find rewarding.

The impact on marriage appears to increase with severity and time since injury. Oddy and Humphrey (1980) found that most relationships were intact at 12 months in severe head injury, but problems were common at 2 years in a very severe group (Tyerman, 1987) and few relationships remained intact in a 10–15-year follow-up of people with extremely severe injuries (Thomsen, 1984). In two of the few studies on the quality of marriage, wives of husbands with severe head injury rated their relationship less positively than wives of husbands with moderate or mild

head injury or spinal cord injury in terms of expression of affection, satisfaction and cohesion (Peters *et al.*, 1990, 1992). In an exploratory study, Young (1994) revealed that persons with severe head injury often both overestimate the state of the marriage compared with spouses (in terms of satisfaction, communication and intimacy) and underestimate the changes desired of them by their partner. The sexual relationship is also often affected, with reduced drive and difficulties in sustaining erections and reaching orgasm commonly reported (Kreutzer and Zasler, 1989).

Severe head injury clearly has a major impact on marriage: some couples remain close but with the spouse under stress and less fun in the relationship; some spouses remain caring and supportive but can no longer reciprocate their partner's intimacy; in other cases the effects of the injury are such that the spouse is unable to cope and the marriage fails.

Family effects

Head injury also has a major impact upon the whole family, who are all too frequently left to cope with little support, especially where the person is left with subtle changes in cognition and personality which may not be apparent to extended family and friends and are noticed even less by professional staff. As life is tailored to meet the needs of the injured person, the occupational, leisure and social lives of family members often falter. For ageing parents there is the added worry about long-term needs.

The high stress and distress amongst relatives in the first year is well established (Oddy, Humphrey and Uttley, 1978; McKinlay *et al.*, 1981; Livingstone, Brooks and Bond, 1985). This does not diminish, with a marked increase in stress at 5 years (Brooks *et al.*, 1986). Whilst less is known about the impact on other family members, children have been reported by the uninjured parent to have a poor relationship with the injured parent or to exhibit acting out behaviour or emotional problems (Pessar *et al.*, 1993).

There have also been very few studies of overall family functioning. However, substantial difficulties were found in a study of 62 persons with injuries of variable severity at 1–60 months, with over half in the 'unhealthy' range in communication, affective involvement and general functioning (Kreutzer, Gervasio and Camplair, 1994). In a recent follow-up of persons with very severe injuries, primary carers rated families as less cohesive, to have more conflict, to be less active socially, to have a more external locus of control, to be less like the ideal family and to have increased enmeshment and decreased disengagement post-injury. Marked changes in family roles were reported for couples, with the injured persons contributing much less to practical, social and parenting roles and spouses struggling to compensate. A marked reduction in mutual marital roles of 'lover' and 'friend' were also evident (Tyerman, Young and Booth, 1994).

The consequences of head injury can therefore be quite devastating for the person with major restrictions on their independence, occupational, leisure and social lives. This is often mirrored by substantial psychological and social impact upon the family, with couples also experiencing marital and sexual difficulties. However, this depressing catalogue of restrictions must be viewed in the context of available health, social and vocational services.

REHABILITATION SERVICES

Services in the UK have concentrated on acute care with little rehabilitation to assist the person in returning to an independent and productive role in society (Greenwood and McMillan, 1993). Rehabilitation post-discharge is very patchy, with all treatment tending to diminish dramatically after 6 months (Murphy *et al.*, 1990). The contribu-

tion of vocational rehabilitation services has been equally disappointing. For example, only 8 of 134 severely injured persons attended employment rehabilitation centres in Glasgow (Brooks *et al.*, 1987) and most of those returning successfully to work in Cambridge did so without employment rehabilitation services (Johnson, 1989).

This is in marked contrast with the networks of post-acute rehabilitation programmes in the USA. Cope *et al.*, (1991a), for example, report on a coordinated system of residential, community and home programmes. Results for 115 persons with head injury admitted at on average 15 months and receiving on average 6 months' treatment show decreased requirement for treatment and increased numbers living at home, independent in daily care and in competitive employment or study (Cope *et al.*, 1991b). This was achieved at an average cost of $50 000 per person. Comparable positive results are reported by Teasdale, Christensen and Pinner (1993) for a 4.5 month programme of 'psychosocial rehabilitation' at the Centre for Hjerneskade in Copenhagen. However, Johnson (1991) draws attention to the high cost of residential 'community re-entry' programmes in the USA (e.g. $108 000 per person), especially as the majority did not return to employment. As such, a number of specialist vocational programmes have been developed.

The New York University Head Trauma Program, for example, has three phases: remedial intervention; guided occupational trials; and vocational placements. Of 94 selected persons with very severe injuries, 56% were in competitive and 23% sheltered work at 6-month follow-up, with outcome holding up well at 3 years (Ben Yishay *et al.*, 1987). An alternative model is the supported placement model, characterized by intense one-to-one on-site training, counselling and support by a job coach. Of 43 persons with severe injuries, over 70% were competitively placed in employment at 6 months (Wehman *et al.*, 1993). This required an average of 290 hours of specialist intervention at a cost of $6000–12 000 per person. A detailed cost–benefit analysis is reported for the specialist Work Re-entry Program at Sharp Memorial Rehabilitation Center, San Diego, which combines elements of work rehabilitation, supported placements and an adjustment/support group. The total operational costs over 5 years were $4377 per person, but taking into account taxes paid and savings in state benefits, the average payback period was just 20 months (Abrams *et al.*, 1993).

In summary, there is accumulating evidence of the benefits of post-acute rehabilitation. However, it is questionable whether this is best undertaken on a residential basis. As previously noted, inpatient rehabilitation is costly and does not guarantee good community outcome. The focus of such units tends appropriately to be on restoring independence for the most severely disabled. This results in improved mobility and self-care, but leaves many languishing at home with no regular occupation or social life (Tyerman, 1987). It highlights the need for community rehabilitation services to promote further recovery, to guide and support appropriate resettlement plans and to facilitate personal, family and social adaptation (Tyerman and Humphrey, 1988).

The British Psychological Society Working Party Report (1989) outlined a community model. This acknowledges the need for acute rehabilitation, specialist (regional) inpatient rehabilitation for the most severely injured and behavioural treatment units for those with marked behavioural disturbance. However, the heart of the envisaged model is a local day rehabilitation facility providing:

1. outpatient assessment and advice;
2. coordination of rehabilitation;
3. treatment/re-training;
4. an occupational/social outlet;
5. advice, training and support for families and professionals.

The need for a range of other services is stressed:

1. respite care;
2. supported living;
3. work centres for those unable to return to previous work or training.

Whilst it is unrealistic to imagine that such a model could be adopted in all districts, our experience in Aylesbury is that local community services can be developed.

DEVELOPING A COMMUNITY HEAD INJURY SERVICE

Rayners Hedge is home to a physical rehabilitation service in a community healthcare NHS trust, providing assessment, rehabilitation, relief care and support for adults with a physical disability. The primary diagnostic groups are multiple sclerosis, stroke and head injury. Whilst most of the work is on an outpatient basis, some inpatient assessment, relief care and rehabilitation is also provided.

When the unmet needs of persons with head injury and their families were first highlighted in 1988, there were no specialist services. Since then, community head injury service has been built up. This has involved five stages of development requiring some redeployment of resources, plus additional funding from Joint Finance, the Department of Health and Employment Service. The current specialist service, summarized in Figure 31.1, comprises: a head injury clinic; individual treatment programmes; weekly cognitive and communication group; weekly personal issues group; family counselling/support; specialist relatives' group programme; vocational assessment/rehabilitation; and marital/family counselling.

The specialist service will now be described. Routine formal assessments and rating scales adopted or developed for use in the head injury service are listed in Table 31.1.

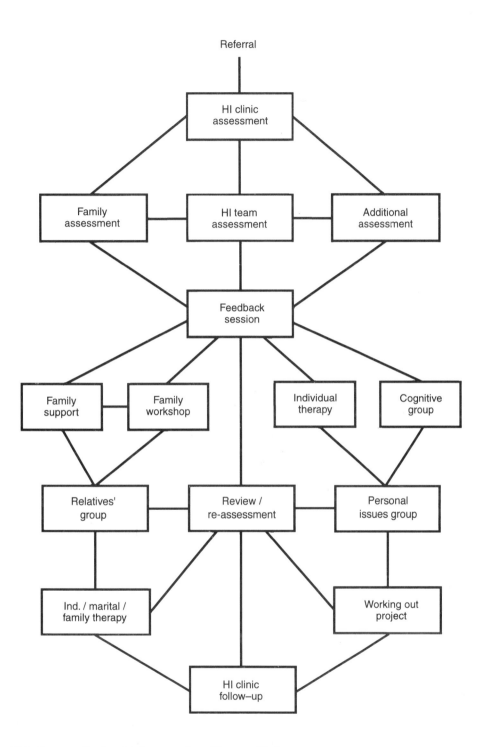

Figure 31.1 Community head injury services, Rayners Hedge.

Table 31.1 Head injury clinic assessment measures

	Person	*Family*
Initial assessment	HIBIS HIPS HISD HAD	(HIBIS) HIPS HISD RHSFI
Further assessment	Neuropsychology COTNAB Physiotherapy Medical Nursing Speech and langauge therapy	FBI FIQ AFRQ GRIMS/FACES
Review + (re-assessment)	HIRI RHSFI HISD HAD (Neuropsychology) (COTNAB) (Physiotherapy) (Speech and language therapy)	HIRI RHSFI HISD AFRQ
Follow-up	HIFUI HIPS RHSFI HISD HAD	HIFUI HIPS RHSFI HISD FIQ AFRQ GRIMS/FACES

AFRQ = Aylesbury Family Roles Questionnaire; COTNAB = Chessington OT Neurological Assessment Battery; FACES = Family Adaptability and Cohesion Scales; FBI = Family Background Interview; FIQ = Family Impact Questionnaire; GRIMS = Golombok Rust Inventory of Marital State; HAD = Hospital Anxiety and Depression Scale; HIBIS = Head Injury Background Interview Schedule; HIFUI = Head Injury Follow-up Interview; HIPS = Head Injury Problem Schedule; HIRI = Head Injury Review Interview; HISD = Head Injury Semantic Differential; RHSFI = Rayners Hedge Scales of Functional Independence.

Referrals

Currently, the service receives about 50 new referrals per annum from Buckinghamshire and neighbouring counties, most with very severe or extremely severe injuries. As a community service some referrals come direct from hospital, but over half are from community sources, principally general practitioners, social services, employment services and local physical disability and mental health teams. Many of the community referrals are of longstanding injuries, some 10 or more years postinjury.

Assessment

New referrals are seen first along with a relative for an initial assessment within a weekly Head Injury (Assessment) Clinic, staffed by the consultant clinical psychologist and specialist social worker. Given the common loss of self-awareness and insight after head injury, the presence of the family member is essential to gain as full and accurate an account as possible. However, this also provides initial impressions of how the family is coping.

Having introduced the service, the head injury background interview schedule is completed, covering family, educational, occupational and clinical history, course of recovery and current situation. Questions are addressed as far as possible to the person, with the relative helping out as necessary. This also enables us to assess the extent of retrograde and post-traumatic amnesia, as well as gauge informally the extent of memory and other cognitive difficulties. Then the person and relative are interviewed separately on a Head Injury Problem Schedule (HIPS) (adapted from Tyerman, 1987), which covers physical, sensory, cognitive, behavioural, emotional and social problems. Both the person and relative also rate change in the person on a Head Injury Semantic Differential Scale (HISD) (adapted from Tyerman, 1987). Whilst the person is screened on the Hospital Anxiety and Depression Scale (HAD), the relative also rates the level of mobility, self-care and cognitive function of the injured person on the Rayners Hedge Scales of Functional Independence (RHSFI) (adapted from Tyerman, 1987).

This process provides us with a detailed clinical and social history and profile of current problems, as perceived by the person and relative. After a brief recess to compare notes, we discuss further assessment and rehabilitation needs, provide general information and advice and address any pressing needs. This initial assessment takes at least 2 hours for those recently injured but longer for those with longstanding injuries and a more complex course of recovery. In their interview relatives often break down in relief at finding someone who at last takes seriously and understands the difficulties with which they have been struggling.

After discussion in our weekly head injury team meeting, further assessments are arranged as required. This routinely includes neuropsychological assessment; Chessington Occupational Therapy Neurological Assessment Battery (COTNAB); physiotherapy assessment; and, where appropriate, a medical examination and speech and language assessment. Nursing care and activities of daily living (ADL) assessments are undertaken as required on an inpatient basis. Psychiatric assessment is occasionally required, but mental health services tend to be involved already for those with severe behavioural or other major psychiatric difficulties.

The social worker may also undertake a family assessment, where indicated. This involves background family information and assessment of the impact on individual family members and changes in family roles on the Aylesbury Family Roles Questionnaire (AFRQ) (Tyerman, Young and Booth, 1994). The overall functioning of the family or the marriage may also be screened on the Family Adaptability and Cohesion Scales (FACES) (Olson *et al.*, 1992) or the Golombok and Rust Inventory of Marital State (GRIMS) (Rust *et al.*, 1988), as appropriate. Where marital counselling is undertaken subsequently the Personal Assessment of Intimacy in Relationships Inventory (Schaefer and Olson, 1981) may be administered with both partners.

The results of these assessments and the recommendations of the team are discussed first at a Head Injury Team Meeting and then with the person and family at a feedback/planning session back in the Head Injury Clinic and arrangements made for any ongoing rehabilitation.

Rehabilitation programmes

Those requiring ongoing rehabilitation are generally offered a programme of individual therapy (cognitive rehabilitation, occupational therapy, physiotherapy), a weekly Cognitive and Communication Group programme and a Personal Issues group. (Acute referrals with multiple and severe disability may be referred to Rivermead Rehabilitation Centre for intensive inpatient treatment before returning to us on discharge for further inpatient or day rehabilitation.) The cognitive and communication group combines group educational/coping sessions on areas of cognitive difficulty with individual goal-directed treatment, feedback/summary sessions, peer group support and occasional social outings. The group runs for 16 weeks and serves as a focal point for our rehabilitation programmes. Individual psychological therapy for emotional and/or behavioural difficulties is also provided, as necessary. The personal issues group and individual psychological therapy provide an opportunity for people to express their frustrations and worries about the head injury and to explore, understand and cope emotionally with their new selves and new situation.

Progress is reviewed with the person and family back in the Head Injury Clinic and monitored through re-administration of clinic rating scales (see Table 31.1). Formal reassessments are arranged routinely for those in the first year or so post-injury and, where indicated, for those with longer-standing injuries. Re-assessment results and any further rehabilitation or resettlement needs are then discussed with the person and family. Some may require a further period of rehabilitation, referral to the Leisure and Lifestyle Group at Rayners Hedge or to the local Headway House, others may be ready for a guided return to work or referral to Working Out, our specialist vocational rehabilitation project.

Vocational rehabilitation

Working Out is a specialist vocational rehabilitation project for persons with severe head injury, funded originally by the Department of Health, as part of the Brain Injury Rehabilitation Initiative (Department of Health, 1994), and now jointly with the Employment Service.

On referral to the Working Out project people are seen for an initial month's assessment. As all referrals have been assessed fully within the Head Injury Clinic, the thrust of the month's assessment is observation of the person within discussion groups and work-related group activities in the community. This allows us to assess work potential using specialist ratings scales: Functional Assessment Inventory (Crewe and Athelstan, 1984), Work Personality Profile (Bolton and Roessler, 1986), as well as overall employment potential.

In the rehabilitation phase the person is helped to prepare for a return to employment or alternative productive occupation. This is achieved through community projects; individual counselling/project work; work preparation group; and personal issues group. The community projects allow us to observe people in the real world away from the structure and security of the rehabilitation centre and to help them to develop greater understanding of the effects of their injury and their implications for employment. The work preparation group and individual project work/counselling help people to re-evaluate their strengths and weaknesses, explore suitable jobs, and consider how to handle issues related to the head injury in the workplace.

In the third phase of the project we work with the person to find a suitable voluntary or training placement, carefully selected and set up to meet the needs of the individual and closely monitored and evaluated by project staff. Where possible, people graduate to therapeutic earnings, supported placements or open employment or training. Such placements are again carefully set up by project staff, working with employment services and other agencies as appropriate, with ongoing advice and support for the individual and employer.

Family rehabilitation

Whilst the person is undergoing a rehabilitation programme, the family may be receiving individual counselling and support from the specialist social worker and may also join the head injury relatives' group programme. This programme combines educational workshops on aspects of head injury with ongoing fortnightly coping sessions and peer group support. Ongoing consultations with the family are arranged as necessary, especially where the person is an inpatient, to maintain close contact and provide advice and support inbetween formal reviews. Couples may be seen by the consultant clinical psychologist and social worker for specialist marital counselling, as appropriate. This latter work tends to be later in rehabilitation, most commonly when the person is on the Working Out project. It is vital that such marital work is set appropriately within the framework of the effects of the head injury.

Follow-up

After discharge the person and the primary carer are followed-up routinely at 6 months, or as soon as possible thereafter, within a weekly Review/Follow-up Clinic. This is essential to monitor progress and respond to emergent long-term difficulties which may arise as the person and family seek to take steps forward in re-building their lives.

Commentary

The Community Head Injury Service, implemented in pilot form in April 1992, has been in development for 3 years at the time of writing. For those referred early postinjury the service has provided continuity of care from assessment through rehabilitation to long-term adaptation. This helps to facilitate optimal recovery, promote insight and guide/support appropriate resettlement. For the most severely injured, referred first to Rivermead Rehabilitation Centre for intensive inpatient treatment, this service provides a further stage of community rehabilitation and the opportunity to work with the family to explore and implement chosen resettlement plans. The integrated vocational rehabilitation project has greatly extended our rehabilitation input, thereby allowing us to support both the person and the family through the long process of recovery and adaptation. For those with longstanding injuries, the service provides an assessment of the residual effects of the head injury and guidance and support to stabilize an often fraught home situation whilst long-term options are considered.

The service has not, of course, been without various teething problems. These have included: securing funding for the expanding service; establishing and refining our operational procedures; implementing effective referral protocols and developing joint working and decision-making with the many statutory, voluntary and independent agencies involved. An over-riding need is to increase the awareness of the effects of head injury in both health and other professional groups.

Whilst this service is community health service led, close collaboration with other services is essential: with acute hospitals to ensure appropriate referrals; with the regional inpatient rehabilitation facility to ensure smooth transfer of care; with the independent sector to ensure specialist treatment for the more behaviourally disturbed; with social services to set up appropriate care packages; with the local Headway group for specialist day care provision; with the local college for both special needs and mainstream courses; and with employment services for the development of the specialist vocational assessment and rehabilitation project. Working in partnership with these agencies, it is our experience that a community head injury service can develop a range of services that address many of the needs of persons with head injury and their families.

CONCLUSIONS

To summarize, research has catalogued a depressing array of social problems for the person with head injury and their family. However, this has to be seen in the context of inadequate health, employment and social services provision, highlighted by the number of persons seen in the rehabilitation service provided at Rayners Hedge who have struggled with the effects of their injuries over many years without specialist assessment, rehabilitation or support. The evidence accumulating from postacute and specialist vocational rehabilitation abroad suggests that social outcome can be improved for the person, thereby reducing stress on the family. The experience in the UK is that a community rehabilitation service has much to offer.

Community rehabilitation requires a network of health, social, employment, educational and voluntary services, working in partnership with the person and family. Health services need to provide acute care, short-term inpatient rehabilitation and long-term community rehabilitation. Whereas medical and nursing care, physiotherapy and speech therapy have the major role in acute rehabilitation, the key personnel in community rehabilitation are from clinical psychology, occupational therapy and social work, working in partnership with other agencies: with social services to secure appropriate day care and residential care; with employment services to address vocational assessment and rehabilitation needs; with education services for those wishing to continue with former or alternative studies; with voluntary agencies (Headway in the UK), in disseminating information about head injury, in providing specialist day care and in supporting families. Head injury specialists will need both to provide training and support for less experienced professionals and to seek opportunities to educate purchasers, employers, teachers, politicians and the general public about the needs but also the unrealized potential of persons with head injury.

There will remain a need for long-term support to respond to difficulties or changes that emerge late post-injury, such as marital/sexual problems, starting a new job, developing new relationships or moving out to live independently. A commitment to community rehabilitation and long-term support appears costly. However, this investment needs to be offset against the high costs of personal and/or family breakdown and major potential savings in service provision and state benefits, as well as the prospect of additional tax revenues for those who make it back to paid employment.

Large-scale multi-centre research will, of course, be required to evaluate which is the most effective model of service provision. However, the experience reported here of a specialist community service is that it is possible to develop rehabilitation programmes and a network of services which offer persons with severe head injury and their families the opportunity to optimize recovery, resettlement and adaptation and, thereby, lay the foundation for re-building their shattered lives.

REFERENCES

Abrams, D., Barker, L.T., Haffey, W. and Nelson, H. (1993) The economics of return to work for survivors of traumatic brain injury: Vocational services are worth the investment. *Journal of Head Trauma Rehabilitation*, 8, 59–76.

Ben-Yishay, Y., Silver, S.M., Piasetsky, E. and Rattok, J. (1987) Relationship between employability and vocational outcome after intensive holistic cognitive rehabilitation. *Journal of Head Trauma Rehabilitation*, 2, 35–48.

Bolton, B. and Roessler, R. (1986) *Manual for the Work Personality Profile*, University of Arkansas: Arkansas Research and Training Center in Vocational Rehabilitation.

British Psychological Society Working Party Report (1989) *Services for Young Adult Patients with Acquired Brain Damage*, British Psychological Society, Leicester.

Brooks, N., Campsie, L., Symington, C. et al. (1986) The five year outcome of severe blunt head injury: a relative's view. *Journal of Neurology, Neurosurgery and Psychiatry*, **49**, 464–470.

Brooks, N., McKinlay, W., Symington, C. et al. (1987) Return to work within the first seven years of severe head injury. *Brain Injury*, **1**, 5–19.

Cope, D.N., Cole, J.R., Hall, K.M. and Barkan, H. (1991a) Brain injury: analysis of outcome in a post-acute rehabilitation system. Part 1. General analysis. *Brain Injury*, 5, 111–125.

Cope, D.N., Cole, J.R., Hall, K.M. and Barkan, H. (1991b) Brain injury: analysis of outcome in a post-acute rehabilitation system. Part 2. Subanalysis. *Brain Injury*, 5, 127–139.

Crewe, N.M. and Athelstan, G.T. (1984) *Functional Assessment Inventory Manual*, University of Wisconsin-Stout, Stout Vocational Rehabilitation Institute.

Department of Health (1994) Report of the Brain Injury Rehabilitation Conference, Peterborough, March 1994.

Greenwood, R.J. and McMillan, T.M. (1993) Models of rehabilitation programmes for the brain-injured adult. 1. Current provision, efficacy and good practice. *Clinical Rehabilitation*, 7, 248–255.

Johnson, M.V. (1991) Outcomes of community re-entry programmes for brain injury survivors: Part 2. Further investigations. *Brain Injury*, 5, 155–168.

Johnson, R. (1989) Employment after severe head injury: do Manpower Services Commission schemes work. *Injury*, **20**, 5–9.

Kreutzer, J.S., Gervasio, A.H. and Camplair, P.S. (1994) Primary caregivers' psychological status and family functioning after traumatic brain injury. *Brain Injury*, **8**, 197–210.

Kreutzer, J.S. and Zasler, N.D. (1989) Psychosexual consequences of traumatic brain injury: methodology and preliminary findings. *Brain Injury*, **3**, 177–186.

Livingstone, M.G., Brooks, D.N. and Bond, M.R. (1985) Patient outcome in the year following severe head injury and relatives' psychiatric and social functioning. *Journal of Neurology, Neurosurgery and Psychiatry*, **48**, 876–881.

McKinlay, W.W., Brooks, D.N., Bond, M.R., *et al.* (1981) The short-term outcome of severe blunt head injury as reported by relatives of the injured persons. *Journal of Neurology, Neurosurgery and Psychiatry*, **44**, 527–533.

Murphy, L.D., McMillan, T.M., Greenwood, R.J. *et al.* (1990) Services for severely head injured patients in North London and environs. *Brain Injury*, **4**, 95–100.

Oddy, M., Coughlan, A., Tyerman, A. and Jenkins, D. (1985) Social adjustment after closed head injury: a further follow-up severe years after injury. *Journal of Neurology, Neurosurgery and Psychiatry*, **48**, 564–568.

Oddy, M. and Humphrey, M. (1980) Social recovery during the year following severe head injury. *Journal of Neurology, Neurosurgery and Psychiatry*, **43**, 798–802.

Oddy, M., Humphrey, M. and Uttley, D. (1978) Subjective impairment and social recovery after closed head injury. *Journal of Neurology, Neurosurgery and Psychiatry*, **41**, 611–616.

Olson, D.H., McCubbin, H.I., Barnes, H. *et al.*, (1992) *Family Inventories*, University of Minnesota (Family Social Science), St Paul.

Pessar, L.F., Coad, M.L., Linn, R.T. and Willer, B.S. (1993) The effects of parental traumatic brain injury on the behaviour of parents and children. *Brain Injury*, **7**, 231–240.

Peters, L.C., Stambrook, M., Moore, A.D. and Esses, L. (1990) Psychosocial sequelae of closed head injury: effects on the marital relationship. *Brain Injury*, **4**, 39–47.

Peters, L.C., Stambrook, M., Moore, A.D. *et al.*, (1992) Differential effects of spinal cord injury and head injury on marital adjustment. *Brain Injury*, **6**, 461–467.

Rust, J., Bennun, I., Crowe, M. and Golombok, S. (1988) *The Golombok Rust Inventory of Marital State (GRIMS)*, NFER-Nelson, Windsor.

Schaefer, M.T. and Olson, D.H. (1981) Assessing intimacy: the PAIR inventory. *Journal of Marital and Family Therapy*, **7**, 47–60.

Tate, R.L., Lulham, J.M., Broe, G.A. *et al.* (1989) Psychosocial outcome for the survivors of severe blunt head injury the results of a consecutive series of 100 patients. *Journal of Neurology, Neurosurgery and Psychiatry*, **52**, 1128–1134.

Teasdale, T.W., Christensen, A.L. and Finner, E.M. (1993) Psychosocial rehabilitation of cranial trauma and stroke patients. *Brain Injury*, **7**, 535–542.

Thomsen, I.V. (1984) Late outcome of very severe blunt head trauma: a 10–15 year second follow-up. *Journal of Neurology, Neurosurgery and Psychiatry*, **47**, 260–268.

Tyerman, A. (1987) Self-concept and psychological change in the rehabilitation of the severely head injured person. Univ. London. Doctoral thesis.

Tyerman, A. and Humphrey, M. (1988) Personal and social rehabilitation after severe head injury, *New Developments in Clinical Psychology*, Vol. 2 (ed. F.N. Watts), John Wiley, Chichester.

Tyerman, A., Young, K. and Booth, J. (1994) Change in family roles after severe traumatic brain injury. Paper presented at The Fourth Conference of the International Association for the Study of Traumatic Brain Injury. St. Louis: September.

Weddell, R., Oddy, M. and Jenkins, D. (1980) Social adjustment after rehabilitation: a two year follow-up of patients with severe head injury. *Psychological Medicine*, **10**, 257–263.

Wehman, P., Kregel, J., Sherron, P., Nguyen, S., Kreutzer, J., Fry, R. and Zasler, N. (1993) Critical factors associated with the successful supported employment placement of patients with severe traumatic brain injury. *Brain Injury*, **7**, 31–34.

Young, K. (1994) The quality of marriage after head injury: investigating both partners views. British Psychological Society, Leicester. Unpublished Dissertation.

USEFUL ADDRESS

Headway, 1 King Edward Court, King Edward Street, Nottingham NG1 1EW, UK.

32 Stroke

D.T. Wade

INTRODUCTION

Stroke is an important disease because it is common and often leaves long-term problems. Many patients may have their lives completely disrupted; many families suffer intolerable stress; health services and social services devote huge resources to the management and care of patients with stroke; and society pays for the consequences through taxes and, to an extent, through lost employment. It has been demonstrated beyond reasonable doubt that a well-organized stroke service focusing on the management of disability (dependence) is cost effective, reducing morbidity and expenditure. Therefore it is essential that all clinicians managing patients with stroke are familiar with this information, and are prepared to argue their case.

This chapter covers the overall management of patients who have suffered a stroke. There is a vast literature now available, and readers in search of detailed references should consult the texts given in the list of Further Reading at the end of this chapter.

Two major advances have occurred since this chapter was written for the first edition of this book. The first is the recognition of the power of the World Health Organization model of illness which conceives of four levels of illness: pathology; impairment; disability; and handicap. This has allowed a systematic model of rehabilitation to be developed based on the definition:

'Rehabilitation is an active, educational, problem-solving process which focuses on disability and aims to optimise a patient's social role functioning, to minimise a patient's somatic and emotional distress, and to minimise the stress on and distress of the family.'

The second major advance has been the development of an intervention which reduces mortality by 25%, reduces the level of dependence experienced by patients in the long-term, and does so at less expense than previous interventions. The 'intervention' is for the patient to be managed by a well-organized specialist stroke service which focuses on disability. (It is interesting to speculate on the contrast between the low profile achieved by this advance compared with the attention likely to be given to a drug which might, if lucky, achieve a 10% reduction.)

The main thesis of this chapter is to suggest that effective management depends upon:

- An integrated specialist service which covers all aspects of stroke care for all patients from stroke onset to arranging and monitoring long-term care; which is...
- staffed by clinicians who are expert in, interested in and able to cover the range of problems faced; and who pay...
- close attention to clinical details by clinicians; and...
- the use of standard measures.

Rehabilitation of the Physically Disabled Adult. Edited by C. John Goodwill, M. Anne Chamberlain and Chris Evans. Published in 1997 by Stanley Thornes (Publishers) Ltd, Cheltenham. ISBN 0-7487-3183-0.

THE PROBLEM

In a typical British Health District of 250 000 people there will be about 1 500 people who have suffered a stroke, 750 of whom will have significant problems as a result of their stroke. Each year 400 more people will suffer an acute stroke, of whom approximately 200 will die within the year. In British acute hospitals, patients with acute stroke alone account for nearly 5% of all expenditure in any one year. Stroke is perhaps the single commonest cause of long-term severe disability (excluding mental illness), and about half of all long-term nursing home patients have suffered a stroke. Similar statistics apply to most countries.

In traditional medical systems, stroke is too common to allow all patients to be concentrated under the care of a few specialists, and too rare to allow all doctors to gain great experience. Instead, patients with stroke are managed by a wide variety of doctors, most of whom are not neurologists and many of whom may not be interested in stroke. Consequently some patients may receive sub-optimal care. This chapter covers the major aspects of stroke management from the medical point of view; other aspects are covered elsewhere.

Stroke is also a very different disease to manage because patients:

- present with a wide variety of problems
- show a wide variation in the severity of those problems
- have an uncertain prognosis individually (though not statistically in groups)
- come from a wide variety of social and cultural backgrounds.

PRINCIPLES OF STROKE REHABILITATION

In order to manage stroke successfully it should be possible to apply a single set of principles. Good stroke management both requires and depends upon the following.

- An accurate medical diagnosis, separating stroke from other causes of the stroke syndrome (i.e. an accurate diagnosis of pathology).
- The provision of immediate support and nursing care, together with specific treatment when available and where appropriate.
- A thorough early assessment using a structured approach and standard assessment protocols as far as possible in order to identify all problems (i.e. an accurate disability diagnosis). There needs to be triage at this stage so that the response meets the needs of the patient, and must include thoughts about prevention of another stroke.
- Full and accurate knowledge of the natural history of stroke, and how to make a prognosis.
- Patient-centred goal planning from the early stages (McGrath et al, 1995).
- Planned, coordinated active early intervention to:
  - reduce complications
  - enable 'natural recovery' to occur without hindrance
  - teach adaptive techniques for overcoming any difficulties
  - ensure that appropriate aids are given and used correctly, and possibly
  - encourage intrinsic neurological recovery.
- The immediate involvement of:
  - a coordinated team of helpers (therapists, social workers, doctors, etc.)
  - who should be readily available to all patients wherever they are, and
  - who should specialize in and have expertise in stroke care.
- Active monitoring of progress and the effectiveness of any intervention, and early identification of any new problems.
- Forward planning, especially concerning all major changes and transitions such as hospital discharge.

- Active early involvement of relatives, with stress upon providing them with accurate, understandable and appropriate information and emotional support.
- Always leaving a telephone 'life-line' for recovered or discharged patients to use, to ask for help and advice if circumstances change.

Some of these principles will be discussed within this chapter, but the detail is necessarily limited. Further information and evidence for most statements can be obtained from the texts given at the end of this chapter.

DIAGNOSIS

The clinical diagnosis of stroke (in distinction to 'not stroke') is usually easy and reliable. It is important to establish that the onset was relatively sudden. One good way is to try to discover the time of onset of symptoms: if the patient or the family cannot fix the onset then doubt the diagnosis. Most strokes come on in under an hour, but some can evolve over a day or more. Further, there may be some fluctuation during the first few days in up to 25% of all patients. The second important aspect of diagnosis is to ensure that there is no other reasonable explanation for the neurological deficit.

The conditions most commonly misdiagnosed as acute stroke are post-epileptic (Todd's) paresis, transient ischaemic attacks and non-specific alterations in consciousness. Tumours, subdural haematoma and other surgically treatable causes are rare, as is hypoglycaemia.

Diagnosis of the type of stroke (haemorrhage or thromboembolic) is unreliable on clinical grounds. Atrial fibrillation, for example, is as common in cerebral haemorrhage as it is in non-haemorrhagic stroke, and other clinical features are equally unreliable at distinguishing the type of stroke. Identification of cerebral haemorrhage becomes of importance if the patient is already on anti-coagulant drugs, or if anticoagulation is being considered (see later). A computerized tomographic scan (CT scan), preferably done within 10–14 days, is the only reliable way to identify cerebral haemorrhage: lumbar puncture with simple inspection of the CSF cannot reliably exclude haemorrhage. It is unlikely that thrombotic and embolic strokes can be separated.

INVESTIGATION

There are four reasons for investigating a patient presenting with a clinical diagnosis of acute stroke. The first is to exclude other causes of the acute stroke syndrome. As stated above, clinical diagnosis is usually correct and the majority of other causes are revealed by the passage of time rather than by any specific test. Any patient suspected of having a cerebral mass needs a CT scan. Routine blood tests will help in excluding temporal arteritis, subacute bacterial endocarditis and other medical causes of unconsciousness, a blood glucose is wise, especially in anyone on hypoglycaemic drugs (e.g. insulin, chlorpropamide).

The second possible reason for investigation is to establish more detail about the stroke, such as its site and size, or the presence of haemorrhage. This rarely affects management and is not useful prognostically in comparison with clinical prognostic indicators discussed later. The only type of stroke which may need identification is a cerebellar haemorrhage or infarction causing hydrocephalus, when surgical intervention might save life. In practice cerebellar haemorrhage is rare (less than 1%). Moreover not all cases need surgical treatment, and so CT scan should be reserved for those cases where the clinical suspicion is strong (predominantly cerebellar symptoms/signs with little weakness), where someone is deteriorating, and where neurosurgical intervention is a realistic option.

Third, investigation could reveal some underlying cause for the stroke. For example some strokes occur after myocardial infarction; the proportion is disputed but is probably less than 5% of all strokes. The major preventable cause of stroke is hypertension, which is easily detected; anaemia and polycythaemia rubra vera are rare but treatable other causes. This avenue is only worth pursuing if management might be altered. Routine blood investigations can be justified, as they are not expensive; but each case should be considered individually. It is helpful to know the lipid status as treatment to lower lipids may reduce the risk of recurrence.

Enthusiastic searching for an occult cause is often fruitless, even in patients under 55 years. In most patients the cause is generalized arterial disease secondary to aging, hypertension or diabetes. There is often other evidence of arterial disease. A few patients develop stroke as a recognized complication of a disease which has already been diagnosed, such as aortic valve disease. Very few patients have a hidden treatable cause, but it is most important that they are identified.

The last reason for investigation is to detect some potential complication of stroke, preferably one which is treatable. For example, some patients develop hyperglycaemia (or may have undiagnosed diabetes); other patients may become uraemic.

A CT scan cannot always prove the diagnosis as it is normal in about 20% of patients with stroke. However, it is essential in four specific circumstances.

1. When there is serious suspicion that the patient has an intracranial mass (tumour, subdural haematoma, abscess).
2. When it is important to exclude cerebral haemorrhage, notably when a patient is already on anticoagulant or antiplatelet therapy or is about to be given some.
3. When hydrocephalus due to a cerebellar haemorrhage or infarction is suspected, particularly if the patient's level of consciousness is dropping and surgical intervention is possible.
4. When the patient's course is atypical, which should always raise doubt as to the correct diagnosis.

The major use of CT scans is to exclude haemorrhage before starting anticoagulation. There is good evidence that anticoagulation reduces the risk of a recurrent stroke in patients who are in atrial fibrillation. Thus it would be reasonable to perform a CT scan to exclude cerebral haemorrhage in all patients in atrial fibrillation before anticoagulation is started. This applies in the case of an apparently embolic stroke, and in progressing stroke as the diagnosis of embolism cannot be made with certainty. Moreover, anticoagulation can lead to haemorrhage into infarcted brain tissue.

Carotid endarterectomy reduces the risk of recurrent stroke in some patients who have suffered a Transient Ischaemic Attack (TIA) or minor (i.e. fully recovered) stroke and who have a carotid stenosis of 70–99%. Consequently, rapid assessment of the carotid arteries is needed. Carotid endarterectomy is only indicated in patients who:

1. have undoubted carotid territory stroke
2. have made a reasonably complete recovery
3. are prepared to take the immediate risk associated with surgery.

Investigation by arteriography should not be initiated unless carotid endarterectomy is an available option agreed by the patient and which can be carried out within 6 months of the initial incident. The surgical team involved should undertake over 60 operations a year with a documented morbidity and should have a mortality rate of under 5%. Arteriography carries a significant if low morbidity and is rarely needed in the diagnostic investigation of definite stroke, but Doppler studies carry much less risk, so help in selection of those who may go on to arteriography.

DRUG TREATMENT

No routine drug regime has yet been proved to benefit all patients with stroke. There are no reliable guidelines to select patients for the specific treatments sometimes recommended, and no proof that any treatment is effective even for selected patients. In particular there is currently no evidence that steroids (e.g. dexamethasone), intravenous dextran or mannitol, immediate anticoagulation with heparin, hyperbaric oxygen, naloxone or other drugs are of benefit.

Surgical intervention is only of benefit to patients with a cerebellar infarction or haematoma causing hydrocephalus with a progressive deterioration in consciousness. Evacuation of intracerebral haematoma has yet to be proven beneficial.

IMMEDIATE CARE

After diagnosis, the doctor's main early task is to ensure that satisfactory nursing care is available. Often this will require hospital admission but not inevitably so. If the patient and/or the family wish for home care and the general practitioner (family doctor) agrees, then this can be undertaken. The principles are similar, though the solutions to practical problems may differ.

Specific details are outside the remit of this chapter. Comatose patients need the usual care, with special consideration given to swallowing, as about 10% of conscious patients choke on attempting to swallow in the first few days. There is a place for the use of percutaneous endoscopic gastrostomy (PEG), which should be considered earlier rather than later. Speech and languages therapists often offer this assessment and support (see Chapter 39). Excretion may provide problems, usually overcome using a commode, pads and patience; early catheterization should be avoided. Paralysis will necessitate careful positioning and handling of the patient. Fear, both in the patient and in the family, should not be overlooked; explain what has happened.

SURVIVAL AND RECURRENCE: NATURAL HISTORY AND INTERVENTION

About 30% of patients die within three weeks and about half will be dead within a year of their stroke. Indicators of a poor prognosis include incontinence of urine for whatever reason, loss of consciousness, severe paralysis, and inability to look towards the paralysed side. Most patients die directly or indirectly from their stroke, but an appreciable number die from a further stroke or heart disease.

Considering early (three-month) survivors, about 16% die each year, an increased rate when compared with age-matched controls. Some of these deaths can be attributed to the original stroke, but cardiac disease is the commonest cause, followed by dying from another stroke. Recurrent stroke (fatal or non-fatal) occurs in about 10% of survivors each year. The major prognostic indicators of long-term risk of death and/or recurrent stroke are any manifestations of cardiac or vascular disease, such as major ECG abnormalities.

Control of hypertension even after a stroke may reduce the risk of death or recurrence. Before initiating treatment one should ensure that the raised blood pressure is not simply a response to the stroke. Unless there is independent evidence of hypertension it is wise to wait three weeks before diagnosing someone as suffering hypertension. Decisions upon the level of blood pressure warranting treatment are difficult; it is best to treat only those normally treated using the standard criteria and reduction should be done in a controlled manner.

Aspirin reduces the risk both of death and of recurrent stroke. Dipyramidole (Persantin) as an addition to aspirin has not yet been shown to increase the protection, and is no more effective than aspirin alone. The best dose of aspirin is uncertain, but it need be no more than 300 mg/day. The duration of treatment is also unknown but, as the risk remains high for life, life-long treatment would seem logical. Anticoagulation should be considered in anyone in atrial fibrillation because it reduces the risk of stroke; however, it should only be initiated if the patient is likely to comply with instructions and if there is an effective system in place to monitor and control the dose of warfarin.

RECOVERY

Planning intervention depends upon knowing the natural history of stroke, and on knowing the specific prognosis if possible.

Natural history

That most survivors of acute stroke show some recovery is well known. More recently the speed and extent of that recovery has been studied in detail, and it is now possible to give guidelines as to the natural history of recovery. It should be stressed that most of this information has been gained from groups of patients. Individual patients may not conform exactly to the general rules; prognosis is considered later. On the other hand, the rules about to be described probably apply to all types of loss seen after stroke.

About half of all recovery occurs in the first 14–21 days, with many patients making an apparently complete recovery in that time. This applies to such activities as walking independently and being able to dress, and probably applies to recovery of language, visual field loss and sensation.

Four qualifications should be noted. First, this statement is based upon research conducted upon people who survived at least three months, and often longer. Therefore one cannot necessarily conclude that patients who are so severely affected that they are destined to die within a month or so are going to recover in the same way. Second, some patients may deteriorate (or even have a

further stroke), which will tend to reduce the apparent rate of recovery in studies based on groups of patients. Third, a proportion of patients will never lose independence in some spheres: for example, not every patient loses the ability to dress. Last, most studies have used a dichotomous classification, with patients being either dependent or independent. No account is taken of speed or ease of performance once independence has been achieved. For example many patients may 'walk independently' but many of these will stop visiting shops alone because of fear, embarrassment or poor endurance and a slow gait.

Recovery can continue for at least six months, with 2–9% of patients making an appreciable recovery of independence between six months and one year. Published information on later qualitative improvements in performance is scarce. It is quite likely that patients continue to improve their performance in recovered functions for well over six months. For example, few patients regain independent mobility after six months, but possibly walking becomes easier in those who have become independent.

Prognosis

Two questions arise after an acute stroke. Will the patient survive and if so, how good will the recovery be? A single observation at 24–48 hours can give good guidance. Patients who are incontinent of urine for whatever reason (e.g. in coma, unable to get attention of nurse, previously incontinent) are both more likely to die within the first six months and, if they survive, to be left seriously disabled and often needing long-term care. This single factor is more powerful than complicated prognostic scores derived from multiple variables.

An important distinction should be drawn between variables which are important in giving a prognosis, and variables which may influence rehabilitation. For example, urinary incontinence is important as a prognostic indicator but specific treatment of incontinence (e.g. using a catheter) is unlikely to influence outcome. On the other hand, apraxia is not a good prognostic indicator because it is uncommon but if present may have a major influence on the pattern of rehabilitation.

When considering any particular function (e.g. speech, use of the arm) then the more severe the original loss in that sphere, the less good will be the final outcome. For example, the first measure of language function taken at (say) three weeks is the major prognostic factor determining language function at six months. Similarly the best predictor of arm function is the initial severity of arm paralysis. In practice, urinary incontinence will allow an early estimate of overall recovery, but specific measures of each function will probably give a better indication of recovery in each individual ability.

ASSESSING THE PATIENT

Just as an accurate medical diagnosis precedes effective medical management, so effective rehabilitation depends upon accurate assessments of disability and the cause(s) of that disability. No single test or assessment can 'measure' or 'assess' stroke. Rather each aspect of stroke needs to be tested separately and interpreted in the light of other tests. Details of what to assess when, and how, are discussed later. First some important general principles need to be stated.

Use standard measures wherever these are available. Stroke management has long been frustrated by the wide variety of measures used by therapists and doctors. If there is no common language, communication between team members is inhibited. Communication is also hampered between teams which use different assessments.

Some recommended measures are given in Table 32.1. Details and full references are in Wade (1992).

Perform a thorough assessment. Too often important problems are overlooked simply because no-one formally tests for them. A common example is the failure to recognize aphasia (this term will be used to cover all grades of language disturbance, and is synonymous with dysphasia). Obviously there is a limit to the detail which can be achieved, but each aspect should be covered. The other impairment commonly not recognized is amnesia (i.e. forgetfulness, difficulty in learning or visio-spatial problems).

Case history

A 58-year-old woman, Mrs. W, was discharged from hospital to her flat after a two-week stay in hospital, most spent attending for rehabilitation. She spent the first 24 hours at home in great distress as she was unable to find her way around the kitchen, could not use any equipment, and kept knocking against things. She could not read. No-one in hospital had detected her hemianopia and her apraxia. After spending four weeks with her sister she was able to return home.

Monitor progress, auditing the effectiveness of any interventions. One advantage the doctor has is that of a relatively objective involvement, seeing the patients less frequently than most others involved. By monitoring progress the doctor can evaluate whether any treatment initiated has had any effect. Moreover, failure to progress might be due to some unidentified problem itself amenable to treatment.

Use appropriate assessments. For example, when screening for language loss soon after stroke, a short test should be used, reserving more detailed assessments for those patients found to have aphasia (dysphasia). In addition the aspects needing assessment will change with time. For example depression is an important long-term complication but does not need to be searched for within the first few days.

Table 32.1 Some recommended routine assessments (see also Chapter 9)

Measure	When?	Why?
Urinary incontinence	2–3 days	Best prognostic indicator
Motricity Index	2–3 days	Measures motor loss
Trunk Control Test	2–3 days	Prognostic importance
Frenchay Aphasia Screening Test	2–3 days	Detects aphasia; if present refer to speech and language therapist
Short Orientation-Memory-Concentration Test	2–3 days, at 6 months and at discharge	Culture-free, simple measure of cognition; a common impairment, often missed
Barthel ADL Index	2–3 days, weekly to discharge, 6 months	Measures dependence; identifies important areas of disability
Rivermead Mobility Index	2–3 days, at discharge and at 6 months	Mobility is one of the most pressing problems for patients
Gait speed	During therapy	Most sensitive measure of mobility
Hospital Anxiety and Depression Scale	At discharge and at 6 months	Prompts attention to any emotional problems
Frenchay Activities Index	At 6 months	Outcome of importance to patient

INITIAL ASSESSMENT

The first full assessment of any stroke patient should be carried out as soon as the diagnosis is certain and any immediate investigations and treatment have been completed. This will often be within 24 hours, and should not be delayed beyond three days if possible. Early assessment is useful for several reasons. It can identify otherwise undiagnosed deficits which may modify initial management. For example, it is quite common for mild aphasia to be unrecognized for several days or even weeks. Second, initial deficits might be of prognostic importance. Last, an early assessment provides a useful objective measure against which future progress can be gauged.

Two competing requirements influence the first assessment. On the one hand it is important to cover all likely areas of deficit, and not simply to concentrate upon those already diagnosed. On the other hand the assessment is constrained by the patient's clinical state, and the assessor's time and patience. The major functions which should be assessed are cognition, communication, motor and sensory function, and probably, activities of daily living.

LATER ASSESSMENTS

Once the immediate crisis is over then it is important to assess the social background of the patient. This includes obtaining information on his lifestyle and abilities before stroke, assessment of his housing and the problems it might pose, and evaluation of the social support available. Emotional disturbance is common after stroke. While this is often recognized in the first weeks, it is not always taken into consideration later. It might be worth considering the use of formal assessment of mood as an adjunct to clinical judgement.

Ideal rehabilitation would probably include formal assessments at four weeks, six months and possibly one year after stroke. These assessments allow monitoring of general progress and can be used to audit the overall standard of care given to the generality of patients. In addition it is probably useful to interpolate assessments at one week after discharge from hospital and one month after the end of formal rehabilitation. These help to ensure that no major difficulties are left at these points. It is less certain that this ideal can ever be achieved, and as yet it is unproven that it actually benefits patients (but see Friedman, 1996).

Several advantages might accrue from a policy of routine follow-up. Deficiencies in the rehabilitation service are more likely to be identified and thus remedied. Patients may feel less abandoned. Staff will become more aware of the natural history of stroke, in particular that many people do make good recoveries. On the other hand, it has to be accepted that routine follow-up is expensive. Until evidence is produced to show that there are benefits, some doctors might prefer simply to discharge patients as soon as possible without follow-up, performing regular assessments simply on patients still under active rehabilitation.

COGNITION

Coma and confusion will affect about half of all patients in the first few days. A record of the lowest level of consciousness reached is useful for prognostic reasons: it is associated with an increased fatality rate and a less good outcome. A record of the current level of consciousness and cognitive function is important, especially to help interpret other findings (a confused patient may not cooperate with other tests). Last, a routine assessment of memory and orientation is useful in management.

The level of consciousness is best measured using the Glasgow Coma Scale (GCS). This assesses a patient's best response to stimulation in three sections: opening of eyes, verbal response and motor (limb) movement. Because patients with aphasia will score badly on the verbal section it is important to show the individual section scores, not simply the total. If brevity is vital then the motor scale alone should be used. Memory and orientation should be tested using the Short Orientation–Memory–Concentration test because it is culture free and probably more sensitive than the widely used Hodkinson mental test. Other more detailed cognitive tests are available, but may not be needed in most patients.

COMMUNICATION

Dysarthria (slurring of speech) occurs in at least one-third of conscious patients in the early stages. This rarely causes a persisting difficulty with communication and in this situation other forms of expression are feasible.

Aphasia* occurs in about a further one-quarter of conscious patients, and about 15% of survivors are left with some aphasia. It is important to identify aphasia as soon as possible so that a speech therapist can identify a patient's capabilities thoroughly, thus allowing staff and relatives to communicate with the patient in the most effective manner. The Frenchay Aphasia Screening Test (FAST) has been developed specifically for use with patients after an acute stroke. It is a reliable method of detecting aphasia, although certain precautions are needed in interpreting the results in patients with confusion or hemianopia. This test should be used routinely after stroke if there is any possibility of aphasia (e.g. in all patients with right-sided weakness). The test covers expression, comprehension, reading and writing.

---

* **Aphasia** is the 'inability to express thought in words, or an inability to understand thought expressed in the spoken or written words of others' (*Chambers Dictionary*). **Dysphasia** implies difficulty rather than inability. Common usage has corrupted both definitions, and they are even used synonymously by some.

Aphasia needs only to be tested for once. If absent, then no further assessments of language are needed. If present, more complete assessment by a speech therapist is required, and she should perform further follow-up assessments as needed.

MOTOR AND SENSORY TESTING

Although it is the most obvious manifestation of stroke, weakness is discussed third because testing depends upon adequate cognitive and communicative ability. Detection of weakness is not usually a problem, but describing its severity is often ignored. A simple rapid measure is the 'Motricity Index' which gives a 0 (total paralysis) to 100 (normal) score, reflecting the extent of paralysis in the arm and in the leg. Although less detailed than other available measures, it has the great advantages of brevity and simplicity.

Sensory testing is much more difficult, and often unreliable. The one sensory modality which should be tested routinely is the visual fields. Confrontation testing using both individual and simultaneous stimuli (usually moving fingers) should be carried out to detect both complete hemianopia and visual inattention. Where possible an orthoptist should be involved (see Chapter 21).

ACTIVITIES OF DAILY LIVING

Information about a patient's activities of daily living (ADL) function is central to the management of all disabling diseases, including stroke. The Barthel ADL Index has been used in more research than any other ADL index, and should be adopted as the standard.

More detailed information on individual aspects of function does not need to be recorded routinely. Measures do exist, but they should probably be used selectively on patients who have particular problems and where significant effort or resources are being devoted to treatment. For example, anyone

whose walking is affected should have his speed measured by timing it over a 10-metre walk using whatever aid is needed and walking at his own preferred speed.

It is important to consider 'Extended' activities of daily living in most patients (EADL). This term covers the patient's ability to undertake necessary domestic (household) activities and community activities such as shopping. Formal assessment is possible using, for example, the Nottingham EADL measure or the household sections of the Rivermead ADL assessment.

SOCIAL AND EMOTIONAL ASPECTS

It could be argued that formal assessments are unnecessary in this field because the clinical (i.e. unstructured) approach is adequate and possibly more adaptable. This may be true when there are sufficient numbers of experienced and conscientious staff but the use of a standard approach helps to ensure that all major areas are covered, and that other people involved in the team understand these aspects.

These are perhaps the most difficult areas to assess formally. The only short simple index of 'non-ADL' activities available is the Frenchay Activities Index (FAI), which covers 15 different activities. Information on pre-stroke functioning should be gathered as soon as possible. At any time from six months on, a patient's performance on the FAI should be checked. An explanation should be sought for any reductions observed; often there will be an obvious case for stopping an activity, but it is quite common for the FAI to reveal unnecessary changes in lifestyle. For example, someone may not go shopping, even though they are capable, simply because no-one has 'given permission'.

About one-third of survivors feel depressed at any one time after stroke; some have clinical depression. The important point is to look for depression, particularly in relation to people who have restricted their lifestyle without good (physical) cause. Clinical diagnosis is not always easy, and the use of questionnaires might help. Several exist. One self-assessment questionnaire designed for use on hospital patients with physical disorders is the Hospital Anxiety and Depression Scale (HADS). It is a useful screening test for significant emotional disturbance later after stroke. It has only 14 questions, which should enhance its acceptability (see Chapter 9).

Housing is still more difficult to assess, and is covered in more detail in Chapter 54. A problem-orientated approach is probably the simplest, considering six problems: numbers of living levels (one floor or two?); toilet arrangements; bathing and kitchen arrangements; mobility within the house; and mobility out of and outside the house.

INTERVENTION

Texts on rehabilitation traditionally concentrate upon what to do to (or for, or with) the patient, yet this chapter has scarcely mentioned intervention. There are several reasons for this. First, most techniques are practical, being learnt most easily by experience with patients and not from books. Second, there is little scientific evidence as yet that any specific intervention necessarily improves upon natural recovery. Last, and most important, it is quite likely that the major defects in current practice are the poor organization of care in its widest sense, and the failure to detect remediable problems.

Despite the lack of hard evidence, the following actions are likely to be beneficial:

1. Ensure rapid, early mobilization (i.e. within hours or days). It is certainly not contraindicated and may be beneficial.
2. Give good physical (nursing) care. This is vital to avoid such complications as bedsores or contractures.
3. Actively involve the patients, their family, all nursing and ward staff, and anyone else concerned with the patient throughout the waking day. Even 'intensive therapy' can only occupy 5% of a patient's waking hours. Therefore the need is for a rehabilitative milieu to be in effect at all times, rather than episodic 'treatment' in isolation from normal daily care.
4. Maintain motivation and interest. Every achievement should be praised. Listen to their wishes.
5. Be pragmatic and patient centred. Relate therapy to a patient's needs and abilities. Do not stop someone from walking in an odd way if it enables him to be mobile. The increase in morale outweighs most other considerations.
6. Identify and treat all relevant problems: not only the difficulties arising from the stroke, but also any incidental disabling problems such as arthritis, blindness or deafness.
7. Use a uniform approach. All team members treating an individual patient need to use a consistent method, and their answers to questions (e.g. on prognosis) need to be consistent.
8. Be curious. If someone is not progressing as expected, find out why. Patients who put clothes on wrongly or get lost in the department may have visuo-spatial (perceptual) problems. Other patients lack drive, usually due to depression but sometimes specifically from frontal lobe damage.

Some particular aspects of intervention need discussing. As mentioned initially, all professional staff involved should work as a team, with as little demarcation as possible. All team members should work towards the same goal; consequently their distinct roles will overlap to a considerable degree. Each profession represented in the team should see each patient at lest once, to assess whether their expertise is needed. The approach to the patient should be sensible and not dictated by some all-enveloping theory. There is no evidence yet to support any particular approach (e.g. Bobath); even the importance of 'positioning' has not been investigated scientifically. Each therapist should use the methods they have experience of, adapting the approach as necessary. It is important, though, that each team member uses the same approach, and that family and friends use the same approach at home. Further, whatever the theoretical basis, it seems cruel to place patients with hemianopia so that they cannot see the rest of the ward, or to place their belongings on the neglected side. There is no evidence that this approach improves recovery.

Spasticity has been described as 'the fable of the neurological demon and the emperor's new therapy'. There is no evidence that regular use of antispastic drugs is useful. On rare occasions such drugs (baclofen, dantrolene) may be needed to reduce tone which is painful or obstructive, but they are unlikely to benefit patients who are still recovering. Spasticity reflects poor motor control, rather than causing it (see Chapter 34).

One aspect of stroke care sometimes overlooked is the need for long-term social support. Too often patients who appear to have made a good recovery or a good adaptation to their residual disability are discharged only to fester at home, lonely and depressed. Most areas, but by no means all, of Britain and other countries have voluntary and state-run organizations (e.g. Stroke Clubs) which can provide help and support for people left with problems after stroke. Medical social workers are the usual source of information on this topic. Every patient should have a reason to get out of bed each morning, and rehabilitation is incomplete until this is ensured.

ORGANIZATION OF STROKE CARE SERVICE

There is now much good evidence that a well-organized stroke service with expert clinicians is cost effective. It leads to a better patient outcome (fewer deaths, a reduced level of dependence, and less likelihood of being in a nursing home) and at the same time it uses fewer health resources (the length of stay is shorter). This evidence comes from many randomized trials, and it has been confirmed that the trial evidence does translate into normal clinical practice.

The research has not identified which specific components of the service are vital and which are unnecessary, and at present it would seem best to aim for a specialist service which is responsible for all patients. The team should be responsible for all aspects of rehabilitation including leisure, and longer term problems with mobility as both of these can be improved.

Audit of stroke management is in its infancy. A package has been developed for the acute phase, the first few days, and this should be used wherever possible. There are no methods for ensuring quality control of rehabilitation which have been shown to be practical and effective at improving quality.

CONCLUSIONS

The most important recent advance in stroke management has been the demonstration that a well-organized service, focusing on disability, can reduce mortality by 25% and can reduce morbidity and long-term care needs at less cost than standard management. It is likely that the well-organized service will use the general principles and approaches discussed in this chapter. This approach will become even more important when an effective acute treatment is discovered. This treatment is likely to bring everyone to hospital and though it may increase the total number of independent people, it is unlikely to reduce the number of disabled people needing rehabilitation (instead, everyone will be shifted up the curve, with people who would otherwise have died being left disabled). A good standard of care requires constant attention to detail, and will be further facilitated by the use of standard assessment procedures.

REFERENCES

Friedman, P.J. (1996) Stroke rehabilitation in the elderly: analysis of six years experience. *Clinical Rehabilitation* 1996; **10**: in press.

McGrath, J.R., Marks, J.A., Davis, A.M. (1995) Towards interdisciplinary rehabilitation: further developments at Rivermead Rehabilitation Centre. *Clinical Rehabilitation* **9**, 320–6.

Wade, D.T. (1992) *Measurement in Neurological Rehabilitation*. Oxford University Press, Oxford.

FURTHER READING

Bamford, J., Sandercock, P., Dennis, M., Burn, J. and Warlow, C. (1991) Classification and natural history of clinically identifiable subtypes of cerebral infarction. *Lancet*, **337**, 1521–6.

Freemantle, N. (1992) Stroke Rehabilitation. Effective Health Care: Bulletin 2: School of Public Health, University of Leeds and Centre for Health Economics, University of York.

Freemantle, N., Pollock, C., Sheldon, T.A., Mason, J.M., Song, F., Long, A.F. and Ibbotson, S. (1992) Formal rehabilitation after stroke. *Quality in Health Care* **1**, 134–7.

Gariballa, S.E., Robinson, T.G., Parker, S.G. and Castleden, C.M. (1995) A prospective study of primary and secondary risk factor management in stroke patients. *Journal of the Royal College of Physicians of London*, **29**, 485–7.

Mackey, F., Ada, L., Heard, M.A. and Adams, R. (1996) Stroke rehabilitation: are highly structured units more conducive to physical activity than less structured units? *Archives of Physical Medical Rehabilitation*, **77**, 1066–70.

Norton, B., Homer-Ward, M., Donnelly, M.T., Long, R.G. and Holmes, G.K.T. (1996) A randomised prospective comparison of percutaneous endoscopic gastrostomy and nasogastric tube feeding after acute dysphasic stroke. *British Medical Journal* **312**, 13–15.

Partridge, C.J., Johnston, M. and Edwards, S. (1987) Recovery from physical disability after stroke: normal patterns as a basis for evaluation. *Lancet*. Feb 14; 373–5.

Partridge, C.J., Morris, L.W. and Edwards, M.S. (1993) Recovery from physical disability after stroke: profiles for different levels of starting severity. *Clinical Rehabilitation*, **7**, 210–17.

Post-Stroke Rehabilitation Clinical Practice Guideline (1995). Available from Agency for Health Care Policy and Research, Willco Building, Suite 310, 6000 Executive Boulevard, Rockville, MD 20852, USA.

Rothwell, P.M., Slattery, I. and Warlow, C.P. (1996) A systematic comparison of the risks of stroke and death due to carotid endarterectomy for symptomatic and asymptomatic stenosis. *Stroke* **27**, 266–9.

Samuelson, M., Soderfeld, B. and Olsson, G.B. (1996) Functional outcome in patients with lacunar infarction. *Stroke* **27**, 842–6.

Sandercock, P. (1993) Managing stroke: the forward way: Organising stroke care saves lives. *British Medical Journal* **307**, 1297–8.

Stone, S.P. and Whincup, P. (1994) Standards for the hospital management of stroke patients. *Journal of the Royal College of Physicians* **28**, 52–8.

Wade, D.T. and the Rivermead Speciality Team (1993) Services for people with stroke. *Quality in Health Care* **2**, 263–6.

Wade, D.T. (1994) Stroke: Acute cerebrovascular disease, in *Health Care Needs Assessment. The epidemiologically-based needs assessment reviews.* Stevens, A., Raftery, J. (eds), *Radcliffe Medical Press Ltd* **1**, 111–255.

33 Parkinson's disease and other forms of Parkinsonism

A.M.O. Bakheit and D.L.L. McLellan

INTRODUCTION

Parkinson's disease is a relatively common condition, having an incidence of approximately 20/100 000 and prevalence of some 160–200/100 000. In Britain approximately 74/100 000 people are severely disabled due to Parkinson's disease (Sutcliffe *et al.*, 1985; Fahn, 1986; Mutch *et al.*, 1986a). The mean age at onset is 65 years and the male to female ratio is 3:2. The disease is commoner in the elderly, some estimates suggesting that one in 10 of all those over the age of 80 have Parkinsonism.

The main pathological finding in Parkinson's disease is severe degeneration of the pigmented substantia nigra cells. More than 80% of these cells are usually lost before the first symptoms of the disease are noticed. Parkinson's disease starts insidiously and progresses slowly. In the pre-levodopa era death would be expected 12–15 years after the first symptom due to complications of immobility, notably bronchopneumonia. Levodopa has improved the prognosis in these patients considerably, restoring life expectancy to near normal.

Terminology

The terminology of Parkinson's disease is confusing. Parkinson's original description in 1817 is usually held to apply to the idiopathic progressive form of the disease so the term Parkinson's disease (or idiopathic Parkinsonism) is reserved to this clinical entity.

'Parkinsonism' is used to embrace the whole spectrum of neurological disorders in which **bradykinesia** is accompanied by one or more of the other classical clinical features of the disease.

Rarely, some of the clinical features of Parkinsonism coexist with further neurological deficits suggesting lesions in other parts of the nervous system. These conditions are identified by their additional features, and are grouped under the rubric ' Parkinson Plus' syndromes (Fahn, 1986).

CAUSES OF PARKINSONISM

The cause of Parkinson's disease is not known. Causes of Parkinsonism include viral encephalities and exposure to drugs and toxins. Most cases of postencephalitic Parkinsonism were produced by pandemics of encephalitis lethargica in 1918 and 1922 but obvious postviral cases are now very unusual. Phenothiazine drugs (which block dopamine transmission) can induce Parkinsonism with persistence of the symptoms for up to 2 years. Recently a number of cases of acute, severe Parkinsonism have occurred in young intravenous drug addicts poisoned with MPTP (N-methyl-4-phenyl-1-1,2,3,6-tetrahydropyridine), a contaminant of inexpert attempts to manu-

Rehabilitation of the Physically Disabled Adult. Edited by C. John Goodwill, M. Anne Chamberlain and Chris Evans. Published in 1997 by Stanley Thornes (Publishers) Ltd, Cheltenham. ISBN 0-7487-3183-0.

facture heroin, which selectively destroys nigrostriatal dopaminergic neurones.

CLINICAL FEATURES OF PARKINSONISM

The core features of Parkinson's disease are bradykinesia, tremor, rigidity, gait disturbances and postural instability. Other complaints include fatigue, muscle aches, disturbances of speech and swallowing. Symptoms of autonomic failure also occur.

Bradykinesia

The fundamental clinical disorder in Parkinsonism, bradykinesia, is thought to reflect more than any other feature of Parkinson's disease the consequences of striatonigral degeneration (Marsden, 1984); the diagnosis cannot be made in absence of this symptom no matter what other features are present. Bradykinesia is slowness of voluntary movements, referring both of the initiation of movement and its execution. Its earliest manifestation in the hands is impairment in the performance of fine skilled tasks such as writing or handling delicate tools; later it may be increasingly difficult to button or unbutton clothing or to use a knife and fork effectively. The most sensitive test for bradykinesia of the hands is to place the palmar surface of the wrist on a table and to drum the middle and index fingers alternately as fast as possible, ensuring that as one finger extends the other flexes concurrently and that these movements simultaneously reverse. In bradykinesia this sequence can only be performed slowly, and both fingers tend to move in the same direction or each finger makes a succession of taps while the other fails to move. In the legs bradykinesia presents as difficulty in rapid movements of the feet (as in drumming or dancing) or a tendency to shuffle. Slowness of cognitive processes also occurs and has been termed bradyphrenia.

Formal studies of the nature of bradykinesia have shown that the simple reaction time may be normal, but that more complex responses in which a decision or choice has to be made are delayed. There is a characteristically slow build-up of muscle activation and the burst of activity achieved when attempting to perform a ballistic movement is of a lower amplitude than normal. Complex sequences (such as grasping with the hand at the same time as flexing the elbow) are conducted much more slowly than either component would be if undertaken singly. This has led to the suggestion that superimposing and sequencing of simple basic motor 'programmes' is defective bradykinesia.

Tremor

Tremor does not occur in all cases of Parkinsonism, and in an untreated patient, tremor unaccompanied by bradykinesia is not due to Parkinsonism. At least two types of tremor are seen, which are described below.

Tremor 'at rest' when the subject is awake but not having to move or maintain a posture so that the limb is relaxed. In the upper limb this is the 'pill-rolling' tremor in which the forearm is partially supinated and the thumb extends as the fingers flex, mimicking the movement of rolling a small object in the palm of the hand. It is slow, with a frequency of 4–5 Hz, and may be suppressed when a voluntary movement is made, but returns after a few moments (in severe cases) even though voluntary activity continues.

'Action' or 'postural' tremor brought out by maintaining a posture such as holding the arm out to the front. This resembles a physiological tremor but its frequency at 7–8 Hz is intermediate between resting tremor and physiological tremor, and coincides with the frequency of cogwheeling described below. Finally some patients quite clearly have mild intention tremor, but by common consent this fact is ignored, since it is incompatible with the clinical categorization of tremors as taught to medical students.

Rigidity

Rigidity is the term given to 'plastic' or 'velocity-independent' resistance to passive stretch which is seen especially in the flexor muscle groups in the arms and legs. The resistance is usually broken up into bursts of activity at a rate of 7–8 Hz, i.e. similar to the frequency of postural tremor, whether or not overt tremor is present, and is due to a specific and characteristic abnormality in the passive stretch response.

Rigidity expresses itself by altering the posture of the patient; since it is most pronounced in flexor muscles both upper and lower limbs (and the neck and trunk) tend to assume a flexed posture. In mild cases this tendency can be readily overcome by voluntary effort. Impoverishment of movement is much more likely to be due to bradykinesia than rigidity, for the mechanism of reciprocal inhibition is unimpaired in mild and moderate rigidity so that there is little or no mechanical constraint by antagonist muscles during voluntary movements.

Gait abnormalities

Gait disturbances in Parkinson's disease are complex and cannot be entirely explained on the basis of bradykinesia. Failure to swing one arm when walking is usually the earliest deviation from normal gait. Stride length is reduced at this stage and becomes progressively shorter as the disease advances. In the later stages of the disease patients experience difficulties initiating gait and in more severe cases a step that cannot be initiated voluntarily may be initiated in a reflex-like way by pushing the subject forward or rocking him/her from side to side. Such a stimulus can initiate a sequence of short steps ('festination') over which the subject has only a tenuous voluntary control, and he/she may continue to festinate forwards or backwards until meeting an obstacle or something to grasp hold of.

Visual cues may either help or hinder the ability to walk. Parkinson reported of his sixth case, 'it was observed by his wife, that he believed, that in walking across the room, he would consider as a difficulty the having to step over a pin' (Parkinson, 1817). Patients with advanced disease tend to 'freeze' as they approach doorways and may be assisted by the presence of horizontal lines across the surface over which they are walking. It is uncertain whether these observations are best interpreted as signs of poor sensory-motor integration, or whether these visual cues simply facilitate or inhibit the complex process of voluntary initiation of movement by acting as targets. Some patients develop complex stereotyped mental strategies to reinforce their ability to initiate movement. Under extreme emotional stress (such as immediate physical danger) the ability to move may for a few moments be restored almost to normal; a phenomenon known as kinesia paradoxica. Similar short-lived periods of mobility sometimes occur in the first few minutes after waking from sleep.

Other features

Infrequent blinking, hypomimia (facial immobility) and the 'reptilian stare' which result from a combination of muscular rigidity and bradykinesia may occur. Another group of frequently reported symptoms comprise excessive fatigue, fleeting muscular pain (often described by patients as rheumatism), intermittent paraesthesiae and burning skin sensations, urinary symptoms, postural dizziness, depression and impairment of cognitive function.

Associated pains

Somatic pains are common. Muscle cramps and tightness in the neck, paraspinal and calf muscles are the most frequently reported complaints. Painful dystonias occur mostly in the mornings, though a few are related to times at which dopaminergic drug action is at its peak. Radicular pains may also occur. All these features are associated in time with the severity of bradykinesia and, to a lesser extent, rigidity.

Abnormalities of swallowing and speech

Dysphagia and speech disorders are present in the vast majority of patients with Parkinson's disease. Dysarthria with hoarseness, decreased volume and monotonous tone are common. Consonants may be imprecise and the patient finds it increasingly difficult to gain and sustain the attention of the listener (Robbins, Logemann and Kirshner, 1986).

Autonomic features

Mild symptoms of autonomic failure, for example postural dizziness, urinary frequency, urgency and a sensation of incomplete bladder emptying, impotence and excessive or reduced sweating are compatible with a diagnosis of Parkinson's disease. However, when present in the early stages of the disease these symptoms are usually a manifestation of a Parkinson plus syndrome (see below).

Cognitive dysfunction

Impairment of memory and other aspects of cognitive function are common in some of the diseases associated with Parkinsonism. In Parkinson's disease there are subtle impairments of visuospatial function, associative learning and recent memory, and also in tests of order-dependent short-term memory (Mayeux, 1981).

The literature relating to dementia in Parkinson's disease is confusing, partly because of the difficulty in allocating patients to this category and partly because of the confounding effects of increasing age. In patients presenting before the age of 65 years the likelihood of developing subsequent dementia is probably 10–15%.

Atypical features

Erectile impotence, excessive sweating, a feeling of incomplete bladder emptying, constipation and orthostatic hypotension are common symptoms in Parkinson's disease, but are usually mild and late. Severe early autonomic failure in patients with extrapyramidal signs suggests the diagnosis of Shy–Drager syndrome. The presence of an extensor plantar response in these patients is an indication of coincidental cerebrovascular disease or a widespread neurodegenerative disorder such as multisystem atrophy or progressive supranuclear palsy.

Neuroradiological investigations are useful in distinguishing Parkinson's disease from other Parkinsonian syndromes and magnetic resonance imaging (MRI) is particularly helpful. Stern and colleagues (1989) have found that a combination of low levels of signal from the putamen and atrophy of the brainstem on MRI is a consistent finding in Parkinson's plus syndromes and, when taken with other clinical features, virtually excludes Parkinson's disease.

Focal and segmental dystonias are rare but well-recognized features of untreated Parkinson's disease (Nausieda, Weiner and Klawans, 1980). However, in a young patient dystonia is more likely to be a manifestation of levodopa-responsive dystonia or Wilson's disease. A detailed family history, ophthalmic examination for Kayser–Fleischer rings and copper studies are mandatory in these patients.

Idiopathic Parkinsonism is almost invariably a unilateral disease in its early stages and when the disease is advanced it is nearly always asymmetrical. Bilateral or symmetrical extrapyramidal tract signs should raise the suspicion of a Parkinson plus syndrome.

Occasionally some patients with normal pressure hydrocephalus present in this way and these patients may even partially respond to levodopa drugs (Clough, 1987). Presentation with bradykinesia in the lower limbs but no impairment in either of the upper limbs is extremely unusual in idiopathic Parkinsonism.

DIAGNOSIS

Early diagnosis is difficult, but can be facilitated by diagnostic clinical criteria and radiological and laboratory tests.

A confident diagnosis of Parkinson's disease can be made if, in addition to bradykinesia, and in the absence of a typical features (see above), a history of encephalitis or treatment with neuroleptic drugs, one or more of the core features are present. It is arguable whether the use of more stringent diagnostic criteria such as those adopted by the United Kingdom Parkinson's Disease Society Brain Bank (Gibb and Lees, 1988) confers any additional advantage in clinical practice, as they may exclude genuine cases of Parkinson's disease and can deny them effective treatment.

The sequence in which the cardinal features of Parkinson's disease occur is often helpful in distinguishing it from other extrapyramidal disorders. Resting tremor of one hand tends to be the earliest sign of Parkinson's disease in the majority of patients and it seldom extends to other extremities in the first 2 years. The onset of tremor is usually followed by rigidity and/or bradykinesia. By contrast, the 'midline' features, i.e. disturbances of gait, speech, phonation and righting reactions, are late manifestations of the disease.

WHEN TO INVESTIGATE?

Onset at a young age, rapid disease progression, presentation with atypical symptoms or a poor response to dopaminergic drugs all suggest an extrapyramidal disorder other than Parkinson's disease. Radiological and laboratory investigations often help to discriminate.

Early onset Parkinsonism

In a large community survey (Mutch *et al.*, 1986a) the disease prevalence in those aged 40–44 years old was 12.5 per 100 000 of the population compared to an overall prevalence of 164.2. Patients presenting with extrapyramidal features before the age of 40 require a careful evaluation to exclude metabolic and other basal ganglia disorders.

Inadequate response to dopaminergic drugs

A significant response to levodopa and dopamine agonists is an essential diagnostic criterion of Parkinson's disease. An initial sustained symptomatic improvement of 70% or more of the baseline assessment with the introduction of these drugs is confirmatory. This response is not affected by disease severity or the patient's age (Diamond *et al.*, 1989), nor is it influenced by the disease duration when therapy is commenced (Markham and Diamond, 1981). The slowness and poverty of movements and muscle stiffness that occur in old age do not improve with levodopa therapy (Newman *et al.*, 1985).

The response of patients with Parkinson's disease to levodopa therapy can be predicted by measuring the motor function 90 minutes after the subcutaneous administration of a single dose of apomorphine (50 µg/kg body weight). Studies on the sensitivity and specificity of the apomorphine test (Hughes, Lees and Stern, 1990; D'Costa *et al.*, 1991; Bonuccelli *et al.*, 1993;) have shown that 95% of patients with Parkinson's disease respond to apomorphine compared to 25% of those with Parkinson plus syndromes. Severe drowsiness during the test occurs in all patients with Parkinson plus syndromes but not in those with Parkinson's disease (D'Costa *et al.*, 1991). The apomorphine test may give false negative results in a minority of patients with Parkinson's disease.

In summary, Parkinson's disease is essentially a clinical diagnosis. Investigation with MRI scans is indicated in patients presenting with symmetrical or bilateral disease and the those with early severe autonomic failure or rapid disease progression. A trial of levodopa therapy or an apomorphine test is also very helpful in these situations. When cerebrovascular disease or normal pressure hydrocephalus is suspected a computerized tomographic (CT) brain scan is the investigation of choice. Finally, the diagnosis of Wilson's disease should be considered in young patients with extrapyramidal tract signs, especially if there is a family history or other unusual signs.

DRUG TREATMENT

Initial management

At the time of diagnosis a full explanation of the nature and prognosis of the disease should be given. It is not easy to predict the time-course of deterioration in an individual patient, but patients may be encouraged by knowing that there are treatment options, and that they can exercise their judgement in the dose of medication used. Obesity should be avoided; exercise should be encouraged. An occupational therapist can advise about alternative ways of undertaking particular physical tasks, and the selection and use of physical aids and adaptations.

Patients often ask what the cause of Parkinsonism is, and whether their way of life has brought it on or will affect prognosis. They want to know if it is familial or transmittable, and whether any measures are available that will slow down the rate of deterioration. Booklets such as those published by the Parkinson's Disease Society (Franklyn, Perry and Beattie, 1982) are helpful and should be routinely available, enabling the patient to contact the Parkinson's

Disease Society if desired. Follow-up consultation after an interval of a few days ensures that the patient has a clear understanding of the condition, and should also confirm that the stress of learning the diagnosis has not been made worse by inadequate information or misunderstanding. Sometimes a nurse or other professional holds a brief for informing and counselling patients with Parkinson's disease.

Drugs available

There are five groups of drugs currently available:

- anticholinergic drugs
- levodopa preparations
- selegiline
- dopamine agonists
- amantadine.

Anticholinergic drugs

Centrally acting anticholinergic drugs such as benzhexol, benztropine and orphenadrine have been used in the treatment of Parkinson's disease for more than a century. They are believed to correct the imbalance between the cholinergic and dopaminergic neurotransmitter systems that results from dopamine depletion. Anticholinergic drugs are modestly beneficial and are used to improve tremor without having much effect on bradykinesia. In patients unable to tolerate levodopa or other dopamine agonists, anticholinergic drugs may also provide helpful reduction in rigidity and stiffness of the axial musculature. In high doses they often cause serious adverse effects, especially in elderly subjects (Table 33.1).

Levodopa

Dihydroxyphenylalanine (DOPA) is the precursor of the neurotransmitter dopamine. It is converted in substantia nigra neurones to dopamine by a pyridoxine-dependent en-

Table 33.1 The adverse effects of antiparkinsonism drugs

Drug	Adverse effects
Levodopa	Anorexia, nausea, vomiting, weight loss, postural hypotension, arrhythmias, flushing, mental confusion, hallucinations, insomnia, chorea, dystonia
Dopamine agonists	As above but greater tendency to confusion and postural hypotension
Selegiline	Potentiates effects of levodopa
Anticholinergic drugs	Dry mouth, blurring of vision, prostatism, constipation, mental confusion
Amantadine	Anorexia, nausea and vomiting, peripheral oedema, skin rashes, levido reticularis

zyme, DOPA decarboxylase (DDC). Dopamine deficiency can be corrected with the administration of the synthetic compound levodopa which is the levo-isomer of DOPA. As DDC is a ubiquitous enzyme levodopa is metabolized to dopamine in many tissues of the body. To achieve optimal concentrations in the brain, the drug must therefore be taken in large doses which result in serious cardiovascular and gastrointestinal adverse effects. However, the combination of levodopa with a peripheral DDC inhibitor, such as carbidopa (as in Sinemet) or benserazide (as in Madopar), prevents peripheral metabolism without affecting the intracerebral concentration of levodopa (DDC inhibitors do not cross the blood–brain barrier). The combined preparations also increase the turnover of dopamine in the nigrostriatal system more selectively than levodopa alone. For these reasons, the use of levodopa alone s become obsolete. The optimal ratio of levodopa to DDC inhibitor is 4:1 (as in Sinemet Plus and Madopar), a ratio of 10:1 (as in Sinemet 110) is less satisfactory. Some patients with brittle Parkinsonism may benefit from small doses of levodopa and a DDC inhibitor given separately (McLellan and Dean, 1982).

The absorption of levodopa is erratic but this has no practical significance until the later stages of the disease.

Levodopa drugs may cause a number of dose-dependent early adverse effects. With chronic use, there are often long-term complications such as peak-dose dyskinesia, peak-dose delirium and diphasic dyskinesia.

Peak-dose or persistent confusion or psychosis can occur especially in the later stages of levodopa therapy or in elderly patients. This consists of mainly visual hallucinations. This may be caused or exacerbated by anticholinergic drugs or by selegiline and these should be stopped. If the confusion is induced by levodopa itself then it should be reduced or stopped. Changing to controlled release formulation may achieve this. Treatment can then be gradually resumed after 2–4 weeks. If the patients is acutely confused, agitated and needs some sedation, benzodiazepines should be used initially, but if a neuroleptic drug is required then one of the newer agents with less extrapyramidal side-effects, such as risperidone, should be used to limit any worsening of their Parkinsonism. (Selby, 1990).

Controlled-release formulation of levodopa aim to achieve sustained plasma levodopa levels. They improve the motor 'on–off' fluctuations, increase the time 'on' and reduce the daily dosing frequency (Hutton *et al.*, 1989) but are less effective than conventional levodopa and they increase the incidence and severity of dyskinesias.

Selegiline

Selegiline, a selective monoamine oxidase (MAO) type B inhibitor, was an important milestone in the treatment of Parkinson's disease. A single daily dose of 10 mg results in almost complete and irreversible inhibition of MAO-B, though only 30% inhibition of MAO-A. The result is a high concentration of dopamine in the central nervous system without a significant increase in the levels of noradrenaline or 5-HT. However, this selectivity is lost when doses exceed 10 mg per day. There is no advantage to be gained by further increase in the dose of selegiline; because the biological half-life of the drug is 24 hours a similar length of time is required to regenerate the inhibited enzyme. Selegiline also increases the postsynaptic pool of dopamine by inhibition of its re-uptake. It does not interfere with the protective effect of MAO in the gut and, therefore, does not precipitate hypertensive crises when taken with tyramine-rich food. No serious adverse effects of selegiline have been reported.

Selegiline potentiates the action of levodopa and is a useful adjunvant to levodopa therapy. The dose of levodopa should be reduced by a third with the addition of selegiline in order to avoid dose-related adverse effects.

Selegiline has possible neuroprotective effect. It prevents the development of Parkinsonism in animals exposed to MPTP (Heikkila *et al.*, 1984) and delays the need for levodopa therapy by up to 18 months when used alone in de novo Parkinsonian patients, presumably by slowing nigrostriatal degeneration (Tetrud and Langston, 1989). There is a strong case for the use of this drug routinely in patients with early Parkinson's disease.

Dopamine agonists

The dopamine agonists in clinical use at present are bromocriptine, lisuride, pergolide, ropinirole and apomorphine (the latter for parenteral administration only). These drugs have strong affinity for both D1 and D2 receptors. By acting directly on dopaminergic postsynaptic receptors, dopamine agonists have the advantage over levodopa of not requiring dopa decarboxylase for metabolic conversion or storage in the brain (the latter enzyme is deficient in Parkinson's disease). These agents have a longer plasma half-life than levodopa, and are therefore useful in improving end-of-dose deterioration, on–off motor deficits and off-dose painful dystonias. Dopamine agonists are more effective when combined with levodopa.

The adverse effects of dopamine agonists are similar to those of levodopa (Tables 33.1 and 33.2) and occur in about 15% of patients. They are usually dose-dependent and reversible. They are uncommon if treatment is started with a small dose which is increased gradually. Dopamine agonists should be taken with or immediately after food. Hepatic disease, psychiatric disorders and severe ischaemic heart disease are contraindications to the use of these drugs.

Amantadine

Amantadine is an antiviral agent which stimulates dopamine release, blocks its re-uptake, and has a central anticholinergic effect. The therapeutic value of amantadine is small as the drug loses its efficacy in 4–8 weeks in a third of patients but in some patients a good response is sustained for up to a year. It may be used in early Parkinson's disease to delay the introduction of levodopa.

When should drug treatment start?

Drugs used for the treatment of Parkinson's disease control symptoms, improve the patient's quality of life and probably prolong life expectancy, but do not reverse the underlying pathological process. There is no point in treating signs or symptoms if the patient is not inconvenienced by them.

Table 33.2 Phenomena associated with long-term use of levodopa

Phenomena	Clinical signs
End-of-dose deterioration	Bradykinesia, rigidity and tremor 3–4 hours after each dose of levodopa. Occurs progressively earlier as the disease advances
'Freezing' episodes	Unpredictable periods of akinesia occurring for variable lengths of time
Painful dystonias	Painful limb postures, usually affecting the feet. Not associated with tremor, rigidity or bradykinesia
'On–off' motor fluctuations	Unpredictable, sudden and extreme changes in motor function
Peak dose dyskinesia	Chorea, orofacial dyskinesia or dystonia occurring 1–2 hours after administration of levodopa
Peak dose akinesia	Dysphonia and immobility 1–2 hours after the administration of levodopa. No rigidity
Peak dose delerium	Toxic confusional state correlating with high levodopa blood levels
Diphasic dyskinesia	Very rare. Characterized by involuntary movements which appear 1 hour after the administration of levodopa, disappear 1–2 hours later, and reappear when the effects of levodopa wears off

Experimental evidence also suggests that prolonged treatment with levodopa itself induces changes in synaptic function leading to poor clinical response and unpredictable fluctuations in motor function (Spina and Cohen, 1988). The introduction of levodopa should therefore be delayed for as long as possible to postpone the development of these complications.

The decision to start drug therapy should always be negotiated with the patient but it is not a good idea to wait until function is seriously compromised. Sometimes patients may deny symptoms because they do not associate certain difficulties they have experienced (like turning over in bed) with the obvious signs of the disease (such as tremor). It is useful to go through the following checklist of functions with the patient: writing, using a knife and fork, eating soup with a spoon, using a small screwdriver, rising from a chair, walking through doorway, turning over in bed at night, getting comfortable in a chair, going for a walk and speaking in company.

Having identified a goal for treatment it is essential to adjust the dose of medication until this goal is reached. Both the individual doses and the overall daily dose need to be titrated against the beneficial result and adverse effects; requirements change as the disease progresses, so that the dose should be reviewed regularly even in patients who appear stable.

Treatment strategies

Early stages of the disease

Early treatment should probably be by a non-dopamine agent. Treatment with levodopa drugs should be commenced only when Parkinsonian symptoms are causing significant functional disability. Selegiline probably has neuroprotective properties and its use alone in the early stages of the disease has also been recommended, especially for young patients. Another common treatment strategy in early Parkinsonism is to combine a small dose of levodopa with a dopamine agonist, such as pergolide. Anticholinergic drugs have also been used in this way, especially for young patients when tremor is the predominent symptom but should be avoided in elderly subject. Some physicians advocate the use of amantadine initially to postpone the introduction of levodopa, sometimes achieving a good response for up to 12 months.

Later stages of the disease

The later stages of Parkinsonism are characterized by end-of-dose deterioration and unpredictable on–off motor fluctuations. **End-of-dose deterioration** is predictable and results from disease progression. It manifests as worsening of symptoms of Parkinsonism when the effects of the drug begin to wear off, typically 2–3 hours after each dose of levodopa. End-of-dose effect is usually improved by small, frequent doses of levodopa, by the addition to the treatment regime of a dopamine agonist, a slow-release formulation of levodopa or selegiline.

The **unpredictable motor fluctuations**, i.e. periods of rigidity and severe bradykinesia alternating with mobility and dyskinesia, occur in advanced disease and are more refractory to treatment. Treatment strategies similar to those used for end-of-dose deterioration are only partly effective. A more successful strategy is to use subcutaneous apomorphine injections as a 'rescue medication'. Domperidone should be started a few days before the commencement of apomorphine to reduce the risk of adverse effects. Doses of 0.5–4 mg of apomorhine can then be given using a Penjet intermittently in anticipation of or at the onset of the off periods. More complex fluctuations are usually improved with continuous all-day subcutaneous infusion of apomorphine delivered via a small battery-operated syringe-driver pump. The pump delivers bolus doses of the drug and patients should be encouraged to use the pump's

booster function in off periods. Apomorphine infusion is usually started at a dose of 1 mg/hour and the dose is titrated to achieve an optimal clinical response. In addition to the systemic adverse effects common to other dopamine agonists, apomorphine also causes skin reactions at the site of injections such as itchy or painful subcutaneous nodules (Figure 33.1), bleeding and infection at the injection site. These skin reactions are reduced when apomorphine is diluted with normal saline e.g. 40 mg of apomorphine in 6 ml normal saline). The recommended injection sites are below the umbilicus, on the upper outer arms and the upper outer parts of the thighs. The injection site is rotated daily.

'Drug holidays' for levodopa-induced dyskinesias

Levodopa drug holidays, that is withdrawal of levodopa for a short period and its reintroduction in small doses, have been advocated for the treatment of levodopa-induced dyskinesias. It is thought that post-denervation supersensitivity of the surviving dopaminergic neurones partially compensates for the nigral depigmentation seen in Parkinson's disease. When high doses of levodopa are used, these receptors are down-regulated. Interruption of treatment should, in theory, allow desensitization of these receptors, improve the response to smaller doses of levodopa and abolish dyskinesias, but this hypothesis is not supported by experimental or clinical evidence. **Withdrawal of levodopa drugs can be dangerous** and may lead to complications of immobility including bronchopneumonia, pulmonary embolism and pressure sores. Several cases of the potentially fatal neuroleptic malignment syndrome have also been reported following sudden withdrawal of levodopa. Levodopa drug holidays are associated with a high risk of complications and are not recommended.

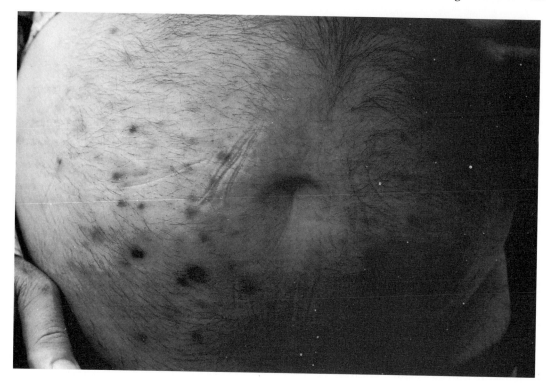

Figure 33.1 Subcutaneous nodules in a patient treated with apomorphine injections. These are usually itchy and may be painful.

Management of symptoms of autonomic failure

With advanced Parkinson's disease mild autonomic failure occurs and may require symptomatic treatment. Symptoms include postural hypotension, abnormalities of urinary bladder function, constipation, sexual impotence and excessive sweating. **Postural hypotension** is often aggravated by antiparkinsonism medication. When orthostatic hypotension is symptomatic physical measures such as the use of elastic stockings may be tried first. Sudden change of posture from supine to erect accentuates postural hypotension, especially early in mornings and after meals, and should be avoided. Domperidone (10–20 mg tds) reduces the peripheral adverse effects of levodopa and dopamine agonists, including postural hypotension. In severe cases fludrocortisone in doses of 0.1–0.2 mg is often effective and, in this dose, does not cause ankle oedema or potassium loss. Indomethacin also enhances sodium and fluid retention. Early morning postural hypotension which is refractory to the above measures usually responds to a combination of fludrocortisone and intranasal desmopressin (5–40 μ at night), especially when it is accompanied by nocturnal polyuria.

Urinary frequency, urgency and nocturia in patients with Parkinson's disease may result either from detrusor instability or sphincter dysfunction. Urodynamic studies may be helpful. The commonest abnormality is that of detrusor hyperactivity and bladder neck obstruction. Imipramine, propantheline and oxybutanin are effective but intermittent catheterization or sphincterotomy may be necessary in severe cases. In patients with detrusor hypoactivity alpha-adrenergic drugs, for example phenoxybenzamine or prazocin, are useful. Intranasal spray of desmopressin at night is sometimes prescribed for troublesome **nocturia**.

Constipation is a common complaint in patients with Parkinsonism. Increased physical activity, high fibre diet and adequate fluid intake may be sufficient in younger subjects. Bulking agents and laxatives may be needed. Cisapride, a cholinomimetic drug which increases gut motility, may cause worsening of the symptoms of Parkinsonism.

Excessive sweating usually occurs in the later stages of Parkinsonism and is frequently aggravated by levodopa-induced dyskinesias. It improves with better control of these involuntory movements and the use of betablockers.

SURGICAL TREATMENT

The value of surgery is limited, most of the procedures used are still experimental. They can be classified into functional procedures that modify the basal ganglia-transcortical reflex loops and tissue transplantation surgery which aims to restore dopaminergic neurotransmission. The established functional procedures are stereotactic thalamotomy, ventromedial pallidotomy and chronic stimulation of the ventral intermediate nucleus of the thalamus. The sources of neural cells for transplantation are the adrenal medulla and mesencephalic tissue from aborted fetuses. The results of adrenal medullary tissue transplantation are modest and transient (Olanow *et al.*, 1990l; Diamond *et al.*, 1994). This form of treatment has now been abandoned and will not be discussed further.

Stereotactic thalamotomy

Lesions in the ventrolateral nucleus of the thalamus not only abolish contralateral tremor, but also abolish or greatly reduce levodopa-induced dyskinesia. Stereotactic thalamotomy is rarely performed now because of the effectiveness of drug treatment, although it can still be valuable in a few young patients with severe unilateral drug-resistant tremor. Its beneficial effect may be short-lived. The possible complications of stereotactic thalamotomy include hemiplegia (5% risk), hemisensory loss, limb apraxia and dystonia. Bilateral thalamotomies should be avoided because of the high risk of severe speech disturbances.

Ventromedial pallidotomy

A few Parkinsonian patients with severe bradykinesia have had this procedure and the reported results were impressive (Laitinen, Bergenheim and Hariz, 1992). However, there are no long-term follow-up data of these patients.

Stimulation of the ventral intermediate thalamic nucleus

This method has been shown to be useful in patients with Parkinsonian and essential tremor (Benabid *et al.*, 1991), but the experience with this treatment is limited and no long-term follow-up results are currently available.

Fetal neural tissue transplantation

Laboratory experiments have demonstrated that dopamine-rich mesencephalic fetal cells transplanted into the caudate nucleus survive, form connections with the host brain and produce dopamine. Furthermore, this procedure restored function in rodents and monkeys rendered Parkinsonian with stereotactic chemical destruction of substantia nigra neurones. These observations have encouraged the use of neural tissue transplants in humans. To date very few patients had this operation and were studied in depth to allow full evaluation of this treatment (Lindvall *et al.*, 1992).

In summary, the help of an experienced neurosurgeon should be sought when surgery is thought to be a possible therapeutic option.

GENERAL MANAGEMENT AND THERAPIES

Many measures other than drugs can improve the quality of life in Parkinsonism (Montgomery *et al.*, 1994). The future should be discussed with the patient so that realistic plans are made, and activities that depend on full mobility are not postponed until the progression of the disease has made them impossible. The patient may need to plan for changes at work or for moving house. In Britain local placement and counselling teams (PACT) based at job centres can provide funds for equipment to the employer of a physically disabled person to help them remain at work, and it is essential to inform the patient of this possibility (Chapter 54).

Physiotherapy

Regular physical exercise should be encouraged, and obesity avoided. The role of physiotherapy in Parkinsonism is controversial (Franklyn and Stern, 1981; Perry and Das, 1981; Johnson and Pring, 1990). There is little evidence that bradykinesia can be improved by training, but there is considerable anecdotal evidence that periods of immobility (e.g. being confined to bed after a limb fracture) leave the patient significantly more impaired than before, while regular spells of exercise promote a sense of physical confidence and well-being (Doshay, 1962; Gordon and Oster, 1974; Formisano *et al.*, 1992). Physical therapy has also been credited with reduction in mortality associated with Parkinson's disease. Kuroda *et al.* (1992) have demon-

strated a lower observed to expected mortality ratio in patients who exercised regularly than in those who did not. However, the authors did not compare disease severity in the two groups and their findings could be explained by there being milder disease in the study group.

Very few objective trials have been undertaken, and they have mostly been small, technically unsatisfactory and inconclusive (Gibberd *et al.*, 1981; Robertson and Thomson, 1984). Negative trials of physiotherapy have tended to use either very crude outcome measures or refined measurements totally different from the functions that the therapy was designed to improve (Gibberd *et al.*, 1981; Formisano *et al.*, 1992). There is no convincing evidence that the specific techniques employed by physiotherapists, for example the use of predictive strategies and cuing (Homberg, 1993; Yekutiel, 1993), have a specific effect upon the type of disability that occurs in Parkinsonism, but the encouragement provided by therapists in setting goals and specifying exercises may kindle interest and enthusiasm in the patients' relatives also, which probably help to keep the patient active.

A minority of patients with Parkinsonism themselves develop mental strategies for initiating movement such as ritual preparatory movements or 'mental countdowns'. This has encouraged some therapists to employ 'rhythmic intention' introduced as one of the techniques of 'conductive education' to improve mobility in children with cerebral palsy. This approach is worthy of research, but at present there is insufficient evidence to recommend it as standard practice in the management of Parkinson's disease.

Mobility

Bradykinesia poses unique problems for mobility. Where there is difficulty turning over in bed or getting out an electrically operated cushion or 'sit-up' bed will be useful. The difficulty in rising from low chairs can be avoided by the use of firm high chairs, and electrically operated standing chairs which achieve the upright posture more gradually are well tolerated in the more severely affected subjects. Walking frames are difficult to use because a ballistic movement is required to lift and replace them; trolleys are more useful but the subjects' poor balance may allow them to run out of control. The most useful walking aid is a three-wheeled frame with two handles and a handbrake, that can also be folded for ease of transport (Chapter 48).

A technique for getting up after falling needs to be worked out for all patients whose ability to walk is becoming compromised. Many physiotherapists include this in their treatment programmes. Physiotherapy may help to improve the slowness of movement (Franklyn and Stern, 1981; Gibberd *et al.*, 1981) and reduces shuffling, leading to a more normal heel-strike toe-off gait. It is not clear whether these gains require continuous conscious effort by the patient or whether they are at a 'semi-conscious' level of awareness, leaving the subjects' mind free to think of something else.

Activities of daily living

The value of independence training as practised by occupational therapists is difficult to assess in patients with Parkinson's disease. Although in laboratory conditions the execution of everyday skilled tasks, such as doing up buttons, improved with practice (Soliveri *et al.*, 1992), it is not clear whether these gains were transfered to real-life situations. Nonetheless, the help of an occupational therapist should be enlisted to assess the nature of practical difficulties encountered by the patient and to recommend strategies such as alterations in clothing, the provision of special equipment and adaptations of the patient's home environment which may make life easier.

Significant improvements in independence and lifestyle can be achieved especially when the therapist visits the patient at home. Bathing and feeding are activities most widely helped (Beattie and Caird, 1980; Beattie, 1981). In one study of a group of severely disabled Parkinsonian patients living at home, as many as 25% needed additional equipment (Beattie and Caird, 1980). The need for equipment appears to increase over time so that routine visits every 6 months could be justified for many cases, correcting the 'gross underprovision of equipment' found by Beattie and Caird (1980), but their recommendations have not been widely adopted; 5 years later Mutch *et al.*, (1986b) reported that only a quarter of patients in the community had seen an occupational therapist.

Communication and feeding

Dysphonia, dysarthria and swallowing difficulties are common in patients with Parkinson's disease (Scott *et al.*, 1985). Speech and language therapists can teach the patient strategies to deal with the rigidity and bradykinesia which underlie the articulatory disorder and are helpful in advising on the prevention of aspiration (Chapter 22). It is also important to recognize the response which is likely to be provoked in therapists, doctors and carers by the patient's facial immobility. Pentland and collaegues (1987) showed that lack of smiling and facial movement bring forth a negative response on the part of the observer which is likely to produce an unconscious bias against the patient with Parkinson's disease, even in the absence of any depression or dementia.

Driving

Public transport is often inaccessible to people with disabilities and independence of these subjects for outdoor mobility often hinges on their ability to drive. Only 18% of patients with Parkinson's disease are able to drive (Oxtoby, 1982), and although patients with Parkinson's disease have a record of lifetime accidents similar to that of control subjects, they have more accidents per mile and the frequency of these accidents correlates with disease severity (Dubinsky *et al.*, 1991).

The disability score is a poor predicter of the driving ability of these patients and assessment of driving skills using simulators is appropriate. It has confirmed that patients with Parkinsonism commit more directional errors, have a reduced accuracy of steering and increased reaction time (Lings and Dupont, 1992). In those whose mobility is subject to frequent fluctuation it is important to time driving periods so that they fall within safe periods of mobility. Fatigue may impair driving so driving long journeys should be shared or interrupted frequently. Mental confusion, poor concentration or dementia are contraindications to driving. In some cases power-assisted brakes and steering may improve the safety record of these patients, and an automatic gearbox is an advantage but experience suggest that many patients with Parkinsonism receive inappropriate advice with respect to driving (Pentland *et al.*, 1992). There is no substitute for a road test and it is advisable that in doubtful cases patients are referred for a formal assessment (Chapter 50).

Leisure activities

The Glasgow survey of Manson and Caird (1985) showed much reduction of gardening and other social activities, patients restricting themselves to televisions, reading and sedentary pursuits. These findings are in agreement with previous reports (Singer, 1973; Oxtoby, 1982) and suggest that there may be difficulties occupying time pleasurably. Local self-help groups, such as the Parkinson's Disease Society, can offer advice and also practical help in these circumstances.

Counselling and social support

The effects of Parkison's disease on the social life of patients and their families can be profound. It is often difficult for patients to engage in activities or make social contacts outside the house because of limitations in mobility and transport; and speech disturbances may lead to problems with social relationships (Oxtoby, 1982). Counselling is an essential part of the management of Parkinson's disease. A model developed in Romford has gained the approval of patients and their carers (Pentland *et al.*, 1992). Counselling starts at diagnosis when the physician discusses the disease, treatment options and prognosis with the patient in the presence of a counsellor. Four weeks later the counsellor meets again with the patient to give further information about the disease and discuss the role of statutory and voluntary organizations in providing practical and emotional support. Any questions that the patient may have can be answered then or in counselling sessions as required.

Practical support improves mood and helps Parkinsonian patients to develop adequate coping strategies (MacCarthy and Brown, 1989; Ehmann *et al.*, 1990); Fleminger, 1991). However, although early and intensive social support is often welcomed by patients and their carers, professionals must be careful not to interfere with the patient's autonomy. Excessive reliance on professionals, instead of one's own social network, may adversely affect the patient's coping stratgies (Jahan-shahi, 1991).

THE CARER

The burden of care on the patient's spouse or companion may be heavy, particularly if the patient is suffering from dementia; the carer too is likely to be of the age at which some degree of physical disability is common. An important priority for the physician is to ensure that the carer obtains regular periods of relief from care and supervision of the patient, in order to help maintain a cordial relationship between them and to reduce the risks of serious symptoms of stress and depression in the carer. In Britain the Parkinson's Disease Society provides many patients and their families with valuable support, and similar associations or societies exist in the USA, Canada, Australia and several other countries.

REFERENCES

Beattie, A. (1981) Aids to daily living for the patient with Parkinson's disease. *British Journal of Occupational Therapy*, **44**, 53–56.

Beattie, A. and Caird, F.I. (1980) The occupational therapist and the patient with Parkinson's disease. *British Medical Journal*, **280**, 1354–1355.

Benabid, A.L., Pollak, P., Gervason, C. *et al.* (1991). Long-term suppression of tremor by chronic stimulation of the ventral intermediate thalamic nucleus. *Lancet*, **337**, 403–406.

Bonuccelli, U., Piccini, P., Del Dotto, P. *et al.* (1993) Apomorphine test for dopaminergic responsiveness: a dose assessment study. *Movement Disorders*, **8**, 158–164.

Clough, C.G. (1987) A case of normal pressure hydrocephalus presenting as levodopa-responsive Parkinsonism. *Journal of Neurology, Neurosurgery and Psychiatry*, **50**, 234.

D'Costa, D.F., Abbott, R.J., Pye, I.F. and Millac, P.A.H. (1991) The apomorphine test in Parkinsonian syndromes. *Journal of Neurology, Neurosurgery and Psychiatry*, **54**, 870–872.

Diamond, S.G., Markham, C.H., Hoehn, M.M. *et al.* (1989). Four-year follow-up of adrenal-to-brain transplants in Parkinson's disease. *Archives of Neurology*, **51**, 559–563.

Doshay, L.J. (1962) Method and value of exercise in Parkinson's disease. *New England Journal of Medicine*, **267**, 297–299.

Dubinsky, R.M., Gray, C., Husted, D. *et al.* (1991) Driving in Parkinson's disease. *Neurology*, **41**, 517–520.

Ehmann, T.S., Beninger, R.J., Gawel, M.J. and Riopellel, R.J. (1990) Coping, social support and depressive symptoms in Parkinson's disease. *Journal of Geriatric Psychiatry and Neurology*, **3**, 85–90.

Fahn, S. (1986) Parkinson's disease and other basal ganglia disorders, *Diseases of the Nervous System* (eds A.K. Asburg *et al.*), Heinemann, London, pp. 1217–1228.

Fleminger, S. (1991) Left-sided Parkinson's disease is associated with greater anxiety and depression. *Psychological Medicine*, **21**, 629–638.

Formisano, R., Pratesi, L., Modarelli, F.T. *et al.* (1992) Rehabilitation and Parkinson's disease. *Scandinavian Journal of Rehabilitation Medicine*, **24**, 157–160.

Franklyn, S. and Stern, G.M. (1981) Physiotherapy in Parkinson's disease, in *Research Progress in Parkinson's disease*, (eds Rose, C. and Capildeo, R.), Pitman Medical, London, pp. 397–400.

Franklyn, S. Perry, A. and Beattie, A. (1982) *Living with Parkinson's Disease*, Parkinson's Disease Society, London.

Gibb, W.R.G. and Lees, A.J. (1988) The relevance of the Lewy body to the pathogenesis of idiopathic Parkinson's disease. *Journal of Neurology, Neurosurgery and Psychiatry*, **51**, 745–752.

Gibberd, F.G., Page, N.G.R., Spencer, K.M. *et al.* (1981) Controlled trial of physiotherapy for Parkinson's disease. *British Medical Journal*, **282**, 1196.

Gordon, V.C. and Oster, C. (1974) Rehabilitation of the patient with Parkinson's disease. *Journal of the American Osteopathic Association*, **74**, 307–315.

Heikkila, R.E., Nauzio, L., Cabbat, F.C. and Duvoisin, R.C. (1984) Protection against dopaminergic neurotoxicity of 1-methyl-4-phenyl-1,2,3,6-tetrahydropyridine by monoamine oxidase inhibitors. *Nature*, **311**, 467–469.

Homberg, V. (1993) Motor training in the therapy of Parkinson's disease. *Neurology*, **43**, (Supple. 6), S45–S46.

Hughes, A.J., Lees, A.J. and Stern, G.M. (1990) Apomorphine test to predict dopaminergic responsiveness in Parkinsonian syndromes. *Lancet*, **336**, 24–32.

Hutton, J.T., Morris, M.A., Bush, D.F. *et al.* (1989) Multicenter controlled study of Sinement CR vs Sinemet (25/100) in advanced Parkinson's disease. *Neurology*, **39**, 67–72.

Jahanshahi, M. (1991) Psychological factors and depression in torticollis. *Journal of Psychosomatic Research*, **35**, 493–507.

Johnson, J.A. and Pring, T.R. (1990) Speech therapy in Parkinson's disease: a review and further data. *British Journal of Disorders of Communication*, **25**, 183–194.

Kurodo, K., Tatara, K., Takatorige, T. and Shinsho, F. (1992) Effect of physical exercise on mortality in patients with Parkinson's disease. *Acta Neurologica Scandinavica*, **86**, 55–59.

Laitinen, L.V., Bergenheim, A.T. and Hariz, M.I.H. (1992) Leksell's posteroventral pallidotomy in the treatment of Parkinson's disease. *Journal of Neurosurgery*, **76**, 53–61.

Lindvall, O., Winder, H., Rehnocorna, S. *et al.* (1992) Transplantation of foetal dopamine neurones in Parkinson's disease: one year clinical and neurophysiological observations in two patients with putaminal implants. *Annals of Neurology*, **31**, 155–165.

Lings, S. and Dupont, E. (!992) Driving with Parkinson's disease. A controlled laboratory investigation. *Acta Neurologica Scandinavica*, **86**, 33–39.

MacCarthy, B. and Brown, R. (1989) Psychological factors in Parkinson's disease. *Journal of Clinical Psychology*, **28**, 41–52.

Manson, C.D. and Caird, F.I. (1985) Survey of the hobbies and transport of patients with Parkinson's disease. *British Journal of Occupational Therapy*, **48**, 199–200.

Markham, C.H. and Diamond, S.G. (1981) Evidence to support early levodopa therapy in Parkinson's disease. *Neurology*, **31**, 125–131.

Marsden, C.D. (1984) Motor disorders in basal ganglia disease. *Human Neurobiology*, **2**, 245–250.

Mayeux, R. (1981) Depression and dementia in Parkinson's disease, in *Movement Disorders* (eds C.D. Marsden and S. Fahn) Butterworths, London, pp. 75–95.

McLellan, D.L. and Dean, B. (1982) Improved control of brittle Parkinsonism by separate administration of levodopa and benserazide. *British Medical Journal*, **284**, 1001–1002.

Montgomery, Jr. E.B., Liberman, A., Singh, G. and Fries, J.F. (1994) Patient education and health promotion can be effective in Parkinson's disease: a randomised controlled trial. PROPATH Advisory Board. *American Journal of Medicine*, **97**, 429–435.

Mutch, W.J., Dingwall-Fordyce, I., Downie, A.W. *et al.* (1986a) Parkinson's disease in a Scottish city. *British Medical Journal*, **292**, 534–536.

Mutch, W.J., Strudwick, A., Roy, S.K. and Downie, A.W. (1986b) Parkinson's disease: disability, review and management. *British Medical Journal*, **213**, 675–677.

Nausieda, P.A., Weiner, W.J. and Klawans, H.L. (1980) Dystonic foot response of Parkinsonism. *Archives of Neurology*, **37**, 132–136.

Newman, R.P., LeWitt, P.A., Jaffe, M. *et al.* (1985) Motor function in the normal aging population: treatment with levodopa. *Neurology*, **35**, 571–573.

Olanow, C.W., Koller, W., Goetz C.G. *et al.* (1990) Autologous transplantation of adrenal medulla in Parkinson's disease. 18-months results. *Archives of Neurology*, **47**, 1286–1289.

Oxtoby, M. (1982) *Parkinson's Disease Patients and their Social Needs*, Parkinson's Disease Society, London.

Parkinson, J. (1817) *An Essay on the Shaking Palsy*, Sherwood, Nelly & Jones, London.

Pentland, B., Barnes, MP., Findley, L.J. *et al.* (1992) Parkinson's disease: the spectrum of disability. *Journal of Neurology, Neurosurgery and Psychiatry*, **55**, 32–35.

Pentland, B., Pitcairn, T.K., Gray, J.M. and Riddle, W.J.R. (1987) First Impressions of Parkinson's Disease Patients. Paper presented at the meeting of the Society for Research in Rehabilitation, 1987.

Perry, A.R. and Das, P.K. (1981) Speech assessment of patients with Parkinson's disease, in *Research Progress in Parkinson's Disease* (eds F. Clifford Rose and R. Capiledo), Pitman Medical, London, 1981, pp. 373–383.

Robbins, J.A., Logemann, J.A. and Kirshner, H.S. (1986) Swallowing and speech production in Parkinson's disease. *Annals of Neurology*, **19**, 283–287.

Robertson, S.J. and Thomson, F. (1984) Speech therapy in Parkinson's disease: a study of the efficacy and long-term effects of intensive treatment. *British Journal of Disorders of Communication*, **19**, 213–224.

Scott, S., Caird, F.I. and Williams, B.O. (1985) *Communication in Parkinson's Disease*, Croom Helm, Beckenham.

Selby, G. (ed.) (1990) Neuropsychiatric changes in Parkinson's disease, in *Parkinson's Disease*, Chapman & Hall, London.

Signer, E. (1973) Social costs of Parkinson's disease. *Journal of Chronic Disorders* **2**, 243–254.

Soliveri, P., Brown, R.G., Jahanshahi, M. and Marsden, C.D. (1992) Effect of practice on performance of a skilled motor task in patients with Parkinson's disease. *Journal of Neurology, Neurosurgery and Psychiatry*, **55**, 454–460.

Spina, M.B. and Cohen, G. (1988) Exposure of striatal synaptosomes to L-dopa increases levels of oxidized glutathione. *Journal of Pharmacology and Experimental Therapeutics*, **247**, 502–507.

Stern, M.B., Braffman, B.H., Skolnick, B.E. *et al.* (1989) Magnetic resonance imaging in Parkinson's disease and parkinsonian syndromes. *Neurology*, **39**, 1524–1526.

Sutcliffe, R.L., Prior, R., Mawby, B. and McQuillan, W.J. (1985) Parkinson's disease in the district of the Northampton Health Authority, UK. A study of the prevalence and disability. *Acta Neurologica Scandinavica*, **72**, 363–379.

Tetrud, J.W. and Langston, J.W. (1989) The effect of deprenyl (selegiline) on the natural history of Parkinson's disease. *Science*, **245**, 519–522.

Yekutiel, M.P. Patient's full records as an aid in designing and assessing therapy in Parkinson's disease. *Disability and Rehabilitation*, **15**, 189–193.

USEFUL ADDRESS

The Parkinson's Disease Society,
22 Upper Woburn Place, London WC1H 0RA,
UK Tel: 0171 383 3513

PART SIX
COMMON MEDICAL PROBLEMS

34 *The management of spasticity*

B. Bhakta and J.A. Cozens

DEFINITION

Spasticity is a form of pathological muscle tone, identified clinically as resistance to passive muscle stretch that increases with the velocity of stretch. It has been formally defined as 'a motor disorder characterised by velocity dependent increase in tonic stretch reflexes with exaggerated tendon jerks, resulting from hyperexcitability of the stretch reflex' (Young, 1994). It is one component of the upper motor neurone syndrome. The velocity dependence in particular distinguishes spasticity from **extrapyramidal rigidity**. Other clinically relevant features of spasticity are clonus, exaggerated cutaneous reflexes (nocioceptive and flexor withdrawal reflexes), autonomic hyperreflexia, dystonic posture and contracture. In severe spasticity, the muscles may be very stiff throughout the range of movement. In this situation the term **spastic dystonia** is used. Spasticity, paresis, lack of dexterity and fatiguability constitute the upper motor neurone syndrome.

Traditionally spasticity is assessed with the patient resting, but this may not be representative of tone present during voluntary movement. This is important, since the functional significance of spasticity is often more relevant in the context of voluntary movement.

CLINICAL SYNDROMES

Cerebral spasticity

The cerebral cortex and basal ganglia modulate muscle tone. It is not known, however, which descending tracts must be damaged in order to cause spasticity. Lesions restricted to corticospinal tracts (as in patients with pure motor hemiplegia caused by damage to the medullary pyramids) cause muscle weakness, loss of dexterity and a Babinski response without spasticity. Conversely, lesions of the parasagittal regions can cause severe spastic paraparesis. The pattern and extent of spasticity are not only dependent on the site of the lesion but also on concurrent damage to the extrapyramidal tracts (medullary reticulospinal, rubrospinal and vestibulospinal fibres). Stroke affecting the motor cortex or the internal capsule commonly produces initial hypotonia and absent tendon jerks, followed several days or weeks later by spastic hypertonia in the antigravity muscles. The upper limb adopts an adducted posture at the shoulder and a flexed posture at the elbow and wrist, with the fingers flexed into the palm. In the lower limb there is hip and knee extension, with plantarflexion at the ankle. The appearance of spasticity immediately after stroke is unusual but may occur following basal ganglia haemorrhage (Steiner *et al*, 1985).

Rehabilitation of the Physically Disabled Adult. Edited by C. John Goodwill, M. Anne Chamberlain and Chris Evans. Published in 1997 by Stanley Thornes (Publishers) Ltd, Cheltenham. ISBN 0-7487-3183-0.

Spinal spasticity

Following spinal cord injury rostral to the conus medullaris, initial hypotonia (part of the syndrome of spinal shock) is gradually replaced by spastic hypertonia. However, the pattern of spasticity differs from that seen in cerebral disease. Labile flexor reflexes are seen in the lower limbs, often causing the hips and knees to become flexed and adducted. Extensor spasticity tends to replace flexor spasticity in the lower limbs after about 6 months. However, the exact pattern of spasticity in the limbs is determined by the level and extent of injury (anterior cord syndrome, central cord syndrome, complete spinal injury). In general, patients with incomplete spinal lesions have more spasticity and associated muscle spasms than patients with complete spinal cord injury. Cervical cord injury can result in severe bilateral upper limb spasticity with adduction, flexion and internal rotation of both shoulders, flexion of the elbows and flexion and pronation of the wrists.

PATHOPHYSIOLOGY

Neurophysiology/neurochemistry

The tension developed in a non-contracting muscle when passively stretched is dependent on the reflex muscle contraction and inherent viscoelasticity of the contractile elements and the tendons and connective tissue within muscles. Initially after cerebral or spinal damage, tonal abnormalities arise through release of intact segmental reflexes from higher motor control. Subsequently, secondary changes in the viscoelastic properties become important in maintaining tension in patients with longstanding spastic hypertonia.

Of the neural circuits involved in spastic hypertonia, the segmental myotatic reflex is the most important. This circuit is best known for its monosynaptic connections between primary afferent (Ia) fibres from muscle spindles and the alpha–moto neurone pool. However, most of the activity contributing to spasticity is mediated via polysynaptic pathways involving afferents from secondary spindle endings, cutaneous receptors and golgi tendon organs. Overactivity of the myotatic reflex in spasticity appears to be a central phenomenon, causing exaggerated reflex response to normal afferent input.

Several mechanisms appear to contribute to the exaggerated excitability of the myotatic reflex in spasticity. The best documented are reductions in the inhibitory mechanisms that normally regulate the myotatic reflex. These mechanisms are dependent upon descending pyramidal and extrapyramidal control (via vestibulospinal, reticulospinal and rubrospinal tracts) and therefore operate less effectively when it is disrupted. In particular, reduced effectiveness of presynaptic inhibition (mediated by gamma amino butyric acid (GABA)) and reciprocal Ia inhibition (mediated via glycine) have been demonstrated in man. Presynaptic inhibition modulates the reflex effects of spindle afferents from the same muscle; group Ia reciprocal inhibition is elicited by spindle afferents of antagonist muscles. Reciprocal Ia inhibition prevents co-contraction of antagonist muscles. Following stroke, inappropriate co-contraction may arise through reduced reciprocal Ia inhibition; this may reduce the effectiveness of voluntary movement.

Exaggerated excitability of the myotatic reflex may also arise through changes in intrinsic electrical properties of alpha-neuronal cell body membranes. For example, serotonin and substance P can change the properties of voltage-dependent ionic channels in the neuronal cell membrane. The intraspinal release of these substances is known to be controlled by descending brainstem pathways, raising the possibility of involvement in spasticity.

Cutaneous and nociceptive afferents converge on interneurones that, in turn, can excite alpha-motorneurones. Spinal or supraspinal damage may disrupt control of these interneurons, allowing cutaneous stimuli (particularly if noxious) to facilitate the myotatic reflex. This is seen clinically when spasticity is provoked by discomfort, for example through rough handling or from joint problems. There is considerable overlap between neurotransmitters involved in pain modulation and those involved in motor control (inhibition via GABA acting on GABA$_A$ and GABA$_B$ receptors; excitation via glutamate acting on NMDA (N-methyl-D-aspartate) receptors). This suggests that nociceptive neuronal circuits and motor pathways have considerable influence on each other, emphasizing the clinical importance of pain management in the prevention and treatment of spasticity.

Musculoskeletal sequelae

Spastic hypertonia may cause contractures as a result of prolonged limb immobility. Contractures are characterized by an increase in stiffness and shortening of joint and muscle connective tissue, thereby preventing a full range of passive joint movement even under anaesthesia. Associated heterotopic calcification in the tendons and joint ligaments may result in pain and persistence of limb contracture, despite standard antispastic treatment. Direct pathological studies of spastic contractures are few. Contracture formation has been mainly examined in animal models (where splintage is used to immobilize limbs) and human autopsy specimens from patients who have had therapeutic immobilization of joints. In these studies, there is evidence of fibrofatty connective tissue proliferation and adhesion formation obliterating the joint synovial space and causing joint cartilage damage. There is reduction in water content, collagen and matrix proteoglycans in the joint connective tissue following immobilization. Prolonged immobility in patients with long-standing spasticity may cause muscle fibre atrophy as a result of disuse.

MEASUREMENT OF SPASTICITY

The characteristics of spastic hypertonia during passive and active movement are complex. Measuring the phenomenon is therefore difficult. Spasticity measurement may be clinical, or involve biomechanical and electrophysiological techniques. Ideally any measurement technique should be applicable in routine clinical practice; at present, only the clinical scales described below are used routinely, whereas current biomechanical and electrophysiological measurements are confined to research.

Clinical scales

Clinical scales may be categorized into those assessing spasticity itself and those measuring its functional consequences. The former includes the Ashworth Scale (Bohannon and Smith, 1987). The modified Ashworth Scale is a 5-point rating that quantifies spasticity in terms of the resistance felt to passive stretching of the relaxed muscle. Inevitably, any clinical assessment is not only subject to inter- and intra-observer variability, but may also vary with the muscle tested and the disease process. The Ashworth scale has been shown to have good reliability in assessing the spasticity of muscles acting at the elbow and ankle joints. This assessment may also be supplemented by grading the frequency of muscle spasms in the affected limbs. The Ashworth scale is easy to administer and is therefore employed widely.

Spasticity may also be described in terms of associated reactions. Associated reactions are involuntary movements of affected body parts elicited by voluntary movement elsewhere in the body. These involuntary movements become more pronounced as muscle tone increases. In stroke patients, when the unaffected arm is flexed against resistance, the hemiplegic arm may flex involuntarily at the elbow. It is though that associated reactions only occur in the presence of spasticity. They may be described in terms of changes in limb or body posture but are not easily quantifiable.

Assessing the functional consequences provides an indirect method of measuring spasticity; for example, global measures of function such as the Barthel Index are widely used. Functional grading may also be applied to more specific tasks, such as the ease of perineal hygiene or ability to walk.

Biomechanical measurements

The simplest of the biomechanical assessments is the pendulum test. Use of this measurement is confined to the muscles acting at the knee joint. Damping of the passive oscillation of the lower limb under gravity is used as an index of stiffness in the flexors and extensors of the knee. Although easy to implement, this measure is modelled upon the assumption that the passively oscillating knee is a simple system of springs and masses. Its value as a measure of spasticitiy is limited because it does not take into account the variation in muscle excitation and length. A more detailed analysis of the resistance felt during passive muscle stretch can be obtained by measuring the amount of force required to move the limb at a specified angular velocity over a range of joint angles (Katz and Zev Rymer, 1989). Simultaneous surface electromyography from the agonist and antagonist provides information about timing of muscle activation. These measurements require laboratory equipment and are therefore usually confined to research.

Electrophysiological measurements

Electrophysiological assessments aim to (1) explore the segmental reflex arc and associated neuronal circuits and (2) the timing and amount of electrical muscle activity during passive or voluntary limb movements.

A variety of electrophysiological investigations (Davidoff, 1992) may be used to quantify the neural abnormalities associated with spasticity; for example, by comparison of H and M reflexes. These, however, do not measure the disordered tone itself. The H reflex is the electrophysiological equivalent of the tendon reflex and is usually elicited by a submaximal stimulus to the afferent nerve in the monosynaptic arc and recording the response in the effector muscle (e.g. stimulating the tibial nerve and recording over the soleus muscle). The M response is the compound action potential measured in a muscle when the corresponding efferent nerve has been maximally stimulated. Increase in the ratio of the H reflex to the M response has been found in spastic hemiplegia, but unfortunately this ratio neither correlates with treatment effect nor the clinical assessment of spasticity. There is evidence that the failure to suppress the H reflex following tonic vibratory stimulation relates to reduced presynaptic inhibition. Although these measurements may add to the understanding of spasticity, they have a limited role in the routine assessment of spasticity, because of wide variation between individuals and lack of correlation with clinical assessment.

During voluntary movement the distinction between spasticity and inappropriate or unwanted muscle activity becomes blurred as both the timing and amount of muscle activity are important for effective movement. Surface electromyography allows timing of muscle activation to be measured while voluntary movements are performed. Inappropriate antagonist activity that hinders smooth movement may arise from either reduction in reciprocal inhibition at the spinal level or altered supraspinal drive. At the elbow this may be manifest by inappropriate coactivation of both biceps and triceps muscles during elbow flexion and extension, with loss of the normal phasic activation of biceps and triceps. During walking this may be manifest by unwanted coactivation of knee flexors and extensors during the swing phase of gait.

In the future, a combination of biomechanical and electromyographic measurements (gait analysis, treadmill analysis and arm trajectory analysis) may define the role of spastic hypertonia in abnormal voluntary movement

CONSEQUENCES OF SPASTICITY

Although paresis, fatiguability and loss of motor control are the main causes of functional disturbance after upper motor neurone damage, spasticity often contributes significantly.

In patients with no voluntary limb movement, spasticity and subsequent contracture formation can cause considerable disability. In the arm, severe spasticity may interfere with hand hygiene and dressing. In the lower limbs, spasticity around the hips and knees may cause difficulty with wheelchair seating and transferring, as well as popliteal fossa and groin hygiene. In severe cases the heel may be in contact with the buttock, with the risk of pressure sores developing. Hip adductor spasticity, particularly if bilateral, can cause difficulty with perineal hygiene, catheter care and sexual activity. An exaggerated reflex response to cutaneous stimuli may result in painful flexor or extensor spasms. This causes difficulty with seating, transferring, and sleep disturbance. These problems are commonly encountered in patients with severe multiple sclerosis or following spinal injury.

In patients with voluntary limb movement, spasticity may prevent useful limb activity, for example inappropriate coactivation of both agonist (triceps) and antagonist (biceps) muscles can impede reaching movements. In the lower limb dynamic equinus deformity of the ankle restricts toe clearance during the swing phase of walking: patients may fall as a result of their toe catching on uneven surfaces (e.g. carpets). Also in the lower limb, hip adductor spasticity may cause difficulty with weightbearing and walking because of scissoring of the affected limb.

Spasticity can be reinforced by voluntary movement of another part of the body. In the clinical assessment of spasticity, tendon reflexes can be augmented by deliberate reinforcement (Jendrassik manoeuvre). Physiotherapists observe this phenomenon as a form of associated reaction. Certain functional activities increase these associated reactions. In particular, self-propelling a wheelchair can increase spasticity in some patients (Cornall, 1991).

Not all the consequences of spasticity are negative. Following stroke, hip and knee extensor spasticity may allow weightbearing with the affected limb acting like a splint. Pain in some patients can be an important consequence of spasticity. Articular and periarticular pain are due partly to the abnormal resting position and immobility of the joint and partly to adjacent muscle spasticity causing spasm. The importance of pain as a factor that can increase spasticity and thus affect function should not be underestimated. The interaction of nociceptive pathways and segmental reflexes has been discussed.

MANAGEMENT

The management of spasticity can be broadly divided into strategies to discourage the development of spasticity and treatments to manage established spasticity and prevent its complications (e.g. contractures). Factors promoting spasticity include pain and poor posture.

Prevention

Pain may result from intercurrent disorders such as urinary tract abnormalities (infections, retention of urine, renal calculi), constipation, soft tissue rheumatism (shoulder capsulitis, contracture, ligamentous injury, myositis ossificans), pressure sores and deep venous thrombosis. Pain may also result as a direct consequence of the neurological insult in terms of abnormal perception to normal cutaneous sensation (e.g. 'poststroke pain syndrome'). Nociceptive stimuli are well recognized as potent promoters of spasticity and consequently attention to pain management and prompt treatment of intercurrent illness is of paramount importance. In addition, bladder filling and voiding can have a direct effect on spasticity by increasing segmental stretch reflex activity (Mai and Pederson, 1991).

Positive influences on spasticity via attention to careful positioning of the patient from the earliest stage of rehabilitation can reduce spasticity (Carr and Kenney, 1992). Therapeutic positioning of the patient aims to manipulate primitive reflexes (e.g. tonic neck reflexes and labyrinthine reflexes) released from higher motor control. After stroke, patients are encouraged to adopt a 'reflex inhibiting' posture. While lying on the affected side, the head is held in a symmetrical position, the shoulder flexed and protracted, elbow extended, wrist in neutral, fingers extended, trunk straight and knee flexed. In sitting, the midline position of the head, neck and trunk should ideally be maintained, with the shoulder protracted, wrist pronated, fingers extended, hips and knees flexed to 90° with the body weight equally distributed between both hips with the feet flat on floor. There is some controversy about the type of shoulder positioning needed to counteract the tendency for adduction and internal rotation due to shoulder girdle spasticity. Abduction and external rotation of the shoulder has been advocated. After spinal cord injury, positioning of the patient using a tilt table has also been shown to reduce spasticity (Bohannon, 1993).

Treatment of established spasticity

The effective management of spasticity requires a multidisciplinary approach both for assessment and treatment and must be appropriate to concurrent motor and perceptual impairments. The presence of spasticity in itself is not a reason for treatment, rather its functional implications must be defined and appropriate treatment goals planned. The treatment of established spasticity first depends on effective treatment of the factors mentioned above. The aims of treatment are to improve function, reduce direct and indirect consequences such as contracture formation and pressure sores, respectively, and to alleviate pain.

Specific treatments for spasticity

Physical treatment

Physiotherapy is felt to be effective in improving control of movement mainly through the treatment of spasticity, although specific evidence for this is scarce (Corriveau *et al*, 1992). There are several physical techniques used to improve motor control during rehabilitation. There is little evidence showing significant advantage in terms of functional outcome of using any particular approach (Brunnstrom, 1970; Bobath, 1990). However, the different methods influence spasticity to varying degrees, some even exacerbating muscle hypertonia.

The Bobath approach advocates techniques to reduce spasticity and primitive postural reflexes prior to facilitating voluntary movement of paretic muscles. Attention to trunk posture is emphasized, not only if walking is to be regained but also to optimize upper limb function. In the upper limb, muscles are slowly stretched in a proximal to distal progression, beginning with outward rotation and abduction of the shoulder then extension of the elbow, wrist, fingers and abduction of the thumb. There is some evidence that this approach reduces segmental reflex hyperexcitability. Distal limb spasticity often reduces as slow proximal muscle stretch is performed. This is believed to occur through inhibition of distal segmental reflexes via Ib inhibitory interneurones.

The Brunnstrom approach advocates techniques to promote flexor and extensor synergistic movements, in conjunction with manipulation of the postural reflexes mentioned above. Activity in weak agonists is encouraged by maximal stimulation of corresponding muscles in the unaffected limb or proximal weak muscles on the paretic side. This technique focuses on individual muscle groups with the underlying concept that stimulation of the weak agonist muscle will result in Ia-mediated reciprocal inhibition in the spastic antagonist muscle. Unfortunately, reduction in Ia reciprocal inhibition often accompanies spastic hypertonia, and therefore this avenue of reflex suppression may not be available. It would appear that this technique is more suited to flaccid muscles rather than reducing spasticity, as the techniques involved promote associated reactions (Brunnstrom, 1956).

Other techniques as suggested by Rood can be used to reduce spasticity (Stockmeyer, 1967). This treatment uses manipulation of the somatosensory system to influence neck, trunk and limb muscle activity. Sensory stimulation is applied using heat, cold and brushing the skin.

Contracture prevention and treatment also require manipulation of limbs through the full range of movement. It is recommended that this should be performed for 2 hours during a 24-hour period. There is however no evidence as to the frequency of repeated movement required to prevent contractures.

Local cooling of affected muscles can reduce spasticity (Price *et al*, 1993). Cooling is applied by placing ice packs on the spastic muscles for 15–20 minutes. There is rapid reduction of skin temperature to approximately 20°C. There is a rapid reduction in segmental reflex excitability, probably related to a fall in skin receptor sensitivity. There is evidence to suggest that subsequent intramuscular cooling depresses muscle spindle sensitivity, further reducing segmental reflex excitability. Patients most likely to benefit from muscle cooling are those with voluntary limb movement hampered by spasticity, rather than those with a completely paralysed spastic limb. Although reductions in spasticity are often short lived with local cooling alone, cooling spastic antagonist muscles can facilitate treatment of weak agonists. Repeated cooling treatments in conjunction with other physiotherapy may produce long-term beneficial effects.

Orthoses offer another avenue of physical treatment. Orthotic management of spasticity aims to accommodate and reduce the musculoskeletal consequences of limb spasticity or manage limb posture during physiotherapy. Splintage of limbs in a functional position can reduce disability regardless of spasticity. Concern has been expressed that splintage may increase spasticity, however there is no evidence that this occurs. Indeed some orthoses, as developed by Snook, are designed to reduce spasticity (Snook, 1979). The use of wrist splintage may reduce the amount of permanent finger and wrist flexion contracture of the forearm finger flexor muscles. Similarly, an ankle–foot orthosis may be used to correct spastic equinovarus deformity during the swing phase of walking. Serial plaster casts can be used to treat established contractures, particularly at the knee and elbow. Use of orthoses requires close collaboration between the medical staff, physiotherapist, occupational therapist and orthotist. Inflatable pressure splintage has been advocated by Johnstone as an adjunct during physiotherapy (Johnstone, 1989). The aim is to reduce unwanted muscle tone and provide adequate limb stability for early weight-bearing exercises both in the upper and lower limbs. This treatment is undertaken in conjunction with the neurodevelopmental techniques suggested by Bobath.

Drug treatment

Pharmacological manipulation of spasticity can be undertaken systemically, regionally or locally. Systemic treatments include baclofen, dantrolene, diazepam, tizanidine and clonidine (Young and Delwaide, 1981a, b). Regional treatments include intrathecal phenol and intrathecal baclofen. Local treatments consist of either nerve or motor point blocks with alcohol/phenol or intramuscular botulinum toxin.

Baclofen selectively activates presynaptic and postsynaptic GABA receptors in the spinal cord. Activation of presynaptic receptors decreases calcium conductance, thereby reducing the amount of excitatory amino acids released by the afferent fibre terminals. Postsynaptically, baclofen causes an increase in K^+ conductance producing slow inbibitory postsynaptic potentials. Both these mechanisms depress segmental reflex excitability thus reducing spasticity particularly following spinal cord injury. In addition to its antispastic action, oral baclofen also has an antinociceptive action particularly on episodic pain rather persistent pain (Fromm, 1994). This dual action is likely to benefit patients who have both pain and spasticity (e.g. spinal cord injury or multiple sclerosis patients with painful limb muscle spasm). A potential problem with any systemic treatment is its effect on muscles with normal tone as well as muscles that are spastic. The resulting unwanted muscle weakness may affect function (e.g. ability to transfer or stand). **The dosage of baclofen must be increased slowly**. Baclofen is rapidly and almost completely absorbed after oral administration (up to $100\,mg\,day^{-1}$ in divided dosage), with peak serum concentration occurring in about 2 hours. It is excreted unchanged mainly by the kidney. Dizziness, fatigue or sedation, and occasionally nausea, depression, hallucinations or seizures, may occur in high doses or when dose is not increased slowly. **Withdrawal of baclofen must be done gradually,** as abrupt dicontinuation after prolonged use may cause psychosis and seizures. Attention to concurrent medication is also important. Newer non-tricyclic antidepressants, such as fluoxetine acting via $GABA_B$ receptors, may antagonize the antispastic effect on baclofen.

Dantrolene acts directly on the muscle by reducing Ca^{++} release from the endoplasmic reticulum in response to stimulation of the muscle membrane. This reduces skeletal muscle fibre contraction in response to alpha-motorneurone activity. Dantrolene is effective in all types of spasticity. Unfortunately, however, it has a non-selective action, acting on normal as well as spastic muscles. Its use may be limited by liver toxicity, diarrhoea, and sedation. Fatal hepatic injury may occur rarely and therefore it is paramount that liver function is monitored during treatment.

Diazepam has an antispastic effect which is thought to be mediated by facilitation of the presynaptic inhibitory effect of GABA on the Ia afferent terminals. Diazepam is most effective in incomplete spinal cord lesions and has little effect on muscle spasticity caused by supraspinal lesions. Its use is limited by central effects, particularly sedation, ataxia and fatigue. There is a risk of dependence. As with baclofen, abrupt cessation of long-standing treatment with diazepam may cause depression and seizures.

Tizanidine is an alpha$_2$ adrenergic receptor agonist (Delwaide and Pennisi, 1994). Its antispastic effects occur at both the spinal and supraspinal levels. The mechanism of action is thought to be related to reduction in firing rate of the adrenergic neurones in the locus ceruleus and stimulation of inhibitory spinal interneurones normally under reticulospinal descending control. Like baclofen, tizanidine also appears to have an independent antinociceptive effect which would have obvious theoretical benefits for patients with painful muscle spasms. Clinical studies using doses between 12 and 36 mg/day in divided doses demonstrate that the antispastic effect of tizanidine is comparable to baclofen and superior to diazepam. Tizanidine appears to be better tolerated: the most frequent adverse effects are fatigue, sedation and dry mouth. It is suggested that unwanted muscle weakness is also less common with tizandine than baclofen.

Clonidine is another alpha$_2$ adrenergic receptor agonist, with similar antispastic and antinociceptive action to tizanidine (Yablon and Sipski, 1993). Unfortunately the use of clonidine is limited because of its hypotensive effects. Other antispastic drugs such as NMDA antagonists. L-threonine (gylcine precursor) and progabide (GABA agonist) remain experimental.

INTRATHECAL ADMINISTRATION

Administration of antispastic agents directly into the cerebrospinal fluid is based on the rationale that drugs delivered to the site of action are likely to be more effective at lower doses, thus reducing the risk of adverse effects. Initially intrathecal morphine used for pain control was found to reduce lower limb tone. This highlights the close association between pain and segmental reflexes. Currently both phenol and baclofen are administered intrathecally.

Intrathecal phenol

Intrathecal phenol can also be effective in reducing severe lower limb spasticity and painful muscle spasms, particularly when nursing care and seating is affected. The treatment causes chemical neurolysis to both the sensory and motor components of the spinal nerve roots. This treatment is reserved for patients with no voluntary bladder or bowel control, no functionally useful voluntary movement, loss of sensation and, where standard antispastic treatments have failed, 2–4 ml of 5% phenol is administered intrathecally throughout a lumbar puncture at L3/L4 level. Phenol is viscous at room temperature

and the vial must be warmed prior to injection. Positioning of the patient is critical. The patient is positioned lying on their side with the lumbar spine the most dependent part of the axial skeleton, with the head, chest and pelvis highest. This position is used to prevent intrathecal phenol from migrating rostrally after injection and thus reducing the risk of unwanted damage to the cervical and thoracic spinal roots. The patient should be maintained in this position for at least 2 hours. The antispastic effect usually develops between 1 and 2 days and can last for several months. This treatment is inexpensive and easy to administer. However its use is limited in all but the most severely affected patients by potential adverse effects, including painful dysaesthesia and loss of sensation in the limbs, loss of bowel and bladder control.

Intrathecal baclofen

This can certainly be very effective where physical treatment and oral medication have failed to control lower limb spasticity and painful muscle spasms (McLean, 1993). Intrathecal baclofen also improves bladder function in terms of increased bladder capacity and reduced residual volume (Ochs, 1993). This treatment is more effective in spinal causes of spasticity than supraspinal causes. It is important to stop oral antispastic medication prior to administering intrathecal baclofen.

All patients require a trial of intrathecal baclofen (25–50 μg) which is given via an indwelling intrathecal catheter usually inserted at L3/L4 level. If an effect occurs it has a rapid onset and is maintained for 6–8 hours. The bolus can be titrated until an effective dose is reached. Signs of overdosage must be monitored. Adverse effects include hypotension, clouding of consciousness, progressive arm weakness and respiratory arrest. The daily dose required is usually about one to two times the effective bolus dose.

The continuous intrathecal delivery of the

baclofen is achieved with a pump that is surgically implanted over the chest or abdominal wall. There are two types of pump available. The manually controlled pump depends on the patient, who delivers boluses of baclofen intrathecally. The electronic pump allows continuous delivery of baclofen to the patient. The dosage injected per day can be altered electronically. The reservoir in both pumps needs to be filled every 4–5 weeks by transcutaneous injection into the reservoir port. The main advantages of the electronic pump compared to the manual pump are:

1. larger baclofen reservoir;
2. continuous infusion;
3. control of delivery independent of the patient;
4. it can be sited over the abdominal wall, which is often more comfortable.

The manual pump is usually sited over the chest so that the ribs can support the pump when pressure is applied to deliver the bolus. Problems may arise later, particularly if there is subsequent loss of subcutaneous tissue. For both systems during the first weeks after implantation it is important that the baclofen dosage is increased slowly and adverse effects are carefully monitored.

The surgical complications (local sepsis, wound erosion, haematoma, meningitis) are low if the procedure is carried out by experienced personnel. Mechanical complications such as catheter displacement as well as medical complications such as deep venous thrombosis may occur.

Intrathecal baclofen has considerable advantages over intrathecal phenol. In particular, sensation is not affected, the dose may be easily regulated to the patient's needs and bladder function in some patients may be improved. The disadvantages of intrathecal baclofen include the need for a delivery system, the risks of surgical procedures and the potential life-threatening complications. Use of intrathecal baclofen may also be limited because of the cost of pump implantation, although the baclofen solution itself is inexpensive.

Local blocks

Local drug treatment aims to reduce spasticity in individual muscles, or a group of muscles innervated by a single peripheral nerve. It comprises either percutaneous nerve and/or motor point blocks using phenol or alcohol, or intramuscular botulinum toxin. Phenol and alcohol are non-selective treatments in that they can affect both motor and sensory nerve fibres. Botulinum toxin affects only the motor nerve fibres.

Percutaneous phenol nerve blocks

These have been used in both upper and lower limb spasticity successfully (Copp and Keenan, 1972). In the lower limbs, nerves treated include the posterior tibial nerve (to reduce equinovarus deformity), both branches of the obturator nerve (to improve perineal hygiene and gait by reducing hip adductor spasticity) and the sciatic nerve (to relieve hamstring spasticity) (Petrillo and Knoploch, 1988). This treatment requires electromyography to localize the nerve to be treated. The approximate position of the nerve innervating the spastic muscles is identified using a surface stimulator and the overlying skin is anaesthetized. A Teflon-insulated needle which allows nerve stimulation at the tip as well as injection of phenol is inserted at this site. The nerve is stimulated through an insulated Teflon-coated needle. The needle position and stimulating current are adjusted until maximum muscle contraction is seen with minimal stimulation. The phenol is injected through this needle, ensuring that no blood vessels have been punctured. The quantity of phenol used varies between 1 and 6 ml of 3–6% phenol diluted in water. There is usually some immediate relaxation of target muscles, with the full effect occurring over 3–4 days. A long-acting anaesthetic may be injected first, if there is concern about the likely antispastic effects of phenol, for example when there is voluntary activity in the target muscles. Obviously this should not be performed immediately prior to the phenol treatment as the site of phenol injection will not be identifiable.

Occasionally painful dysaethesia may occur through damage of the sensory fibres by phenol. This can be a particular problem when the median and ulnar nerves are treated. Rarely vascular damage such as arterial occlusion can occur in adjacent blood vessels. Motor point blocks have been used to reduce the incidence of sensory disturbance. The technique of localizing the injection site is similar but the site of maximal muscle contraction by minimal stimulation is identified on the muscle itself (i.e. the motor point). It is believed that this technique allows targeting of primarily motor nerve fibres innervating the target muscle. The duration of action of phenol motor point and nerve blocks generally lasts between 3 and 8 months, but occasionally can last up to 2 years (Skeil and Barnes, 1994). The effectiveness of this treatment depends on accurate localization of the nerve to be treated, as injection of phenol even a few millimetres off target may not be effective. 50% alcohol has been used as an alternative to phenol, but it is generally less effective.

Intramuscular botulinum toxin A

This offers the possibility of local treatment of spasticity without affecting sensation (Jan-çovic 1994). It is an established treatment for squint, blepharospasm, hemifacial spasm, torticollis and focal dystonias. More recently it has been used successfully on an unlicensed basis, in the treatment of limb spasticity following stroke, traumatic brain injury and multiple sclerosis. Botulinum toxin irreversibly blocks the release of acetylcholine from the nerve endings at the neuromuscular junction thus preventing neuromuscular

transmission. When used in treating limb spasticity it therefore has a selective action on motor nerves without affecting sensory nerve conduction. Since perception is an integral part of motor function, treatments that preserve sensation have a theoretical advantage over less specific local treatments (alcohol and phenol nerve blocks). The two preparations of botulinum toxin currently available are Dysport and Botox. The 'dose' of botulinum toxin is measured in mouse units. This is a bioassay, 1 mouse unit representing the median lethal intraperitoneal dose of botulinum toxin given to a mouse. Unfortunately the bioactivities of the mouse unit of the two commercially available preparations are different. There is no agreed ratio between the bioactivities of the two preparations, although it is generally believed that 1 mouse unit of Botox is equivalent to 3–4 mouse units of Dysport. Botulinum toxin is injected directly into the spastic muscle. Distant unwanted muscle weakness (e.g. resulting in dysphagia) may occur as a result of diffusion of toxin across muscle fascial boundaries and also by systemic spread. Fortunately this problem is rare when botulinum toxin is used to treat limb muscles. The duration of benefit is usually between 3 and 6 months. Loss of effect occurs as new nerve growth forms new neutromuscular junctions.

SURGICAL TREATMENT

Surgical intervention can be broadly divided into procedures that interfere with the neuronal pathways and procedures that correct musculoskeletal deformity secondary to spasticity (Leland Albright, 1992).

Surgical ablation of neural pathways

This is usually reserved for patients in whom conservative antispastic treatments have failed. Where regional reduction in spasticity is required, controlled lesions to the nerve can be made at the spinal root level. Both anterior and posterior rhizotomies have been used. Currently, microsurgical techniques are used to perform more selective dorsal root entry zone (DREZ) lesions to minimize the risk of sensory disturbance and maximize antispastic effect. More extensive procedures such as myelotomies and cordotomies are rarely performed due to their significant adverse effects (Putty and Shapiro, 1991). Neurectomies (e.g. of the obturator nerve) are performed for local relief of spasticity, usually in combination with tenotomies.

Surgical treatments targeted at the musculoskeletal system can be used to improve function and reduce disability in patients with voluntary movement as well as in those with complete paresis. Fractional lengthening of forearm finger flexors in the spastic upper limb can improve grasp in selected patients. Similarly, voluntary elbow movement may be improved in some patients by proximal release of the brachioradialis, and lengthening of the biceps and brachialis tendons. However, surgical intervention is more commonly used for contracture release in a non-functioning limb (e.g. biceps, brachioradialis, brachialis tendons for flexion deformity at the elbow and Achilles tendon lengthening in spastic equinus deformity at the ankle). Serial splintage postoperatively maximizes benefit and prevents damage to the contracted neurovascular bundle. In patients with no voluntary wrist or finger extension, tenodesis may be performed to stabilize the wrist in extension. Some surgical treatments are carried out in conjunction with neurectomies to maximize benefit from surgery. In the lower limb, hip adductor spasticity may cause difficulty with perineal hygiene and urinary catheter care and in the ambulant patient reduce walking ability because of scissoring. Adductor tenotomy in conjunction with selective obturator nerve neurectomy can produce good results in these patients.

ELECTRICAL TREATMENT

Electrical stimulation of peripheral and central pathways are used to treat limb spasticity. Afferent stimulation seems to modulate the segmental reflexes. Efferent stimulation is used to compensate for the lack of appropriate efferent output from the segmental motor reflexes. In addition, cutaneous electrical stimulation has been used directly over the antagonist muscles to relieve agonist spasticity presumably by reciprocal inhibition. Cerebellar stimulation has also been employed to reduce spasticity.

Transcutaneous nerve stimulation (TENS)

This is commonly used for chronic pain (Levin and Hui-Chan, 1992; Ji-sheng, Xiaohong and Shang-cheung 1994). Although the exact mechanism of its action is not known, it is believed that cutaneous afferent impulses modulate spinal cord nociceptive pathways. In addition, a generalized central effect may occur through endorphin release. Owing to the close relationship between nociceptive and segmental motor reflex modulation. TENS has been used to treat spasticity. Cutaneous stimulation (80–100 Hz) is applied over the dermatome corresponding to the nerve supply of the spastic muscle. Although electrophysiological changes have been noted following TENS, there is not conclusive evidence of lasting functional benefit. Nevertheless, a small proportion of patients do show improvement and therefore it is worth trying as it is safe and easy to administer. **Dorsal column stimulation** has also been used to reduce spasticity, although the mechanism of action is unknown (Koulousakis, Buchhaas and Nitter, 1987). This treatment may be beneficial particularly when pain is a prominent feature. **Functional electrical stimulation** is an experimental technique primarily used for patients with muscle weakness in whom there is a lack of central drive (Stefanovska et al, 1989). It also appears to have a paradoxical effect in reducing spasticity in stimulated spastic muscles, although the mechanism for this action is unclear.

CONCLUSION

Spasticity can influence function in patients with complete muscle paresis as well as those with voluntary movement. As muscle tone measurement during active movement is often more informative than during passive limb movement, spasticity should be viewed in the context of inappropriate muscle activity. There is a wide range of treatments designed to reduce spasticity, but it is important to define the effect of spasticity on function prior to any intervention. A variety of concurrent impairments such as pain may exacerbate spasticity, requiring prompt identification and treatment. Physiotherapy, attention to posture and seating, and drug treatment with baclofen and dantrolene remain the mainstays of treatment and are appropriate for most patients. Nerve blocks and intrathecal antispastic medication can produce good results in selected patients. Newer treatments such as botulinum toxin show promise but need further evaluation. Although electrical stimulation techniques can reduce spasticity, they are currently confined to experimental use. Existing treatments in combination with newer antispastic drugs (botulinum toxin, tizanidine) and improved modes of delivery (intrathecal baclofen) make it likely that the number of patients with refractory spasticity requiring surgical intervention will diminish. Despite this, refractory spasticity will occur in some patients and therefore there is continued need for expertise in specific antispastic surgical procedures such as DREZ lesioning.

REFERENCES

Bobath, B. (ed.) (1990) *Adult Hemiplegia: evaluation and treatment*, Heinemann, London.

Bohannon, R.W. (1993) Tilt table standing for reducing spasticity after spinal cord injury. *Archives of Physical Medicine and Rehabilitation*, **74**, 1121–2.

Bohannon, R.W. and Smith, M.B. (1987) Inter-rater reliability of a modified Ashworth scale of muscle spasticity. *Physical Therapy*, **67**, 206–7.

Brunnstrom, S. (ed.) (1970) *Movement Therapy in Hemiplegia*, Harper and Row, New York.

Brunnstrom, S. (1956) Associated reactions of the upper extremity in adult patients with hemiplegia. *Physical Therapy Review*, **36**, 225–36.

Carr, E.K. and Kenney, F.D. (1992) Positioning of the stroke patient: a review of the literature. *International Journal of Nursing Studies*, **29**, 355–69.

Copp, E.P. and Keenan, J. (1972) Phenol nerve and motor point block in spasticity. *Rheumatology and Physical Medicine*, **11**, 287–92.

Cornall, C. (1991) Selfpropelling wheelchairs: the effect on spasticity in hemiplegic subjects. *Physiotherapy, Theory and Practice*, **7**, 13–21.

Corriveau, H., Bertrand Arsenault, A., Dutil E. *et al.* (1992) An evaluation of the hemiplegic patient based on the Bobath approach: a reliability study. *Disability and Rehabilitation* **14**, 81–4.

Davidoff, R.A. (1992) Skeletal muscle tone and the misunderstood stretch reflex. *Neurology* **42**, 951–63.

Delwaide, P.J. and Pennisi, G. (1994) Tizanidine and electrophysiologic analysis of spinal control mechanisms in humans with spasticity. *Neurology* **44**, 21–77.

Fromm, G.H. (1994) Baclofen as an adjuvant analgesic. *Journal of Pain Symptom Management*, **9**, 500–9.

Jancovic, J. (1994) Botulinum toxin in movement disorders. *Current Opinions in Neurology* **7**, 358–66.

Johnstone, M. (1989) Current advances in the use of pressure splints in the management of adult hemiplegia. *Physiotherapy*, **75**, 381–4.

Ji-sheng, H., Xiao-hong, C., Yu, Y. and Shang-cheung, Y. (1994) Transcutaneous electrical nerve stimulation for treatment of spinal spasticity. *Chinese Medical Journal*, **107**, 6–11.

Katz, R.T. and Zev Rymer, W. (1989) Spastic hypertonia: mechanisms and measurement. *Archives of Physical and Medical Rehabilitation*, **70**, 144–5.

Koulousakis, A., Buchhaas, U. and Nitter, K. (1987) Application of SCS for movement disorders and spasticity. *Acta Neurochirurgica*, **39**, 112–6.

Leland Albright, A. (1992) Neurosurgical treatment of spasticity: selective posterior rhizotomy and intrathecal baclofen. Proceedings of the meeting of the American Society for Stereotactic and Functional Neurosurgery, vol **58**, 3–13.

Levin, M.F. and Hui-Chan, C.W.Y. (1992) Relief of hemiparetic spasticity by TENS is associated with improvement in reflex and voluntary motor functions. *Electroencephalography and Clinical Neurophysiology*, **85**, 131–142.

Mai, J. and Pederson, E. (1991) Central effects of bladder filling and voiding *Journal Neurology, Neurosurgery and Psychiatry*, **39**, 171–7.

McLean, B.N. (1993) Intrathecal baclofen in severe spasticity. *British Journal of Hospital Medicine*, **49**, 262–7.

Ochs, G.A. (1993) Intrathecal baclofen. *Bailliere's Clinical Neurology* **2**, 73–86.

Petlillo, C.R. and Knoploch, S. (1988) Phenol block of the tibial nerve for spasticity: a long term follow up study. *International Disability*, **10**, 97–100.

Price, R., Lehmann, J.F., Boswell-Bessett, S. *et al.* (1993) Influence of cryotherapy on spasticity at the human ankle. *Archives of Physical Medicine and Rehabilitation*, **74**, 300–4.

Putty, T.K. and Shapiro, S.A. (1991) Efficacy of dorsal longitudinal myelotomy in treating spinal spasticity: a review of 20 cases. *Journal of Neurosurgery*, **75**, 397–401.

Skeil, D.A. and Barnes, M.P. (1994) The local treatment of spasticity. *Clinical Rehabilitation*, **8**, 240–6.

Snook, J.H. (1979) Spasticity reduction splint. *American Journal of Occupational Therapy*, **33**, 648–51.

Stefanovska, A., Vodovnik, L., Gros, N. *et al.* (1989) FES and spasticity. *IEEE Transactions on Biomedical Engineering*, **36**, 738–745.

Steiner, I., Argov, Z., Gomori, J.M. *et al.* (1985) Immediate spasticity with acute hemiplegia is a sign of basal ganglia haemorrhage. *Acta Neurologica Scandinavica*, **71**, 168–70.

Stockmeyer, S.L. (1967) An interpretation of the approach of Rood to the treatment of neuromuscular dysfunction. *American Journal of Physical Medicine*, **6**, 900–55.

Yablon, S.A. and Sipski, M.L. (1993) Effect of transdermal clonidine on spinal spasticity. *American Journal of Physical Medicine and Rehabilitation*, **72**, 154–7.

Young, A. (1994) Spasticity: a review. *Neurology*, **44**, (Suppl. 9), 13–19.

Young, R.R. and Delwaide, P.J. (1981a) Drug therapy: spasticity. Part I. *New England Journal of Medicine*, **304**, 28–33.

Young, R.R. and Delwaide, P.J. (1981b) Drug therapy: spasticity. Part 2. *New England Journal of Medicine*, **304**, 96–9.

FURTHER READING

Delwaide, P.J. and Young, R.R. (eds) (1985) *Clinical Neurophysiology in Spasticity*, Elsevier, Amsterdam.

Thilmann *et al*, (eds) (1993) *Spasticity: mechanisms and management*, Springer Verlag, Berlin.

35 The management of urinary incontinence

J. Malone-Lee

The prevalence of urinary incontinence in the UK increases from 2% of men and 9% of women aged 15–64 years, to 7% of men and 12% of women aged 65 years and over (Thomas *et al.*, 1980). The main primary causes are urethral sphincter incompetence, detrusor instability and idiopathic late nocturnal enuresis. In people with neurological disease, particularly multiple sclerosis, concomitant, chronic urinary retention frequently features. The important secondary causes are impairment of mobility, or of cognitive function, sufficient to preclude self-toileting. The secondary causes are the more common.

One of the most attractive aspects of the treatment and management of incontinence, associated with physical disability, is that usually it is possible to achieve extremely good results regardless of age, aetiology or sex. Additionally, it is not necessary to have a detailed knowledge of the sciences of incontinence in order to treat patients successfully. This chapter contains the information necessary for the management of the vast majority of continence problems.

ANATOMY AND PHYSIOLOGY

The smooth muscle fibres of the bladder, termed the detrusor, funnel at the bladder neck to be continued into the urethra as longitudinal fibres forming a tube. In the male these fibres are inserted into the verumontanum, but in the female they terminate in the distal urethra. The contraction of the detrusor results in a rise in bladder pressure associated with shortening of the urethra. The trigone forms a triangular base-plate with its apex at the bladder neck, and base running between both ureters. Contraction of the muscle of the trigone results in funnelling of the bladder neck. Some fibres are inserted into the external surface of the trigone distally. These pull the distal margins of the trigone apart, thus opening the bladder neck.

The detrusor has the ability to stretch considerably without developing an increase in tension. This means that it is normal for a bladder to be filled to 500 ml, and more, without an increase in intravesical pressure, other than the pressure head resulting from the height of the fluid in the bladder. If, during the filling phase of a urodynamic study, the detrusor contracts spontaneously, despite attempts to inhibit this, and thereby increases the pressure in the bladder, the detrusor is said to be 'unstable'. If the tension of the detrusor increases in association with filling, irrespective of any contractions, then the bladder is said to lack compliance. Low compliance may result from fibrosis, detrusor hypertrophy or increased resting tone sec-

Rehabilitation of the Physically Disabled Adult. Edited by C. John Goodwill, M. Anne Chamberlain and Chris Evans. Published in 1997 by Stanley Thornes (Publishers) Ltd, Cheltenham. ISBN 0-7487-3183-0.

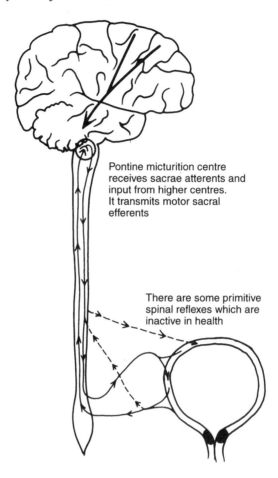

Pontine micturition centre
receives sacrae atterents and
input from higher centres.
It transmits motor sacral
efferents

There are some primitive
spinal reflexes which are
inactive in health

Figure 35.1 The sacral reflex mediates bladder relaxation during filling and long spinal reflex mediates the initiation of voiding.

ondary to reduced neural inhibition (Brading and Turner, 1994).

The normal mechanism for activating contraction of the detrusor is the release of acetylcholine from parasympathetic nerves, stimulated by the spinobulbospinal micturition reflex, the main micturition reflex. Tension receptors in the detrusor activate afferents travelling in the pelvic nerves. These afferents pass through the lumbosacral dorsal roots to ascending tracts up to the pons. At this level the pontine micturition centre provides the site at which connections are made with descending motor tracts,

destined for the sacral parasympathetic nuclei. The preganglionic, sacral parasympathetic axons originate in the sacral parasympathetic nuclei, leave the spinal cord through ventral roots, and travel in the pelvic nerves to ganglia in the pelvic plexus, Lincoln and Burnstock, 1994; De Groat, 1995).

Since higher cerebral centres tend to inhibit the pontine micturition centre, lesions above this are associated with detrusor overactivity (Figure 35.1). Subpontine lesions are more complex. There are some spinal micturition reflexes located below the pons which are weak in the adult and probably inactive in health. Therefore, lesions of the spinal cord below the pons, but rostral to the sacral nuclei, result in bladder areflexia **initially.** Subsequent to the injury, over weeks or months, reflex mechanisms in the spinal cord become active resulting in some uncoordinated and poorly sustained reflex bladder activity. However, if a spinal lesion involves complete destruction of the sacral nuclei, bladder areflexia will be permanent. Spinal injury may also be associated with the evolution of some primitive C-fibre (pain) mediated reflexes. These promote contraction of the detrusor, particularly in association with cystitis, but also cause arterial pressor responses induced by bladder distension and contraction. The latter can cause dangerous hypertension and is termed **autonomic dysreflexia** (Hoyle, Lincoln and Burnstock, 1994; De Groat, 1995).

The internal urethral sphincter is only present in the male, forming a circular collar continuous with the smooth muscle of the prostate. This sphincter is not part of the continence mechanism but contracts during ejaculation to prevent the retrograde flow of semen into the bladder. Failure of this sphincter leads to infertility, dry ejaculation and seminuria. The internal sphincter is cut during transurethral resection of the prostate; however, continence is maintained.

The external urethral sphincter is the principle mechanism for maintaining urethral continence in both sexes. The circularly arranged muscle fibres are striated and predominantly slow twitch. The striated muscles of the pelvic floor and the external sphincter are supplied by somatic efferents originating in the anterior horns of the sacral cord segments S2–S4. The motor neurones are grouped in a specific region called Onuf's nucleus. This nucleus differs from other somatic motor nuclei, with histochemical appearances similar to sacral parasympathetic nuclei along with evidence of adrenergic innervation. The axons, originating from Onuf's nucleus, pass to the periphery through the pudendal nerve and the pelvic nerves. External sphincter activity is supported by the adrenergic smooth muscle of the urethra.

The sympathetic innervation for the lower urinary tract comes from postganglionic nerves travelling in the hypogastric plexus, the pelvic nerves and the pudendal nerves. The sympathetic innervation inhibits the detrusor and stimulates the urethral smooth muscle and the sphincters. The stimulatory receptors on urethra and sphincter myocytes are alpha-1_c. The inhibitory noradrenergic receptors on detrusor cells are sparse and beta-2 in type. The stimulatory action of noradrenaline on the smooth muscle of the prostate has precipitated an interest in selective alpha-1_c receptor antagonists in the treatment of prostatism (Hoyle, Lincoln and Burnstock, 1994; De Groat, 1995).

The acetylcholine acts on muscarinic receptors, which when stimulated activate second messengers which cause release of Ca^{++} ions from intracellular stores in the sarcoplasmic reticulum. The rise in intracellular Ca^{++} ion concentration activates the actin and myosin, thereby promoting contraction. It is known that the detrusor cell can depolarize with the inward current consisting of Ca^{++} ions passing through L-type channels in sufficient magnitude to support depolarization. The calcium influx may then trigger further intracellular Ca^{++} ion release. However, it seems that acetylcholine does not cause depolarization. The role of detrusor depolarization is as yet unexplained. It may be that its limited role would explain the lack of efficacy of calcium channel blockers in the treatment of detrusor instability (Palfrey, Fry and Shuttleworth, 1984; Montgomery and Fry, 1992; Wu, Kentish and Fry, 1994).

The muscarinic receptor itself is the focus of much current interest. Molecular biological studies have identified five subtypes of the muscarinic receptor (m1 to m5) (Rosario *et al.*, 1995), which are distributed throughout the central nervous system and in the periphery.

Selective agonists and antagonists have identified three pharmacological subtypes (M1–M3) which correspond to the cloned M1–M3 receptors. M1 activity is detected in the autonomic ganglia and central nervous system. M2 activity is found in the heart and M3 activity is found in glandular tissue and smooth muscle. mRNA activity for m4 receptors has been identified in rat striatum and rabbit lung. Nothing is known about the role of m5 receptors.

Studies of M2 and M3 receptors have shown that in the bladder the greater proportion (85%) are M2 receptors, with only 20% being M3. However, pharmacologically the M2 receptor appears redundant and all of the contractile activity can be attributed to the M3 receptor. As a consequence, current pharmacological research and development is centred on antagonists of the M3 receptor. It has been found that some antagonists, despite the wide distribution of the M3 receptor in the body, prove highly selective for the bladder. Such organ-selective properties have yet to be explained (Jurgen, 1993; Andersson *et al.,* 1991; Eglen *et al.,* 1994).

It is now known that acetylcholine and noradrenaline are not the only significant neurotransmitters in the lower urinary tract. Non-adrenergic non-cholinergic (NANC) neurotransmitters are neuropeptides which modulate the actions of the classical transmitters and may act as transmitters themselves. Neuropeptide-Y (NPY) and vasoactive intestinal polypeptide (VIP) are important neuromodulators which are released at neuromuscular junctions so as to influence the release and uptake of acetylcholine and noradrenaline. Adenosine triphosphate (ATP) is thought to be an important neurotransmitter. It is known to cause depolarization of the detrusor. There is some evidence that in diseased states the activating mechanisms of the detrusor change and that NANC transmitters exert a much greater influence on the bladder (Andersson *et al.,* 1991, Jurgen, 1993; Eglen *et al.,* 1994).

CLINICAL SYNDROMES

Detrusor instability is an important cause of incontinence amongst disabled people, particularly in the elderly, affecting 75–85% of women and 85–95% of men aged 75 and over with incontinence (DuBeau and Resnick, 1991; Malone-Lee, 1992). Detrusor instability in the presence of neurological disease is termed **detrusor hyperreflexia.**

Genuine stress incontinence, resulting from urethral sphincter incompetence, is probably the most common problem in women. The main cause is damage to the sphincter mechanism during childbirth, although 15% of women with genuine stress incontinence are nulliparous. Some patients with spinal injuries have surgically induced sphincter incompetence which was carried out to counter urinary retention when intermittent catheterization was not an option. If the external sphincter is damaged during a transurethral prostatectomy, then serious genuine stress incontinence will be experienced by the man.

Lower motor neurone lesions, affecting the somatic motor supply to the striated muscles of the pelvic floor and external urethral sphincter will lead to genuine stress incontinence. Because such lesions may also affect the parasympathetic efferent nuclei to the detrusor, as in spina-bifida, neurogenic genuine stress incontinence is often associated with chronic urinary retention caused by detrusor underactivity.

Lesions of the central nervous system, causing detrusor hyperreflexia, are associated with voiding contractions which are poorly sustained and also inadequately coordinated with sphincter relaxation (detrusor-sphincter dyssynergia). This results in incomplete emptying and chronic urinary retention, coincident with detrusor overactivity. These neurogenic voiding disorders are particularly associated with diseases of the spinal cord, notably multiple sclerosis and spinal injury. The clinical presentation results from loss of suppression of more primitive voiding reflexes, active in the absence of influence from higher centres. It should be noted that idiopathic detrusor instability is associated with higher urethral opening pressures, so there is some abnormal sphincter activity, without overt detrusor-sphincter dyssynergia, in this situation (Chapter 28).

Afferent pathway lesions will interrupt the sensory component of the normal voiding reflex and lead to urinary retention. This typically occurs in diabetics with peripheral neuropathy. Additionally, distension of the bladder results in damage to the voiding reflex and thereby promotes areflexia of the detrusor.

Chronic urinary retention will always be associated with a higher incidence of urinary infection. It is notable that some patients are more susceptible to this than others.

DIAGNOSIS AND URODYNAMIC ASSESSMENT

The clinical assessment requires a history describing frequency, nocturia, urgency, the characteristics of incontinence and the quality of voiding. One must ask about infection and haematuria, bowel function, previous urogynaecological surgery and current medication. Information on sexual life should only be explored where appropriate. It is necessary to perform a proper pelvic and rectal examination. Check the action of the periurethral striated muscle by asking a female to contract the muscles 'as if trying to stop passing urine' whilst your finger palpates the posterior urethra. Vaginal prolapse, particularly of the anterior wall, may effect voiding function but prolapse and stress incontinence are not causally related. Rectal examination should include an assessment of a sphincter contraction. The anal, bulbocavernous and cough reflexes help in the examination of sacral reflex activity. Lumbar and sacral motor and sensory function should also be checked.

A dipstick test of the urine is advisable but not urine culture. It is important to check the postmicturition residual urine volume by catheter or ultrasound. Renal tract ultrasound should be considered in those with obstruction or recurrent infection.

Disabled patients presenting with incontinence tend to describe symptoms which could be attributed to different aetiologies. Frequency, nocturia, urgency and urge incontinence are typical of **detrusor instability;** hesitancy, a reduced stream, straining, terminal dribbling and postmicturition dribbling would be considered typical of a **voiding problem**; incontinence on coughing, sneezing and laughing might be considered to be due to **sphincter incompetence**. In truth, the symptoms prove very unhelpful in pointing to the diagnosis.

The bladder empties more efficiently from a higher capacity (Griffiths, 1974; Griffiths *et al.*, 1992). With a full bladder, you start micturition with the advantage of a bladder pressure head which helps to open the urethra. Additionally, elongation of the detrusor fibres in response to filling promotes optimum contact between the actin and myosin so that a better contraction can be obtained. Flow rates are well known to be related to the voiding bladder volume. People with frequency, therefore, often describe the symptoms of poor voiding even though obstruction or detrusor underactivity may not be present.

Loss of bladder compliance in association with detrusor instability may push the resting bladder pressure up towards the urethral threshold. In these circumstances, coughing will lead to stress incontinence which is not due to sphincter incompetence.

Genuine stress incontinence results from a failure of sphincter function. If, on bladder filling, the hydrostatic pressure head approaches a reduced sphincter threshold the patient will experience frequency, urgency and urge incontinence even though the bladder is stable.

The doubt about the significance of symptoms has promoted a great interest in diagnostic methods. The **urodynamic study** has been used for some time to characterize the behaviour of the lower urinary tract in incontinence. It certainly has the potential to clarify ambiguous symptoms and one should understand the method (Griffiths, 1980).

On presentation, patients are asked to empty their bladders whilst the urine flow rate is measured by means of a flow meter positioned in an adapted commode. A Jaques catheter (French gauge 10) and a nylon catheter (16G) are placed in the bladder via the urethra, which is anaesthetized with 2% lignocaine gel. The postmicturition residual urine is drained off and measured. Another catheter (French gauge 10) tipped with a perforated latex sheath, to avoid faecal plugging, is introduced into the rectum. The smaller bladder catheter and the rectal catheter are filled with normal saline and then connected to force displacement transducers mounted at the level of the superior ramus of the pubic bone. This reference point is used to establish atmospheric pressure. The detrusor pressure, generated by the walls of the bladder, is calculated by subtracting the intra-abdominal pressure (measured via the rectal catheter) from the intravesical pressure (measured via the urethral catheter). The bladder is filled with a fluid (usually normal saline at $20°C$) at a rate of between 50 and 100 ml min^{-1}. Sadly, the filling rate, fluid temperature and content are not standardized and vary with department preference.

The analogue data obtained from the transducers may be digitized and collected on magnetic disk. The bladder is filled until either a maximum of 500 ml has been infused; or unstable detrusor activity prohibits further filling; or the patient is found to be unable to tolerate any further infusion. On completion of the filling study the Jaques catheter, which was used for filling is withdrawn from the bladder leaving the pressure measuring catheter *in situ*. The patient is then asked to void to completion. During voiding the bladder and rectal pressure and the flow rate are recorded simultaneously.

During normal filling to 500 ml the detrusor pressure rises to around $8\ cmH_2O$ consequent on the pressure head of infused fluid and the relaxation of the detrusor in response to filling (Figure 35.2).

The detrusor pressure, recorded during filling at 60 ml s^{-1}, from a woman with detrusor hyperreflexia is shown in Figure 35.3. This patient demonstrates hyperreflexic contractions occurring on a background of poor compliance caused by persistent muscle tone. This differs from the pattern shown in Figure 35.4, from a woman with detrusor instability, where the contractions are less consistent on a background of compliance.

TESTING THE URINE

Urinanalysis frequently causes some confusion over interpretation and management. This needs to be avoided, since properly conducted it is a most useful tool.

Bacteriuria means the isolation of bacteria colonizing the urinary tract. **Significant bacteriuria** means that there is a high probability that the isolated bacteria came from the urinary tract. It does not mean that this has clinical significance. Significant bacteriuria in asymptomatic women is 10^5 colony forming units (CFU) of a single species per ml. In symptomatic women this threshold has a very low sensitivity. It has now been shown that a midstream urine specimen (MSU) culture from a symptomatic woman of 10^2 CFU ml^{-1} of a single species of a known urinary pathogen is significant. In symptomatic men the threshold is 10^3 CFU ml^{-1} of a single species. Most automated culture systems have a sensitivity threshold of 10^4 CFU ml^{-1}. Given the difficulties with specimen collection and storage, it has been found that almost half of urine specimens from people with definite urinary tract infections prove culture negative. Urine culture, therefore, is an insensitive

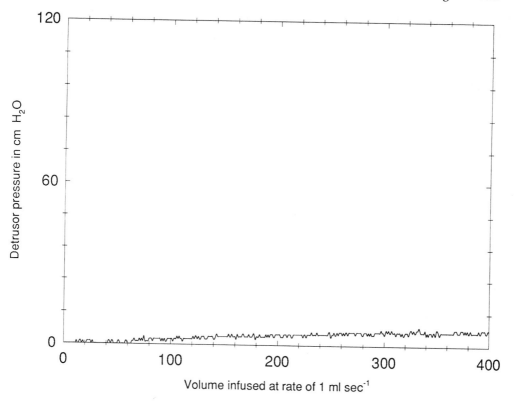

Figure 35.2 Detrusor pressure against infusion volume. Record obtained from non-disabled adult with a stable bladder.

but very specific diagnostic instrument (Stamm, 1988).

Pyuria remains a useful diagnostic test. Leucocyte counts of eight cells per mm^3 point to infection, and where cultures are negative in the presence of pyuria a chlamydial infection should be suspected. **Absence of pyuria on microscopy suggests that infection is not a feature.** Leucocyte counts by haemocytometer are time consuming and expensive, so simpler techniques have been explored. A simple count of more than 10 leucocytes per high-powered field only correlates with colony counts of 10^5 CFU ml^{-1}. Similarly, a positive leucocyte esterase test, using chemical urine dip sticks (Ames Multistix 8SG, Bayer Diagnostics), correlates with 10^5 CFU ml^{-1} So the simpler methods of

screening for pyuria are highly specific but insensitive. Testing for urine nitrite using urinary dipsticks proves similarly sensitive and specific (Pappas, 1991; Faro, 1992; Maskell, 1995).

Haematuria can be detected in 50% of patients with acute urinary infection and it is a useful confirmatory finding. It should always be followed up in order to confirm resolution. The chemical test on a dipstick is highly sensitive and asymptomatic haematuria, found chemically, should be confirmed by microscopy before investigating by cytology, ultrasound and cystoscopy so as to exclude malignancy (Pappas, 1991).

Albuminuria is a pointer to renal disease. It is quite possible to have acute urinary infection without proteinuria on dipstick analysis.

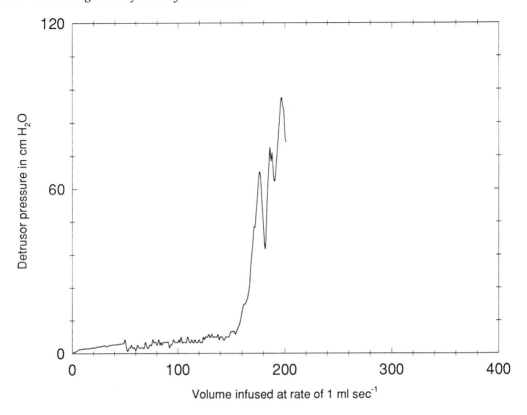

Figure 35.3 Detrusor pressure against infusion volume. Record obtained from the hyperreflexic bladder of a patient with multiple sclerosis.

If albuminuria is detected, it should be quantified by means of a 24-hour excretion test, characterized for an orthostatic pattern, and examined by electrophoresis for selectivity. Renal function should be assessed simultaneously (Pappas, 1991).

Measuring urinary pH is no longer considered to be a valid means of screening for urinary infection.

The limitations of our investigation techniques have resulted in it becoming accepted that the most sensitive indicators of urinary infection are the patients' symptoms. This means that it is important to ensure that patients with lower urinary tract dysfunction become adept at identifying the symptoms, particular to themselves, which point to infection. It is quite wrong to delay treatment

of a symptomatic patient whilst awaiting culture results. Patients at particular risk should be provided with a supply of antibiotics to self-administer when indications present (Pappas, 1991; Hooton *et al.*, 1995; Maskell, 1995).

TREATMENTS

Whilst attempting to treat urinary incontinence the aim is to achieve one or all of the following goals:

1. The reduction of bladder sensitivity.
2. The stabilization of the detrusor.
3. The promotion of adequate bladder emptying during voiding.
4. The competence of the urethral sphincter.

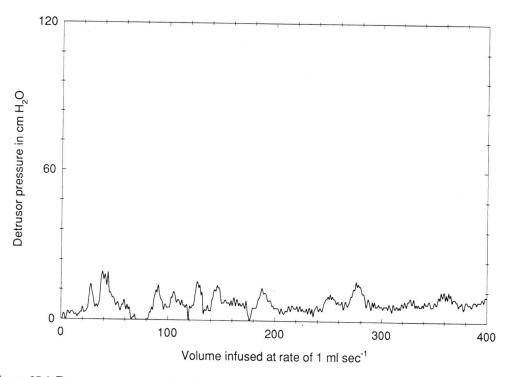

Figure 35.4 Detrusor pressure against infusion volume. Record obtained from a patient with instability.

Since a number of the therapeutic options will promote more than one of these objectives, it is easier to consider treatment modalities individually.

Bladder retraining uses a protocol designed to encourage the patient to reduce the frequency of micturition. Several methods are proposed and none have been shown to be any better than others. There are a number of different bladder-retraining charts available, many of which are distributed by manufacturers of continence drugs or aids. The patient uses the chart to keep a record of episodes of micturition. During this time efforts are made to delay micturition long after the urge to urinate is experienced. It has been found that whilst practising the technique the frequencies of micturition tend to reduce (Jarvis and Millar, 1980; Frewen, 1982; Wiseman, Malone Lee and Rai, 1991). In an outpatient department we have found that the

period of change, in a patient who is responding, lasts up to 4 weeks (Szonyi *et al.*, 1995).

Patients with sensory urgency, who experience inappropriate desires to micturate at low bladder capacities in the absence of detrusor activity, may use this to reduce their frequency. However, it is not necessarily easy and the patient needs to be warned of this and persuaded of the great importance of compliance if there is to be any hope of recovery. An unstable bladder will tend to become less reactive if stretched by higher bladder volumes. This principle is used to treat detrusor instability where the frequency will be promoting very low bladder capacities. Some patients with detrusor instability will experience pain whilst delaying micturition and there is a real possibility of urge incontinence whilst working with the regime. Because one is attempting to stretch the bladder the process can be augmented by encouraging higher fluid intake whilst at home and not in danger of public scrutiny should an episode of incontinence occur.

If the urethral sphincter is incompetent, the greater pressure head applied to the bladder neck by larger bladder volumes will result in a strong sense of pending incontinence. This results in frequency being a feature of sphincter incompetence. For this reason it is appropriate to use a bladder-retraining regime as part of the treatment of genuine stress incontinence, provided, of course, that attention is also applied to the sphincter lesion.

The bladder empties more efficiently from a higher capacity (Griffiths, 1974; Griffiths *et al.*, 1992). Frequency will result in bladder fatigue, since the chemistry of the detrusor muscle is probably not well suited to the rapid regeneration of energy stores. People with frequency often describe the symptoms of poor voiding; hesitancy, a reduced stream, straining to void, terminal dribbling and postmicturition dribbling. It is therefore logical to use a bladder-retraining regime to treat voiding problems secondary to detrusor muscle lesions. A proviso is to avoid excessive delay such that the bladder capacity rises substantially above 400 ml when there will be a danger of reducing detrusor power by overextension of the detrusor muscle fibres.

Detrusor stabilizing drugs are used to reduce the frequency and efficacy of unstable bladder contractions, thereby allowing a patient a greater chance of cooperating with a bladder-retraining regime. It takes approximately 10 years to develop a new molecule from the basic science laboratory to licensing for prescription. Many drugs fail to retain their licences after launch because of post-marketing identification of toxicity or questionable efficacy. Drugs used in the elderly are particularly prone to this problem. Until recently, drugs for incontinence were not seen as lucrative investments. It is not surprising, therefore, to learn that there are few drugs for treating detrusor instability and many of them have been around for a long time. In addition, in all cases their efficacy has been tested by small-scale studies with questionable conclusions.

There is a need for some well-organized, large-scale multicentre studies to examine the efficacy of the popular methods of treating the unstable bladder. In the meantime, we have to rely on data from less satisfactory smaller studies. These will have some probability of accuracy, albeit limited and unquantified.

Oxybutynin hydrochloride (Ditropan, Cystrin) seems to be the first choice drug of most centres in the treatment of the unstable bladder, although evidence for efficacy remains weak (Malone-Lee, 1995; Szonyi *et al.*, 1995; Yarker, Goa and Fitton, 1995). It is a tertiary amine with powerful anticholinergic and papaverine-like properties which is very well absorbed from the gastrointestinal tract, reaching a maximum plasma concentration 30 minutes after ingestion. It is excreted by the kidneys and has a plasma half-life of about 3 hours. This is very slightly increased in the elderly. The side-effects involve a dry mouth, constipation, reflux oesophagitis (the usual reason for withdrawal of this medication), dry skin, visual accommodation problems and minor ankle swelling. Recent work indicates that a lower dose than recommended in the data sheet is efficacious in all age groups. The authors start all patients on 2.5 mg b.d. and titrate the dose in response to efficacy and side-effects (Malone-Lee, Lubel and Szonyi, 1992). It is probably best to wait at least 4 weeks between dose alterations, as the dynamics of the drug seem to be slower than the kinetics would suggest. In a recent clinical trial, a drug effect evolving 6 weeks after starting treatment was detected. A new slow-release formulation of oxybutynin is currently undergoing clinical trials.

The tricyclic antidepressant imipramine (Tofranil) has anticholinergic, alpha-agonistic, antihistaminic and anti 5-HT properties (Castleden *et al.*, 1981; Battcock and Castleden,

1990). Most patients respond to a single dose of between 10 mg and 25 mg at night. Some patients with troublesome daytime symptoms require an extra dose in the morning. The side-effects are similar to oxybutynin but milder, although postural instability and drowsiness may be experienced by the elderly. Imipramine is probably not as effective as oxybutynin but there is some observational data which suggests that it may have useful synergistic properties when combined with oxybutynin, both drugs being administered in low dose, when treating particularly resistant patients.

The quaternary ammonium compound propantheline (Probanthine) is recommended by some workers. It is not well absorbed from the gastrointestinal tract and therapeutic levels are difficult to achieve. Evidence of efficacy in published works is not convincing and doubt exists as to what dose should be used. It is probable that a dose higher than that recommended in the data sheet would be required in order to achieve a response (Holmes, Montz and Stanton, 1989; Thuroff *et al.*, 1991). Emepromium bromide (Cetiprin), another quaternary ammonium compound, is no longer available in the UK. There are considerable doubts about its efficacy and gastrointestinal absorbtion is not good. It has a reputation for causing oesophageal ulceration (Battcock and Castleden, 1990).

There was an interest in the calcium channel blocking drugs for use with detrusor instability. Terodiline (Micturin) was the best known of this group (Wiseman, Malone Lee and Rai, 1991). However, it was withdrawn from the market in 1991 following reports of serious cardiac problems, in particular the arrythmia of Torsade de point (van der Klaw, van Ray and Stricker, 1992). Terodiline had anticholinergic properties as well but it is highly likely that the cardiac effects were caused by the calcium channel blocking properties. Other anticholinergics used to treat the unstable bladder have not been linked to this problem. It is probable that calcium channel blocking properties are not of significance to the bladder since depolarization does not appear to be important for contraction.

Flavoxate hydrochloride (Urispas) is a drug with papaverine-like properties. At one time this was used extensively for treating the unstable bladder but doubts arose as to its efficacy and these were confirmed by data from controlled clinical trials (Milani *et al.*, 1993). It is no longer considered to be an effective drug for the unstable bladder.

Two new drugs, which have been developed specifically for the bladder, are currently undergoing phase three clinical trials. Darifenasin, developed by Pfizer, has selective M3 antigonistic properties and is thought to be efficacious with fewer side-effects than other antimuscarinics (Rosario *et al.*, 1995). Tolterodine, developed by Pharmacia, is not receptor subset selective but does demonstrate a remarkable organ selectivity for the bladder. It also shows evidence of efficacy (Naerger, Fry and Nilvebrant, 1995; Nilvebrant, Stahl and Andersson, 1995).

About 2% of the adult population suffer from **nocturnal enuresis** and the prognosis for recovery after puberty is not good. Persistent nocturia is a disabling symptom associated with a chronic fatigue state which may not be evident until after successful treatment. Nocturia and nocturnal enuresis feature in a number of neurological diseases particularly multiple sclerosis. In a number of patients both these symptoms may prove resistant. DDAVP (Desmopressin) has been an important advance in this area. A dose of 10 µg nocte, intranasally, will usually produce a gratifying response with no ill effects. Some patients may prove very sensitive to the drug and rapidly develop a water intoxication with the symptoms of headache, a sense of fullness, nausea and confusion. These people will need to be managed with a lower dose (5 µg nocte) which can only be dispensed in the dropper format as opposed to the spray. It is possible to prescribe DDAVP in tablet form in a dose of 100–600 µg nocte, most people responding to between 200 and 400 µg. The oral form is less reliable than the intranasal administration but, in those who respond to this form, it is much more convenient (Hilton and Stanton, 1982; Eckford *et al.*, 1994).

DDAVP is useful for children whilst they are staying away from home and it may be used for this indication from the age of five. It is not recommended that this drug be used continuously in children at the moment. Our experience has made it clear that it should **not** be used in patients over the age of 65. It can be quite dangerous for this age group due to the side-effects noted above.

Surgery for detrusor instability and hyperreflexia has been the focus of a number of procedures. Cystodistension is a discredited procedure, as is subtrigonal phenol injection.

The **Clam cystoplasty** has proved to be a most important operative intervention for incontinence resistant to other treatment. The procedure is simple with a low morbidity. The bladder is cut open like a clam by means of a coronal incision and a patch of ileum is sutured between the two halves of the bladder so as to prevent these parts rejoining. The bladder, therefore, remains functionally transected and can no longer contract effectively. This stops the incontinence but, in most cases and particularly with neurological disease, voiding is ineffective and must be achieved by the use of intermittent self-catheterization. The main complications include an increased risk of urinary stone formation, occurring in 6%. This results from urinary infection and the mucous secreted by the intestinal patch. There is a risk of metabolic acidosis resulting from absorption of ammonium (NH_4^+) and chloride (Cl^-) ions by the bowel segment which may lead to a hyperchloraemic acidosis, as was the case with ureterosigmoidostomy (transplantation of the ureters into the colon). The acidosis may be undetected on electrolyte analyses but evident on blood gas analysis. The calcium resorption from bone, due to acidosis, may

lead to growth retardation in children. There is a risk of malignancy, particularly at the junction of the gut segment with the bladder. The precipitants are thought to be nitrosamines released as a result of bacterial activity in the urine. It is not possible at present to quantify this risk. Anecdotal cases have been reported. In ureterosigmoidostomy it generally required 15 years for the tumour to develop. The procedure has not been in existence for 15 years. (George *et al.*, 1991; Malone-Lee *et al.*, 1994)

The Brindley Anterior Root Stimulator can be used to treat some neuropathic bladders very successfully. The method is best suited to patients with complete cord transections that leave the sacral segments of the cord intact and those with incomplete cord lesions and no pelvic sensation. The stimulator electrodes are applied to the anterior roots of S2 to S4, but this depends on individual anatomical variation. The electrodes are stimulated by a magnetic activator held by the patient over a stimulator box placed subcutaneously. Intermittent stimulation, particularly of the S3 root, results in a sustained rise in bladder pressure with intermittent contraction and relaxation of the external sphincter. As a result the patient is able to void. At the time of surgery the posterior roots (S2–S4 usually) are cut, thus destroying afferent function and thereby preventing reflex contractions of the bladder. The result is that a patient who previously suffered from troublesome hyperreflexic contractions and poor voiding, secondary to dyssynergia and unsustained voiding contractions, becomes continent and is able to void to completion. The operation is a long process. Genital sensation, if previously present, would be lost, as would reflex erection. In patients with intact pelvic pain sensation, stimulation has been found to cause unpleasant dysaesthesia (Brindley *et al.*, 1986; Brindley, 1988).

The Continent Ileal Reservoir (Kock Pouch) was first introduced in the 1970s.

The operation requires technical skill. A 70-cm segment of ileum is isolated and folded into a U shape. In the well of the U the two segments of ileum are fused so as to form a bag which will act as the reservoir which has two ileal tubes leading from it. Both tubes are intussuscepted and the ureters anastomosed with one of them, the afferent tube. The efferent tube is passed through a channel in the abdominal wall and attached to the rectus muscle. The stoma is flat. Because the intussusception causes a valve action the stoma is continent and the reservoir is emptied by means of intermittent catheterization. The afferent intussusception provides a valve action which protects the kidneys from back flow (Davidsson, Barker and Mansson, 1992). Possible complications include necrosis of the anastomoses, failure of the valve functions causing urinary leakage and reflux, prolapse of the stoma, parastomal hernia and stomal strictures (Norlen, Philipson and Kock, 1988; Shull 1991).

Patients empty the reservoir four or five times a day. They must maintain a routine since they do not experience sensations. It is preferable, wherever possible, to preserve the bladder as the receptor of the ureters. A Kock Pouch is therefore infrequently used and reserved for patients with gross neurogenic bladder dysfunction, interstitial cystitis, carcinoma of the bladder, congenital abnormalities and troublesome fistulae.

INTERMITTENT CATHETERIZATION

Voiding problems are most commonly managed by this method. It has gained general acceptance in the management of voiding disorders associated with neurological disease (Kuhn, Rist and Zaech, 1991; Pearman, Bailey and Riley. 1991). Additionally, it is known that the elderly of both sexes have an increased tendency towards incomplete bladder emptying and this frequently coexists with detrusor instability (Malone-Lee, 1992). Voiding disorders in the elderly may occur in the absence of symptoms. Treating detrusor instability in the presence of a voiding disorder may exacerbate the incomplete bladder emptying. The latter can be managed by intermittent catheterization.

The author's policy is to identify patients with voiding disorders by including an assessment of the postmicturition residual urine volume as part of the standard assessment protocol. When significant problem is discovered, which is defined as a residual of 150 ml or more, a temporary, once-daily, intermittent catheterization programme is instituted. If this results in a rapid and significant improvement in symptoms, a more permanent regime is then established, otherwise no further action is taken.

The technique involves a clean non-sterile catheterization of the bladder using a CH10 or CH12 Jaques catheter lubricated with KY jelly. There are shorter catheters for women, called 'female-length' catheters. The catheters should be washed and dried after use. Dryness is a better antiseptic than many chemical solutions. There is little justification for using self-lubricating catheters because these cannot be reused and are expensive. However, Lofric do produce a very useful composite self-lubricating catheter and collecting bag for travelling purposes.

These are practical difficulties in administering the procedure in the presence of **impaired manual dexterity.** In such circumstances it is more usual for the services of a spouse or partner to be enlisted to administer the procedure initially. This allows the patient time to learn to self-administer the catheter at home without pressure. It is very important that the instructor be well trained, confident and firmly encouraging during the early introduction of the procedure. Infection, haematuria and failed catheterization attempts are more common during the early days and can be very discouraging. The instructor needs experience and confidence, and to be sensitive to the patient's feelings.

Once the technique has been established the

patient works out a regime which satisfies his or her needs. This usually involves a catheterization twice daily with the odd extra one before special events. The residual volume does not need to drive the frequency of catheterization. If the procedure is working there is a very marked effect on symptoms. Whilst intermittent catheterization frequently reduces urinary infection, secondary to retention, an increased incidence of cystitis must be expected. This should be managed on symptoms. There are no indications for routine urine cultures in the absence of acute symptoms. Asymptomatic bacteriuria should be left well alone.

URINE INFECTION

In order to treat a urinary infection a drug which is well absorbed from the gastrointestinal tract, and therefore does not accumulate in the colon, needs to be chosen. It must be excreted in the urine rapidly, not be associated with high resistance rates and inexpensive. Nitrofurantoin (Furadantin) fits this bill. Some patients experience nausea with nitrofurantoin and in these circumstances the macrocrystals (Macrodantin) prove useful. Trimethoprim (Monotrim) is a useful urinary antibiotic. Amoxycillin (Amoxil) continues to be recommended for urinary infections and it is effective but particularly associated with the development of vaginal thrush infections. These occur in 25% of women prescribed amoxycillin. Nalidixic acid (Negram) is also a useful urinary antibiotic which is worth considering as a non-toxic first-line treatment. The newer quinolones such as ciprofloxacin (Ciproxin) should really be used as second-line therapies for resistant infections (Hooton and Stam, 1991).

The dose and duration should be designed to limit the period of treatment. Clinical trials have shown that uncomplicated cystitis will respond usually to a single dose of 3 g of amoxycillin or 400 mg of trimethoprim. Recurrent, postcoital cystitis usually responds

to 100 mg nitrofurantoin immediately after intercourse. If the bladder is abnormal this may be less efficacious. The authors' policy is to prescribe the antibiotic in a generous dose to be taken 12 hourly from the first hint of symptoms until they have cleared. This is an easy protocol for patients to follow and results in short courses of around 2 days (Stamey, 1987). Nitrofurantoin is preferred as first-line therapy and ciprofloxacin as second line if a urine culture has not provided sensitivity data. In the rare circumstances of needing to use prophylactic therapy because of recurrent urinary infections, this is given as nitrofurantoin 50 mg nocte for 3 months. Long term nitrofurantoin may, very rarely, cause peripheral neuropathy and pulmonary fibrosis. Since nitrofurantoin's action depends on rapid renal excretion, it is of limited value in renal impairment.

Pelvic floor exercises are a popular means of non-surgical therapy for patients with urethral sphincter incompetence. The evidence for their efficacy is far from established and is based on data from open studies or within group analyses of comparative trial data (Mantle and Versi, 1991; Mouritsen, Frimodt Moller and Moller, 1991). Pelvic floor exercises have not been found to be superior to surgery (Cardozo, 1991). There is little consistency in the techniques which are adopted by different centres. Whilst they have been advocated for the treatment of stress incontinence in older women, there is evidence which may suggest that they are less effective. It is regrettable that no large-scale studies of efficacy, which include age comparisons, have been conducted so that doubt hangs over their application (Fantl, 1989; Cammu *et al.*, 1991 Wells, Buick and Diokno, 1991; Wijma, Tinga and Wisser, 1991).

For women, the most effective means of dealing with genuine stress incontinence is **colposuspension.** During this procedure the bladder neck is identified through a suprapubic incision and sutures are placed in the paravaginal fascia either side of the bladder neck. These are then used to approximate the paravaginal fascia to the ileopectineal ligament. This results in elevation of the bladder neck in the pelvis, lengthening of the urethra, and apposition of the anterior vaginal wall behind the urethra. The result is a relative urethral obstruction which stops the stress incontinence over 90% of the time. Complications are unusual but include urinary retention and postoperative voiding problems, detrusor instability and dyspareunia (Jarvis, 1994; Monga, 1994; Alcalay, Monga and Stanton, 1995).

The **AS artificial urinary sphincter** is an option for the management of urethral sphincter failure in both sexes. It is best suited to people who do not have unstable bladders, The operation involves the insertion of a cuff around the urethra which is passively inflated from a reservoir of fluid placed in the pelvis. The cuff can be deflated, so as to allow voiding, by activating a pump placed in the scrotum or labia major. After voiding the cuff reinflates spontaneously. Complications include infection, displacement of the device and mechanical failure. Some manual dexterity is required. These devices have been in use since 1972. In correctly selected patients this prosthetic sphincter is highly effective (Mundy, 1991).

Incontinence pads continue to play an important role in the management of uncontrolled urinary or faecal incontinence. They are best suited to patients with dementia and severe progressive disability. However, ambulant patients will need to use these devices whilst awaiting a permanent cure. The design, technology, function and performance of incontinence pads have been reviewed with meticulous detail elsewhere (Cottenden *et al.*, 1987b; Cottenden, Malone-Lee and Butchers, 1988). Nowadays, there are some very effective products available, but care needs to be taken when choosing a suitable range. There is now considerable data on which to base an informed judgement of the most suitable products for a service.

Too often decisions on the aids to provide for people are not given sufficient importance and tend to be hurried and ill-conceived. It is worth auditing the criteria adopted by local organizations when purchasing incontinence aids (Cottenden *et al.*, 1987a, b; Cottenden, Malone-Lee and Butchers, 1988)

Permanent indwelling catheters still have a role in the management of some patients. They are not suitable for those with uncontrolled instability or hyperreflexia, since they will cause pain and bypassing. They are best reserved for those with voiding problems, with or without controllable instability, who are unable to manage intermittent catheterization. Urethral catheters in women run the risk of inducing a vesico-vaginal fistula. A **suprapubic catheter** is by far the better option. It is easier to maintain and does not traumatize the urethra. If the bladder is impalpable the suprapubic catheter must be inserted under cystoscopic scrutiny.

Recurrent blocking and infections are complications of permanent catheterization. Anecdotal reports favour the use of vitamin C, 1 g qds, and cranberry juice to combat blockage, but there is no clinical trial data to support this. The former acidifies the urine and the latter reduces the tenacity of mucous. Suby G bladder washouts do protect against blocking. A successful indwelling catheter need be changed only once every 3 months. Asymptomatic bacteriuria should be left untreated.

External sheath drainage is an option in some men. The old cumbersome latex contraptions have given way to penile sheaths, derived from the condom, which are fixed to the penis using adhesives specifically developed for this purpose. The urine drains from a tube connected at the apex of the sheath. The main problem is difficulty in fixation caused by penile retraction. Additionally, some patients have problems with displacement in response to the physical stresses of movement. There is an increased incidence of urinary infection from organisms ascending in the urinary column. Whilst skin ulceration has reduced with the advent of better adhesives, it remains a complication. A retractile penis can be splinted internally by implanting the Small Carrion prosthesis which is normally used for managing erectile failure (Pryor, 1988).

Continence advisors have become a regular part of most continence services. They are usually nurses who have chosen to take a particular interest in managing incontinence and are often referred to as clinical nurse specialists. Unsupported by medical staff their role becomes limited to the administration of the supply of incontinence aids. With medical support they are able to participate substantially in the diagnosis and treatment of the patient population. Their experience is of particular value in screening patients, teaching techniques such as intermittent self-catheterization, providing support to patients with difficult problems and offering preoperative counselling.

REFERENCES

Alcalay, M., Monga, A. and Stanton, S.L. (1995) Burch colposuspension: a 10–20 year follow up. *British Journal of Obstetrics and Gynaecology*, **102** , 740–5.

Andersson, K.E., Holmquist, F., Fovaeus, M. *et al.*, (1991) Muscarinic receptor stimulation of phosphoinositide hydrolysis in the human isolated urinary bladder. *Journal of Urology*, **146**, 1156–9, (abstract).

Battcock, T.M. and Castleden, C.M. (1990) Pharmacological treatment of urinary incontinence. *British Medical Bulletin* **46**, 147–55.

Brading, A.F. and Turner, W.H. (1994) The unstable bladder: towards a common mechanism. *British Journal of Urology*, **73**, 3–8, (abstract).

Brindley, G.S. (1988) Nerve-stimulating implants for bladder control in patients with spinal cord injury or disease, in *Controversies and Innovations in Urological Surgery* (eds C. Gingell and P. Abrams), Springer-Verlag, London, pp. 253–8.

Brindley, G.S., Polkey, C.E., Rushton, D.N. and Cardozo, L.D. (1986) Sacral anterior root stimulators for bladder control in paraplegia: the first 50 cases. *Journal of Neurology, Neurosurgery and Psychiatry*, **49**, 1104–14.

Cammu, H., Van Nylen, M., Derde, M.P. *et al.* (1991) Pelvic physiotherapy in genuine stress incontinence. *Urology*, **38**, 332–7.

Cardozo, L. (1991) Urinary incontinence in women: have we anything new to offer? *British Medical Journal*, **303**, 1453–7.

Castleden, C.M., George, C.F., Renwick, A.G. and Asher, M.J. (1981) Imipramine a possible alternative to current therapy for urinary incontinence in the elderly. *Journal of Urology*, **125**, 318–20.

Cottenden, A.M., Fader, M.J., Barnes, K.E. *et al.* (1987a) The clinical performance of incontinence pads in relation to their design and constitutent materials. *Proceedings of TAPPI*, **1**, pp. 155–68.

Cottenden A.M., Fader, M.J., Barnes, K.E. *et al.* (1987b) The clinical performance of incontinence products in relation to technical testing. *Proceedings of INSIGHT* **2**, 1–30.

Cottenden, A.N., Malone-Lee, J.G. and Butchers, D. (1988) Technical testing and user requirements for adult incontinence products. *Proceedings of INSIGHT*.

Davidsson, T., Barker, S.B. and Mansson, W. (1992) Tapering of intussuscepted ileal nipple valve or ileocecal valve to correct secondary incontinence in patients with urinary reservoir. *Journal of Urology*, **147**, 144–6.

De Groat, W.C. (1995) Neurophysiology of the pelvic organs, in *Handbook of Neuro-Urology*, (ed. D.N. Rushton), Marcel Dekker, New York, pp. 55–93.

DuBeau, C.E. and Resnick, N.M. (1991) Evaluation of the causes and severity of geriatric incontinence. A critical appraisal. *Urological Clinics of North America*, **18**, 243–56.

Eckford, S.D., Swami, K.S., Jackson, S.R. and Abrams, P.H. (1994) Desmopressin in the treatment of nocturia and enuresis in patients with multiple sclerosis. *British Journal of Urology*, **74**, 733–5.

Eglen, R.M., Reddy, H., Watson, N. and Challis, J.R.A. (1994) Muscarinic acetylcholine receptor subtypes in smooth muscle. *Trends in Pharmacological Science*, **15**, 114–9 (abstract).

Fantl, J.A. (1989) Genuine stress incontinence: pathophysiology and rationale for its medical management. *Obstetrics and Gynaecology Clinics of North America*, **16**, 827–40.

Faro, S. (1992) New considerations in treatment of urinary tract infections in adults. *Urology*, **39**, 1–11.

Frewen, W.K. (1982) A reassessment of bladder training in detrusor dysfunction in the female. *British Journal of Urology* **54**, 372–3.

George, V.K., Russell, G.L., Shutt, A. *et al.* (1991) Clam ileocystoplasty. *British Journal of Urology,* **68**, 487–9.

Griffiths, D.J. (1974) The mechanical functions of the bladder and urethra in micturition. *International Journal of Urology and Nephrology,* **6**, 177–82.

Griffiths, D.J. (1980) *Urodynamics: the mechanics and hydrodynamics of the lower urinary tract,* Adam Hilger, Bristol.

Griffiths, D.J., van Mastrigt, R., van Duyl, W.A. and Coolseat, B.L.R.A. (1992) Active mechanical properties of the smooth muscle of the urinary bladder. *Medical and Biological Engineering and Computing,* **17**, 281–90.

Hilton, P. and Stanton, S.L. (1982) The use of Desmopressin (DDAVP) in nocturnal urinary frequency in the female. *British Journal of Urology:* **54**, 252–5.

Holmes, D.M., Montz, F.J. and Stanton, S.L. (1989) Oxybutinin versus propantheline in the management of detrusor instability. A patient-regulated variable dose trial. *British Journal of Obstetrics and Gynaecology,* **96**, 607–12.

Hooton, T.M., Winter, C., Tiu, F. and Stamm, W.E. (1995) Randomized comparative trial and cost analysis of 3 day antimicrobial regiments for treatment of acute cystitis in women. *Journal of the American Medical Association,* **273**, 41–5.

Hooton, T.M. and Stam, W.E. (1991) Management of acute uncomplicated urinary tract infection in adults. *Medical Clinics of North America* **75**, 339–57.

Hoyle, C.H.V., Lincoln, J. and Burnstock, G. (1994) Neural control of pelvic organs, in *Handbook of Neuro-Urology,* (ed. D.N. Rushton), Marcel Dekker, New York, pp. 1–54.

Jarvis, G.J. (1994) Surgery for genuine stress incontinence. *British Journal of Obstetrics and Gynaecology,* **101**, 371–4.

Jarvis, G.J. and Millar, D.R. (1980) Controlled trial of bladder drill for detrusor instability. *British Medical Journal,* **281**, 1322–1333.

Jurgen, W. (1993) Molecular basis of muscarinic acetylcholine receptor function. *Trends in Pharmacological Science,* **14**, 308–13 (abstract).

van der Klauw, M.M., van Rey, F.J. and Stricker, B.H. (1992) Polymorph ventricular tachycardia with torsades de pointes caused by administration of terodiline (Mictrol). *Nederlands Tijdschrift vool Geneeskunde,* **136**, 91–3.

Kuhn, W., Rist, M. and Zaech, G.A. (1991) Intermittent urethral self-catheterisation: long term results (bacteriological evolution, continence, acceptance, complications). *Paraplegia,* **29**, 222–32.

Malone-Lee, J.G. (1992) Incontinence. *Reviews in Clinical Gerontology,* **2**, 45–61.

Malone-Lee, J.G. (1995) The clinical efficacy of oxybutynin. *Reviews in Contemporary Pharmacotherapy,* **5**, 195–202.

Malone-Lee, J.G., Lubel, D. and Szonyi, G. (1992) Low dose oxybutynin for the unstable bladder. *British Medical Journal,* **304**, 1053.

Malone-Lee, J.G., Wagg, A., Mundy, A. *et al.* (1994) Science of urinary incontinence *Lancet,* **344**, 311–15.

Mantle, J. and Versi, E. (1991) Physiotheraphy for stress urinary incontinence: a national survey [see comments] *British Medical Journal,* **302**, 753–5.

Maskell, R. (1995) Management of recurrent urinary tract infections UTI in adults. *Precribing Journal,* **35**, 1–11.

Milani, R., Scalambrino, S., Milia, R. *et al.* (1993) Double-blind cross-over comparison of flavoxate and oxybutynin in women affected by urinary urge syndrome. *International Urogynecology Journal,* **4**, 3–8.

Monga, A. (1994) Female urinary incontinence and gynaecological surgery. *British Journal of Obstetrics and Gynaecology,* **101**, 1096–8.

Montgomery, B.S.I. and Fry, C. (1992) The action potential and net membrane currents in isolated human detrusor smooth muscle cells. *Journal of Urology,* **147** 176–84, (abstract).

Mouritsen, L., Frimodt Moller, C. and Moller, M. (1991) Long-term effect of pelvic floor exercises on female urinary incontinence. *British Journal of Urology,* **68**, 32–7.

Mundy, A.R. (1991) Artificial sphincters. *British Journal of Urology,* **67**, 225–9.

Naerger, H., Fry, C.H. and Nilvebrant, L. (1995) Effect of Tolterodine on electrically induced contractions of isolated human detrusor muscle from stable and unstable bladders. *Neurourology and Urodynamics,* **14**, 76–7.

Nilvebrant, L., Stahl, M. and Andersson, K.E. (1995) Interaction of Tolterodine with cholinergic muscarinic receptors in human detrusor. *Neurourology and Urodynamics,* **14**, 75–6.

Norlen, L.J., Philipson, B.M. and Kock, N.G. (1988) The continent ileal reservoir (Kock Pouch) in urinary diversion, *Controversies and Innovations in Urological Surgery* (eds C. Gingell and P. Abrams), Springer-Verlag, London, pp. 271–81.

Palfrey, E.L.H., Fry, C.H. and Shuttleworth, K.E.D. (1984) A new *in vitro* perfusion technique for the investigation of human detrusor muscle. *British Journal of Urology,* **56**, 635–40.

Pappas, P.G. (1991) Laboratory in the diagnosis and management of urinary tract infections. *Medical Clinics of North America*, **75**, 313–325.

Pearman, J.W., Bailey, M. and Riley, L.P. (1991) Bladder instillations of trisdine compared with catheter introducer for reduction of bacteriuria during intermittent catheterization of patients with acute spinal cord trauma. *British Journal of Urology*, **67**, 483–90.

Pryor, J.P. (1988) Penile prostheses, in *Controversies and Innovations in Urological Surgery* (eds C. Gingell and P. Abrams), Springer-Verlag, London, pp. 365–72.

Rosario, D.J., Leaker, B.R., Smith, D.J. and Chapple, C.R. (1995) A pilot study of the effects of multiple doses of the M3 muscarinic receptor antagonist darifenasin on ambulatory parameters of detrusor activity in patients with detrusor instability. *Neurourology and Urodynamics*, **14**, 36–7.

Shull, B.L. (1991) Urologic surgical techniques. *Current Opinions in Obstetrics and Gynecology*, **3**, 534–40.

Stamey, A. (1987) Recurrent urinary tract infections in female patients: an overview of management and treatment. *Reviews of Infectious Diseases*, **9**, S195–208.

Stamm, W.E. (1988) Protocol for diagnosis of urinary tract infection: reconsidering the criterion for significant bacteriuria. *Urology*, **32**, 6–25.

Szonyi, G., Collas, D.M., Ding, Y.Y. and Malone-Lee, J.G. (1995) Oxybutynin with bladder retraining for detrusor instability in elderly people: a randomized controlled trial. *Age and Ageing*, **24** 287–91.

Thomas, T.M., Flymat, K.R., Blannin, J. and Meade, T.W. (1980) The prevalence of urinary incontinence. *British Medical Journal* **281**, 1243–5.

Thuroff, J.W., Bunke, B., Ebner, A. *et al.* (1991) Randomized, double-blind, multicentre trial on treatment of frequency, urgency and incontinence related to detrusor hyperactivity: oxybutynin versus propantheline versus placebo. *Journal of Urology*, **145**, 813–17.

Wells, T.J., Buick, C.A. and Diokno, A.C. (1991) Pelvic muscle exercises for stress incontinence in elderly women. *Journal of the American Geriatrics Society*, **39**, 785–91.

Wijma, J., Tinga, D.J. and Visser, G.H. (1991) Perineal ultrasonography in women with stress incontinence and controls: the role of the pelvic floor muscles. *Gynecologic and Obstetric Investigation*, **32**, 176–9.

Wiseman, P.A., Malone Lee, J. and Rai, G.S. (1991) Terodiline with bladder retraining for treating detrusor instability in elderly people. *British Medical Journal* **302**, 994–6.

Wu, C.U., Kentish, K.J. and Fry, C.H. (1994) The effects of pH on Ca^{2+} activated force in 2-toxin permealised detrusor smooth muscle isolated from guinea-pig bladder. *Journal of Physiology*, **477**, 42.

Yarker, Y.E., Goa, K.L. and Fitton, A. (1995) Oxybutynin: a review of its pharmacodynamic and pharmacokinetic properties, and its therapeutic use in detrusor instability. *Drugs and Aging*, **6**, 243–62.

FURTHER READING

Report of Royal College of Physicians (1995) *Incontinence: management and provision of services*, Royal College of Physicians, London.

USEFUL ADDRESS

Association for Continence Advice,
Winchester House, Kennington Park, Cranmer Road, The Oval, London, SW9 6EJ, UK. Tel: 0171 820 8113.

36 *The maintenance of tissue viability*

E. McClemont, H. Henderson and J. Phillips

INTRODUCTION

Pressure sores are localized areas of dead or devitalized tissue resulting either from direct pressure on the skin causing pressure ischaemia or from shearing forces causing mechanical stress to the tissues. They are painful, unsightly, difficult to treat and costly, both in terms of human suffering and finance. Their occurrence is still all too frequent a complication of illness or deterioration, especially in the old or neurologically compromised.

EPIDEMIOLOGY

Pressure sores typically occur in severely disabled, elderly, immobile, unconscious or paraplegic patients, especially in the presence of toxaemia or malnutrition. The formation of a pressure sore is a complex process involving many factors. The pathophysiology remains poorly understood. The state of the patient and their illness, and the condition of the superficial tissues are important intrinsic variables. Unphysiological loads acting on the skin and subcutaneous tissues are also major causes of the initiation of tissue damage.

Pressure sores most often occur in people with disabilities at two specific times in the course of their illness. At the onset of acute disability as in spinal injury, paralysing infection or tumour, the damage can occur whilst attention focuses on lifesaving measures or diagnostic procedures. The rehabilitation process is then delayed while sores heal, adding to the burden of disability (Figure 36.1).

Later in the course of disability, an alteration in the circumstances of the patient adapted to his/her altered tissue viability may lead to the occurrence of pressure sores. Physical problems such as intercurrent infection, weight loss or increased spasticity, or the strain of moving a disabled body with increasing age, are common causes of pressure sores. Psychological problems such as family bereavement, depression or a changed daily routine may alter the constant vigilance necessary for pressure sore prevention and leave an additional burden for the individual to bear. Hospitalization can lead to sores when staff are not prepared to listen to care needs.

Amongst younger patients, sores are commonest in multiple sclerosis, spinal injury and spina bifida, although as disability and age increases, rheumatoid arthritis and diabetes begin to cause problems, when intercurrent illness or exacerbation of disease occurs. Children with disabilities rarely suffer from sores, although the author remembers a girl with spina bifida who sat for longer than her able-bodied school mates on a hot classroom radiator with disastrous consequences.

Rehabilitation of the Physically Disabled Adult. Edited by C. John Goodwill, M. Anne Chamberlain and Chris Evans. Published in 1997 by Stanley Thornes (Publishers) Ltd, Cheltenham. ISBN 0-7487-3183-0.

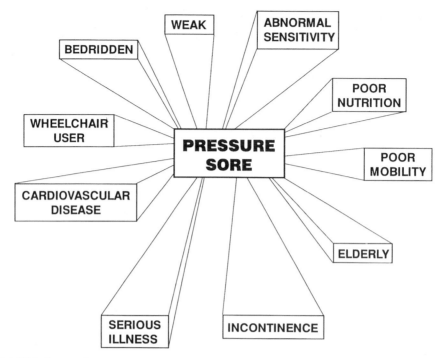

Figure 36.1 Risk factors for pressure sores.

Particular attention must be paid to the fitting of new boots or orthoses (calipers) and the application of plaster of Paris or splints after surgery. Equally hazardous are hot water bottles on a cold winter evening or untested bath water.

Extent of the problem

The incidence and prevalence of pressure sores increases with age, the majority occurring in people over 60 years. Prevalence rates of 30–40% are not uncommon for elderly care units and incidence rates as high as 66% have been recorded for elderly patients with fractured neck of the femur (Versluysen, 1986). A survey of hospital patients showed a prevalence of 18.6% (O'Dea, 1993), whilst a Health Authority survey found a figure of 9.6% over all units (Bond, 1993).

In a survey of 50 well-documented cases of deaths in patients attending the Stoke Mande-ville Spinal Injuries Unit between 1964 and 1980, 47 had pressure sores, 36 being present on admission to the Unit from another hospital. Twenty patients had sores for more than two-thirds of their clinical lifetime. Death from renal amyloid due to pressure sore sepsis was a major cause (Baker, Silver and Tudway, 1984).

Many authorities have tried to establish the extent of the pressure sore problem. Some measure incidence, others prevalence. Some include minor sores, others do not. Even consensus about pressure sore classification and grading has not been achieved (National Pressure Ulcer Advisory Panel, 1989). Until consensus is reached about the definition and inclusion of Stage 1 damage, it will remain difficult to establish a footing on which to base clinical outcomes, audit and research.

There is also a need to standardize routine data collection in respect of pressure sores. It is important to establish incidence studies, not just prevalence, as this will highlight development of new sores. This should be done as part of a general quality assessment process. Data needs to be collected which recognizes at-risk patients and this information passed on to all involved in their care. Information on the presence of pressure sores or the risk of their development should also be included on all medical and nursing discharge summaries. Increasing awareness in this way should be a positive factor in procuring required resources for prevention and management rather than a negative criticism, implying failure of care, (Dealey, 1995).

As the costs of health care increase and resources become limited, managers are becoming increasingly aware of the huge financial costs of pressure sores and the necessity to invest in prevention. The estimated lowest cost of treating pressure sores is £180 million in English hospitals and more than $3 billion in the USA. This, and the growing numbers of cases of successful litigation for pressure damage against hospitals, has finally taken pressure sores out of the 'nursing problem' category and made it everybody's business. The cost of treating a single, deep pressure sore in hospital has been estimated at £25,000 (West and Priestley, 1994) and an extra £340 000 to the average district hospital over 1 year. In one of the few community studies (Preston, 1991) excess annual costs, based on additional visits by district nurses, were put at between £100 000 and £200 000 for the treatment group visited. Whatever the true figures, it is all too apparent that scarce resources could be better spent with consequent immeasurable improvement in the quality of life for people with disabilities.

AETIOLOGY AND PHYSIOLOGY

It is well established that a combination of intrinsic and extrinsic factors leads to the development of pressure sores (Table 36.1). The most critical are prolonged downward

Table 36.1 Factors causing pressure sores

Intrinsic	Disease, medication, malnourishment, age, dehydration, lack of mobility, incontinence, skin condition, weight
Extrinsic	External influences causing: skin distortion, pressure, shear, friction

pressure causing capillary occlusion and hence ischaemia, friction, shear or a combination of all three.

Pressure causes tissue necrosis from impaired capillary perfusion. There is no evidence that a critical closing pressure analogous to the capillary blood pressure of 32 mm Hg at the arteriole end can be identified. Higher pressures undoubtedly produce more disruption of the microcirculation and reduce the time needed for tissue necrosis to occur. Surface pressure causing local capillary occlusion, with resulting ischaemia and tissue necrosis, has been described as a Type One pressure sore (Barton and Barton, 1981).

There are various definitions of types, stages or grades of pressure sores; it is perhaps best to use the grades defined in the Effective Health Bulletin:

Grade 1   Discoloration of intact skin, including non-blanchable erythema, blue/purple and black discoloration.

Grade 2   Partial-thickness skin loss or damage involving epidermis and/or dermis.

Grade 3   Full-thickness skin loss involving damage or necrosis of subcutaneous tissues; but not through the underlying fascia and not extending to the underlying bone, tendon or joint capsule.

Grade 4   Full-thickness skin loss with extensive destruction, and tissue necrosis extending to the underlying bone, tendon or joint capsule.

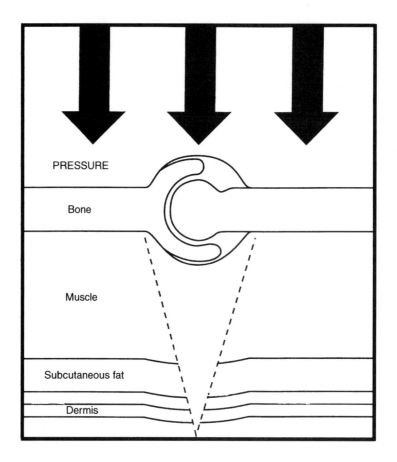

PRESSURE

Bone

Muscle

Subcutaneous fat

Dermis

Figure 36.2 Cone of pressure.

Interface pressure is the only variable that has been routinely measured and shown to be of practical importance, although it is important to realize that capillary closing pressure varies from patient to patient regardless of interface pressure. (Burman and O'Dea, 1994). Simple electropneumatic or fluid-filled sensors may be constructed in sheets to produce pressure mapping systems, which can be used to evaluate different support surfaces such as cushions or mattresses (Barbanel and Sockalingham, 1990) (Figure 36.2).

Shear and friction can be generated by patients, attendants or gravity and sacral sores have been shown to develop more readily when the head of the bed is raised. Lower pressures can result in tissue damage if friction is also present. The subcutaneous fat lacks tensile strength and is particularly susceptible to these shearing forces.

The **general condition** of ageing skin, with its loss of subcutaneous tissue, diminished pain perception, slowed wound healing and altered barrier properties, is fundamental to the problem. Combined with impaired mobility, poor mental state or reduced sensation, the effect of pressure on compromised tissues will be increased. Elderly stroke patients or those with orthopaedic injury, such as hip fracture, anaemia or diabetes, are thus particularly at risk.

Poor nutrition is frequently present in patients with pressure sores (Dickerson and Wright, 1986). Following starvation prior to theatre and sedation with analgesia afterwards, the elderly patient may be in serious negative nitrogen balance. Cancer cachexia, prolonged pyrexia or hypermetabolic states also prevent efficient cellular repair, whilst the chronic inflammation and infection due to the sore itself will aggravate the hypoproteinaemia and anaemia (McLaren, 1992).

Tissue oxygenation is vital to healthy tissue and depends on efficient oxygenation in the lungs and an adequate circulating haemoglobin. Patients with arterial disease are especially prone to develop sores and hypotension from any cause must be considered an at risk factor.

PREVENTION

Prevention and management of pressure damage must not be regarded as solely a nursing responsibility. (North Lincolnshire Pressure Sores Policy, 1990)

Prevention is the main aim of anyone involved in pressure sore management, although this may not be the cheap option it has been promoted as being in the past.

The Touche Ross report showed prevention programmes to be as costly as treatment, benefits only being apparent when the physical and psychological damage to the patient, the cost of possible litigation and the releasing of resources (beds, staff, equipment) were also considered (Touche Ross, 1993).

The three essentials for a successful prevention and management programme are:

1. A comprehensive policy relevant to the area where it is to be implemented.
2. An on-going interdisciplinary education programme.
3. Management commitment to the provision of resources.

Policy

An interdisciplinary group should compile the policy with particular reference to all areas handling at-risk patients; for example, X-ray department, emergency services and theatres. The policy should include all physiological factors such as sleep, nutrition and wound healing. Standards within policies also provide a means of auditing performance and compliance with the policy. Historically, pressure sores have been seen as a result of bad nursing. Fortunately, as knowledge of causative factors has increased, more disciplines have become involved in prevention strategies, but there are still pockets of resistance where people refuse to consider the full aetiology.

Risk assessment

Nursing assessment for identifying at-risk patients should be the first step in planned management. Many tools exist, including the Norton, Braden-Bergstrom, Waterlow (Figure 36.3 and Table 36.2), Andersen, Knoll, Douglas and Goswell assessment scales (Effective Health Care Bulletin, 1995), but not all of them are validated (Clark and Farrar, 1991). Indeed it has been stated that 'the evidence on the accuracy of pressure sore risk scales is confusing' (Effective Health Care Bulletin, 1995). Some do not consider key factors such as nutrition, others have been criticized for over or under-predicting. Choosing a tool should include looking at its reliability and validity as well as the patient groups to be assessed. These are only tools, however, and should be used in conjunction with professional judgement of the care team, particularly if risk factor is being matched to choice of pressure-relieving equipment. Bridel (1994) looks at some of the issues related to these tools, and summary of the more commonly used ones can be found in the Effective Health Care Bulletin (1995)

Managers and staff need to recognize the

Waterlow pressure sore prevention / treatment policy
Ring scores in table, add total.   Several scores per category can be used

BUILD/WEIGHT FOR HEIGHT		SKIN TYPE VISUAL RISK AREAS		SEX AGE			SPECIAL RISKS	
AVERAGE	0	HEALTHY	0	MALE	1		TISSUE MALNUTRITION	
ABOVE AVERAGE	1	TISSUE PAPER	1	FEMALE	2			
OBESE	2	DRY	1	14-49	1		E.G.:TERMINAL CACHEXIA	8
BELOW AVERAGE	3	OEDEMATOUS	1	50-64	2		CARDIAC FAILURE	5
		CLAMMY (TEMP)	1	65-74	3		PERIPHERAL VASCULAR	
		DISCOLOURED	2	75-80	4		DISEASE	5
CONTINENCE		BROKEN/SPOT	3	81+	5		ANAEMIA	2
							SMOKING	1
COMPLETE/ CATHETERISED	0	MOBILITY		APPETITE			NEUROLOGICAL DEFICIT	
OCCASION INCONT.	1	FULLY	0					
CATH/INCONTINENT OF FAECES	2	RESTLESS/ FIDGETY	1	AVERAGE	0		e.g.: DIABETES, M.S.,CVA,	
DOUBLY INCONT.	3	APATHETIC	2	POOR N.G. TUBE/	1		MOTOR/SENSORY	4-6
		RESTRICTED	3	FLUIDS ONLY	2		PARAPLEGIA	
© J. Waterlow 1988		INERT/TRACTION	4	NBM/ANOREXIC	3		MAJOR SURGERY/	
		CHAIRBOUND	5				TRAUMA	

SCORE	10+ AT RISK	15+ HIGH RISK	20+ VERY HIGH RISK

ORTHOPAEDIC- BELOW WAIST, SPINAL ON TABLE>2 HOURS	5 5
MEDICATION	
STEROIDS, CYTOTOXICS, HIGH DOSE ANTI-INFLAMMATORY	4

OBTAINABLE FROM: NEWTONS, CURLAND, TAUNTON, TA3 5SG

PEGASUS
A I R W A V E

Presented by Pegasus Airwave Ltd.
Pegasus House, Kingscroft Court, Havant, Hants. PO9 1LS
Telephone: 0705 451444. Fax: 0705 4511121

REMEMBER: TISSUE DAMAGE OFTEN STARTS PRIOR TO ADMISSION, IN CASUALTY.

ASSESSMENT   IF THE PATIENT FALLS INTO ANY OF THE RISK CATEGORIES THEN PREVENTATIVE
(see Over)   NURSING IS REQUIRED. A COMBINATION OF GOOD NURSING TECHNIQUES AND
                 PREVENTATIVE AIDS WILL DEFINITELY BE NECESSARY.

PREVENTION:
PREVENTATIVE AIDS:
Special Mattress/Bed...   10+ Water Mattresses, e.g. Dyson, Topper   Mechanical Aids:........ Real sheepskin-sacral, heel/
                          Spenco, Vaperm.   elbow pads, e.g. `pegasus Lamb
                          15+ Large cell ripple, e.g. Huntleigh, Water beds.   Pads. Gel-Protection Bed Cradle
                          20+ Pegasus Airwave, Clinitron, Mediscuc.

Chair:.................................Correct for patient protection-sides/seats,   Patient Aids:.............. Monkey Pole Hand Lifts
                          movement, e.g.: Nestor, Roho.

Bed Clothing:........................ i) Cotten cellular blanket   Operating Table/   e.g.:'Moulding Top'
                          ii) Duvet   Theatre Trolley:.......... Topper
                          iii) Vapour permeable draw sheet Bead pillow

NURSING CARE: .... Pain control   Skin Care: ....General Hygiene, NO rubbing.
                          Turning   Prevent shearing force damage
                          Passive movements   e.g.: correct lifting & positioning
                          Nutrition-High protein, minerals, vitamins   Dress with inert covering e.g. Opsite

IF TREATMENT IS REQUIRED, FIRST REMOVE PRESSURE
WOUND CLASSIFICATION:

BLANCHING HYPERAEMIA	STAGE 1	is wound RED?	→ YES	Semi-occlusive dressing e.g. Opsite
NON-BLANCHING HYPERAEMIA	STAGE II	is wound RED, clean but not healed?	→ YES	Granuflex, Scherisorb, Sorbsan, Silastic Foam (deep)
ULCERATION PROGRESSES	STAGE III	is wound YELLOW/ infected/inflamed?	→ YES	Sorbsan, Scherisorb, Debrisan Silastic Foam, Granuflex
ULCERATION EXTENDS	STAGE IV	Infected?	→ YES	Sorbsan Packing, Iodosorb, Actisorb, Flammazine (for pseudomonas), Debrisan.
INFECTIVE NECROSIS	STAGE V	is wound BLACK/ Necrotic?	→ YES	Debride-surgical excision saline swabs, Granuflex, Scherisorb.

Figure 36.3 Waterlow risk assessment scoring system.

Table 36.2 Use of risk calculators for development of pressure sores

Score[a]	Category	Proportion of study population	Incidence of pressure sores
<10	Not at risk	50%	0%
10–14	At risk	26%	15%
15–19	High risk	16%	41%
20+	Very high risk	8%	66%

[a]Related to Waterlow Risk Assessment Scoring System.

limitations of any chosen methodology and ensure that information obtained results in action rather than mere recording.

Equipment

They spent a fortune hiring this expensive bed, but they sat me in a chair all day, and I still got a pressure sore. (Department of Health, 1993)

Providing equipment has not been shown on its own to reduce pressure sores, however highly technical. Education is needed on Who?, How?, When? and Where? to use equipment. This also results in effective use of resources. Lack of clinical trials has been identified as a problem with equipment and certainly manufacturers could do more to address this. But good quality new equipment may be missed if this is rigidly applied as a purchasing pre-requisite. More relevant would be that a small interdisciplinary group select equipment based on the patient's needs using established criteria (Young 1990):

- effectiveness
- ease of use
- maintenance
- ease of nursing procedures
- cost.

All areas should have as a minimum good pressure relieving mattresses. Cushions for sitting patients are also essential. After this, choice from the ever increasing number of systems should be determined by the patient group and selection team. Disabled patients in particular need to be individually assessed for lying and sitting surfaces if problems are to be avoided. Maintenance of electrical mattresses is extremely important and must be considered along with the purchase price. Purchase or leasing of equipment is often more cost-effective than hiring. Good liaison with other providers of equipment, for example wheelchair services for wheelchair cushions, is essential.

Education

Education and training is probably the single most effective way of reducing the incidence of pressure sores. (Department of Health, 1993)

An education programme alone, without any other changes, has been shown to reduce the incidence of pressure sores in elderly patients by 63% (Moody *et al.*, 1988). For any prevention strategy to work, education of all disciplines is essential. This needs to be on-going to allow for staff changes and also to combat the change resisters who operate throughout the health field. Carers and patients also need to be included in the education programme, which should include practical advice on moving and handling. In addition, educational programmes need to be developed for the private and voluntary sectors and social services staff. Education needs to be available in many forms – lectures, updating sessions, leaflets and videos are all necessary. Policies need to state clearly how staff are to receive education – mandatory annual lectures or link nurse systems are both possible methods.

Although not universally accepted, the specialist advisor role properly utilized provides the educator – this should be the main part of the role – and a person who can liaise with the different groups, purchasing, policy makers, managers and carers, to provide an effective cohesive service for pressure sore prevention and management. They facilitate and enable others to improve their practice and thereby reduce the incidence of pressure sores by taking ownership of the problem and developing good multidisciplinary team working. Liaison between services is particularly important if discharge planning is to be effective in reducing pressure damage (Figure 36.4).

MEDICAL MANAGEMENT

This is based upon three principles:

1. improving tissue resistance to pressure;
2. preventing further skin damage;
3. eliminating damaging pressure.

The viability of the skin and its ability to withstand insults is often compromised further at times of ill-health. Practices such as routine sedation or prolonged periods of starvation before theatre are to be avoided and close attention paid to fluid balance, nutritional state and cardiac output. Anaemia

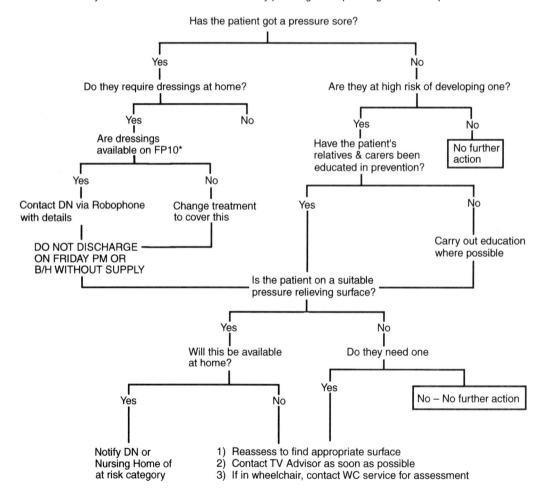

Figure 36.4 Pressure damage discharge list.

must be corrected – the haemoglobin level must be at least 10 g/dl if wound healing is to occur. Specific medical problems such as diabetes or infection should be rapidly brought under control. Meticulous attention to skin care and hygiene is imperative. Skin can be damaged by contact with urine and faeces and delay in attending to any soiling is harmful. Any lifting or handling of the patient must be done without shearing or friction and all members of the health care team must be aware of good practice.

Further pressure damage can be avoided by careful planning and management. Agreement must be reached on the length of periods spent out of bed, and equipment found which is appropriate for visits to X-ray and other departments. An audit of sores found patients sitting in dayrooms whilst expensive hired mattresses lay empty on their beds (McClemont and Phillips, 1993). Medical management of sores is a team approach. Listening to the opinion of the disabled patient with the sore is often a salutary experience, but too often that opinion goes unheard.

Dressings

Dressings are an aid to wound healing which will assist the process providing all other factors have also been considered, such as nutrition and treating or removing the cause of the wound. The concept of moist wound healing should now have been embraced by all professionals and is supported by research and clinical trials (Simpson, 1987).

The ideal wound dressing is one which:

1. absorbs exudate;
2. maintains high humidity but is not wet;
3. allows gaseous exchange;
4. demonstrates impermeability to microorganisms;
5. insulates the wound from low temperatures;
6. keeps the wound free from particulate contamination.

Table 36.3 Choosing a dressing

Wound type	Aim	Dressing
Necrotic	Rehydrate and debride	Hydrocolloid or hydrogel
Sloughy	Rehydrate and deslough	Hydrogel: hydrocellular foam
Granulating	Promote re-epithelialization	Alginate: hydrocolloid: hydrocellular foam

The choice of modern dressings is extensive and increasing all the time, and it is best practice to become familiar with a selection from a comprehensive guide to the many which are available (Thomas, 1994). To rationalize usage and choice, a wound protocol based on clinical research and devised by a multidisciplinary group can be a useful tool. For this wounds should be divided into categories, the type of wound influencing the choice of dressing (Table 36.3).

Additionally, factors such as pain, amount of exudate, control of odour and infection need to be taken into account. All malodorous wounds are not infected, but are often treated unnecessarily with antibiotics. Wound swabs are generally a waste of time, as pressure sores are open wounds colonized with bacteria. Only if spreading cellulitis or systemic signs of infection are present should swabs be taken and systemic antibiotics given. Malodorous wounds will cease to smell as soon as the slough or necrotic tissue is removed. Some control can be provided by carbon dressings (not available in the community) or oral administration of metronidazole.

A knowledge of the stages of wound healing is essential for anyone prescribing or using dressings and will help in correct selection. An argument often presented against modern dressings is their cost, when in reality it is inappropriate dressing choice which is the problem. A hydrocolloid dressing which requires changing daily represents a poor and expensive choice of dressing for that wound and patient. One which remains *in situ* for 3 days or more shows appropriate use. Use of gauze next to granulating and epithelializing wounds should no longer be sanctioned, whether dry or wet, as it achieves none of the criteria for an ideal wound dressing and on removal frequently tears away the newly formed capillary buds within the tissues which are attempting to heal. It is also often painful for the patients, requiring warm soaks, analgesia or Entonox before the dressing can be changed, indicating a highly questionable quality of care, especially when modern pain-free alternatives exist.

A problem which still exists is restrictions on dressings available on the Drug Tariff in the UK. With more patients being discharged early into the community with unhealed pressure sores, as well as other wounds and pressure sores acquired in the primary care setting, this anomaly compromises the patient and his/her care.

SURGICAL APPROACH TO PRESSURE SORES

In the past, the interest of the reconstructive surgeons has focused on the state of the sore and the technical problems of the type of plastic surgery needed to close the wound securely. Follow-up studies of recurrence rates have attempted to relate the speed and frequency of breakdown following surgery to the type of repair, rather than the non-surgical preventative measures in the postoperative recovery period.

Pressure damage can be compared to a high-speed bullet wound injury on a slow time scale. Prolonged pressure causes damage beyond the immediate macroscopic injury, with the pressure sore as the central zone of concentric rings of pressure damage.

Relief of pressure allows the outer rings of pressure damage to recover, but this may take several weeks. Thus, the timing of surgery must take account of the amount of hidden healing that has been achieved since pressure relief was first instituted. There are two types of surgery which may be synchronous if appropriate. The first is thorough debridement, the second is repair and reconstruction.

Debridement

Debridement means the surgical removal of dead tissue. This may simply require the lifting of a skin scab with a pair of forceps or the use of a pair of scissors to cut through the remaining tethering fibres of a chunk of slough. At times a major operation to cut out all tissue of dubious viability with a scalpel, together with shaving of bony prominences with osteotomes and bone instruments, is needed as a separate event, but in most cases adequate debridement can be achieved in the bed in the ward (Figures 36.5 and 36.6). The purpose of debridement is to enhance contraction and healing of the wound. The surgeon should be called in when the wound has been debrided and is cleaning up well.

Debridement has to be radical if there has been only a short time allowed for recovery of the outer zones of pressure damage to recover. If the type of repair is one which introduces new blood supply to the pressure sore area, as with a healthy muscle flap, the debridement may not need to be quite so radical because the new blood supply provided by the flap helps the outer zones of damage to recover more quickly. Debridement can be life-saving in that an infected pressure sore containing a large mass of infected material may be the source of bacteraemia and septicaemia and it should then be done under appropriate antibiotic cover.

All sores are, to a greater or lesser extent,

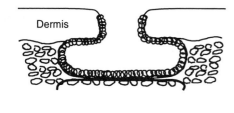

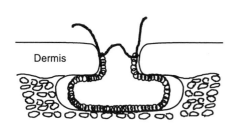

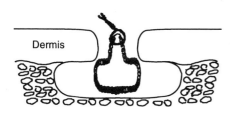

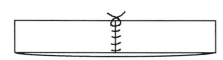

Figure 36.5 The Guttman method of treating the sore and its granulation tissue as though it were a malignant tumour – excising all of it.

contaminated by organisms. The bacteria which surgeons worry about most are the Streptococci Lancefield Group A and *Pseudomonas* which interfere with wound healing and can ruin any surgical repair. Methicillin-resistant Staphylococcus aureus (MRSA) organisms are an increasing hazard in the European scene and attempts to get rid of this organism before repair should be strenuous. MRSA may linger in slough and may only be controlled once thorough debridement has been carried out.

Recent publicity focusing on the dangers of synergistic gangrene has led to the referral of several cases of Grade 4 pressure sores as possible examples of synergistic gangrene. Patients with synergistic gangrene are usually very much sicker and show evidence of crepitus around the wound and have no history of pressure damage. Most cases follow routine abdominal surgery.

PHILOSOPHY OF SURGERY OF PRESSURE SORES

There are two main types of pressure sore patient referred for surgery. Firstly, the patient without permanent physical deformity or loss of function who develops a sore when very ill or injured. Such mobile individuals do not have an underlying problem of wound healing and almost any form of surgical repair will achieve wound healing. The emphasis with such a patient must be speedy debridement and repair, with consideration given to the cosmetic result and minimal sacrifice of functional muscles to effect the repair. No special effort will be needed to ensure future prevention, provided recovery from the initial precipitating illness occurs.

The second type of patient has a chronic underlying illness or disability such as paraplegia, multiple sclerosis, stroke, head injury, rheumatoid disease or terminal cancer and usually develops pressure sores because of intercurrent illness or complications. Thus

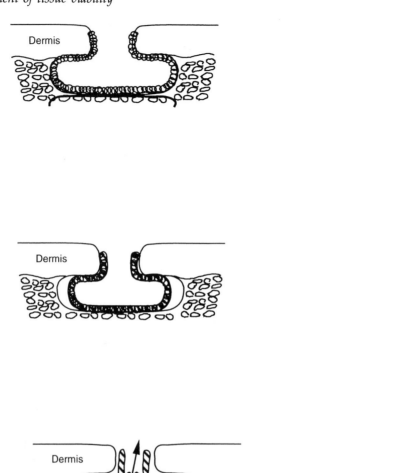

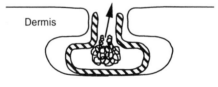

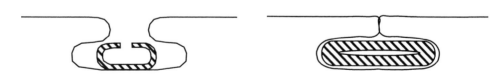

Figure 36.6 Preservation of the lining fibrous base and walls of the sore, but removal of the lining granulation tissue. This preserves padding and base.

surgery in this context can be viewed as a minor part of the overall care of the patient and should be resorted to only when proper conservative forms of therapy and prevention have been instituted.

The monetary costs of surgery are equivalent to approximately 2–3 weeks of bed occupation in a British hospital and so becomes cost effective if more than this length of time can be saved. Nevertheless, the risks of surgery are greater than conservative treatment and the psychological toll of surgery which fails to achieve closure of a pressure sore is considerable. Once a patient has undergone surgery there will be fewer options open if there is a recurrence of the sore and so it is imperative that the patient and carers do not gain the impression that surgery is an easy option and an answer to suboptimal preventative measures.

SURGICAL APPROACHES

Nearly all pressure sores will heal spontaneously if pressure is relieved. However, the speed with which they do this is often so slow, or the quality of the scar following spontaneous healing so poor, that surgery offers a quicker and more secure wound repair which is cost and comfort effective.

The authors' preference is for an operation when the wound shows signs of healing and is starting to contract. There may be evidence of re-epithelialization at the margins and the amount of discharge and exudate from the wound is lessening. Healthy granulation tissue is present in the wound.

Under these circumstances healing of a surgical wound can be expected, whereas an operation at a much earlier stage before evidence of granulation tissue and wound contraction requires much more radical debridement and a more complicated repair. This may run a high risk of wound dehiscence.

The range of plastic surgery repairs for the different types of sore have increased in the last decade with increasing knowledge of the anatomy of the blood supply of the skin via the underlying muscles.

Pressure sores can be closed by direct apposition of the margins of the wound, but this frequently leads to rapid breakdown once pressure is re-applied to the area because of the relatively weak scar tissue and poorly vascularized supporting tissue. Wounds can be closed by shifting the better vascularized adjacent soft tissues, either skin and fat, or muscle, skin and fat, into the wound. Thus, a large sacral sore is often best closed by rotating a segment of a circle of skin and fat adjacent to it in the form of a rotation flap

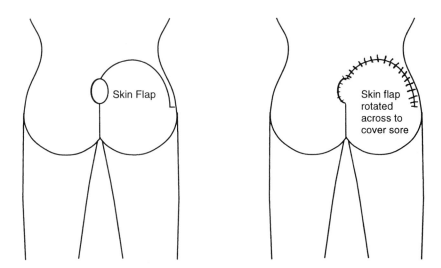

Figure 36.7 Sacral sore excised and repaired by a large rotation flap.

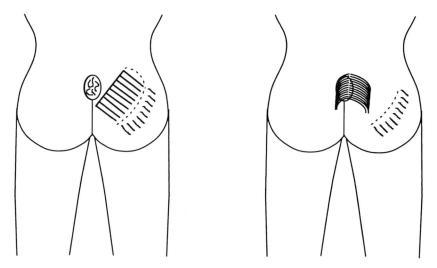

Figure 36.8 Sacral sore. Turnover flap of gluteus maximus muscle. This can be covered by a skin flap or skin graft.

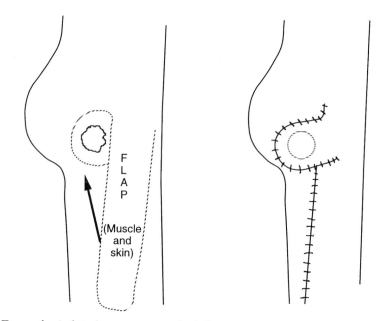

Figure 36.9 Tensor fascia lata (myocutaneous flap) flap to cover a trochanteric sore.

(Figure 36.7). Sometimes it is necessary and worthwhile to incorporate part of the gluteus maximus muscle in this procedure (Figure 36.8).

A trochanteric wound is often best closed by swinging part of the tensor fascia lata myocutaneous flap into the wound after thorough debridement and removal of the outer part of the greater trochanter (Figure 36.9).

An ischial sore is often the most difficult sore to close successfully and may require

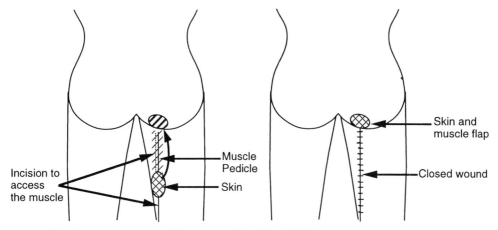

Figure 36.10 Gracilis myocutaneous flap to resurface the ischial sore.

transfer of muscle or muscle and skin from the posterior thigh up into the wound (Figure 36.10).

A further alternative technique of closure for shallow wounds with no overhanging margins is simple split skin grafting. This presupposes that the wound will not be subject to frictional forces afterwards and may, therefore, be appropriate for pressure sores which have developed in the less classical sites, such as the back of the head, the chest wall and the knee area.

Heel and ankle sores are often the most difficult of all to treat surgically because of the paucity of local skin flaps available to resurface the area. The only alternative may be complex operations involving free tissue transfer and microvascular surgery which may be totally inappropriate in the elderly and infirm who can withstand a prolonged operation less easily. If the ulcer is very painful and not capable of healing, amputation may be necessary.

Where there is an inherent problem in wound healing, such as rheumatoid arthritis or vasculitis, intravenous prostacylin may sometimes be effective. This gives brief restoration of the normal processes of wound healing for a sufficient time to get skin grafts to take, or wounds to heal. Other physical agents have included hyperbaric oxygen, ultrasound and electrotherapy.

SOME SUGGESTIONS FOR PHYSICIANS NEEDING SURGICAL HELP

1. Show the surgeon that the cause of the sore has been established and that appropriate measures have been taken to try and prevent recurrence of this.
2. The patient's overall general health should be improved as far as possible.
3. The help of a dietitian should be sought if appropriate.
4. The patient's haemoglobin and protein level should be restored to normal as far as possible.
5. A wound swab should be taken and show absence of MRSA or other important pathogens.

Note: The type of dressing of the wound in the early stages of slough formation is largely irrelevant and only becomes important once debridement has been completed.

Invite the surgeon to see the patient and to inspect the wound once these measures have been instituted so that he/she can make any additional suggestions and plan ahead for the timing of any surgery, including order of the special pressure relieving equipment for his ward or the operating theatre. Agreement must also be reached about responsibility for postoperative care.

Sinograms and X-rays of bony prominences may help determine the extent of likely surgery, but simple probing of a wound is usually sufficient to indicate the direction of a sinus or a cavity. The injection of methylene blue into a sinus at the time of surgery is the most effective way of locating it and ensuring its complete removal.

Occasionally X-rays show the presence of bony sequestra which will need removal, or osteitis which will require bone to be shaved down until healthy, bleeding, cancellous bone is achieved.

The development of a recurrence of a sore after surgery is an indictment of the care plan for that person which must be the responsibility of all the medical carers, not least the surgeons and physicians looking after the patient.

REFERENCES

Baker, J., Silver, J. and Tudway A. (1984) Late complications of pressure sores. *Care, Science and practice*, **3**, 56–9.

Barbenel J. and Sockalingham S. (1990) A device for measuring soft tissue interface pressure *Journal of Biomedical Engineering*, **12**, 519–20.

Barton, A.A. and Barton, M. (1981) *The Management and Prevention of Pressure Sores*, Faber & Faber, London.

Bond, M. (1993) North Derbyshire Health Authority pressure sore survey. *Journal of Tissue Viability*, **3**, 114–22.

Bridel, J. (1994) Risk assessment. *Journal of Tissue Viability*, **4**, 84–5.

Burman, O. and O'Dea, K. (1994) Measuring pressure. *Journal of Wound Care*, **3**, 83–6.

Clark, M. and Farrar, S. (1991) *Comparison of Pressure Sore Risk Calculators*. Proceedings of 1st European Conference of Wound Management. MacMillan, Basingstoke.

Dealey, C. (1995) Pressure sore audit. *Journal of Tissue Viability* **5**, 29–30.

Department of Health (1993) *Pressure Sores – a key quality indicator*, HMSO, London.

Dickerson, J. and Wright, J. (1986) *Hospital Induced Malnutrition. Nutrition in Nursing Practice*, University of Surrey Publications, Guildford.

Effective Health Care Bulletin (1995) *The Prevention and Treatment of Pressure sores*, vol. 2 Nuffield Institute for Health, University of Leeds NHS Centre for Reviews and Dissemination, University of York, pp. 1–16.

McClemont, E. and Phillips, J. (1993) Medical and nursing audit of a patient group with pressure sores – a quality initiative. *Journal of Wound Care*, **3**, 346–8,

McLaren. S. (1992) Prevalence of pressure damage in hospital patients in the UK. *Journal of Wound Care*, **2**, 221–5.

Moody, B., Fanale, J. and Thompson, M. (1988) Impact of staff education on pressure sore development in elderly hospitalised patients. *Activities of Internal Medicine*, **148**, 2241–3.

National Pressure Ulcer Advisory Panel, (1989) Pressure ulcers prevalence, cost and risk assessment: consensus development conference statement. *Decubitus*, **2**, 24.

O'Dea, K. (1993) Prevalence of pressure damage in hospital patients in the UK. *Journal of Wound Care*, **2**, 221–5.

Preston, K. (1991) Counting the cost of sores. *Community Outlook*, **11**, (9), 19–24.

Simpson, G. (1987) Assessment and choice. *Community Outlook*, 16–18.

Thomas, S. (1944) *Handbook of Wound Dressings*, MacMillian, Magazines Ltd., London.

Touche Ross (1993) *The Cost of Pressure Sores, Department of Health*, London.

Versluysen, M. (1986) How elderly patients with femoral fractures develop pressure sores in hospital. *British Medical Journal*, **292**, 1311–13.

West, P. and Priestley, J. (1994) Money under the mattress. *Health Services Journal*, **104**, (5398), 20–2.

Young, B. (1990) Aids to prevent pressure. *British Medical Journal*, **300**, 1002–4.

FURTHER READING

Bader, D.L. (1990) *Pressure Sores: clinical practice and scientific approach*, Macmillian, London (a key textbook).

Department of Health (1993) *Pressure Sores – key quality Indicator*, HMSO, London.

Journal of Wound Care (has many useful articles).

The Kings Fund Document (updated 1993) *The Prevention and Management of Pressure Sores within Hospital and Community* (single copies available free from: Department of Academic Medicine for the Elderly, Chelsea and Westminster Hospital, Fulham Road, London SW 10 9NH, UK).

Liischer, N.J. (1992) *Decubitus Ulcers of the Pelvic Region*, Hogrefe and Huber, Toronto.

US Department of Health and Human Services guidelines on pressure sores:

Pressure Ulcers in Adults: Prediction and Prevention – a clinical practice guidelines (substantial text).

Pressure Ulcers in Adults: Prediction and Prevention – a quick reference guide for clinicians.

Preventing Pressure Ulcers – a patient's guide (a snappy information booklet). (Contact: US Department of Health and Human Services, Public Health Service, Agency for Health Care Policy and Research, Rockville, Maryland, USA.)

Your Guide to Pressure Sores (a leaflet for patients issued by the Department of Health, June 1994).

EQUIPMENT

Equipment evaluations: e.g. Evaluation No PS1 on pressure-relieving mattresses are available from Medical Devices of the Department of Health. Directorate Room 222, 14 Russell Square, London WC1B 5EP, UK.

How To Get Equipment for Disability 3rd edn. (1993) published for the Disabled Living Foundation by Jessica Kingley and Kogan Page (provides extensive details of available equipment).

VIDEOS

Focus on Pressure Sores: £35.19 from the Tissue Viability Society, Wessex Rehabilitation Association, Salisbury District Hospital, Salisbury, Wilts SP2 8BJ, UK. Tel: 01722 336262.

Pressure Sores – the hidden epidemic: £47 plus p+p for sale, or £14 plus p+p for hire from Concord Video and Film Council, 201 Felixstowe Road, Ipswich IP3 9BJ UK. Tel: 01473 715754.

A Sore Point – Managing the stages of pressure sores: £27.46 from Healthcare, 2 Stucley Place, Camden Lock, London NW1 8NS, UK. Tel: 0171 267 8757.

Understanding Pressure Sores (a helpful guide for carers) by Fosse Health NHS Trust): video and Booklet £19.95 from Blaze Advertising and Marketing Ltd, Oakley Hay, Corby, Northamptonshire NN18 94S, UK. Tel:01536 744515.

37 Surgical management in neurological disability

T. Morley and R. Birch

INTRODUCTION

Surgery will be unnecessary for most patients with neurological disability. Yet for some it may result in substantial gains, prevent or correct deformity, or enable patients to get to a higher level of function. Sometimes this gain may be quite specific; a person unable to write may be enabled to do so and thus hold down a job. On other occasions the benefit will accrue mainly to the carer, making nursing less arduous or preventing sores. This chapter is not exhaustive, but is written to illustrate the use which may be made of surgery in common disabilities. Timing may be crucial.

Skeletal deformity may be caused by many factors, including:

1. Paralytic muscle imbalance;
2. Spastic muscle imbalance;
3. Shortening of structures crossing a joint.

The aim should be to prevent deformity by physiotherapy, stretching and splintage. Sometimes deformity develops despite every effort. In this event surgery may have to be considered.

The aim of surgery should be:

1. To improve function, remembering that this can only work within the confines of the neurological condition.

2. To prevent further deformity when conservative measures fail.
3. To allow the maintenance of hygiene.
4. To improve cosmetic appearance.

The indications for surgery and the type of surgical intervention in neurological disability can cause considerable disagreement; this is mainly due to a lack of objective preoperative assessment, resulting in inappropriate surgery. The situation is also made worse by the lack of careful objective follow-up. Neurological disability amenable to surgical intervention can be divided into flaccid or spastic paralysis, the latter being responsible for the majority of unpredictable results.

FLACCID PARALYSIS

Disability and deformity in flaccid paralysis result from the unopposed pull of antagonist muscle, or from total paralysis resulting in a flail deformity in which joint position is solely the result of body weight and gravity. The surgical approach is either tendon, or occasionally muscle, transfer, or by stabilization of a flail joint by arthrodesis. An orthosis may be an alternative method of treatment (Chapter 47).

Rehabilitation of the Physically Disabled Adult. Edited by C. John Goodwill, M. Anne Chamberlain and Chris Evans. Published in 1997 by Stanley Thornes (Publishers) Ltd, Cheltenham. ISBN 0-7487-3183-0.

Tendon transfers

In selecting tendons for transfer the principles originally laid down for the treatment of poliomyelitis still remain valid:

1. The muscle to be transplanted must be strong enough for its new function, remembering that it will lose a grade of power when transferred, and should be at least grade 4 initially.
2. The transferred tendon should be inserted as close as possible to the paralysed muscle being replaced.
3. Transfer through tunnels in fascia or bone may cause adhesions and should be avoided.
4. The nerve and blood supplies to the muscle need to be protected.
5. The joint on which the tendon transfer acts should be mobile and free from deformity.
6. The muscle excursion should remain unchanged as far as possible.
7. Agonists are preferable to antagonists. Antagonists may work voluntarily but rarely in a functional pattern, and require extensive retraining.

Bearing in mind these principles, the results are both predictable and valuable. Excluding poliomyelitis, flaccid paralysis results from traumatic lower motor neurone lesions, a variety of cord compressive lesions and from peripheral neuropathies. Due consideration should be given to the long-term prognosis and, if progressive, the rate of progression and also the pattern should be borne in mind. There is no point in transferring a muscle which is almost certainly going to become involved in the paralytic process.

The **technical details** were admirably set out by Brand (1987) and Tubiana and Brockman (1993). Tissues must be handled gently, the transferred musculotendinous unit is passed through a gliding plane such as subcutaneous fatty tissue, avoiding scar tissue. The tendon should be re-routed to its destination in as direct a course as possible. Tendon to tendon suture is stronger than tendon to bone and the transferred muscle can be asked to act across one joint only.

The foot and ankle

Operations around the foot and ankle are the most frequent and rewarding. **Clawing of the toes** can be treated by joint excision and fusion, or if the toes are still mobile by Girdlestone's flexor/extensor tendon transfer (Taylor, 1951). The commonest foot deformities which need surgery are **cavovarus** and **equinovarus**. If there is no osseous deformity then procedures such as the transfer of extensor hallucis longus into the neck of the first metatarsal (Jones, 1916) or extensor digitorum longus into the third cuneiform may be justified. Equinovarus deformity may be appropriately treated by lengthening the tendo Achilles, plantar fasciotomy and either lengthening or transfer of the tibialis posterior.

The **common peroneal nerve** is particularly prone to damage in its subcutaneous pathway at the knee, resulting in foot-drop. Despite the fact that anterior transfer of the tibialis posterior tendon breaks all the rules, by being brought through a fascial plane and being an antagonist, results are often gratifying, functioning mainly as a tenodesis. Transfer aims to dorsiflex the ankle in a neutral position, avoiding undue inversion or eversion.

Surgical intervention at the knee or hip is rarely required.

JOINT STABILIZATION

Joints which either have fixed deformity or are flail cannot be treated by tendon transfer. In this case arthrodesis may be considered. Examples of this are fixed clawing of toes treated by interphalangeal arthrodesis, or cavovarus deformity treated by triple arthrodesis (talocalcaneal, talonavicular and calcaneocuboid). Flail joints such as ankle and shoulder may be fused in the position of function.

The spine

Deformity in the spine, secondary to neurogenic lesions, is essentially similar in both flaccid and spastic conditions. A neurogenic curve is typically a long C curve with a tendency to associated kyphosis. In adults, because the ribs afford some form of stability, the deformity is most marked in the lumbar area and may be associated with severe pelvic tilting.

The deformities so produced cause:

1. loss of sitting balance;
2. difficulty with seating;
3. skin pressure sore problems;
4. cardiorespiratory failure, if deformity is affecting the chest;
5. difficulty with controlling hip stability;
6. loss of body image, particularly in adults;
7. renal obstruction and problems with urinary diversion.

Adults developing neurological disability rarely develop fixed spinal curvatures, because growth has ceased. However, children with neurological disability such as spina bifida develop kyphoscoliosis and may need continuing treatment for this in adult life. The basis of surgical treatment, when required, is that the correction must be complete, and instrumentation and fusion must be extensive, including both the front and back of the spine, it must extend over the whole length of the deformity otherwise correction will be lost (Figure 37.1).

SPASTIC PARALYSIS

Because of the unpredictable results, there remains disagreement about the overall value of surgery in adult spastic paralysis. This unpredictability is due to difficulty with assessment of muscle control, patterns of weakness and individual muscle weakness (Roper, 1982). Surgery can be complicated by associated soft tissue contractures requiring extensive soft tissue release. Arthrodesis is more difficult to achieve, and with osteotomies union may be delayed with subsequent loss of correction. Postoperative rehabilitation is difficult because the simplest surgery may upset patterns of function. There may be loss of correction, and the patient may find it difficult to cooperate with attempts at rehabilitation if there is brain damage.

The commonest causes of spastic disability in adults are stroke, multiple sclerosis or head injury. The initial prognosis in stroke may appear poor because intercurrent complications and associated diseases are common and the average age is high, so relatively few patients are considered for surgery (Chapter 32). These factors are less marked following severe head injuries, which are more prevalent in young males. The aim is to start conservative treatment as soon as possible, and surgery is usually only considered once the patient has achieved a steady neurological state and any residual deformity or obstructive spasticity has been identified. There is a complex interaction of normal muscles, spastic muscles, stretch reflexes and reflex action. These are difficult to evaluate on routine clinical examination but by watching the patient walk, by discussion with therapists, by video-recording and by gait analysis, the interpretation of typical patterns of action is more accurate, with a greater understanding of the effects of surgery. Assessment has also been aided by selective blocking of peripheral nerves with the use of intramuscular botulinum toxin and the use of dynamic electromyography (Chapter 34). With a head-injured patient surgery may be consider earlier on, where it is clear that spasticity and/or contracture will impede recovery of function.

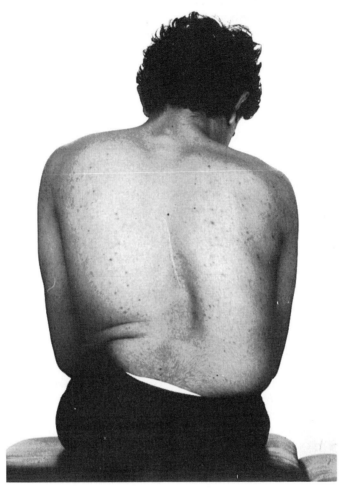

Figure 37.1 Typical neurogenic scoliosis. The curve was treated by segmental spinal instrumentation and fusion.

Surgery is generally more useful in the lower limbs and consists of:

1. release of tendons;
2. lengthening and thus weakening muscles;
3. occasional tendon transfer;
4. neurectomies;
5. soft tissue release;
6. bony operations, with osteotomy or joint fusion.

Different considerations apply depending on whether the patient is chairbound or ambulant. Where there is severe hemisphere and/or spinal cord damage leaving primitive reflex arcs, surgery may be of value in aiding nursing care and in the maintenance of simple hygiene. In this circumstance the problems are usually *hip adduction and flexion, and knee flexion.* For the hip, release should be of the iliopsoas and the adductor muscles, with obturator neurectomy and sometimes release of the anterior capsule of the hip joint. Knee flexion contracture is treated by hamstring tenotomy, sometime augmented by posterior capsulotomy of the knee joint, followed by serial plastering or reverse traction.

THE AMBULANT DISABLED PATIENT

Surgery may be indicated where there is usable reflex activity, or when the muscles have usable voluntary control but function suffers from interference from excessive spasticity or from contracture.

The commonest deformity in these patients is **equinovarus**. This is caused by a relative overaction of the plantar flexors and invertors over the power of dorsiflexion and eversion. The Silfverskiold test to differentiate equinus caused by gastrocnemius or soleus is unreliable, and here the use of dynamic electromyography is useful (Perry and Waters, 1975). In most instances the tendo Achilles requires lengthening. This may be done by the percutaneous slide with the tendon being divided percutaneously through half its bulk, medially proximally and anteriorly distally. The ankle is then forcibly dorsiflexed against the spastic muscles (White, 1943). If the equinus is very severe then the tendon can be lengthened by the open slide method; if there is varus at the heel the tibialis posterior may be divided or elongated at the same time (Roper, Williams and King, 1978). For **foot varus** which cannot be controlled by bracing with an orthosis, and where tibialis anterior is strong enough to allow clearance in the swing phase of gait, split tibialis anterior transfer may allow the orthosis to be discarded. Part of the tibialis anterior tendon is detached from its insertion and passed through a bony canal in the lateral tarsus.

Clawing of the toes, where these are still mobile, can be corrected by Girdlestone flexor to extensor tendon transfer. The severe clawing of the toes caused by imbalance of the intrinsic muscles of the foot is a more difficult problem and there is no satisfactory answer.

The commonest problem in **the knee** in the ambulant patient with spasticity, is a persistent stiff leg gait. Selective tenotomy of one of the heads of the quadriceps based on electromyographic criteria improves knee flexion, but usually only by about 20° (Waters *et al.* 1979). Knee flexion contracture is usually less of a problem in the ambulant and rarely needs surgical treatment. If required, hamstring tenotomy is used, followed by serial plastering or reverse traction.

Hip deformity is usually flexion and adduction causing scissoring of gait, this is treated by flexor/adductor release from the public bone.

UPPER LIMBS

Musculotendinous transfers and allied operations have a useful role in the palliation of loss of function following irreparable neurological lesions. However they are only one element within the process of rehabilitation which aims to reduce or abolish dependence. There are four main groups of operations:

1. release of contracture;
2. transfer of musculotendinous units to regain a specific motor activity;
3. nerve transfer to restore cutaneous sensibility;
4. arthrodesis or osteotomy to correct skeletal deformity and stabilize joints.

The principles underlying muscle transfer will be considered here. Results from these procedures are always inferior to the normal state and in peripheral nerve lesions always less successful than the outcome of good nerve regeneration. They are most successful in the treatment of loss of function from paralysis of the muscle or groups of muscles and are usually preferred to orthoses. Few patients

Table 37.1 Simplified version of Pulvertaft's classification of paralytic disorders. (Source: Pulvertaft, 1983)

---

1. Upper motor neurone disorders
a. Extrapyramidal tract lesions: ataxia, athetosis
b. Pyramidal tract lesions
   Congenital
   Trauma (cerebral palsy, head injury)
   Vascular
   Infection
   Neoplasm
2. Lower motor neurone disorders
a. Spinal cord and roots
   Congenital (craniovertebral anomaly)
   Trauma
   Vascular
   Infection (poliomyelitis, herpes zoster)
   Neoplastic
   Hamartoma (haemangioma)
b. Brachial plexus
   Trauma
   Neoplasia
   Compression syndromes
   Miscellaneous (irradiation)
c. Peripheral nerves
   Trauma
   Vascular (Volkmann)
   Infection (leprosy)
   Metabolic (diabetic neuropathy)
   Compression syndromes

---

really use dynamic extension splints for wrist-drop, only a minority of patients with lesions of the brachial plexus find the flail arm splint valuable, and a surprising number of patients with foot-drop discard the ankle–foot orthosis, preferring to wear boots.

Pulvertaft (1983) presented a useful classification of paralytic disorders which bring together cause, pathology, symptoms and anatomical considerations. This is set out in a simplified way in Table 37.1.

This classification is useful in drawing attention to the particular difficulties facing patients and those attending them in each group. Spasticity is a feature of the pyramidal lesion, uncontrolled movement is a disorder of the extrapyramidal. Some of those with lesions of the central nervous system have severe defects of cognition. The functional needs of someone with transection of the spinal cord at C6 are wholly different in scale and in detail from one with irreparable injury of an isolated peripheral nerve trunk. Elbow extension is exceptionally valuable in the wheelchair user, the otherwise healthy person can manage without. Injury to the brachial plexus causes widespread loss of power and sensation and, usually, significant pain; results of muscle transfer in these patients are usually inferior to those performed for isolated injury to peripheral nerves.

The scale of the problem is immense. Antia, Enna and Daver (1992) suggest that 15 million people experience significant loss of function from leprosy. Huckstep, writing in 1975 of his experience in Uganda, estimated that 90 000 people from a population of 10 million suffered residual paralysis from poliomyelitis and estimated several million untreated patients existed in the developing countries. Both of these excellent volumes are strongly recommended to the reader.

The experience of the Peripheral Nerve Injury Unit of the Royal National Orthopaedic Hospital is almost entirely drawn from treatment of injuries to the brachial plexus and peripheral nerves. It is summarized in Table 37.2. Musculotendinous transfers are proposed for patients with a clearly defined deficit from paralysis of muscles. Obvious examples include **wrist-drop, foot-drop, paralysis of flexor muscles of the elbow and of extensor muscles of the knee**. These are defects of motor function and the defect can be remedied if there is an available muscle to transfer which is truly spare and of full power. All transfers must 'rob Peter to pay Paul' and the price must not be too high. Muscles act to move joints and their transfer aims to restore dynamic balance across a joint within a functional

Table 37.2 Some musculotendinous transfer and allied operations in the Peripheral Nerve Injury Unit of the Royal National Orthopaedic Hospital: 1979–94

---

1. Upper motor neurone lesion, pyramidal tract lesion
   a. Trauma
       Adult 71
       Children 48
2. Lower motor neurone lesion, spinal cord lesion
   a. Trauma
       Adult 31
       Child 14
   b. Infection (Polio)
       Adult 4
       Child 7
3. Lower motor neurone lesion, brachial plexus lesion
   a. Trauma
       Adult 585
       Child 310
4. Lower motor neurone lesion, peripheral nerves
   a. Trauma
       Adult 355
       Child 87
   b. Vascular
       Adult 78
       Child 45
   c. Peripheral neuropathy
       Adult 14

---

range of movement. A common example of this principle is regaining wrist extension by transfer of a wrist flexor. At least one wrist flexor must be left to avoid a fixed hyperextension posture.

An accurate understanding of the diagnosis and the prognosis of the underlying condition is an essential prerequisite. Success from these operations depends almost entirely on the motivation and cooperation of the patient who has to do most of the work. The operation itself is only one incident in the course of rehabilitation and what happens in the postoperative period is particularly important. A good outcome follows careful assessment of the patient's needs, correct choice of the appropriate transfer performed at the right time, careful surgical technique and meticulous attention to splinting and, later, mobilization and retraining under the guidance of the physiotherapist. Most patients have reasonable expectations of what can be achieved. Sadly, in those with severe brain damage, unreasonable hopes of return to near normal function may be entertained by family or those caring for the patient. In such cases the observations of experienced nurses, physiotherapists and occupational therapists are important, functional assessments are always helpful in planning treatment. Some graphical principles of patient selection will now be discussed.

PROGRESSIVE DEFICITS

Considerable caution is necessary before advising on reconstructive operations in patients with hereditary sensory motor neuropathy or radiation neuropathy of the brachial plexus, because the condition will progress. Such operations should not be performed in patients with active and untreated leprosy. Operations in the growing child may achieve only a temporary improvement, as the original deformity may recur with skeletal growth if the cause of the deformity is muscular imbalance and if that imbalance has not been rectified. Some of the most severe instances of progressive deformity within leg and foot are seen in children with injuries to the sciatic nerve. Failure to reinnervate the common peroneal nerve in a young child leads to a severe equinovarus deformity and loss of tibial nerve function leads to a crippling calcaneus deformity. The internal rotation contracture, so common in obstetric brachial plexus palsy, will progress to posterior dislocation of the shoulder with severe consequences for the upper limb if it is not treated.

Age

Retraining of transferred muscles can be difficult in elderly patients with other physical disabilities and perhaps loss of plasticity in the central nervous system.

Fixed deformity

Musclotendinous transfer cannot possibly be performed in the presence of severe deformity. No transferred muscle can overcome that deformity and this must be corrected before any transfer. Three important sources of fixed deformity include **ischaemia, untreated spasticity and muscular imbalance**. Such deformities must be overcome before muscle transfer and there are a number of operations which may prove valuable in such cases, for example, **flexion contracture of the wrist and fingers** from ischaemic fibrosis or spasticity can usually be overcome by flexor muscle slide.

PAIN

Palliative operations are a waste of time in patients with severe neurogenic pain. The cause of the pain must be determined and treated, until then reconstructive operations will not work.

SENSORY LOSS

Although loss of sensation within a paralysed arm is not a contraindication to reconstructive operation, the results of muscle transfer in these cases are inferior. Moberg (McDowell, Moberg and Howe, 1986) described the skin of the thumb and index finger as the 'eyes of the hand' in recognition of the density of cutaneous innervation. When these digits are anaesthetic then the hand is blind and complex operations to restore precise pinch or opposition grip may be disappointing,

although Citron and Taylor (1987) did point out that improvement in motor function brought with it improvement in sensation in many cases.

Some case histories

Brachial plexus lesions

This was an irreparable injury to the Vth, VIth and VIIth cervical nerves. The patient presented with useful function within the hand but paralysis of the extensor muscles of the wrist, of the flexor muscles of the elbow and paralysis of the shoulder. Pain was successfully treated with the transcutaneous nerve stimulator (Chapter 38). After this, the appropriate flexor to extensor transfer restored useful extension of the wrist and of the digits, transfer of pectoralis major regained functional elbow flexion and, finally, glenohumeral arthrodesis enabled this man to return to full-time skilled manual occupation (Figure 37.2).

Femoral nerve lesions

Repair of the nerve improved pain but there was no functional recovery into the extensor muscles of the knee. Hamstring transfer allowed this patient to return to work and lead a normal life without orthosis (Figure 37.3).

Gunshot causing partial injury of the median and ulnar nerves

The patient experienced intense pain, appropriately termed causalgia. Severe contractures within the hand developed, the metacarpophalangeal joints were fixed in extension, the proximal interphalangeal joints in flexion, the thumb was adducted. Pain was treated by removal of the bullet, repair of the median nerve and a course of stellate ganglion blocks.

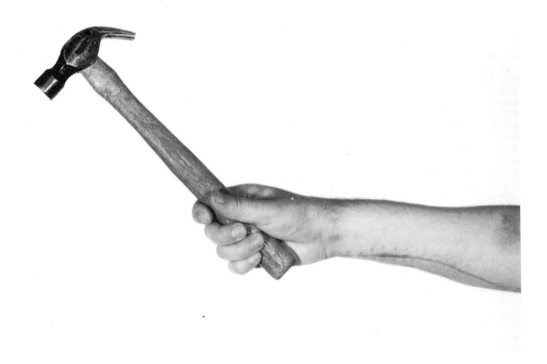

Figure 37.2 Hand function in a patient with C5/6/7 brachial plexus lesion after flexor to extensor transfer, and earlier elbow flexor plasty with arthrodesis of shoulder.

After this, operations were required to release the metacarpophalangeal joints and open out the thumb web space. Finally, muscle transfers were performed to restore flexion to the thumb, index finger and opposition for the thumb metacarpal providing a tripod grip (Figure 37.4).

SPINAL CORD LESION

Lamb (1987) studied 300 cases of cervical cord injury from the Spinal Injury Unit in Edinburgh. He found that 67% of his patients retained function to the sixth cervical segment. These patients retained useful abduction at the shoulder, elbow flexion, pronation and supination. There was good sensation in the thumb and index finger. Usually brachioradialis and radial wrist extensor were available for transfer. Realistic aims of treatment included the restoration of active extension of the elbow using part of the deltoid muscle, and of grasp and thumb index pinch grip using brachioradialis and extensor carpi radialis longus. Lamb emphasized that arthrodesis of the wrist was harmful and it should not be performed in the treatment of the paralysed upper limb.

PYRAMIDAL TRACT LESIONS

Zancolli and Zancolli (1987) and Goldner (1993) reported from their extensive experience in the treatment of children and young

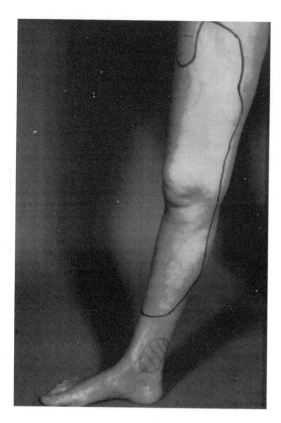

Figure 37.3 Sensory loss in a patient with femoral nerve lesion before quadriceps plasty.

adults. Zancolli's indications for operation were confined to spastic or spastic athetoid hemiplegia. He felt that the patient should have an IQ of 70 or above with reasonable psychological stability and there should be little emotional impact on the spasticity. Functional sensation within the hand with some degree of voluntary control was desirable. He emphasized that, preferably, patients would demonstrate their ability to cooperate, have good motivation and be in a good general condition. Goldner, from his study of 200 children treated between 1950 and 1970, found that careful manual muscle testing with selective local anaesthetic block allowed the surgeon to detect the degree of spasticity in different muscle groups and their

potential value in transfer. Many deformities can be overcome by controlled tendon lengthening. Excessive pronation and flexion contraction of the elbow can be successfully treated and transfers to restore extension of the wrist and digits, abduction and opposition of the thumb and digito-palmar grasp are regularly successful. He also confirmed that multiple procedures can be performed at the same operation.

CONCLUSION

Muscle transfers are mere incidents in the full course of rehabilitation. The surgeon cannot work in isolation nor by remote control. One hesitates to use the term multidisciplinary team as this has been so badly abused, but Wynn Parry (1981) developed this concept at RAF Chessington, and later at the Rehabilitation Unit of the Royal National Orthopaedic Hospital where he developed such a team. **Senior nursing staff** learn of the background of the patient's disability, the patient's own perception of the disability and are responsible for postoperative splinting. **Physiotherapists** work to improve muscle strength before the operation and to retrain muscles after. They are responsible for transcutaneous nerve stimulation in patients with neurogenic pain. **Occupational therapists** have a useful role in the development of orthoses which may be permanent or temporary and in helping patients to adapt to their life circumstances. **The disability employment advisor** is an essential member of the team, for by liaising with employers it may be possible for the patient to return to their work or to be offered retraining (Chapter 52).

Surgery of adult neurological disability is understandably not straightforward, but a relatively small improvement in function can radically improve lifestyle and function. With advances in the preoperative assessment and postoperative treatment, gratifying results can be achieved.

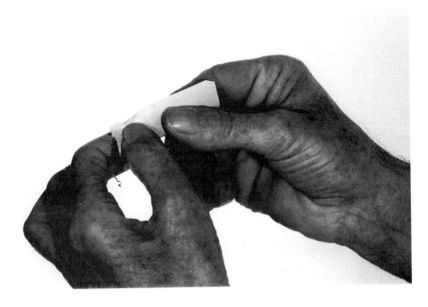

Figure 37.4 The restored thumb to index pinch grip in a patient with gunshot wound of median and ulnar nerves.

REFERENCES

Antia, N.H., Enna, C.D. and Daver, B.M. (1992) *The Surgical Management of Deformities in Leprosy, Bombay,* Oxford University Press, Oxford.

Brand, P.W. (1987) Biomechanics of tendon transfer, in *The Paralysed hand* Lamb, D.W. Churchill Livingstone, Edinburgh, pp. 190–204.

Citron, N. and Taylor, J. (1987) Tendon transfer in the partially anaesthetic hand. Journal of Hand Surgery, **12B**, 14–18.

Goldner, J.L. (1993) Cerebral palsy: assessment and surgical treatment of the upper extremity, in *The Hand*, vol.4 (ed. Tubiana, R) W.B. Saunders Philadelphia, (English translation).

Jones, Sir, R. (1916) The Soldier's foot and the treatment of common deformities of the foot. Part ll: claw foot British Medical journal, **1**, 749–53.

Lamb D.W. (ed.) (1987) The upper limb and hand in traumatic tetraplegia, in *the Paralysed Hand*, Churchill Livingstone, Edinburgh.

McDowell, C.L., Moberg, E. and Howe, J.H. (1986) The Second International conference on Surgical Rehabilitation of the Upper Limb in Tetraplegia (Quadriplegia). *Journal of Hand Surgery*, **2A**, 604.

Perry, J. and Waters, R.L. (1975) *Orthopaedic Evaluation and Treatment of the Stroke Patient. Part ll. la, American Academy of Orthopaedic Surgeons, Instructional Course Lectures*, vol. 24. Mobsy, St Louis.

Pulvertaft, R.G. (1983) Report of the Committee on Paralytic Diseases Including Leprosy. Paralytic Disease Committee of the International Federation of Societies of Surgery of the Hand. *Journal of Hand Surgery*, **8**, 745.

Roper, B.A. (1982) Rehabilitation after a stroke. *Journal of Bone and Joint Surgery*, **64**, 156–63.

Roper, B.A., Williams, A. and King, J.B. (1978) The surgical treatment of equinovarus deformity in adults with spasticity. *Journal of Bone and Joint Surgery*, **60B**, 533–5.

Taylor, R.G. (1951) The treatment of claw toes by multiple transfers of flexor into extensor tendons. *Journal of Bone and Joint Surgery*, **33B**, 539–42.

Tubiana, R. and Brockman, R. (1993) Tendon transfers: theoretical and practical consideration, in *The Hand*, vol. 4 (ed. R. Tubiana, W.B. Saunders, Philadelphia. English translation).

Waters, R.L., Garland, D.E., Perry, J. and Habig, T. (1979) Stiff legged gait in hemiplegia, surgical correction *Journal and Bone Joint Surgery*, **61A**, 917–33.

White , J.W. (1943) Torsion of the Achilles tendon, its surgical significance. *Archives of Surgery,* **46,** 784–7.

Wynn Parry, C.B. (1981) *Rehabilitation of the Hand,* 4th edn, Churchill Livingstone, London.

Zancolli, E.A. and Zancolli, E. (1987) Surgical rehabilitation of the spastic upper limb in cerebral palsy, in *The Paralysed Hand,* (ed. D.W. Lamb), Churchill Livingstone, London, pp. 153–168.

FURTHER READING

Huckstep, R.L. (1975) *Poliomyelitis,* Churchill Livingstone. Edinburgh.

Wynn Parry, C.B. (ed.) (1995) *Management of Pain in the Hand and Wrist,* Churchill Livingstone, London.

Zancolli, E. (1979) *Structural and Dynamic Basis of Hand Surgery,* 2nd edn. J.B. Lippincott, Philadelphia.

38 *The management of chronic pain*

A. Wasti

INTRODUCTION

Pain is a complex subjective experience. It provokes specific emotional, behavioural and psychosocial responses which are unique to each individual. It has a cognitive and an affective component, and the sensation of pain is closely linked to reaction. The responses to pain are determined by pre-morbid personality, psychological and cultural status as well as the socioeconomic impact of pain on the individual. Chronic pain has a profound impact on the patient's life. Sternbach described the contrasting features of acute and chronic pain by suggesting that whereas in acute pain, it is a symptom of a disease, chronic pain itself is the disease. Black (1975) suggested that the term 'chronic pain syndrome' be used for patients who present with complaints of persistent, intractable pain many of which are inappropriate to existing physical problems or illness. Chronic pain which is not a result of malignancy or other chronic aggressive pathological process (see below) is a distinct clinical entity requiring specific management.

DEFINITION AND CLASSIFICATION

Merskey (1964) defined pain as 'an unpleasant experience which we primarily associate with tissue damage or describe in terms of tissue damage, or both'. Subsequently this definition was accepted by the International Association for the Study of Pain (IASP) (1979) following slight modification. It is still the most widely accepted definition and is as follows: 'Pain is an unpleasant sensory and emotional experience associated with actual or potential tissue damage or described in terms of such damage'.

Acute and chronic pain are defined separately. Only chronic pain will be considered here: Bonica, (1990) defined chronic pain 'as pain that persists beyond the usual course of an acute illness or a reasonable time for an injury to heal or that is associated with a chronic pathological process that causes continuous pain or the pain recurs at intervals for months or years'. The IASP set the time for chronicity at 3 months.

Although this definition makes a distinction between chronic pain of a chronic active pathological process and that due to an inactive process or illness, it does not specifically define the entities of chronic intractable malignant and benign pain. This distinction is important to make as it influences the management of chronic pain. Sternbach and associates (1976) introduced the term chronic benign pain to distinguish it from the chronic pain associated with a malignant condition. Pinsky and Crue Pinsky, (1978, Pinsky and Crue, 1984), added the adjective 'intractable' and labelled the chronic pain syndrome as chronic intractable benign pain syndrome (CIBPS).

Rehabilitation of the Physically Disabled Adult. Edited by C. John Goodwill, M. Anne Chamberlain and Chris Evans. Published in 1997 by Stanley Thornes (Publishers) Ltd, Cheltenham. ISBN 0-7487-3183-0.

Table 38.1 Classification of pain

Acute pain

Chronic pain
  Intermittent / episodic
    Benign[a]
    Malignant[a]
  Persistent
    Intractable benign[a]
    Intractable malignant[a]

[a]Here the terms benign and malignant are used to describe the underlying pathological process and not the nature of the pain.

Considerable controversies continue to exist. However from observations noted above, it is possible to develop a simple but practical classification of pain (Table 38.1)

This chapter will discuss chronic intermittent, and persistent, intractable benign pain.

MECHANISMS OF PAIN

Though a detailed description of the physioanatomical background of pain perception would be beyond the scope of this chapter, a brief account of the physioanatomy of pain pathways and their role in chronic pain is given.

There are two types of peripheral pain receptors (nociceptors).

1. **A-delta nociceptors** are small myelinated nerve fibres. These are widely distributed superficially in the skin and its infolding into the mouth and anus. These nociceptors are sensitive to high-intensity mechanical stimuli and to extreme temperature changes.
2. **The unmyelinated nerve fibres** or C-polymodal nociceptors are found in the deeper parts of the skin and all other tissues except the nervous system itself. These nociceptors are sensitive to a wide variety of mechanical, thermal or chemical stimuli, hence the name polymodal.

Nociceptor afferents enter the spinal cord through the dorsal horn and terminate on the dorsal horn neurones. The grey matter of the spinal dorsal horn can be divided into several layers known as laminae. A-delta nociceptors terminate in lamina I and V and the unmeylinated C-polymodal nociceptors terminate in lamina II (the substantia gelatinosa).

The axons of the nociceptive dorsal horn neurones ascend in the spinothalamic tract and terminate in brainstem and thalamic nuclei. This spinothalamic tract partly terminates directly in the nucleus ventralis posterolateralis (VPL) or more diffusely in the brainstem reticular nuclei. Some fibres ascend to the periaqueductal grey matter of the upper brainstem. The direct thalamic connection may be functional in conscious perception of the nociceptive sensations, whereas the diffuse terminations may have a role in mediating the affective and autonomic responses to pain.

Chemical mediators for pain are not clearly defined. However they appear to play an important role in generating pain sensations and promoting a vasomotor response to pain. Several chemical substances are considered to be active in this respect. Some of these are released by the damaged tissue (prostaglandins, serotonin, histamine and potassium). Nerve endings themselves release substance P and others such as bradykinins enter from the circulation.

It is much more complicated to define the mechanisms of chronic pain. The physioanatomy above can explain how a noxious stimulus causes pain, however it does not explain what causes the pain to persist after the stimulus has been removed and when healing has occurred, nor why patients with chronic pain experience severe pain even though the stimulus is mild. Guilbaud, Iggo and Tegner (1985) found that in rats with allergic polyarthritis, nociceptors which are normally silent are continuously active and low threshold (non-nociceptive) mechanoreceptors are activated and discharge at a high rate. Morley suggested that peripheral nociceptors may be chemically altered, and some chemical substances are released in higher amounts at spinal cord and brainstem level, thereby producing pain in response to weak stimuli. Such theories, however, do not take into account the role of the naturally present analgesic system of the human body. This system keeps most of us pain free and is probably also instrumental in defining differing threshold to pain and discomfort in each individual. Why these mechanisms fail or are overrun in patients with chronic pain is not clear.

Aetiology

It is difficult to list all the causes of the chronic intractable benign pain syndrome (CIBPS). Virtually any condition which can cause acute pain can give rise to chronic pain. Any aetiological consideration should therefore deal with pre-or postmorbid factors which put a particular patient at risk of developing, and persistently suffering from CIBPS. Feurstein, Papciak and Hoon (1987) have described the psychosocial and behavioural factors which can influence the development, exacerbation and maintenance of CIBPS. They suggest that reaction to accident or symptoms at an individual and broader-system (family or work environment) level, psychobiological mechanism and subsequent outcome at work and at home, all play a part in the development and maintenance of CIBPS. There are several other theories, to explain this (Lethem *et al*, 1983; and Flor, 1984, Phillips, 1987), but detailed discussion on these theories is beyond the scope of this chapter.

Clinical presentation and manifestations

Patients who present to multidisciplinary pain rehabilitation units will have had many medical and surgical referrals, investi-

gations and treatments. They will be apprehensive and suspicious of any new medical consultations and assessments. It is not only a medical skill but also an art to acquire history from these patients. They have well-established ideas about their illness and their interpretation of important information is often different from that of the members of the team. However, it is important that when taking the history the matters which patients feel are crucial are not brushed aside but are carefully considered. Patients often like to detail the imperfections of past medical and surgical treatments and put the blame for their present condition on the treatments and interventions. These matters require sensitive handling. It is important to be neutral and fair and refrain from passing comments.

A detailed medical history is necessary, with special emphasis on the onset of the symptoms and the circumstances surrounding it. Note should be made of the previous treatments and their effectiveness. Present medications should be recorded with start dates and dosages. Patients should be asked whether any of the medications are helpful. Note should be made of coexisting medical or surgical problems, and any other ongoing treatments or problems, including impending litigation.

A complete and comprehensive social, family, employment and financial history should always be obtained. Patients may be unwilling to provide these details in a clinic where several members of staff are present, so it may help for one member of the team to see the patient in private to acquire this information. The socioeconomic impact of the illness must be ascertained.

A detailed clinical examination is always required. A full assessment of cardiovascular and respiratory state is mandatory. The region of the primary pain should be examined for local signs of inflammation, tenderness and limitation of function. Local and distant soft tissue tenderness, and the pressure required to elicit this tenderness, should be recorded. The patient should be asked to provide an assessment of their pain using one of the methods discussed below.

PAIN MEASUREMENT AND ASSESSMENT

It is good practice to measure and assess pain in all patients at the first consultation and thereafter at regular intervals to determine the response to treatment.

Measurement and assessment are different processes. **Measurement** is ascertaining mass, quantity, extent or degree on a scale of a standardized unit, using instruments or containers. **Assessment** is to critically analyse and judge the nature, significance, merit, effect and other properties of an entity. In the context of pain, measurement quantifies the degree of pain and assessment involves an overall appraisal of the experience of pain (McGuire, 1992). Measurement requires a unidimensional instrument whereas assessment can only be carried out using a multidimensional instrument.

There are two ways to measure pain, subjectively and objectively. Objective methods are complicated and cumbersome to use and are only used for research or experimental purposes. These methods will not be discussed here. For detailed description of these methods readers are advised to refer to a textbook on pain or the article by Melzack and Torgerson (1971). Subjective or self-reporting measurement are the most commonly used measurement scales in clinical practice. There are verbal descriptor scale (VDS), numerical rating scale (NRS) or visual analogue scale (VAS). The VDS is a four-point scale. The patient is asked to describe the level of pain using one of the following adjectives: none, mild, moderate or severe. In the NRS patients are asked to rate the severity of pain using a scale of 0–10, where 0 represent 'no pain at all' and 10 'the worst pain imaginable'. The VAS is an equally

simple and efficient method of measuring pain. 10 cm line is labelled 'no pain at all' at one end and 'worst possible pain' at the other. The patient is asked to mark this line at a point which they best feel corresponds to their pain.

Unidimensional self-reporting scales

Verbal descriptive scale

Descriptions: Choose the word below which best describes how your pain feels right now.

None   Mild   Moderate   Severe

Numeric rating scale

Instruction: Choose one of the numbers below which best indicates how strong your pain is right now.

No pain at all = 0 1 2 3 4 5 6 7 8 9 10 = The worst pain imaginable.

Visual analogue scale

Instruction: Mark on the line below how strong your pain is right now.

No pain at all |_____| The worst pain imaginable

Assessment of pain is more complex. The tools available to assess pain are complicated, often lengthy and time consuming. The most widely used assessment tool is the McGill Pain Questionnaire, which scales pain in three dimensions: sensory, affective and evaluative. Other multidimensional scales available are West Haven – Yale Multidimensional Pain Inventory (WHYMPI) (Huskisson, 1974) and Brief Pain Inventory (BPI) (Joyce and Zutshi, 1975; Melzack, 1975). Other scales pertaining to quality of life and functional ability are being used in the evaluation of patients with pain. These used in conjunction with pain measurement scales can provide a satisfactory assessment of the pain experience. The pain management teams should become familiar with one set of measurement and assessment scales.

TREATMENT AND MANAGEMENT

Fordyce *et al.*, (1973) initially described a multidisplinary programme for patients with chronic non-malignant pain. Since then, there have been reports of successful outcome (Daut, Cleeland and Flanery, 1975; Fordyce *et al*, 1973; Block, 1982, Linton, 1986, Maruta, Swansan and McHord, 1989; Stans *et al*, 1989; Peters Large and Elkin). There has been a rapid proliferation of multidisciplinary pain management programmes over the past few years. This approach has been shown to improve the functional performance of patients both in the short term and the long term (Aronoff, Evans and Enders, 1983). A recent meta-analysis confirmed that the patients treated with this approach, even at a long-term follow-up, function better than 75% of a sample who either receive no treatment or are treated by conventional unimodal treatment approaches (Luscombe, *et al*, 1995). At present a multidisplinary pain management programme (MPMP) is the treatment of choice for chronic pain of non-malignant origin.

The MPMP is specific for patients with chronic pain of non-malignant origin, and is designed to help the patient and the family cope with the pain more effectively. It encourages the patient to reduce the intake of the medications to the minimum. Patients are taught self-treatment methods. It is not the function of the programme to reduce pain through direct intervention but often patients report some improvement in the intensity of pain (see below). Treatment consists of a cognitive conditioning approach, physical rehabilitation measures, medication management, education, group psychotherapy, bio-feedback-relaxation techniques, family member participation and supportive psychological treatment. Each of these will be discussed in detail.

The multidisciplinary pain management programme (MPMP) team should include a medical doctor with interest in pain rehabilitation, a dedicated clinical psychologist, a physiotherapist, and an occupational therapist trained in dealing with patients with chronic pain, and a clinical nurse. Predominantly these programmes are run on inpatient basis but there have been some reports of variable success with outpatient pain management programmes (Flor Fydrick and Turk, 1992). The correct selection of patients for the programme is crucial to its success. Booker (1993) has suggested the following inclusion/exclusion criteria.

(a) Criteria for inclusion

Behavioural – at least two of the following:

- Magnified illness presentation.
- Major interference, due to pain, of activities of daily living (e.g. work, home duties, social life, hobbies and leisure pursuits).
- Long period of resting or lying down during the day.
- Over-activity/under-activity cycles.
- Inappropriate consumption of analgesics or other medications.

Emotional – at least two of the following:

- Major interference, due to pain, of personal relationships.
- Maladaptive pain-related feelings of anger, hostility or anxiety.
- Negative outlook with low mood.
- Disturbed sleep due to pain.
- Other signs of maladaptive coping (e.g. unkempt, dishevelled appearance).

(b) Criteria for exclusion

- Patient has come to end of all possible medical and surgical intervention and MPMP is being used as final disposal ground.
- Further physical investigations/intervention is planned.
- Patient has major structural abnormalities.
- Patient has progressive rheumatological or neoplastic disease.
- Primary drug abuse.
- Patient requires immediate psychiatric intervention.
- Patient aged less than 18 or more than 65 years of age.
- Patient is not willing to accept the approach.

Not all patients who meet the inclusion criteria would invariably benefit from an intensive pain management approach.

Although the team should function as a single unit and remain consistent in its approach towards the individual patient, each member of the team has a specific role. On admission to the programme each patient is seen by individual members of the team on a one-to-one basis. Information relevant to the area of expertise of each individual member is obtained from the patient during these meetings. All this information is collated into a single pool, except for the confidential information given to the clinical psychologist. The role and the duties of each member of the team are given below.

Clinical psychologist

The clinical psychologist has the principal role in counselling patients and overseeing the cognitive–behavioural intervention and carrying out psychometric and behavioural analysis. He or she is also responsible for attitude retraining, anger management and helping patients to develop coping skills. Patients may also need the clinical psychologist's help with information processing, controlling attention and problem solving. Readers who wish to read more about the treatment techniques employed by the clinical psychologist should refer to Booker's chapter in *Psychology, Pain and Anaesthesia* (Booker, 1993).

Doctor

The doctor in the MPMP deals with drug detoxification, pain control and sleep disturbance. Drug detoxification is an important part of the MPMP. All narcotic analgesia should be reduced with a view to total withdrawal. This part of the programme is most feared by the patients. They should be given full details of the purpose of drug reduction/withdrawal. Patients should be taken into confidence at each stage of drug reduction. Drug reduction should accompany active mobilization. Detoxification can be achieved by reducing the narcotic analgesia by small amounts each week. If the patient is on morphine or an equivalent, conversion to methadone may be necessary. Patients should be seen two to three times a week following each reduction to assess pain control. They should be asked to provide a measure of their pain using a unimodal pain measurement scale. If following any reduction pain becomes either unbearable or adversely effects the patient performance unacceptably, alternative methods of pain control should be employed. The temptation to increase the dose of the narcotic analgesia to previously effective levels should be resisted until other methods of pain control have been tried.

Alternative methods of pain control

Transcutaneous electrical nerve stimulation (TENS) The ancient Egyptians were the first to apply electrical stimulation to relieve pain. They used electric eels to treat headaches and gout. Through the centuries this form of treatment has been used to treat pain. In 1965, Melzack and Wall formulated the gate control theory which, with minor alteration, still remains the basis of much of our understanding of the pain mechanism and may explain the therapeutic value of TENS. It stimulates the fastconducting, large-diameter afferent fibres, producing some form of presynaptic inhibition, effectively blocking transmission in the smaller, slower conducting afferent fibres which carry noxious stimuli. Used properly and in discussion with the physiotherapist it is an effective way to gain pain control.

Acupuncture Acupuncture developed as a part of traditional Chinese medicine. Over the past 20 years or so it has become an accepted form of treatment for pain in the west. Its effectiveness can be explained on the basis of gate control theory. In the periphery, needling stimulates A-delta mechanoreceptors. At the spinal level interneurones from the A-delta fibres inhibit pain transmission. The A-delta transmission continues to the thalamus through the spinothalamic tract. This pathway sends a major collateral to the periaquaductal grey matter, which is an area of pain modulation, and produces inhibition of the pain stimuli (Bowsher, 1988). Acupuncture also increases the levels of CSF beta-endorphins (Clement Jones *et al*, 1980) and therefore it is thought that some of its effect is related to endogenous opioid or endorphin secretion. Details of acupuncture techniques are beyond the scope of this chapter.

Other form of alternative treatments, including massage and hypnosis, may also be of value.

To maintain and supplement pain control patients should be offered simple analgesia, for example paracetamol. Medications should always be dispensed at regular intervals and should not be prescribed on an 'as necessary basis'.

In the management of patients with chronic pain, tricyclic antidepressants are an important group of drugs. These are used frequently as pain and sleep modulators. Amitriptyline or other first-generation tricyclics with sedative side-effects are used commonly. The medicine should be started at a small dose and gradually increased until the desired effect is achieved. It is important that the patient should know that the medicine is not being used to treat depression.

Management of sleep disturbance

Sleep disturbance is common in patients with chronic pain. These patients have problems in falling asleep and maintaining sleep. The sleep pattern is lost and deeper stages of sleep, slowwave sleep and dream-sleep are disrupted. Sleep disturbance plays a major role in maintaining the cycle of chronic pain by way of contributing to physical and psychological fatigue. It requires adequate management. Patients should have their hypnotics gradually withdrawn. Stimulants like coffee tea or chocolate should not be allowed several hours before retiring. Patients should have their sleeping arrangements in quiet environment. Time must be spent in finding a comfortable sleeping position. Bed should only be used for sleep and not for resting when awake. Daytime sleep must be discouraged. Patients should practise relaxation prior to retiring. Tricyclic antidepressants should be used to modulate sleep in preference to hypnotic.

Physiotherapist

Physiotherapists involved in MPMP have the important role of encouraging the patient to improve physical fitness and exercise tolerance. He or she will also teach the patient pacing techniques, which means breaking up the day to balance rest or relaxation with activity to avoid severe exacerbations of their symptoms (35). It is essential that the patient should learn pacing techniques, as it will help him or her to avoid pain without compromising functional independence or mobility.

Occupational therapist

Loss of independence in daily living is often distressing both to the patient and the primary carer. The occupational therapist is responsible for helping the patient regain his or her skills in the activities of daily living (ADL) tasks. Using pacing techniques and aids and appliances, it is possible for patients to regain independence in ADL tasks. It is important to involve the primary carer in the treatment sessions. He or she should be encouraged to curb the 'helping instinct'.

Clinical nurse

As the patient spends a large part of his or her stay in the hospital on the ward, the nursing staff often develop a close relationship with them. Nursing staff have varied roles. The primary nurse can become the patient advocate. They can observe the patients on the ward and encourage them to follow the advice of the other members of the team. As they see the family and the patients most often they can act as team communicators. The patient's primary nurse helps the patient and the carer, overcoming toiletting and personal hygiene problems.

Treatment efficacy and maintenance

Several reviews have shown the MPMP to be effective. It has also been shown that patients who improve on the programme will maintain this improvement if, after discharge from the unit, they continue to follow the treatment regime. This must be explained both to the patient and family/carer.

Future of the MPMP

At present the MPMP is the most effective method of dealing with patients suffering from chronic pain of non-malignant origin. Whilst the research must continue to estab-lish the exact pathophysiology of chronic pain, it is of utmost importance to critically analyse the performance of the pain management programmes. Attempts are being made to define the most efficacious aspect of these programmes. At present, in the UK, the availability of pain management programmes is restricted certain areas. More investment is needed to make this form of treatment more widely available, and those of us who are involved with rehabilitation services should make certain that the importance of pain rehabilitation is not underestimated.

REFERENCES

Aronoff, G.M., Evans, W.O. and Enders, P.L. (1983) A review of follow up studies of multi-disciplinary pain units, *Pain*, **16**, 1.

Black, R.G. (1975) The chronic pain syndrome. *Surgical Clinics of North America*, **55**, 4.

Block, A.R. (1982). Multidisciplinary treatment of chronic low back pain: a review. *Rehabilitation and Psychology*, **27**, 51.

Bonica, J.J. (1990). The management of pain, *Pain*, **1**, 19.

Booker, K.C. (1993) Rehabilitation of the chronic pain patient, in *Psychology, Pain and Anaesthesia*, (ed. G.B. Gibson), Chapman & Hall, London, pp. 25.

Bowsher, D. (1988) Modulation of nociceptive input, in *Pain: management and control in physiotherpy* (eds P.E. Wells, V. Frampton and D. Bowsher), Butterworth-Heinemann, Oxford, pp. 30.

Clement-Jones, V., Tomlin, S., Rees, LH. *et al.* (1980). Increased beta-endorphin but not beta-enkephalin levels in human cerebrospinal fluid after acupuncture for recurrent pain. *Lancet*, **ii**, 946.

Daut, R.L., Cleeland, C.S. and Flanery, R.C. (1983) Development of Wisconsin brief pain questionnaire to assess pain in cancer and other diseases. *Pain*, **17**, 197.

Feuerstein, M., Papciak, A.S. and Hoon, P.E. (1987) Bio-behavioural mechanism of chronic back pain. *Clinical and Psychological Review*, **7**, 243.

Flor, H., Fydrich, T. and Turk, DC. (1992) Efficacy of multidisplinary pain treatment centres: a meta-analytic review. *Pain*, **49**, 221.

Fordyce, W.E., Fowler, R.S., Leman, J.R. *et al.* (1973) Operant conditioning in the treatment of chronic pain. *Archives of Physical Medicine and Rehabilitation,* **54,** 399.

Guilbaud, G., Iggo, A. and Tegner, R. (1985) Sensory receptors in ankle joint capsules of normal and arthritic rats. *Experimental Brain Research,* **58,** 29.

Huskisson, E.C. (1974) Measurement of pain. *Lancet,* **ii,** 1127.

International Association for the study of Pain (Sub-committee on Taxonomy) (1979) Pain terms: a list with definitions and notes on usage. *Pain,* **6,** 249.

Joyce, C.R.B. and Zutshi, D.W. (1975) Comparison of fixed interval and visual analogue scales for rating chronic pain. *European Journal of Clinical Phamacology,* **8,** 415.

Kerns, R.D., Turk, D.C. and Rudy, T.E. (1985) The West Haven–Yale multidimensional pain inventory (WHYMPI). *Pain,* **23,** 345.

Lethem, J., Slade, P.D., Troup, J.D.G. *et al.* (1983). Fear avoidance model of exaggerated pain perception. *Behaviour Research Therapy,* **21,** 401.

Linton, S.I. (1986) Behavioural remediation of chronic pain: a status report. *Pain,* **24,** 125.

Luscombe, F.E., Wallace, L., Williams, J. and Griffths, D.P.G. (1995). A district general hospital pain management programme: first year experiences and outcomes. *Anaesthesia,* **50,** 114.

Maruta, T., Swanson, D.W. and McHardy, M.J. (1990) Three year follow up of patients with pain who were treated in multidisciplinary pain management centre. *Pain,* **41,** 47.

McGuire, D.B. (1992) Comprehensive and multidimensional assessment of pain. *Journal of Pain and Symptom Management,* **7,** 312.

Melzack, R. (1975) The McGill pain Questionnaire: major properties and scoring methods. *Pain,* **1,** 277.

Melzack, R. and Torgerson, W.S. (1971) On the language of pain. *Anaesthesiology,* **34,** 50.

Merskey, H. (1964) An investigation of pain in psychological illness. D.M. Thesis, Oxford.

Morley, J.S. (1985) Peptides in nociceptive pathways, in Persistent Pain: modern methods of treatment vol.5. (eds. S. Lipton and J.B. Miles) Academic, London, p.65.

Peters, J., Large, R.G. and Elkind, G. (1992) Follow up results from a randomised controlled trial evaluating in and outpatient pain management programmes. *Pain,* **50,** 41.

Phillips, H.C. (1987) Avoidance behaviour and its role in sustaining chronic pain. *Behaviour Research and Therapy,* **25,** 273.

Pinsky, J.J. (1978) Chronic, intractable, benign pain: a syndrome and its treatment with intensive short-term group psychotherapy. *Journal of J. Human Stress,* **4,** 17.

Pinsky, J.J. and Crue, B.Z. (1984) Intensive group therapy, in *Textbook of Pain,* (eds P.D.Wells and R. Melzack), Edinburgh, Churchill Livingstone, p. 823.

Stans, L., Goossens, L., Van Houdenhove, B. *et al,* (1989) Evaluation of a brief chronic pain management programme: effects and limitations. *Clinical Journal of Pain,* **5,** 317.

Sternbach, R.A. (1981) Chronic pain as a disease entity. *Triangle,* **20,** 27.

Sternbach, R.A. *et al.* (1976) Transcutaneous electrical analgesia: a follow-up analysis. *Pain,* **2,** 35.

Turk, D.C. and Flor, H. (1984) Etiological theories and treatments for chronic pain. *Pain,* **20,** 9.

FURTHER READING

Wynn Parry, C.B. (1995) *Pain in the wrist and hand,* Churchill Livingstone, London.

PART SEVEN

CARE AND THERAPY: A MULTIDISCIPLINARY APPROACH

39 Rehabilitation nursing

S.A. Casley

INTRODUCTION

Nursing rehabilitation patients differs from most other nursing in one particular and important respect. In addition to providing normal care, rehabilitation nurses must be able to stand by and watch patients doing things for themselves and help but not take over. Nursing this way takes longer, as it is usually quicker to do something **for** a patient than help them accomplish a task for themselves. Yet this ability is crucial to the whole process of rehabilitation nursing; it will be required wherever there is a significant rehabilitation component to nursing activity. This will be important for people with disabilities admitted to an acute ward, and in the rehabilitation ward, In the community the philosophy of rehabilitation nursing will influence the team of carers. The nurses are often the link between the family and the general practitioner.

Nursing staff may be involved with individual patients and their families over many years. The trust of the patient and family is often well earned. They will need to help relieve pain and suffering and to maximize independence. The multidisciplinary team(s) of which such a nurse is a part will be more extensive, and may include general practitioners, other professionals from health care, social services and voluntary agencies. It may fall to nurses to call and co-ordinate meetings about the patients.

The nursing student, like the medical student, will have had to learn not only factual information and skills but also attitudes. The qualified nurse deals with patients at their most vulnerable when they are unable to attend to their bodily functions or when procedures invade this territory. There is great potential here for patients to lose their dignity. The nurse will therefore have had to explore her own attitudes and values in relation to dependency and disability and the student or young nurse may need guidance in so doing.

THE PROCESS OF REHABILITATION NURSING

Patients expect their handicaps to be understood and managed competently. The process of rehabilitation nursing is critical during the stay in the **acute general ward**, the **rehabilitation ward**, on a **specialist rehabilitation unit**, during **discharge home** and **in the community** be it at home or in some form of residential accommodation. The practicalities of nursing care will be determined by the situations.

Assessment

A nursing assessment should be comprehensive and take into account any other informa-

Rehabilitation of the Physically Disabled Adult. Edited by C. John Goodwill, M. Anne Chamberlain and Chris Evans. Published in 1997 by Stanley Thornes (Publishers) Ltd, Cheltenham. ISBN 0-7487-3183-0.

tion from other disciplines which may be available. It is important that the nurse has a sound clinical knowledge of the conditions likely to be encountered.

Care plans

The care plan may follow a number of nursing models. The most commonly used models for writing care plans are those of Orem (1980) and Roper, Logan and Tierney (1980). The purpose of a care plan is to identify the individual needs of a patient. These needs should be agreed with the patient and then organized into goals. The goals are then evaluated with the patient, agreed with other staff in the multi-disciplinary team, and developed or changed as progress requires.

The nurse has a statutory duty to provide accurate, current, comprehensive and concise information concerning the condition and care of the patient. Care plans need to be simple so that they can be used as a communication tool for the patient and the team. The nurse should give the patient time to consider what they would like to have written on their care plan. In complex cases care plans can also be used as an informal contract with patients.

Monitoring and maintenance

Care plans need to be evaluated every day to ensure the patient's needs are being met. This is a useful way of recording the patient's progress in a chronological order, which can be encouraging for the patient when their progress is slow. If this happens, one should then question whether the correct aims have been chosen or the right advice given. Other methods can be tried, or perhaps the immediate goal should be changed. Once skills have been developed or relearnt the nurse will need to ensure that the patient maintains his/her independence and moves on to other goals.

Maintaining function in a degenerative disease can be difficult. The nurse needs to be aware of equipment available to the patients which will enable him/her to maintain function, even if functional ability deteriorates. This will help the patient to maintain some quality of life and independence. Great tact may be needed.

Goal planning

Goals set with the patient must be realistic and set in collaboration with the appropriate member of the multidisciplinary team. The ultimate goal is of independence in as many tasks as possible. Total independence is often an unreal aim, as patients may have limited energy, motivation, understanding or needs.

Team work

The multidisciplinary team members need to have mutual respect for and trust in each other. Regular meetings are essential in order to communicate effectively. Nursing staff will benefit from working closely with other members of the multidisciplinary team and gain a greater understanding of the other disciplines involved. Sharing information is essential to the team's effectiveness and helps to ensure that consistent advice is given to the patient and carer.

WHEN IS REHABILITATION NURSING CRITICAL?

There is a need for rehabilitation nursing in many situations: the acute general ward, the acute rehabilitation ward or unit, the community rehabilitation ward and in the community itself.

The acute general ward

Disabling conditions such as rheumatoid arthritis, multiple sclerosis, cerebral palsy, muscular dystrophy, paraplegia or deafness are common. People with such diagnoses are often admitted to acute surgical, medical, gynaecological and obstetric wards whilst being treated for acute conditions such as appendicitis, chest infection, hysterectomy and childbirth. There are many occasions when staff have been unaware of how the disabled person functioned or communicated before admission and, because they did not think to ask, they took over instead. Communication failure can be in two directions. The patients need to explain how they cope at home or they may lose hard-won independence in a few days. For instance, to preserve mobility it is essential that individuals continue to use their own mobility aids, including wheelchairs and communication aids. They also need to understand proposed investigations and the findings, otherwise they may be made needlessly frightened or unhappy.

All possible avenues for communication need to be explored. Simple factors should not be neglected; the disabled person may need his/her hearing aid, spectacles or communication aid or merely be given time to communicate. Although this may seem like a statement of the obvious it is frequently overlooked. For example, patients who have sustained a stroke are sometimes presented with food and drink on the hemiplegic side where there may be sensory inattention and the need for help is neither recognized nor offered. It may even be that the flaccid limb is left hanging over the edge of the wheelchair.

Many patients have learnt individual techniques of managing bowel and bladder and stoma care and should be able to continue these. Lifting and handling can be inexpertly done; it is not unknown for a pressure sore to develop because a patient has been left on a hard trolley in a radiology department albeit, only for a short time. There is evidence from the study by Atkinson and Sklaroff (1987) that much has to be put right.

The key principles governing such admissions are to be found in *A Charter For Disabled People Using Hospitals* (Royal College of Physicians of London, 1992). These are:

- Disabled people who use hospitals must receive appropriate understanding of their individual needs.

- Disabilities must not be aggravated by any procedures, treatment or unnecessary regulations.
- Hospital staff need to distinguish between managing an illness and working with a disabled person.
- A person who has learned to live with a disability is probably better informed about it and the way they have learnt to live with it than anyone else.

Such principles should produce many practical changes on the acute ward which will be driven largely by the ward sister, with nursing management. Successful practice will depend on individual nurses understanding the issues. Ward practice must accommodate the maintenance of the person's normal routines and medication. The initial detailed nursing assessment, together with the care plan produced from this, written with the patient and relative (where appropriate), will ensure these needs are met. This assessment should include baseline observations, including the usual ones of temperature, pulse and blood pressure, and also specialist observations such as the Glasgow Coma Score, body mass nutritional assessment and Waterlow Score (or other method of recording any risk to tissue viability). Such information will be helpful for care on the acute ward and later in the rehabilitation ward and community.

The acute rehabilitation ward

An acute general ward is unsatisfactory for prolonged care for a patient with a recently acquired disability because of conflicting demands on staff as well as an environment which is inappropriate for rehabilitation. Ideally such patients should remain on acute wards only until acute investigation and care is complete. For example, patients who have recently suffered a head injury or stroke should progress to an **acute rehabilitation ward** if there is significant disability remaining. In this type of ward there will be a greater emphasis on promoting individual independence and autonomy. This will influence the nursing process, the functioning and even the design of the ward.

In a **specialist unit** providing intermittent rehabilitation for those adults (aged 16–65 years) with progressive neurological conditions such as multiple sclerosis (MS), motor neurone disease (MND) and Huntington's disease (HD) the aim is to preserve independence over a longer period or at least slow the increase in dependency. The aim of both types of unit is to improve or maintain function so that the quality of life of the patient and family are enhanced.

The specialist rehabilitation unit

The specialist unit (which may be a community rehabilitation unit or young disabled unit) should provide a different environment from the acute ward; its pace should be less hectic and the emphasis of care different, with nurses trained to have a 'hands off' rather than 'hands on' approach. It takes time and patience to allow a patient to become independent but the patient will have a sense of achievement when each skill is mastered, however basic. The unit's philosophy will govern its action.

Rehabilitation unit philosophy

The aims are:

- To provide facilities to enable people with disabilities to develop their maximum potential.
- To maintain the respect, dignity and confidentiality of the person at all times.
- To provide support to patients, relatives and carers by giving attention to physical, spiritual, emotional and social needs.
- To ensure that the service is provided without prejudice.

- To provide quality of care by maintaining the highest possible standards.
- To use a multidisciplinary approach to provide a coordinated service.
- To maintain communication between patients, relatives and carers with **all** members of the rehabilitation team.
- To provide education and act as a resource centre.
- To involve patients, relatives and carers with the treatment and planning of care up to and following discharge.

Nursing is a 24-hour activity unlike all other disciplines. Inevitably nurses get to know patients well and may, on occasion, act as advocates for them. To do this nurses need to understand patients' aspiration and fears. their likes and dislikes and the intricacies of their relationships.

Nurses have a key role in the multidisciplinary team (MDT) as they are often privy to information that other disciplines are not. They will often have had the opportunity to observe which family members visit and how they interact physically and emotionally with the patient. Such information helps with planning for discharge and understanding possible future needs. Individual therapy in the departments is rarely for more than an hour or two daily, often less, and usually insufficient by itself to produce lasting improvement. It is essential that therapists discuss their plans with nurses so that agreed techniques can be used on the ward which will support the aims of therapy. For example, techniques of transferring should be agreed between therapists and nurses. Progress begun in therapy can be consolidated on the wards. This requires discussion at least weekly at team meetings.

The nurse must ensure that the patient's activities are documented each day. These are critically important as they are usually the only daily record. It must also be clear what the individual nurse's role is with each patient and what practical methods, for example of handling, are to be used. It can be helpful to have these written on a board above the bedhead in order that everyone (nurse, therapist or family member) handles and moves the patient in the same way. This avoids confusion and helps the patients and carers to learn the techniques.

Care should also focus on recreation and socialization as well as working to achieve independence. Patients may need to be 'given permission' to rest and relax. They should be encouraged to bring items from home such as their favourite music and should wear their own comfortable, practical clothes and shoes, rather than slippers. Confidence may be boosted by having some personal possessions around them. Patients may need to be encouraged to share activities and socialize whenever possible and congenial day and dining areas are essential. Nurses should wear clothing which puts patients at· their ease and allows them to handle and lift them comfortably. It may be informal when the situation is appropriate.

The value of social activities in the ward should not be underestimated. It is a place where patients feel safe, can try out their new role as a disabled person, and from where they can experience a weekend at home or go out with a friend to a restaurant in the evening. Too often management does not recognize in its allocation of staffing levels the great value of nurses accompanying their patients in some activities for the first time. Providing sufficiently high staffing levels to allow nurses to talk with their patients can be also be a struggle. The patient needs time and this support to adjust to their new circumstances, which can be a very painful process both physically and emotionally. The nurse's role in this setting is challenging. The nurse has to be positive in his/her approach to support patients and families whose lives have changed forever because of an accident or illness.

Community settings.

There are different models of nursing care in the community which may depend on local factors such as geography and the level of services. They may deal with the transition from hospital to home, or be mainly centred in the community.

The liaison health visitor

The principles of health visiting are:

- To liaise and coordinate services in the community for the adequate provision of care and surveillance.
- To assist the patient to maximize opportunities to maintain life skills and independent living.
- To offer support to carers.
- To promote and stimulate awareness of health education and facilitate health-enhancing activities.

In the model of the liaison health visitor described by Firth and Wright (1976), and more recently from the same unit by Geddes, O'Brien, Walker and Chamberlain (1996) the health visitor had the following functions in the rehabilitation unit:

- To bridge the gap between hospital and home.
- To be involved in discharge planning.
- To give patients continuing access to the hospital team's expertise after discharge.
- To monitor progress after discharge.

The survey done by this team was of 48 young patients with stroke who were discharged from a rehabilitation unit over a period of up to 110 weeks postdischarge with a mean of 52 weeks. It showed that during the time the health visitors provided support, a total of over 209 visits was made. Only one patient had no problems at the first visit. Half the patients has medical problems, some arising *de novo*, and the same number had environmental difficulties relating to the provision of aids and adaptations. Twenty had social problems, ten had emotional difficulties and five had financial problems.

By the time of the health visitor's last visit, the incidence of all problems had declined, particularly those related to the acquisition of aids and adaptations. Ideally these should have been prescribed and obtained before discharge, relieving much anxiety, easing the return home, and enabling rehabilitation to continue at home. This study illustrates well the functions of the liaison health visitor (or hospital liaison nurse or hospital discharge nurse).

The community nurse

The role of the nurse when caring for a physically disabled adult at home has a different emphasis. The person is no longer a patient in a ward but an individual living in the community, where the nurse is a guest in the patient's home and where often family life takes precedence. It is important that the community nurse has detailed information about the patient's continuing rehabilitation programme. The nurse will also liaise closely with her colleagues in social services and other health care professionals involved in the patient's care at home.

The nurse's role is to monitor the patient's well-being, support the patient and the family, and initiate intervention as required. This may be as simple as obtaining a piece of equipment or getting advice about continence. Above all it is about maintaining the patient's health at home and should include family members. The general practitioner and other health care professionals involved have to be kept up to date with any changes. The ultimate aim of rehabilitation is independence but sometimes a well-being family wants 'to care' for the relative when they come home. In this situation it may be very difficult for the nurse to intervene.

PROBLEM AREAS FOR THE PATIENT ASSOCIATED WITH PHYSICAL DISABILITIES

Feeding and swallowing

One of the major stigmata for a physically disabled adult is the need to be fed. This can interfere with many social outings. Impairments of swallowing are frequent in neurological disability.

Help is available from the speech and language therapist to decide on the scale and nature of the problem (Chapter 22). In the past, it has often been after a patient has had a stroke associated with language difficulties that swallowing problems have been unrecognized and untreated. The speech and language therapist can assess in detail. Video fluoroscopic examination of swallowing may be required. When a patient is having difficulty with feeding their nutritional state will be compromised unless the deficits are made up. They are more susceptible to infection and pressure sores and the healing process may be slowed. The dietician will help with details of diet.

Some solutions to feeding problems may be as simple as altering the type or texture of food given to the patient who is clumsy or who finds swallowing certain foods difficult. If the meal can be eaten without the need to cut food, the patient may be able to eat independently. The type of plate and cutlery should be reviewed, and care may have to be taken to ensure that food remains hot and its presentation is appetizing. Supplements can also be added to a meal to give it a high nutritional value but small volume. Feeding is much to do with individual preference.

Drinking

Like feeding, as well as being essential, drinking is also a social activity. Recommendations given above apply to both eating and drinking and such matters as thickness and calorie content may need to be discussed.

Assisting a patient to eat and drink is a skilled activity which needs to be taught to inexperienced staff. The nurse should always ensure that he/she sits down at the same level as the patient when feeding him/her. When planning the nursing staffing requirements of a ward, it has to be recognized that ensuring the patient has enough to eat and drink can be time consuming. Carers also have to be taught. Home care plans have to be realistic; the time the carer takes to prepare and feed the patient needs to be known along with other dependency needs. Carers may also need to be instructed on the use of portable suction machines.

Percutaneous gastrostomy (PEG)

There may be times when it is either impossible, or dangerous for patients to be fed orally. For those with swallowing impairments or inadequate oral intake, where feeding is inappropriate, gastric feeding has become an acceptable alternative which is easy to manage and can be maintained for a prolonged period. This used to be by nasogastric tube, but the PEG provides a safe way of treating a patient in a coma as well as those who are unable to swallow.

All nurses on rehabilitation wards, and many in the community, must be able to manage percutaneous gastric feeding. It is important to record accurately what is given (calorie and nutritional content and volume). The nurse, with the support of the dietician, will be able to instruct carers how to use the PEG. Many patients opt to have their feeds overnight so as not to restrict their movements and rehabilitation during the day. Patients who are being fed by a PEG will need to have their weight monitored closely, as without proper supervision there is a tendency for patients to gain excessive weight. High-fibre feeds are available to be given via the PEG. These feeds, together with water, help to prevent the patient becoming constipated. Occasionally patients suffer from

diarrhoea, which necessitates a change in the brand of feeds used.

Oral hygiene

Oral hygiene is of particular importance for patients having feeding problems. The nurse needs to ensure that the patients and/or carers are instructed on how to clean the mouth. This will also include regular resection of the teeth, whether they be real or false. Patients who have suffered a major injury or who have long-term disability are particularly prone to mouth ulcers and infections so monitoring oral hygiene is particularly important.

Elimination

Urinary problems

There are many reasons why the patient may experience urinary problems and those arising from an acute stroke will have a different aetiology from those in longstanding MS (Chapter 37).

The nurse will first need to assess the individual patient's problem by asking the patient to keep a fluid balance chart. Continence advisors are available to help the nurse assess continence and decide which form of treatment he/she should discuss with the medical staff and patient.

Two of the most successful treatments for urinary incontinence which have improved the quality of life for physically disabled patients are intermittent self-catheterization and the insertion of a long-term suprapublic catheter. Both treatments put the patient back in control. Urinary incontinence is a major problem for patients with long-term disabilities. The nurse has a key role to play in promoting continence for his/her patients, otherwise the patient's bladder can rule the patient's life. Often the nurse will be the first person to extract the relevant complaints from the patient.

Bowel problems

These can be equally difficult for the patient. Again the nurse will assess the problem by asking the patient to chart the bowel movements over a number of days together with the diet for this period of time. Once the assessment has been made the nurse will be able to determine what advice is needed. Common problems are lack of fibre in the diet and insufficient fluid intake. Bowel problems may lead to bladder problems if constipation is present. The nurse will need to review the patient's bowel management, particularly if their mobility is decreased and they take regular analgesia. Regular aperients may need to be given. Rectal intervention is the last resort for the patient but particularly in long-term neurological conditions it may be the only effective way of evacuating the bowel.

Menstruation

A regular menstrual cycle may not be seen in a patient with long-term disability. The nurse should be aware of the patient's menstrual cycle and be able to assist and instruct in the use of tampons, pads and liners where manual dexterity is impaired.

Stoma care

Some patients will have established or new stomata. These are of three types: colostomy, ileostomy and urostomy. A colostomy may be an 'end' type, a loop, double-barrelled or divided. It may be, like the ileostomy, permanent or temporary. Ileostomies may be terminal or loop. Urostomies are of ileal conduit or ureterostomy construction and are usually permanent.

Appliances consist of either a one-piece system with a collecting bag or a two-piece system with a flange and pouch. Accessories are available. In a one-piece system the collecting bag adheres directly to the skin.

The appliances have a range of pre-cut openings to enable them to fit closely around the stoma, so protecting the peristomal skin (which is further protected by the skin protective barrier with or without an outer ring of hypoallergenic tape which is part of the system). Frequently the stoma is irregular and the patient has to cut the flange to fit. The completed appliance is discarded after use and replaced.

The two-piece system consists of a base plate which can remain in position for 3–5 days and pouches changed as needed, clipping on or inserted into the flange. Pouches and collecting bags may be drainage appliances, closed or urostomy appliances. Excoriation renders an appliance difficult to fit. Management includes the use of wafers, pastes and powder and topical steroids, antibacterial and antifungal agents.

Diet has a considerable influence on stoma management. Whilst a normal diet is to be encouraged, certain foods regularly cause flatus (onion, pulses, green vegetables), odour (eggs, fish and cheese) and liquid effluent (fruit and salads). Stomata can be blocked by high-fibre foods. The patient should test out a food which appears troublesome on several occasions before deciding not to eat it, but new foods should be tried singly. New stoma patients should know that foods can be retried 3 months or so later. Drugs can easily upset bowel stomata. Whilst some drugs such as opiates cause constipation, the patient's main preoccupation will be with those which cause diarrhoea and potentially dehydration.

Drug treatment for bowel dysfunction should not be tried until dietary management has failed. Diarrhoea can be treated with loperamide 2 mg four times daily or codeine phosphate 30–60 mg four times daily, perhaps with a bulking agent such as ispaghula husk. A stoma care nurse should be consulted where management is proving difficult.

Tissue viability

This is covered more fully in Chapter 36, but the salient points in prevention are:

- nutritional status;
- personal hygiene (or lack of);
- availability of mattress appropriate to the Waterlow Score;
- appropriate seating and positioning;
- adequate methods of lifting and handling;
- age;
- intellectual functioning and state of awareness.

Personal hygiene

Most patients enjoy a bath or a shower which gives the nursing staff an opportunity to assess the skin. The nurse may need to provide skilled assistance with bathing or showering to help the patient progress to higher levels of function. Grooming is also important and advice will be needed about shaving, hair and make-up. Information about easily donned and cared for clothing should be given. Clothing may be adapted to disguise drainage systems and not hinder mobility.

Appropriate mattresses

The nurse should work on the premise that prevention is better than cure. He/she should assess the patient's Waterlow Score and body mass index before deciding which is the most appropriate mattress to use. The ward needs a full range. There are many new mattresses on the market at the moment, but not all take into account the need for the patient to be able to change their own position in bed; the mattress should not make the patient dependent.

Appropriate seating and positioning

Seating and positioning needs to be considered for all types of patients with physical disability and the nurse will work closely with both the physiotherapist and occupational therapist. Seating and positioning needs to be assessed on an individual basis, but factors to consider are the height of the patient in comparison to the height and depth of the seat, the weight of the patient, how to lift and handle the patient and whether a seating cushion required (Chapter 45). Wheelchair seating is a specialist field, but the nurse needs to have a working knowledge of wheelchairs and cushions used frequently by his/her patients (Chapter 44).

Appropriate methods of lifting and handling

Nursing staff must ensure that the method identified to lift and handle the patient not only complies with the local policy but also with the Lifting and Handling Guidance Form of the European Union which identifies specified weights that a nurse may lift. There are many aids to assist the patient and the nurse but all need to be assessed with the patient and their carer. The nurse will demonstrate his/her own personal commitment to using lifting and handling equipment. Carers will say it is quicker to manually lift but do not take in to account the wear and tear on their back. The nurse needs to monitor these situations closely if safe methods of lifting and handling are to be maintained in the community. On the rehabilitation ward the situation is more fluid, with the patient's level of function and handling requirements changing week by week.

Mobility

Walking aids should be prescribed by a physiotherapist. However, the nurse needs a working knowledge of common types in order that he/she can help the patient to use the aid in the correct way. The nurse will encourage patients to keep themselves as mobile as possible in order to maintain functional ability and avoid contractures. Maintaining mobility will also improve both bladder and bowel function and help prevent osteoporosis. Changes of position also help prevent pressure sores.

Sexuality

For some patients the psychosexual aspects of having a physical disability may be as distressing as the physical aspects. Many patients find it helpful to discuss these problems, but not every member of staff will feel confident in the role of listener. The unit should have identified people who are pre-pared to talk through problems when needed. Therefore, at the first contact, which is often with the nurse, frequently all that is required is a sympathetic ear and referral when necessary.

Spiritual needs

Attending to the spiritual needs of the patient may help the patient cope with his/her situation when facing the prospect of living with a disability for the rest of their life. 'Why me?' is a question the patient asks his/herself many times.

If the patient has a religion or beliefs the nurse should where possible enable the patient to practise their religion. An indivi-dual's faith should be respected. Spiritual support for the patient, family and health care professionals is difficult to develop because of the wide range of beliefs and values of all involved but it should not be overlooked.

Safety and risk management

In part rehabilitation is about allowing patients to take some risks so that they can maintain their independence. A rehabi-litation unit that allows no risks is not doing its job properly. The team must know which patients have problems and are likely to take unreasonable risks. These problems may be either physical or cognitive. If the risks are to be taken, they should not be so great that the safety of the patient, other patients or staff is compromised. Advice (e.g. from a psychiatrist) sometimes has to be sought, especially with patients likely to harm themselves.

Self-medication

Many people with new disabilities will have a great number of new skills to learn when they return home. One skill which they can often usually learn in hospital is that of being responsible for their own medication. This process is best worked out on a formal basis, as ward (or hospital) policy with the phar-macy.

Nurses in the UK are required to comply with The United Kingdom Central Council's Standards for the Administration of Medi-cines and The Code of Professional Conduct, as well as their local policies related to health and safety. This is of particular relevance when assessing which patients should be encouraged to self-medicate and which drug dispensers are safe to use.

Health promotion

The nurse has a particular responsibility to the patient with physical disabilities to teach him/her how to preserve his/her health and why it is important to eat a well-balanced diet and drink adequate fluids. Topics such as exercise, smoking, the need for relaxation and weight control need to be discussed. The carer as well as the patient will need this informa-tion.

NURSE EDUCATION

The nurse is a core member of the multi-disciplinary team working with the patient 24 hours a day and needs a positive approach to disability, health promotion and communication with other professionals. To be effective and teach patients and carers the nurse needs to maintain his/her own education. The English National Board has established short and long courses in rehabilitation. The course held at Marie Therese House in Cornwall seeks to ensure that nurses:

- have a core knowledge of neurophysiology to use when assessing the patient;
- are able to plan and implement appropriate care which is research based and evident in daily practice;
- work effectively as part of a multidisciplinary team and apply health promotion models in daily practice;
- utilize expanded activities where appropriate to enhance holistic care;
- advise patients and carers with regard to continuing and future needs;
- apply knowledge to support patients with feeding and swallowing difficulties;
- explore the sociological, emotional, spiritual and psychological aspects of working with people who have physical disabilities.

CONCLUSION

Physical disability is common but is not synonymous with ill health. Much can be done by the nurse trained in the philosophy and techniques of rehabilitation to promote good health, to minimize further disability and provide the person in the nurse's care with skills and opportunities allowing life to be lived fully as possible.

REFERENCES

Atkinson, F. and Sklaroff, S.A. (1987) *Acute Hospital Wards and the Disabled Patient*, Royal College of Nursing, London.

Firth, D., Wright, V. and Chamberlain, M.A. (1976) The assessment of the value of health visitors in the rehabilitation team. *Rheumatism and Rehabilitation*, **15**, 188.

Geddes, J.M.L., O'Brien, A., Walker, C. and Chamberlain, M.A. (1996) The role of the liaison health visitors in rehabilitation. *Health and Social Care in the Community* (in press).

Orem, D. (1980) *Nursing Concepts in Practice*, 2nd ed, McGraw Hill, New York.

Roper, N., Logan, W. and Tierney, A. (1980) *The elements of nursing*, Churchill Livingstone, Edinburgh.

Royal College of Physicians of London (1992) *A Charter for Disabled People Using Hospitals*, 1992) Royal College of Physicians of London.

40 *Physiotherapy*

L.H. De Souza

INTRODUCTION

Physiotherapy is given to many patients with physical disability. They often seek it, and have high expectations of its value (Liversedge, 1977, Partridge 1994). Popular concepts of exercise associate 'fitness' with 'health', and this for some people with disabilities seems to become synonymous with physiotherapy (Forsythe, 1988). Indeed, the main focus of physiotherapy for people with physical disabilities is movement and function, and some type of exercise regimen is often part of treatment. Physiotherapy, however, acts mainly at the level of disability and generally does not modify the majority of pathologies or lesions which cause physical disability. It focuses on improving function in order to enhance the abilities of disabled people to operate in their day-to-day lives.

Notwithstanding the importance of therapeutic exercise as a major component of physiotherapy, those with disabilities and physiotherapists themselves have identified a need to use other skills concurrently as part of therapy. Good communication is considered an essential part of physiotherapy by patients and carers (Partridge, 1994). Ashburn and De Souza (1988) suggest that the supportive and educational roles of physiotherapists should be recognized as integral parts of disability management. This confirms that physiotherapy has a wider focus than just

movement and function. It relates to not only the functional well-being, but also to the social well-being of people with disabilities.

Young physically disabled adults, like their non-disabled peers, have a variety of expectations of life, including relationships, parenthood and employment. The ability to choose appropriate social and cultural roles is critically important (Chapters 51 and 52). Physiotherapy should aim to enhance choices, and therefore quality of life, for those living with physical disability.

APPROACHES TO PHYSIOTHERAPY

It is unlikely that physiotherapy will be the only treatment given to a young physically disabled adult. Many disabled people will be involved in a variety of treatments. Some, such as surgery, medication or counselling, may be provided by other health care professionals, while others, such as alternative therapies, diets or yoga, may be sought by the disabled person for themselves from other sources. Disabled people may therefore be involved in a mixture of therapies, only one of which may be physiotherapy. They must fit all into their lives.

Awareness of the disabled person's diagnoses is essential in planning the approach to physiotherapy. Some people, such as those disabled by coronary disease, asthma and sickle cell disorder, will be apprehensive

Rehabilitation of the Physically Disabled Adult. Edited by C. John Goodwill, M. Anne Chamberlain and Chris Evans. Published in 1997 by Stanley Thornes (Publishers) Ltd, Cheltenham. ISBN 0-7487-3183-0.

about physiotherapy if they feel that the therapist does not understand the condition. An approach which incorporates careful screening for tolerance, close supervision, feedback, and a recognition of vulnerability, will encourage the disabled person to participate with the physiotherapist. Any other therapies that the disabled person may be engaged in need to be taken into account when planning physiotherapy. For example, the timing of physiotherapy is important for diabetics, and planning needs to take account of drug and dietary regimens.

MODELS OF CARE

Two models of care have been suggested by De Souza (1990). The **acute care model** relates to conditions with sudden onset, some resolution and recovery, which are relatively short-lived. This model starts with assessment and goal-setting, followed by intervention and referral to other disciplines if needed. When the goals have been achieved, the client can be discharged. The **chronic care model** is more relevant for conditions which are progressive or have recurrent episodes, such as multiple sclerosis, cerebrovascular accident (CVA) or rheumatoid arthritis. In this model, the initial assessment and goal-setting is followed by care-planning with appropriate reference to other health carers. Intervention and management strategies are implemented within the care-plan, and the client is monitored at intervals and reassessed for change. The care-plan is adjusted on the basis of the reassessment. This model requires a long-term commitment to regular case review and the development of care-planning, but it does not generally require the client to be discharged from treatment.

The frequency of review will depend upon the natural history of the disabling condition; for example, annual review may be sufficient for those with multiple sclerosis, but people with cerebral or spinal tumours may require more frequent re-evaluation. Whichever

model of care is utilized, successful physiotherapy will require the active cooperation of the disabled person and their carers. If the treatment is to evolve, it must remain flexible and responsive to the client's needs and their changing circumstances. In order to achieve this, the approach to physiotherapy must involve discussion and negotiation with the disabled person so that the basis on which treatment will proceed can be clarified. The discussions and negotiations should take place early; the initial assessment affords the best opportunity.

ASSESSMENT

Assesment may be a continuous process. It is used to:

- identify disabilities;
- plan and adjust treatment programmes
- provide a baseline so that changes can be evaluated.

The choice and type of assessment will depend on the needs of the user and the disabilities of the patient. It is generally better to use assessments which are standardized, have a good degree of reliability and have been validated for the purposes they are expected to achieve (Chapter 9). In addition, standardized, reliable and valid assessments have value beyond their immediate clinical purpose, as they provide an objective record of historical data on a person's disability status over time. They can also be used for research and audit, and even though it will not always be possible to do research the quality of data will be improved.

Assessments do not provide answers to problems, they are tools used to inform clinical practice. The skill and experience of the assessor are of equal importance to the tool. Where assessment depends on judgement, and therefore on training and experience, reliability may be compromised. It is therefore advisable to have available instructions, or a protocol, which explains how the

Table 40.1 General areas of physiotherapy assessment in physical disability

Assessment area	Possible features to note
Muscle	Elasticity, stiffness, tone, strength, fatigue, bulk
Range of movement	Active, passive
Joints	Mobility, deformity, stiffness, pain, swelling
Patterns of movement	Range, control, coordination
Sensation	Exteroceptive, interoceptive
Posture	Symmetry, adaptation to supporting surface
Balance	Static, dynamic, equilibrium reactions
Function	Transfers, upper limb skills, gait, activities of daily living
Patient self-assessment	Perception of disability, willingness to change, ability to cope, priorities, choice, expectations

assessment procedure should be carried out. The power of the assessment tool lies mainly in the ability of the assessor to interpret and use the information to formulate an appropriate and feasible plan of treatment (De Souza, 1990). Assessment of physical disability needs to be focused on the purposes for gathering the information. Each assessment component should provide new information, be clinically important and have relevance for the planning of physiotherapy treatment. The expected professional standards for administering tests and taking measurements have been published (Task Force on Standards for Measurement in Physical Therapy 1991: Chartered Society of Physiotherapy, 1994). They should be followed for every assessment.

Irrespective of the need for specificity, the nature of physical disability causes assessments to feature areas common to a majority of conditions, although the exact aspects to be assessed (e.g. body part or system) may differ between conditions. These common areas of physiotherapy assessment are shown in Table 40.1 and illustrate that the main concerns are to identify limitations of movement and function.

The emphasis of a physiotherapy assessment will vary according to the causes of disability. For example, the detailed assessment of joints is more important in conditions such as rheumatoid arthritis and ankylosing spondylitis than in neurological conditions, where more emphasis is generally placed on the assessment of patterns of movement. Many assessments, however, will address issues of the functional impact of disability in everyday life.

Although the major focus of physiotherapy assessment is a detailed and systematic examination of the physically disabled person, other information is needed to put the assessment findings into context. This will influence the treatment plan. Such information may range from prognosis, to social and economic status. This extra information may come from a number of sources, such as referral letters, medical records, the assessments by others, the results of clinical investigations and, most importantly, from the disabled person and their carers.

The use of existing information is preferable to duplicating assessments; all professionals involved should be prepared to share their assessment findings by providing clear, precise documentation in the medical records and by forwarding information with referrals. It is particularly undesirable to repeat, unless absolutely necessary, any assessment procedures which cause physical or emotional distress to the disabled person or their carers. This would include repeating histories of traumatic and disturbing events. Sharing information must, however, be with the consent of the client.

In summary, therefore, physiotherapy assessment for those with physical disability focuses mainly on identifying limitations of movement and function. The major purpose of assessment is to identify the nature and extent of physical disability in order to plan treatment, and to evaluate change that may occur either due to intervention, or to the disease process. Tests used should be reliable, objective and valid for the situation, and each component of assessment should provide clinically important information.

Assessment, however, is a clinical tool and provides information on the standard at which it is used. Solutions to clinical problems are not, therefore, found through assessment, but are resolved by the physiotherapist by interpreting and using the information in clinical practice.

PLANNING TREATMENT

Many adults with physical disabilities will face several years of their future lives with limitations of movement and function. Some may have experienced partial recovery following an acute episode, such as traumatic head injury or spinal cord injury, and have been left with residual disability. Others may have deteriorating conditions, such as multiple sclerosis or rheumatoid arthritis, and cannot look forward to any substantial recovery. Some may come to realize that they have a terminal condition, such as motor neurone disease (or acquired immune deficiency syndrome), and feel that attempts at rehabilitation are a waste of their precious remaining time.

It is within these varied contexts that treatment must be planned and negotiated. Goal-setting is good practice (Chapter 6), but if carried out without the active participation of the disabled person, they will not feel involved. The scenario described by Partridge's (1994) patient-focus groups, where 'treatment goals were "something the physio tells you about, something they decide and then tell you"', should be avoided.

Negotiating a plan of treatment should not mean persuading the disabled person to agree with all the physiotherapist's decisions. Rather, it should mean listening to the patient's expectations and aspirations, and weaving these into the fabric of the physiotherapy programme. In order to negotiate fairly and successfully, physiotherapists should be prepared to compromise on what they believe to be the 'ideal' treatment, in exchange for one which the disabled person and the carers agree to carry out and perceive as being feasible in their circumstances.

During negotiations, the physiotherapist may gain valuable insights into how functional problems are influenced by the person's motivation and social situation. Such factors may have profound influences on the outcome of physiotherapy, as demonstrated in spinal cord injury (Green, Pratt and Grigsby, 1984), amputation (Thompson and Haran, 1984), head injury (Tyerman and Humphrey, 1984) and multiple sclerosis (Robinson, 1988). Information needs to be shared with the team.

A process for negotiating a contract for therapy is suggested in the scheme shown in Figure 40.1. The scheme highlights that both participants, physiotherapist and disabled person have an active role in the planning of treatment. At some point in the negotiations each person's responsibilities for action need to be clarified. It also indicates circumstances when the contract will end and a new one, based on re-assessment, should be re-negotiated.

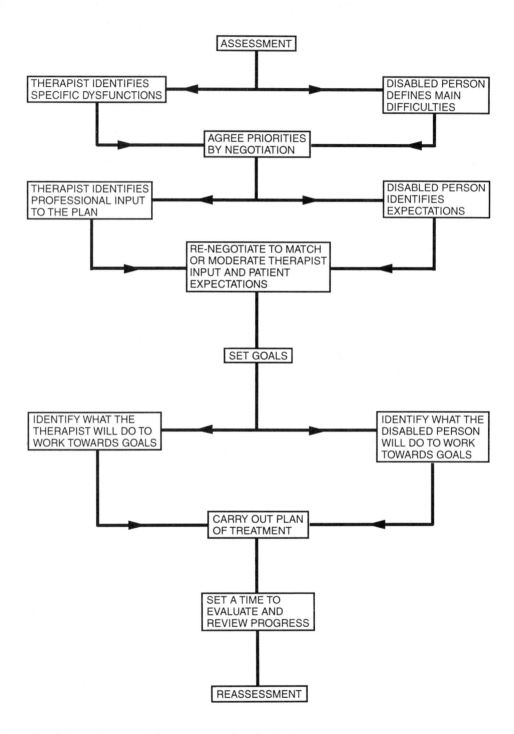

Figure 40.1 Scheme for negotiating a contract for physiotherapy treatment.

Such schemes should be flexible enough to allow for individual needs and preferences. It should also be acknowledged that some disabled people, such as the cognitively impaired, may not be able to participate fully in the process of negotiation. In these circumstances those who carry the major burden of care, such as family members, should be included, but not to the exclusion of the person with the disability, whose views should still be sought.

In summary, therefore, planning physiotherapy treatment should actively involve the person with the disability and the carers, in partnership with the physiotherapist. By utilizing information gained from assessment and evaluation, the focus in planning is on joint goal-setting and discussions of the feasibility of the ways for achieving the goals. During negotiations, each party can apply their expertise to the problems, indicate their expectations of treatment, and agree a plan of action geared to achieving the agreed goals. The process should be flexible to account for individual needs, and requires that the disabled person is encouraged and supported to become a participant in, rather than a passive recipient of, the programme.

APPROACHES TO TREATMENT

There are many different approaches to treatment which may be employed by physiotherapists to help young physically disabled adults. It is beyond the scope of this chapter to detail all the different approaches, and standard texts exist which can fulfil this purpose. For the majority of disorders causing physical disability there is, as yet, little conclusive research evidence to indicate that any one particular approach to treatment is better than any other. In the case of stroke, for example, where a fair amount of research into the effects of physiotherapy has been carried out, studies and trials have been unable to demonstrate that any one particular type of treatment is more beneficial than another.

However, what has been demonstrated by the research is that physiotherapy is significantly more beneficial than no physiotherapy (Ashburn, Partridge and De Souza, 1993).

The disabled person

Physical disabilities, especially those with chronic and continuing pathology, are complex in nature and a range of different approaches to treatment is often required. The physiotherapeutic skill lies in the practitioner's ability to bring together a high level of knowledge about the condition with practical competence in a repertoire of treatment approaches, and to apply them to individual needs.

Flexibility in approach is often the key to successful physiotherapy treatment. In conditions where the initial episode or injury is expected to resolve, some recovery of function is to be expected. Here the approach to treatment has the advantage of riding on a wave of natural recovery, and the physiotherapy programme can be designed to maximize functional recovery in tandem with the natural resolution of the lesion. It is important that the treatment programme neither overestimates nor underestimates the rate and amount of recovery occurring at each stage, and the use of accurate assessment information to guide the programme is required.

In conditions where the person has experienced some recovery, but has residual disability, the approach to treatment changes. The physiotherapy programme must allow for the emotional and psychological distress, and subsequent adjustment, to permanent physical limitations. The treatment programme should also expand to implement maintenance and preventive therapy in order to minimize the likelihood of secondary disability developing. For those who must live with deteriorating conditions, some of which may ultimately cause their death, the approaches to treatment require the most flexibility. For these disabled adults the physical and psychological states are inextricably linked, and the physiotherapy programme needs to address both, as part of the therapeutic team. For instance, in managing motor neurone disease, physiotherapists may be part of the community team from the Macmillan Service. Forward planning is essential in order to initiate therapy for disabling symptoms which arise as the pathology unfolds. For example, respiratory physiotherapy will often be required for those whose disability will progress to leave them chairbound or bedbound, and is best introduced at an earlier stage as part of an overall plan treatment.

The emotional and psychological aspects of progressive disablement also need to be addressed, and the supportive therapeutic role should not be shied away from by therapists who take on this type of caseload. Knowledge of the underlying condition will help in the understanding that these patients live uncertain lives where progressive loss requires constant adjustments and continual reconciliation with ever decreasing physical abilities. Real physical loss should be acknowledged, and therapy introduced to alleviate the functional consequences, for example by exploring alternative strategies, or by providing aids and appliances. Apparent physical loss requires redressing through reassessment and reformulation of the treatment plan. For example, hand skill may be lost due to sensory dysfunction though motor functions remain intact (Rothwell *et al.*, 1982). The approach to treatment should be adjusted to manage the sensory loss and maintain hand skill by encouraging, for example, visual compensation.

Flexible approaches to treatment require a broad range of physiotherapeutic skills to be utilized if physically disabled people are to be offered treatment plans which see each person as a whole individual with both physical and social needs. Treatment plans should focus on that which the disabled person values and identifies as important. Approaches to treatment should seek to open up choices and provide ways and means so that genuine choices can be exercised by enhancing the disabled person's repertoire of movement. The best, feasible, quality of movement is core to most physiotherapy treatment plans, but this should not be pursued at the expense of the disabled person's quality of life.

The carers

For physically disabled adults who live at home the brunt of caring falls on their families. The approaches to treatment should encompass the practical needs of the carers as well as those of the disabled person. Physiotherapy programmes to help carers with, for example, lifting and handling strategies, preventative back care, and the management of fatigue, can have major benefits. Carers, in their turn, may seek the professional advice of the physiotherapist and these exchanges should be encouraged.

However, attention must be given to a number of issues if carers are to be drawn into participating in the treatment plan, and assume a role similar to that of a physiotherapy helper. In these circumstances the physiotherapist will have a similar duty of care for the carer as for the disabled person. Any tasks which are devolved to the carer should be decided on the basis of assessment, negotiation, and a commitment to support and monitor the carer's contribution.

Additional tasks will inevitably add to the burden of care and as such should have a clear duration with an identified point in time when they will cease. This provides carers with an assurance that the added burden will not be forever.

Assessment of the carer's situation needs to overview the nature and extent of the care burden, and determine the impact of new tasks on their quality of life. Issues such as age, sex and family role will help to put into context what tasks are feasible and appropriate for carers to carry out. This is particularly important where the carer is a child, and additional issues of developmental age and understanding will need to be addressed. After an assessment of the carer's situation, it may become apparent that any devolution of tasks from the treatment plan is inappropriate.

The agreement of carers to participate in physiotherapy programmes cannot be assumed, but rather needs to be explored. Neither can it be assumed that the spouse or partner will be the primary carer, as this will not be the case in all families nor socially acceptable to people from some cultures. Family roles and cultural traditions need to be respected in assessing the carer's situation.

Finally, disabled people and their families cope and care within a maelstrom of emotional tensions. Physiotherapists need to become aware of such tensions without being drawn into them, and ensure that the approach to treatment has a neutral or alleviating effect and does not add to the tensions.

COMMUNICATION

For the majority of young physically disabled adults, it is unlikely that physiotherapy will be the only treatment they are receiving. It is important, therefore, that the objectives of physiotherapy are concordant with the objectives of other treatments. Interdisciplinary communication and cooperation are core to the success of a concerted team effort to provide the best available rehabilitation or management programme for an individual.

The objectives of physiotherapy should have a clear focus on the goals and priorities negotiated during treatment planning, but will analyse each to identify the stages and components of treatment needed to achieve

the goal. Once objectives are clear, the specific physiotherapeutic techniques and treatment methods required to fulfil objectives can be decided. The choice of specific techniques is primarily determined by what is judged to be the best intervention to meet the need. It may need to be modified by other issues, such as the patient's tolerance for the intervention. Choice of methods may also be limited by availability of equipment or time, or by the particular environment in which treatment is to be carried out. These issues may require the objectives of treatment to be adjusted.

When treatment objectives have been determined, they should detail the process by which identified goals will be worked towards. The objectives should reflect progression of treatment, and each should be feasible and achievable within available resources and practitioner experience. It is often useful to apply an appropriate time frame to the objectives as a guide for feasibility within the time constraints on treatment, and as a reference for progress. Summary guidelines for setting objectives for a physiotherapy programme are given in Table 40.2.

Table 40.2 Guidelines for setting objectives of physiotherapy treatment

Appropriate to the individual

Appropriate to the treatment environment

Acceptable to the individual, and carers as appropriate

Feasible and achievable within the available resources

Within practitioners' competencies

Able to be operationalized

Progressive in nature, and in time

Orientated towards the agreed goals

Concordant with the objectives of other concurrent treatments

METHODS OF TREATMENT

There are numerous methods of treatment available to the physiotherapist to use as therapeutic interventions. They range from those that require sophisticated equipment, such as electro and electronic therapy, to those which require different modes of communication, such as health education and promotion. Many different media by which treatment is delivered may be employed. Additionally, within the wide gamut of available methods, one modality may effect different therapeutic results depending on how it is applied. For example, the prolonged application of ice to a spastic muscle can reduce tone (Hartviksen, 1962: Knuttson, 1970: Miglietta, 1973), but a fast application such as brushing the skin with ice, can increase muscle activity (Rood, 1956; Goff, 1969). Thus by using the same physical medium (ice) different effects can be achieved by the application of different physiotherapeutic techniques. These various effects are thought to be due to the functional physiology of receptors which are known to respond differently to different stimuli (for a review, see Moore, 1980). The appropriate choice of treatment method and the application of the technique relies on the physiotherapist's knowledge and experience of the pathophysiology of the underlying condition of the disabled person, and knowledge of the contraindications for each method. The treatment method chosen should be the best available to the physiotherapist, and fulfil the criteria set out in Table 40.3.

There are likely to be some choices available for methods which are appropriate to address each aim of treatment. Those which are used should be selected as being the best clinical tool required for the specific purpose and circumstances of the therapeutic intervention. Treatment methods should not be chosen in an 'ad hoc'

Table 40.3 Criteria for choosing treatment methods

Will fulfil aims of treatment (has therapeutic efficacy)
Is not contraindicated by any aspect of the patient's condition
Cautions are known and attended to
Safe for the intended application, the individual patient, and the environment in which treatment will be carried out
Is acceptable to the patient
Is tolerated by the patient for the duration of treatment
Can be applied competently and skilfully by the clinician

manner but where more than one may be equally appropriate, variety and choice within the physiotherapy programme may be offered.

A selection of commonly used treatment methods, their indications and contraindications, are shown for musculoskeletal conditions (Table 40.4) and neuromuscular conditions (Table 40.5). The range of available methods for the physical management and rehabilitation of young physically disabled adults is constantly being added to, subtracted from, or adjusted for content as research findings enhance the understanding of treatment effects, and physiotherapy moves from a base of informed experience to evidence-based practice.

PREVENTIVE TREATMENT

Young physically disabled people who have residual disability, or progressing disablement will need to have a carefully planned preventative regimen of physiotherapy treatment offered to them. Where this is formulated as part of the programme of

Table 40.4 Treatment methods available for musculoskeletal conditions

Method	Indications	Contraindications
Thermal methods		
Ice	Short-term pain relief	Poor circulation
	Soft tissue swelling	Defective skin sensation
	Muscle spasm	Skin lesions
Heat (superficial)	Short-term pain relief	Acutely inflamed joints
	Muscle spasm	Defective skin sensation
Wax	Pain relief	Skin lesions and infections
	A medium for hand exercises	Defective skin sensation
Ultrasound	Acute soft tissue injury	Fracture (local)
		Metal implants
		Neoplasm
Electrical methods		
TENS/acupuncture	Pain relief	Hyperpathia
Therapeutic exercise		
Passive	Maintain or increase range of joint movement	Limited by pain threshold
	Joint and muscle stiffness	
Active/Assisted	Muscle weakness	Limited by pain threshold
	Maintain and increase range of movement	
Gravity counterbalanced	Mobilizing	Acutely painful joints
Free active	Mobilizing	Acutely painful joints
	Strengthening	
	Redress muscle imbalance	
	Improve endurance	
Resisted	Strengthening	Acutely painful joints
	Redress muscle imbalance	
	Increase endurance	
Breathing exercises	Increase mobility/reduce stiffness of thoraco-intercostal joints	
	Improve lung function	
Rest	Acute painful joints	Less active joints
	Acute spinal pain	Osteoporosis
		Anklylosing spondylitis
Manipulations		
Massage	Reduce oedema	Poor skin condition
	Retain tissue mobility	
Spinal	Pain relief	Ankylosing spondylitis
	Joint mobility	Serious bone pathology
		Neurological involvement
Peripheral	Increase range of movement	Serious bone pathology
	Pain relief in stiff joints	

Table 40.4 (continued)

Method	Indications	Contraindications
Movement re-education		
Gross motor skill	Increase functional abilities	Limited by fatigue
	Improve independence in	
Gait	daily living activities	
	Increase opportunity for	
Posture	work and leisure	
	Increase mobility	
Upper limb skill	Improve confidence of	
	movement	
Hydrotherapy	Pain relief	Open skin lesions
	General relaxation	Hydrophobia
	Reduce overall stiffness	Incontinence
	Mobilizing	Myocardial disease
	Strengthening	Urinary tract infection
	(e.g. Bad Ragaz)	Caution: tolerance limited
		by low vital capacity
Splints		
Resting	Acutely painful joints	Ankylosing spondylitis
	Protect and support	
	vulnerable joint deformity	
	Prevent joint deformity	
Serial	Reduce joint deformity	
Working	Pain relief during activities	
'Lively'	Aid for activities	
	Assist movements and	
	strength selective muscle	
	groups	
Collar/corset	Mechanical instability	Caution: ankylosing
	(e.g. spondylolithesis)	spondylitis
	Support during activities	

treatment, attention should be given to introduce the concepts of preventative care in a manner which is sensitive but frank. It is always helpful to determine what the person with disability knows about their condition first, and then to work from their knowledge base. The physiotherapist should be well informed about the most recent relevant research and population studies which have been published about a disabled person's condition. For example, the average life expectancy of a newly diagnosed person with multiple sclerosis is now in the region of 35 years (Kurtzke, 1970), while older studies have reported that it is only about 20 years (Kurland and Westland, 1954). This type of information can have serious impact on the plans and expectations of a 25 year old.

Preventative regimens of treatment have the general aim of eliminating secondary disability. The major disabilities which are

Table 40.5 Treatment methods available for neuromuscular conditions

Method	Indications	Contraindications
Thermal methods		
Ice		
Quick application	Increase reflex muscle tone	
Prolonged application	Reduce spasticity and clonus	Compromised circulation Hyperaesthesia
Heat (superficial)	Reduce spasticity Relief of pain and muscle spasm	Anoxic tissue Reduced thermal sensation
Electrical methods		
Muscle stimulation	Muscle activation Reduction of spasticity Reduction of atrophy Re-education of voluntary movement Strengthening	Hyperaesthesia
Biofeedback	Increase voluntary control of movement Compensate for proprioceptive loss Reduce spasticity Improve weightbearing	Profound cognitive involvement
TENS/acupuncture	Pain relief	Hyperpathia
Manipulation		
Massage	Reduce oedema Sensory stimulation Relaxation	Poor skin condition Broken skin Deep vein thrombosis Hyperaesthesia
Facilitation methods		
Neurodevelopmental	Normalize tone Inhibit abnormal reflex activity Modify afferent input Facilitate normal movement and postural/equilibrium reactions	Caution: inappropriate reduction of spasticity can cause loss of mobility
Neuromuscular	Stimulate postural/ equilibrium reactions Increase voluntary movement by afferent input Encourage active muscle contraction (isotonic and isometric)	

Table 40.5 (continued)

Method	Indications	Contraindications
Conductive education	Improve functional development Independent mobility Develop adaptive and learning ability Skill acquisition Complete continence	Profound mental handicap Uncontrolled epilepsy Deteriorating neurological condition
Functional	Enhance/maximize residual motor and sensory abilities Strengthen muscles Prevent atrophy Reduce sensory deprivation Teach new skills using residual abilities	Spinal instability
Hydrotherapy	Relaxation Reduce muscle spasm Movement re-education Relief of ataxia and tremor Freedom of movement Temporary relief of dystonia Strengthening weak muscles	Open skin lesions Myocardial disease Urinary tract infection Tolerance limited by low vital capacity Multiple sclerosis if temperature more than 33°C
Rest	Acute episode (e.g. MS attack) Fatigue	Pressure sores Contractures
Therapeutic exercise		
Passive	Joint and muscle stiffness Prevent contracture Reduce spasticity by muscle stretching Sensory stimulation	Attention needed to flaccid limbs Limited by pain in some cases (e.g. Duchenne muscular dystrophy)
Assisted	Re-education of voluntary movement	
Active/resisted	Re-education of voluntary movement Increase strength and endurance Reduce atrophy Improve cardiovascular functions Reduce local bone mineral loss	Deep vein thrombosis Fatigue Resisted/weightbearing exercises in longstanding immobility Caution: autonomic dysfunction
Respiratory	Respiratory neuromuscular weakness Re-education/maintenance of respiratory muscles and breathing pattern (e.g. for speech)	

Table 40.5 (continued)

Method	Indications	Contraindications
	Flexibility of thorax Retrain active cough	
Splints		
Resting	Prevention of contractures Protection of vulnerable joints	Broken/fragile skin
Arm sling/support	Swollen hand Painful shoulder	
Orthoses	Flaccid dropped foot Stabilize weak joints Knee hyperextension	Fixed contracture Fragile skin
Working	Improve function Attachments for tool usage	Poor skin condition
Serial	Reduce contracture	Pressure sore
Collar	Weak extensor muscles of head, neck and spine ('head drop')	

Table 40.6 Disabilities for which preventive regimens are appropriate

Disuse atrophy of muscle
Contracture
Pressure sores
Respiratory insufficiency
Oedema
Skin breakdown and ulceration
Painful shoulder

secondary, and therefore preventable with therapy initiated in good time, are shown in Table 40.6.

Preventative regimens should be accompanied with information and education which will enable the disabled person and the carers to be alert for early signs of secondary disability. For those who are at risk of acquiring disability which is not a direct result of their condition health promotion and health education is essential, while shielding disabled people and their carers from what may happen is a disservice.

When important information is given, the carers should be involved. However, the agreement of the person with disability for others to be told is paramount. Disclosing information pertinent to the disabled person's condition or well-being to others, even spouses or partners, without the agreement of the disabled person, is unethical and outwith the confidentiality of the patient–therapist relationship. This needs to be balanced against the ability of the patient to give consent.

Young adults with disability have many expectations of physiotherapy. Treatment must be focused on the needs of the individual, and the aims of therapy must be agreed by negotiation. The process should acknowledge the expertise and potential for contributing to the physiotherapy programme of both the therapist and the disabled person.

The success of physiotherapeutic intervention lies in the active cooperation of the disabled person and carers, and their motivation to engage in the therapeutic process. Through these processes the hopes and fears of the parties involved may be realized. Much physical, psychological and emotional investment is made by both therapists, and patients and their families, for a successful outcome and against failure. Herein lie the core issues of satisfaction, or disillusionment, with treatment. On their own part, physiotherapists should, on occasion, reflect upon their attitudes towards people who have disability and the 'gold standard' of what is considered to be normal. A balanced view has been advocated, which considers disablement as one of the variety of ways in which a normal life may be pursued (Shearer, 1981), and challenges negative attitudes which focus on 'problems' and evoke stereotypes of disabled people. People with disabilities can, and do, live life to the full, including love, marriage, children, work and happiness. An important part of physiotherapy is to facilitate the abilities of people with disability to exercise their rights of self-determination.

REFERENCES

Ashburn, A. and De Souza, L.H. (1988) An approach to the management of multiple sclerosis. *Physiotherapy Practice*, **4**, 13–45.

Ashburn, A., Partridge, C. and De Souza L. (1993) Physiotherapy in the rehabilitation of stroke: a review. *Clinical Rehabilitation* **7**, 337–45.

Chartered Society of Physiotherapy (1994) *Standards for Administrating Tests and Taking Measurements*, The Chartered Society of Physiotherapy, London.

De Souza, L.H. (1990) A therapeutic approach to management, in *Multiple Sclerosis: approaches to management* (ed. L.H. De Souza), Chapman and Hall, London, pp 24–33.

Forsythe, E. (1988) *Multiple Sclerosis: exploring sickness and health*, Faber and Faber, London.

Goff, B. (1969) Appropriate afferent stimulation, *Physiotherapy*, **55**, 9–17.

Green, B.C., Pratt, C.C. and Grigsby, T.E. (1984) Self-concept amongst persons with spinal cord injury. *Archives of Physical Medicine and Rehabilitation*, **65**, 751–754.

Hartviksen, K. (1962) Ice therapy in Spasticity. *Acta Neurologica Scandinavia*, **38**, (Suppl. 3), 79–84

Knuttson, E. (1970) On effects of local coding upon motor functions in Spastic Paresis. *Progress in Physical Therapy*, **1**, 124 –31.

Kurland, L.T. and Westland, K.B. (1954) Epidemiological factors in the etiology of multiple sclerosis. *Annals of the New York Academy of Sciences*, **58**, 682–701.

Kurtzke, J.F. (1970) Clinical manifestations of multiple sclerosis, in *Handbook of Clinical Neurology*, vol. 9. *Multiple sclerosis and other demyelinating diseases*, (eds. D.J. Vliken and G.W. Bruyn), North-Holland, Amsterdam, pp. 1444–1452.

Liversedge, L.A. (1977) Treatment and management of multiple sclerosis *British Medical Bulletin*, **33**, 78–83.

Miglietta, O. (1973) Action of cold on Spasticity. *American Journal of Physical Medicine*, **41**, 198–205.

Moore, J. (1980) Neuroanatonical considerations relating to recovery following brain injury, in *Recovery of Function: theoretical considerations for brain injury rehabilitation*, (eds P. Bach-y-rita), Hans Huber, Bern, pp. 9–10.

Partridge, C. (1994) *Evaluation of Physiotherapy for People with Stroke*, King's Fund Centre, London.

Robinson, I. (1988) Symptoms in chronic disease: some dimensions of patient's experience. *International Disability Studies*, **1**, 112–8.

Rood, M.S. (1956) Neurological Mechanisms utilized in the treatment of neuromuscular dysfunction. *American Journal of Occupational Therapy*, **10**, 220–5.

Rothwell, J.C., Traub, M.M., Day, B.L. *et al.* (1982) Manual motor performance in a deafferented man. *Brain*, **105**, 515–42.

Shearer, A. (1981) *Disability: whose handicap?* Basil Blackwell, Oxford.

Task Force on Standards for Measurement in Physical Therapy (1991) Standards for tests and measurement in physiotherapy practice. *Physical Therapy*, **71**, 589–621.

Thompson, M.I. and Haran, D. (1984) Living with amputation: what it means for patients and their helpers. *International Journal of Rehabilitation Research*, **7**, 283–92.

Tyerman, A. and Humphrey, M. (1984) Changes in self-concept following severe head injury. *International Journal of Rehabilitation Research*, **7**, 11–23.

FURTHER READING

Berger, J.R. and Sheremata, W.A. (1983) Persistent neurological deficit precipitated by hot bath test in multiple sclerosis. *Journal of the American Medical Association*, **249**, 1751–3.

Beverly, M.G., Rider, T.A., Evans, M.J. and Smith, R. (1989) Local bone mineral response to brief exercises that stress the skeleton. *British Medical Journal*, **299**, 233–5.

Brown, A. (1995) The effects of exercise on bone mass: implications for manipulative therapy. *Journal of Manual Manipulative Therapy*, **3**, 3–8.

Campion, M.R. and Twomey, L. (1990) *Adult Hydrotherapy*, Heinemann Medical Books, Oxford.

Goddard, D.H., Revell, D.A., Cason, J. *et al.* (1983) Ultrasound has no anti-inflammatory effect. *Annals of the Rheumatic Diseases*, **42**, 582–4.

Harrison, R.A. (1981) Tolerance of pool therapy by ankylosing spondylitis patients with low vital capacities. *Physiotherapy* **67**, 296.

Kim, C.K., Bangsbo,. J. Strang., S. Karpakka, J. and Saltin, B. (1995) Metabolic response and muscle glycogen depletion pattern during prolonged electrically induced dynamic exercise in man. *Scandinavian Journal of Rehabilitation Medicine*, **27**, 51–8.

41 Occupational therapy

M. Sansom

INTRODUCTION

The aim of this chapter is to provide an outline and supporting evidence for a general approach to occupational therapy (OT) in adult physical disability, to guide doctors and managers, and lead clinicians into further, more detailed investigation of principles and practice. Descriptions of OT treatment, including assessments, checklists and activities for specific conditions, are well documented in detail, by Melvin (1989), Thompson and Morgan (1990), Turner (1987), Trombly (1989), Whalley Hammell (1994) and Wilcock (1986).

Definition

Occupational Therapy is the assessment and treatment, in conjunction with other professional workers in the health and social services, of people of all ages with physical and mental health problems, through specifically selected and graded activities, in order to help them reach their maximum level of functioning and independence in all aspects of daily life, which include their personal independence, employment, social, recreational and leisure pursuits and their interpersonal relationship. (Louis Blom Cooper QC, 1989)

PHILOSOPHY UNDERPINNING OCCUPATIONAL THERAPY IN THE REHABILITATION OF THE PHYSICALLY DISABLED ADULT

The all-encompassing definition quoted above seeks to describe the practice of OT in both general and precise terms. In order to justify the unique role of OT in the rehabilitation of disabled adults, some of these elements require further explanation.

Mayers (1990) summarizes a number of aspects of OT that collectively contribute to a unique philosophy:

- Empowerment of the client in planning and decisions that affect him/her.
- The capacity of the client to be motivated to improve his/her health status.
- The capacity of the client to adapt with help, in order to take control of his/her environment.
- The client prioritizes what is important for him/her, according to individual need.
- Meaningful, purposeful activity is central to practice.
- Treatment focuses on the whole person: physical, psychological, emotional, social and spiritual needs.
- The value of individual roles is acknowledged.

Reilly (1969) suggested 'It is the task of medicine to prevent and reduce illness,

Rehabilitation of the Physically Disabled Adult. Edited by C. John Goodwill, M. Anne Chamberlain and Chris Evans. Published in 1997 by Stanley Thornes (Publishers) Ltd, Cheltenham. ISBN 0-7487-3183-0.

whilst the task of occupational therapy is to prevent and reduce the incapacities resulting from illness'. However, it is not sufficient nowadays to talk of prevention and reduction, without mention of 'quality of life'. Aristotle defines 'quality of life' or the 'good life' as 'a fully rational active life' (Ross, 1915). Aristotle argues further that the relevance of physical disability to 'quality of life' depends on how much the disability constrains or limits the ability of the individual to have a fully active rational life. The central core of OT is a holistic approach to purposeful activity and role through individual empowerment and adaptation. To this end the OT seeks to unite and integrate with other professionals working in the health and social care team. The successful outcome for the individual should therefore result in improvement in his/her 'quality of life'.

RESEARCH UNDERPINNING OCCUPATIONAL THERAPY FOR THE PHYSICALLY DISABLED ADULT

Although there is an accumulating body of research to demonstrate the effectiveness of rehabilitation, there is little evidence to support the individual contribution of different therapies, or models of practice. There are inherent problems in research design in this area due to the complexity of treatments, and lack of sensitive, validated measures. Sometimes research asks inappropriate questions. However, there now exists adequate empirical data to support the conceptual frameworks of a growing number of therapeutic approaches.

Historical data can provide valuable information on the effectiveness of rehabilitation. For example, over 50 years ago 99% of people with spinal injuries survived for less than 20 years (Grundy, Russell and Swain, 1986). Today a person in their twenties with a highlevel quadriplegia can expect a lifespan of 30 years or more (Geisler *et al*, 1983). Improvements in survival rates and function

are due to technological advances in medical treatment and to rehabilitation. The unique contribution of OT in spinal injury rehabilitation will be developed later in the chapter. Throughout the historical documentation of disability there is evidence of catastrophic outcomes for the physically disabled prior to the widespread use of rehabilitation methods, and significant improvements in survival and quality of life since the advent of comprehensive rehabilitation programmes (Rusk, Lowman and Block, 1966).

In the specialist area of neurorehabilitation empirical evidence to support unique approaches is appearing.

Functional training

Smedley *et al*. (1986), Feldman *et al*. (1962) and Johannsen *et al*. (1967) described quasi-experimental studies indicating that stoke patients clearly benefitted from functional training. Ostendorf and Wolf (1981) suggested that patients with a chronic hemiplegia could improve their level of function with functional training. Other studies, by Hayes and Carroll (1986) and Stern *et al*. (1971), reveal initial evidence that functional training should start as early as possible after onset of stroke.

Family participation

Although there is no published research specifically evaluating the effect of family participation in stroke recovery, Garraway *et al*. (1980), Smith *et al*. (1982) and Strand *et al* (1985) both provided initial evidence. They suggested that active family participation may be an important factor enhancing functional recovery.

Perceptual training

Results from a study by Young *et al*. (1983) revealed that visual perception training resulted in improved performance in specific neuropsychological tests, and generalization to reading and writing ability. Basmajian, Regenos and Baker (1977) and Mulder (1985) promoted the use of a 'cognitive' approach to relearning motor control.

Active participation

Reviewing studies of recovery after brain damage, Bach-y-Rita and Wicab Bach-y-Rita (1990) concluded that rehabilitation programmes designed to obtain the active, alert, motivated and consistent participation of the individual were more likely to be successful.

Continuing recovery and rehabilitation

Boyeson and Bach-y-Rita (1989) in a randomized controlled trial, demonstrated that patients who had sustained brain damage 30 years previously and longer, obtained significant recovery with an appropriate late rehabilitation programme.

Vocational rehabilitation

Vocational programmes that combined training with follow-up support, counselling and education continuing in the workplace, have been shown to improve success and continuity of employment by Kreutzer *et al* (1988).

Adaptation

Wilson (1992) followed up survivors of head injury with memory impairment for 5–10 years, and found that none had recovered full memory function. One-third showed improvement since discharge on standardized test performance in specific areas of memory, but for the remainder their performance had not changed or had deteriorated. However, 64% were living independently, and significantly more were using memory aids and strategies than at discharge. Wilson suggested that the demands of daily activities influenced survivors to adapt and make more use of memory aids and strategies, long after they were discharged from formal rehabilitation.

Rehabilitation as a learning process

Trieschmann (1980) and Alexander and Fuhrer (1984) report that in speciality areas such as spinal injury growing emphasis is placed on learning processes. Here rehabilitation becomes an educational process concerned with assisting participants to live in their environments, with enhanced opportunities to lead meaningful lives.

There is growing evidence from clinical research to support the basic principles of an empowering, adaptive and holistic approach to rehabilitation through purposeful, functional activity, and the unique contribution of OT. The following will illustrate how these principles are applied in the treatment of different conditions causing physical disability.

OCCUPATIONAL THERAPY FOR PEOPLE WITH SPINAL CORD INJURY, DUE TO TRAUMA OR A MEDICAL CONDITION

The primary aim is for the person to achieve independence in all features of function as far as he/she is able. As early as possible the person should participate in the assessment and goal-setting process to prioritize treatment activities. Early treatment includes functional communication, and additionally splinting to prevent contractures and deformities as required. Early assistance for the person to regain some control over his/her environment may include a basic environmental control system, if the patient has a high cervical cord lesion.

Once sitting is permitted, independent mobility may be the next goal, with careful attention to pressure relief and postural seating. The level of injury determines the mechanism for controlling a wheelchair, ranging from mouthstick or head control for power chairs, to manual wheelchairs. Self-care activities will extend from some feeding activities to dressing, bathing, grooming, bladder and bowel care, and other activities of daily living (ADL). The OT approach to functional mobility varies from the provision of microswitch-operated power chairs to independent transfers, driving, and activities involving some standing and walking.

Whatever the level of lesion, opportunities for independent activities in self-care, mobility, communication, control over the person's environment, relationships, leisure, community re-entry, housing and employment are jointly negotiated, prioritized and enacted by the spinal-injured person with their family. Working within the shared and delegated responsibilities and support of the integrated multiprofessional team, the OT is able to maximize opportunities for the spinal-injured person to improve his/her quality of life. For thoroughly detailed guidance with OT programmes, see Whalley Hammell (1994), and Trombly (1989) for a general overview.

Sport

Chawla (1994) reviews the challenges and opportunities that sport presents and its will often be the Occupational therapist who will initiate this programme. The cover of this book shows the triumph that can still be felt, the participant had just finished a 1000 mile wheelchair journey from to Paris to Compostella, over the Pyrenees. However, as Chawla discusses, there are many sports available, and many conditions in which the quality of life can be greatly enhanced through sport. He specifically mentions:

- paraplegia;
- amputation;
- other locomotor disorders;
- cerebal palsy;
- learning difficulties;
- visual and hearing impairment.

All these disabilities are recognized for international competition.

OCCUPATIONAL THERAPY FOR PEOPLE WITH ARTHRITIS.

The essential purpose is, in liaison with other services, to enable the person with arthritis to maintain the highest possible quality of life, and by educating the person, to help them cope with their arthritis. The aims include improving the person's independence through an examination of their personal environment, with the provision of equipment, advice on adaptation of their lifestyle, and liaison with employers, social services and benefit agencies. Reducing the level of pain the person experiences during ordinary activity is fundamental to treatment principles, as well as reducing the damaging impact of the arthritis on the joints affected. The OT will help to identify personal priorities in everyday life, so the medical and surgical treatment can be directed towards maintaining maximum quality of life. This reduces fear and anxiety about how they are going to manage their everyday life with a painful and disabling condition.

It has been shown that giving the person a better understanding about their condition improves their ability to 'cope'. Education of relatives, carers or employers generates a better understanding and consequently reduces stress on the individual (Lorig Konkol and Gonzalez, 1987; Mazzuca, 1982). Through the use of splints, special equipment and by learning new ways of carrying out activities, the person is able to reduce the pain experienced during everyday life, and to be less dependent on others. Through adapting everyday activities and using prescribed equipment the person is able to reduce the 'load' on severely affected joints. By reducing the 'load' on affected joints, the person is able to reduce the amount of damage to their joints (Melvin, 1989).

It is important that OT treatment should begin early when arthritis is diagnosed in childhood. Children with arthritis who are splinted correctly and given appropriate special equipment to use at home and at school will develop less deformity of their joints and consequently become less disabled as adults. Early treatment has obvious implications for the future quality of life of adults with arthritis diagnosed in childhood.

OCCUPATIONAL THERAPY FOR SURVIVORS OF HEAD INJURY

Treatment starts in the acute stage of recovery, when the person has regained consciousness. Using programmes to stimulate attention, the therapist aims to increase the survivor's level of alertness. Auditory, tactile, olfactory, visual, vestibular and proprioceptive stimuli are used for short periods, repeated during the day. Stimulation is introduced slowly and at low levels, with careful monitoring of the person's physiological responses. The therapist must observe closely for decreases in neurological response, abnormal reflex activity, pupillary changes, vomiting and changes in pulse rate. Changes may indicate an increase in intracranial pressure or risk of seizure, and treatment must be discontinued immediately, and the medical team alerted. Splinting to prevent contractures or deformity may be required at this stage.

Once the head-injured person is able to respond to commands, basic self-care skills of face-washing and light grooming can be introduced. Dysphagia and inhalation are common, but as soon as adequate swallow, and strong gag and cough reflexes return, light feeding activities are practised, in collaboration with the speech therapist and other professionals. Functional activities are taught at appropriate times of the day in a quiet room, **with minimal distractions**, and regular rest periods, to orientate and decrease agitation. As in all acute-stage interventions, the therapist must be critically aware of precautions and contraindications for treatment. These are detailed by Weber (1989), with

valuable information on early and continuing OT programmes.

OT is needed for survivors with impairments of perception, memory, learning, communication, planning and performance in the functions of mobility, personal care, housework, work, education and leisure activities. During continuing rehabilitation the therapeutic aim is for the survivor to regain functional activities to the highest possible level, including self-care, housework and work tasks, mutually agreed and prioritized to account for the needs and aspirations of the individual. Since difficulties with **planning and organizing daily activities** are frequently encountered by survivors of head injury, the occupational therapist has an important role in inventing strategies for planning and organizing daily routines, that the survivor is able to implement independently. Strategies and cues for planning have been shown to generalize more effectively from one activity to another, unlike more conventional methods of routine training which tend to remain activity specific. Motivation and full attention are critical to relearning meaningful activities, as well as new learning of adaptive strategies that may lead to return to independent living, education, home-making and employment. Long-term intervention at regular intervals may be essential to maximize opportunities for recovery.

Survivors with impaired capacity for information processing, indicated by the Paced Auditory Serial Addition Test (PASAT), benefit from OT. They participate in an outpatient programme designed to increase tolerance to fatigue, noise, resistance to distraction and assist working at speed. The programme introduces increasingly complex and abstract tasks, in a supportive and encouraging environment. The PASAT is used as a serial test sensitive to improvement, that is strongly related to the resolution of postconcussional symptoms. When participants achieve scores within one standard deviation of normal scores, they return to part-time work, with a staged increase to full time. Gronwall (1977) reported a 70% return to work within 2 weeks of injury for participants in this programme.

Rehabilitation for survivors of head injury has been described as a multifactorial 'black box' process (Cope, 1993). The significance of an integrated multiprofessional approach cannot be overstated.

Case history

Work and leisure in rehabilitation after head injury

AD, aged 45, suffered a very severe head injury in a road accident, as she drove to work on the first day of a new job as a microbiologist in the dairy industry. She was unconscious for 4 days and had a fractured skull, and fractures of the radius and ulna in both arms. During rehabilitation for mobility and personal activities of daily living, she made a rapid physical recovery and soon considered herself well enough to return home, with the support of her family.

Follow-up at 12 months identified the following problems: difficulties with standing balance on changing position, accompanied by dizziness; weakness and slight incoordination in hand function; severe fatigue and headaches; peripheral double vision; difficulty remembering essential components of everyday tasks and activities. The occupational therapist encouraged AD to keep a record of specific problems that occurred on a daily basis. Together they prioritized the list of problems and developed a programme that involved adapting functional activities to minimize unnecessary postural changes. Equipment and the provision of orthoses assisted hand function. Checklists, prompt cards and a micro-cassette recorded were used to help with memory difficulties.

AD was an enthusiastic musician, playing with a local orchestra. An additional splint was adapted to assist her playing by supporting the wrist in the optimum posi-tion. Her social and leisure activities were centred around music and the orchestra. AD was also anxious to progress towards return to work in her former occupation. She commenced a distance learning course in food hygiene to brush-up on basic work skills. She experienced difficulties in learning material presented in a table, and legislative information. An evaluation of her learning abilities revealed memory skills retained for graphic and task-related information. Working together, AD and the occupational therapist converted the legislative material into practical examples, and the tabular material into flow-charts and pictorial representation. Learning accelerated in these areas.

AD remained insistent that her goal was to return to her former job. A work placement was arranged in the laboratory of a local dairy. The session was limited to half a day, and alternative opportunities were discussed beforehand should the placement be unsuccessful. AD came away from the placement aware that she could not cope with the physical activities and supervisory responsibilities of the job. Because alternatives had been discussed, she remained positive, and considered the placement an important step in her adaptation to her disabilities.

AD and the occupational therapist reviewed the scope for further education and training. Her enthusiasm for music led her to look at opportunities in that area. A visit to a local college identified a course in professional development for musicians. Discussion with tutors and the special needs advisor confirmed the course was suitable, and their enthusiasm to support AD in her studies. AD's personal goal is to qualify as a music teacher, when she would be able to teach music, working at home, part-time. Her goal is realistically achievable.

The occupational therapist is currently resolving problems of access in the college, and the provision of a computer to assist AD in her course work. Continuing support from the occupational therapist in liaison with other professionals, assists rehabilitation to meaningful roles and satisfying occupations, enhancing quality of life for survivors of head injury.

OCCUPATIONAL THERAPY FOR SURVIVORS OF STROKE

Research into recovery from brain damage, especially stroke, demonstrates areas of effectiveness of specific relevance to OT, in terms of consolidating existing approaches and developing new areas of intervention. Increasing evidence is accumulating for the effectiveness of functional training, either alone or in conjunction with other approaches. Similarly, studies of the neurochemistry and neurophysiology of the recovering brain provide valuable theories to explain the significance of motivation and vigilance in learning, the **bilaterality of the brain and use of ipsilateral pathways**. Evidence is emerging of the growth of the dendritic tree as a compensatory mechanism for loss of neurones, synaptic sprouting and unmasking, occurring in the presence of the neurotransmitter noradrenaline. Increased motivation, vigilance and participation are linked to the greater production of noradrenaline. These recent findings offer a challenge to occupational therapists working with survivors of acquired brain damage to make the link between theory and practice, and to capitalize on the opportunities to facilitate recovery, by using motivating and purposeful activities.

Studies of stroke rehabilitation have not demonstrated that one specialized therapeutic regimen is more effective than any other, in terms of independent function at outcome. However, early intervention in purposeful activities of daily living has acquired supporting evidence (Stern *et al.*, 1970; Hayes and Carroll, 1986). Similarly, authors reviewing the research literature have drawn the conclusion that adaptive processes can lead to improvement in many activities of daily living (Wade *et al.*, 1985).

The aims of OT for survivors of stroke are therefore the maximization of functional independence in daily living requirements, both at an early stage of treatment and continuing into care in the community. Continuing treatment programmes may include food preparation and cooking, shopping and restoration of personal and social activities, social pursuits, and age-appropriate work. All programmes should be prioritized and negotiated to meet the individual needs of the person, in the context of family and environment. Integrated multiprofessional collaboration will hopefully reduce confusing and contractory information for the individual and facilitate adaptation and new learning. For more detailed approaches to OT for persons after stroke, readers are recommended to Wilcock (1986) and Pedretti (1985).

The role of the occupational therapist in stroke rehabilitation (Adapted from Mulley, 1985.)

Functional assessment

To determine the degree of disability and handicap and the potential to overcome problems of daily living:

1. Physical – sensory, perceptual problems; power and range of movement; activity tolerance.
2. Activities of daily living – e.g. eating, dressing, washing, transfers, occupations (leisure and work).
3. Therapeutic activities: to help the patient achieve maximum functional ability.

Home assessment

To plan safe discharge and maximum independence in the community:

1. Predischarge home visit.

2. Provision of equipment.
3. Liaison with community services – e.g. to implement required level of care; for structural adaptations.
4. Education for patient, family, carers and professionals.
5. Continuity of support for patient, family and carers – to assist the patient in establishing a meaningful role within the family and society.

COGNITIVE AND PERCEPTUAL TESTING AND TRAINING

Occupational therapists working in neurology frequently become involved in the assessment of and retraining of cognitive and perceptual problems. A number of assessment packages have been developed to assist in testing these impairments. However, a significant problem with many of these scales is their ecological validity: the degree to which a measure is meaningful or useful in the participant's real life, outside of the clinical setting, through generalization to everyday function. Many neuropsychological tests designed to measure brain dysfunction commonly do not translate into real world performance (Johnston *et al.*, 1991). The functional limitations of people with brain injury may decrease considerably during rehabilitation, whereas intelligence or memory scores change little. Assessments may assist the therapist to identify specific areas of brain dysfunction relating to sensory, motor, cognitive or perceptual performance. This evidence can help carers and other professionals to distinguish between dysfunction caused by the presence of brain damage, and other underlying characteristics of the individual: their motivation, values, beliefs and former abilities. However, the results obtained do not necessarily guide the therapist in the selection of appropriate remedial activities, and serial test results may not correspond with functional improvements (Wilson, 1992).

Soderback (1988) aware of the limitations of psychometric tests in predicting functional outcome, and determining remedial activities devised a valuable household assessment that included opportunities for serial measurement and therapeutic application. The assessment of intellectual function is frequently performed in unfamiliar surroundings, using written, graphic and verbal tasks, specially developed equipment and electronic games. A more realistic recommendation is that assessment methods are arranged so that the patient performs everyday work in a familiar but standardized situation. Soderback presented a valid and reliable method in which the patient performed two standardized, everyday household tasks in a training kitchen. The same tasks used in a training programme demonstrated significant training effects. Using the tools of activity analysis synthesized with a model of intellectual function, tasks and work sequences can be evaluated in conjunction with spatial, verbal, numerical, memory, attention, processing and planning functions. Occupational therapists can extend activity analysis into the cognitive domain, with evidence of functional benefits for their patients.

OCCUPATIONAL THERAPY FOR WITH PERSONS WITH PROGRESSIVE ILLNESSES

The aim of OT with persons handicapped by progressive illnesses is primarily the empowerment of the individual to adapt and compensate for loss of function, in order to maintain a level of independent living and quality of life that is acceptable to them. Treatment may involve adaptation to and management of existing symptoms to maintain functional activities, prevention of deformity and modification of the person's environment. Regular evaluation is essential to identify signs of increasing functional handicap, to compensate for and assist adaptation to changes in level of function. In all areas of intervention an integrated multiprofessional approach is essential from the earliest stages, to ensure consistency and adequacy of the information provided to the individual, their family and carers. A consistent supportive team approach can assist the individual and their family to acquire the coping strategies that are crucial to acceptance and adaptation to the course of progressive illness. Team support is also integral to the effectiveness of team members in their work with the individual and family members.

In the treatment of progressive disease, the guiding OT principle of focusing on the whole person, their physical, psychological, emotional, social and spiritual needs (Mayers, 1990), is nowhere more important. The opportunity for successful intervention is greatly assisted by the timely referral of the person by their medical practitioner. Information about practical support and strategies given by the occupational therapist reduce the anxiety of the individual, caused by concerns over their ability to cope in the future. Whether the occupational therapist is introducing the idea of a stairlift or hoist in the individual's home, suggesting adaptive equipment in the kitchen or providing a hand splint, the successful outcome depends occupational therapist's ability to assist the individual to perceive the advantages and opportunities to be gained in achieving their own needs and goals, that the equipment or treatment may render attainable.

OCCUPATIONAL THERAPY IN THE COMMUNITY

The core of OT in the community is working with people (Levine, 1988). Through the skilled support and guidance of the occupational therapist, carers and families learn how to maximize the client's level of function and quality of life, through practice and adaptation of tasks and roles, and modification of the environment. To be effective, treatment in the client's home must focus on the whole person, in the context of surrounding family,

social networks and environment. This may be in marked contrast to the client's experience of hospital care, where treatment may have been fragmented, alienating and isolating to the individual; a technological medical machine focusing on specific aspects of disease or disability. It may fall to the occupational therapist to explain the fragmented pieces of information and experiences, and help the person to put them together to make a coherent and comprehensible picture of the nature of their handicap, and its effect on them as an individual.

Rehabilitation in hospital is frequently intensive and constrained by time. It therefore has a tendency to focus on aspects of mobility and self-care, short-term goals that have an impact on early discharge. In contrast, rehabilitation in the community may be more effective if carried out over a longer time scale. Bach-y-Rita and Wicab Bach-y-Rita (1990) report evidence to suggest that the emphasis on rehabilitation in the early months following brain damage does not reflect the capacity of the brain to reorganize and relearn over a period of years. They emphasize the need for long-term community programmes, primarily with family involvement. The rehabilitation concerns of the occupational therapist working in the community include the broader issues of lifestyle and roles, employment and leisure, a holistic approach to the quality of life of the disabled person and the family. It is mainly in the community that the occupational therapist has the opportunity to empower the family and carers to participate fully in the treatment programme for an extended period of time.

In addition to the client, carers, family and friends, the important members of the community team may include other appropriate professionals, neighbours, voluntary helpers and organizations, local and central government services. In order for the client's individual needs to be met effectively, all these members must be organized in a unified whole. It may fall to the occupational therapist, whose focus is on the client as a whole person, in the context of their family, social networks and environment, to facilitate effective team work, on behalf of the client. It would be naive to assume that merely calling this diffuse group of people a team, would enable them to behave as a team (Fry, Lech and Rubin, 1974).

The occupational therapist working in the community is a unique generalist, with the ability to solve problems with the people, equipment and materials available in the client's environment. Intervention must lead to functional activities that are relevant to the client's lifestyle and values. Levine (1988) describes five phases for the process of occupational therapy, in the community: referral, building a therapeutic relationship, the treatment programme, discharge planning and aftercare. Specific aspects of the treatment programme include physical and psychosocial assessment, setting goals, teaching strategies and adaptive techniques, and resolving architectural barriers to progress or quality of life.

Recent guidelines (Age Concern, 1995) outline the responsibilities of health and local authorities, for the continuing health care of physically disabled adults in the community. Health and local authorities are required to work together with family practitioners to provide services that meet the following needs: rehabilitation; palliative care; regular and routine supervision of specialist staff and provision of specialist equipment; respite care; specialist support for people in nursing homes and residential care; and reassessment of care needs. Additionally clients, families and carers 'should be kept fully informed...and receive the relevant information they require to make decisions about continuing care' in the community. It is imperative that occupational therapists in the community are well informed of national and local guidelines, and policy decisions which affect their area of work.

Taylor (1977) refers to 'charting the obstacle course', in a survey of agencies providing health and social care for disabled people (Beardshaw, 1988). He described a multiplicity of health, local authority and voluntary organizations, further divided into specialist departments, providing a complex array of services. Overlap, replication of services, absence of provision and repeated assessment were common features of organization, which varied both across and within area boundaries. Harrison reporting on the supply of disability aids in one health district, noted regular suppliers, occasional suppliers and absence of provision, for a range of frequently used and essential equipment (Beardshaw, 1988). In the same health district, manual wheelchairs were provided mainly by the disabled services centre, and occasionally by social services, the health authority and charitable organizations, but no provision existed for communication aids. Recent changes in legislation and administration may not have simplified access to services for the consumer.

The individual occupational therapist in the community is required to continually update their knowledge of availability of resources and services, to meet the needs of their clients. In many cases, it is only through the continuing therapeutic relationships, interventions and knowledge of the community occupational therapist, that some of the benefits of hospital and specialist rehabilitation become effective in a lasting way for people with disabilities and their families in the community.

OCCUPATIONAL THERAPY AND LEGISLATION FOR CARE IN THE COMMUNITY

(The Chronically Sick and Disabled Persons Act (CSDP Act) 1970, the Disabled Persons Act (DP Act) 1986, and the NHS and Community Care Act 1990)

The implementation of the Community Care Act 1990 has brought significant changes in funding for the provision of health and social care for disabled people in the community. An emphasis on reducing length of stay in hospitals, and developing community-based rehabilitation demands extensive local organization of the interface between health and social services. Proposals accentuate the requirement for the individual assessment of people with significant disability to ensure the delivery of appropriate support and resources. Opportunities to establish systematic processes of assessment and case management involving families, carers and multidisciplinary teams, offer the potential to improve the quality of care and rehabilitation for disabled people in their homes. A great deal of work and expertise will be required of occupational therapists and other professionals at local level to establish the effective organization of care and rehabilitation in the community.

Local authorities have a statutory duty, under section 2 of the CSDP Act, to provide the following services for disabled people, if the local authority accepts that the disabled person is in need of a particular service or services. Services which the local authority has a duty to provide include practical assistance in the home, a telephone, adaptations to the home to secure safety, comfort or convenience, and leisure and recreational facilities in the home. Additionally statutory provision includes meals in the home or elsewhere, recreational and educational facilities outside the home, a holiday, and assistance travelling to and from the home in order to take advantage of the listed opportunities. Section 4 of the DP Act 1986 confirms the statutory duty of the local authority to assess the needs of a disabled person for any of these services on request. Section 8 of this Act requires that the abilities of carers to continue to provide care on a regular basis must be taken into account during assessment. Local authorities must also provide information on any relevant services for disabled people available from

themselves, or that they know to be available from other organizations.

The cost of these services provided by local authorities may be recovered from individual clients, either through means testing or flat-rate charges. Clients below a certain income may be exempted from charges. Authorities cannot refuse to provide services, when they have accepted a disabled person's need of them, if the clients is unable to pay. Nor can they withdraw a service already provided. Authorities have the right to recover the cost through the civil courts. It is the duty of the local authority to meet the **needs** of an individual, but not necessarily the person's **preferences**, although these must be taken into account in the assessment. Blanket eligibility criteria are therefore unsuitable, and it is unlawful to withdraw or reduce a service from an individual unless it can be demonstrated that his or her need has diminished (RADAR, 1994).

The implications of the CSDP Act for the occupational therapist in the community are clearly to execute a thorough and comprehensive assessment of the disabled person and the abilities of their carers, and make pertinent recommendations for provision of services. Follow up to evaluate effective and proper use of resources provided is essential for both the care and safety of the consumers, and cost-effective provision. It is inevitable that continuing restraints on public spending put pressures on community occupational therapists that test their professional judgement against local authority policies. However, it is unacceptable for disabled people and carers to be told that staff are not available to make assessment or that services cannot be provided if the client is unable to pay (Community Care Act – HMSO, 1990). Similarly, blanket policies epitomized in such statements as: assistance is no longer given for this, or this service is only provided for certain groups of people, are not adequate, without individual assessment being made. Lack of staff, high demand or limiting provision to specific services are not justifiable reasons for reducing, withdrawing or not providing services when the individual's need has been recognized. The NHS and Community Care Act 1990 also requires local authorities to set up procedures for dealing with complaints about social services.

The role occupational therapists employed by local authorities has changed dramatically in the last three decades, and continues to change. The 'craft advisor for the disabled' is now disability advisor and assessor, and may in the future become adjudicator or inspector of services. An occupational therapist employed by a local authority requires extensive skills in assessment, clinical knowledge of adaptive techniques and processes, knowledge of progression and prognosis of impairments, and a comprehensive understanding of policy guidelines and statutory obligations of local authorities and other providers. Local authority occupational therapists and their clients have this statement by the Secretary of State for Social Services (1975) to support them: '...local authorities are aware of the mandatory nature of Section 2 (CSDP Act, 1970). Once they accept that a need exists in respect of one of the services listed in this section, it is incumbent upon them to make arrangements to meet that need'.

INFORMATION TECHNOLOGY AND MANAGEMENT IN OCCUPATIONAL THERAPY

The use of personal computers in rehabilitation is an area of development and plausible benefit. Three main areas of application are as a treatment technique, in vocational rehabilitation and adaptation of the work environment, and in evaluation and audit of clinical practice.

Proctor (1984) suggests four advantages for using a computer: it does not tire or become frustrated; programs can be selected and modified to suit the abilities and needs of the individual; the speed of operation can be graded; the computer programme maintains a consistency of approach. In practice the modification of programs and operating devices to suit individual ability and speed of operation remains limited, unless considerable time and technological resources are available. Nevertheless, programs and operating systems that match individual needs and abilities can be found.

In the rehabilitation of people with acquired brain damage there is some provisional research evidence that computer-assisted instruction effects improvements in attention, concentration and spatial perception. Gracey (1984) demonstrated increases in selective attention and improved response time for survivors of head injury, using programs on visuospatial, memory and spatial perception skills. Research by Milner (1984) replicated the same study, suggesting that the programs assisted improvement of attention and short-term memory of people with right brain damage. Milner stressed that pencil and paper tasks were equally important in cognitive retraining. Larose *et al.* (1989) used computer games to improve visual scanning and tracking, and results revealed significant improvements in the selected spatial abilities tested.

Schacter and Glisky (1993) described a program using the techniques of 'errorless learning' and 'vanishing cues' to teach amnesic survivors of brain injury how to program and interact with a microcomputer. During the program a severely amnesic young woman was taught to perform a real-world job involving data entry into a computer. She was unable to carry out daily living functions without the availability of consistent prompts and reminders, and could not recall her activities from day to day. Learning the task required the acquisition of over 250 separate pieces of information, but the young woman eventually learned it and was able to perform the job and return to employment. However, information learned during the program appeared to be specific to the tasks required, and there was an absence of generalization to other areas of function. The application of the microcomputer as a treatment media in OT is a promising area that requires continued exploration and evaluation.

In the domain of vocational rehabilitation and adaptation the computer is a valuable resource for the OT. Where physical disabilities restrict hand function, adapting tasks that can be performed using a keyboard or other operating system may achieve continued employment for the individual. Similarly, retraining or adapting existing skills can open new potential opportunities for re-employment, when the person is unable to continue in their former occupation. Students with handicaps and people retraining for work are able to benefit from increasing opportunities of computer-assisted learning. They are also enabled to compete as equals in the presentation of their work, using word processing, desktop publishing and graphic design programs. Appropriate hardware and software can be obtained from disability employment services, and special needs education departments. Recent developments in funding for education and training are improving access for unemployed adults with physical disability, with exemption from tuition fees for accredited courses, and additional funding available to meet individual learning needs.

Finally, the collection of data that is essential to the evaluation of the role of OT in rehabilitation services, and the measurement of outcomes for people with handicaps, will only be achieved through familiarization with, and use of computers. Recording appropriate and relevant data for people with disability, the results of selected assessments, and data describing outcomes in a format that is accessible and retrievable for treatment and programme evaluation is imperative for the future development of the OT profession, and for the enhancement of the individual skills and practice of occupational therapists. Familiarity with the use of computer databases and spreadsheets, and the basic statistical analysis accompanying these programs, will make treatment evaluation more accessible to individual practitioners. There is no justification for the continuing use of rehabilitation techniques and methods that have not been evaluated, or are not in the process of evaluation.

ASSESSMENTS AND OUTCOME MEASURES IN OCCUPATIONAL THERAPY

It is essential for therapists to be able to evaluate and review the effectiveness and appropriateness of their treatment methods, both to assist the people they treat, and for professional development. The evolution of assessment batteries is both time consuming and a highly skilled process, if the essential requirements of reliability and validity are to be met by both personal and peer group evaluation. Hence, the production of assessment measures has become a vast business enterprise in both Europe and the USA, with the accompanying deleterious effects of marketing strategies and 'hype'. The pressures from both consumers (government agencies) and producers (commercial enterprises) have lead to the premature release of measures without proper evaluation. The modification or adaptation of any previously validated measure requires the complete process of re-evaluation. The Functional Assessment Measure (FAM), successor to the thoroughly externally validated Functional Independence Measure (FIM), was released before thorough revalidation. Later external revue indicated poor interrater reliability, and that the revised scale was neither linear nor interval (Hall *et al.*, 1993). The FIM continuous to grow in acceptability with repeated acknowledgement from external evaluation (Ditunno, 1992).

Occupational therapists should be concerned with measures of function. Since the assumptions underpinning quantitative measures of function remain questionable, there still exists an ample role for the qualitative rating of the experienced therapist in negotiation with the individual (Depoy, 1992). Although global measures of function that are not specific to medical conditions have a useful comparative role, their comprehensiveness may reduce sensitivity to changes, and introduce irrelevance when used in the assessment of certain conditions. In the selection of measures to assess and evaluate outcome in OT, there is no substitute for the thorough and critical reading of as many published papers as possible on the development and evaluation, both internal and external, of the proposed scales.

An extensive evaluation of the literature pertaining to neurological handicap has supported the use of the Disability Rating Scale (Rappaport *et al.*, 1982) for survivors of head injury. The use of FIM for stroke, multiple sclerosis and other neurological conditions also has considerable support, providing adequate training in administration is available. The Barthel Activities of Daily Living Index (BI) is one of the best brief assessments of basic activities of daily living currently available. Its validity as a measure of needs of care is well established, and recent studies indicate high levels of interrater reliability, but it has limitations as an outcome measure since it may not detect important changes (Mahoney and Barthel, 1965). The maximum score implies independence in personal activities of daily living and mobility, but not necessarily the ability to function alone. The Extended Activities of Daily Living Scale (Lincoln and Gladman, 1992) has demonstrable validity as an overall assessment of functional independence in stroke patients. It is a valuable extension to the BI, with greater sensitivity, and is suitable for postal surveys.

Reducing handicap is a key goal of rehabilitation, but surprisingly few measures have been developed that address the measurement of handicap. The World Health Organization International Classification of Impairment Disability and Handicap provides a suitable framework for such a scale, but attempts to use the classification as a measure have reported low interrated reliability, and problems with agreement among raters. The London Handicap Scale (Harwood *et al.*, 1994), a self-assessment questionnaire, was developed to address these difficulties. Preliminary validation has revealed its usefulness as a measure of handicap, and further use and evaluation is recommended.

Continued use and evaluation is supported for the Medical Outcomes Study Short Forms (SF-20 and SF-36), as global, health-related 'quality of life' measures (Stewart *et al.*, 1989). For global cognitive function, the Mini-Mental State Scale (Dick *et al.*, 1984), and specific cognitive function the PASAT and the Rivermead Behavioural memory test, merit continued use and evaluation (Wilson, 1992). In the measurement of function for persons with arthritis the HAQ (Fries *et al.*, 1980) is widely accepted.

CONCLUSION

Through this chapter the author has endeavoured to describe the philosophical underpinning, rationale and scientific basis for occupational therapy *with* the physically disabled adult. The use of the word *with* is deliberate throughout the text, in order to emphasize that it is critical to the success of an OT programme that the handicapped adult is 'participant' in the widest sense of the word, in all aspects of assessment, development of objectives, planning, implementation and evaluation. 'Participation' in purposeful occupations and activities is integral to the practice of OT. Batavia (1992), writing from the perspective of both provider and consumer of rehabilitation resources, states 'Consumers ultimately want the process of functional assessment to be dignified, and results of functional assessment to be relevant to their desired outcomes. They want to be informed and have input into the ultimate decision-making process that affect their lives'. This viewpoint is relevant to all professions engaged in rehabilitation.

Rather than provide detailed checklists for the assessment and treatment of specific conditions, which are admirably described in the literature, the author has aimed to provide a framework for intervention, applying philosophical principles and empirical evidence to the practice of OT. It is envisaged that the practising occupational therapist his/her existing knowledge and skills within these frameworks, to develop flexible OT programmes that meet the individual needs of consumers. It is hoped that this chapter will further the understanding of practitioners in complimentary professions of the unique role of occupational therapy in rehabilitation.

Finally, to reiterate the words of Aristotle: quality of life or the 'good life' is 'a fully rational active life'. Bach-y-Rita (1989) suggests that 'Medical advances over the last twenty years have lead to the increased survival of stroke and serious accident patients and those who must contend with the major diseases of childhood, adulthood and aging. However, the increased survival has not necessarily been accompanied by a satisfactory quality of life'. This statement carries serious implications for the future roles of all practitioners in rehabilitation, but a unique standard for occupational therapists.

Acknowledgements

I gratefully acknowledge the help given by Christine Mercer, Head Occupational Therapist, in the preparation of the section on occupational therapy for people with arthritis.

REFERENCES

Age Concern Briefings (1995) *NHS Responsibilities for Continuing Health Care, and Hospital Discharge Arrangements*, No. 0895, Age Concern, London.

Alexander, J.L. and Fuhrer, M.J. (1984). Functional assessment of individuals with physical impairments in *Functional Assessment in Rehabilitation*. (eds A.S. Halpern and M.J. Fuhrer), Paul H. Brooks, Baltimore: pp. 45–59.

Bach-y-Rita, P. (1989) Theory-based neurorehabilitation. *Archives of Physical Medicine Rehabilitation*, **70**, 162.

Bach-y-Rita P. and Wicab Bach-y-Rita, E. (1990) Biological and psychosocial factors in the recovery of brain damage in humans. *Canadian Journal of Psychology*, **49**, 148–65.

Basmajian, J.V., Regenos, E.M. and Baker, M.P. (1977) Rehabilitating stroke patients with biofeedback. *Geriatrics*, **32**, 85–8.

Batavia, A.I. (1992). Assessing the function of functional assessment: a consumer perspective. *Disability and Rehabilitation*, **14**, 156–60.

Boyeson, M.C. and Bach-y-Rita, P. (1989) Determinants of brain plasticity. *Journal of Neurological Rehabilitation*, **3**, 35–7.

Chawla, J.C. (1944) Sports for people with disability. *British Medical Journal*, **308**, 1500–04.

Cope, N. (1993) International Brain Injury Forum: the quest for better outcomes. *Brain Injury Services*, (Abstracts) 13.

Beardshaw, V. (1988) *Last on the list: Community Services for people with Physical Disabilities*. Kings Fund Institute, London.

Depoy, E. (1992) A comparison of standardised and observational assessment. *Journal of Cognitive Rehabilitation*, **10**, 30–3.

Dick, J.P.R., Guiloff, R.J. and Stewart, A. (1984) Mini-mental state examination in neurological patients. *Journal of Neurology, Neurosurgery and Psychiatry*, **47**, 496–9.

Ditunno, J.F. Jr. (1992) Functional assessment measures in CNS Trauma. *Journal of Neurotrauma*, **9**, 301–5.

Feldman, D.J., Lee., P.R., Unterecker, J. *et al.* (1962) A comparison of functionally oriented medical care and formal rehabilitation in the management of patients with hemiplegia due to cerebrovascular disease. *Journal of Chronic Disability*, **15**, 297–310.

Fry, R.E., Lech, B.A. and Rubin, I. (1974) Working with the primary care team: the first intervention, in *Making Health Teams Work* (eds H. Wise *et al.*), Ballinger, Cambridge, M.A., p. 633.

Garraway, W.M., Akhter, A.J., Prescott, R.J. and Hockey, L. (1980) Management of acute stroke in the elderly: preliminary results of a controlled trial. *British Medical Journal*, **281**, 827–9.

Geisler, W.O., Jousse, A.T., Wynne-Jones, M. and Breithaupt, D. (1983) Survival in traumatic spinal cord injury. *Paraplegia*, **21**, 364–73.

Gracey, S. (1984) Computer assisted therapy for brain damaged patients, in *Physical Disabilities Special Interest Section*, vol. (72), American Occupational Therapists Association, Rockville.

Gronwall, D. (1977) Paced auditory serial-addition task: a measure of recovery from concussion. *Perceptual Motor Skills*, **44**, 367–73.

Grundy, D., Russell, J. and Swain, A. (1986) *ABC of Spinal Cord Injury*, British Medical Journal Publications, London.

Hall, K.M., Hamilton, B.B., Gordon, W.A. and Zasler, N.D. (1993) Characteristics and comparisons of functional assessment indices: Disability Rating Scale, Functional Independence Measure, and Functional Assessment Measure. *Journal of Head Trauma Rehabilitation*, **8**, 60–74.

Harwood, R.H., Rogers, A., Dickson, E. and Ebrahim, S. (1994) Measuring handicap: the London handicap scale, a new outcome measure for chronic disease. *Quality in Health Care*, **3**, 11–16.

Hayes, S.H. and Carroll, S.R. (1986) Early intervention care in the acute stroke patient. *Archives of Physical Medicine Rehabilitation*, **67**, 319–21.

HMSO (1990) *Community Care in the Next Decade and Beyond: policy guidance*, HMSO, London.

Johannsen, W.J., Jones, D. and Thilli, M.K. (1967) Effectiveness of homemakers training for hemiplegic patients. *Archives of Physical Medicine Rehabilitation*, **48**, 244–9.

Johnston, M.V., Findley, T.W., DeLuca, J. and Katz, R.T. (1991) Measurement tools with application to brain injury. *American Journal of Physical Medicine and Rehabilitation*, **70**, (I Suppl) S114–30.

Kreutzer, J.S., Wehman, P., Morton, M.V. and Stonnington, H.H. (1988) Supported employment and compensatory strategies for enhancing vocational outcome following traumatic brain injury. *Brain Injury*, **2**, 205–23.

Larose, S., Gagnon, S., Ferland, C. and Pepin, M. (1989) Psychology of computers: XIV – cognitive rehabilitation through computer games. *Perceptual and Motor Skills*, **69**, 851–8.

Levine, R.E. (1988) in *Willard and Spackman's Occupational Therapy*, 7th edn. (eds H. Hopkins and H. Smith), J.B. Lippincott, Philadelphia, p. 633.

Lincoln, N.B. and Gladman, JRF. (1992) The extended activities of daily living scale: a further validation. *Disability and Rehabilitation*, **14**, (4) 41–43.

Lorig, K., Konkol, L. and Gonzalez, V. (1987) Arthritis patient education: a review of the literature. *Patient Education Council*, **10**, pages 207–52.

Mahoney, F.I. and Barthel, D.W. (1965) Functional evaluation: the Barthel Index. *Maryland State Medical Journal*, **14**, 379–80.

Mazzuca, J.A. (1982) Does patient education in chronic disease have therapeutic value? *Journal of Chronic Disease*, **35**, 521–9.

Melvin, J.L. (1989) *Rheumatic Disease in the Adult and Child: occupational therapy and rehabilitation*, 3rd edn., F.A. Davis, Philadelphia, Company.

Milner, D. (1984) Use of a microcomputer in treatment of patients with physical disabilities in *Physical Disabilities Special Interest Section*, vol. 7 (2), American Occupational Therapists Association, Rockville, pp. 1–4.

Mulder, Th. (1985) EMG feedback and the restoration of motor control: a controlled group study with 12 hemiparetic patients, in *The Learning of Motor Control Following Brain Damage: experimental and clinical studies*, Swers and Zeitlinger, Lisse, pp. 67–79.

Mulley, G.P. (1985) *Practical Management of Stroke*, Croom Helm, London.

Ostendorf, C.G. and Wolf, S.L. (1981) Effect of forced use of the upper extremity of a hemiplegic patient on changes in function: a single case design. *Physical Therapy*, **61**, 1808–116.

Pedretti, L.W. (1985) *Occupational Therapy: practice skills for physical dysfunction*, CV Mosby, St Louis.

Proctor, J. (1984) in *Micros for Handicapped Users*. (ed. P. Saunders), Helena Press, Whitby, pp. 119–21.

RADAR. (1994). Obtaining Services Under Section 2 of the Chronically Sick and Disabled Persons Act 1970. Health and Social Security Factsheet 2, The Royal Association for Disability and Rehabilitation, London.

Rappaport, M., Hall, K.M., Hopkins, K: *et al.* (1982) Disability Rating Scale for severe head trauma: coma to community. *Archives of Physical Medicine Rehabilitation*, **63**, 118–123.

Reilly, M. (1969) The Educational Process. *American Journal of Occupational Therapy*, **63**, 118–23.

Ross, W.D., (Ed.) (1915) *The Works of Aristotle*, vol. 9, Oxford University Press, London.

Rusk, H.A., Lowman, E.W. and Block, J.M. (1966) Rehabilitation of the patient with head injuries. *Clinical Neurosurgery*, **12**, 312–23.

Secretary of State for Social Services. (1975) House of Commons Debates, vol. 897, col. 218, in Health and Social Security Factsheet 2, RADAR, London.

Schacter, D.L. and Glisky, E. (1993) How much can an injured brain learn?, in *International Brain Injury Forum: the quest for better outcomes*, Brain Injury Services, Northampton, p. 19 (Abstracts).

Smedley, R.R., Fiorino, A.J., Soucar, E. *et al.* (1986) Slot machines: their use in rehabilitation after stroke. *Archives of Physical Medicine Rehabilitation*, **67**, 546–9.

Smith, M.E., Garraway, W.M., Smith, D.L. and Akhtar, A.J. (1982) Therapy impact on functional outcome in a controlled trial of stroke rehabilitation. *Archives of Physical Medicine Rehabilitation*, **63**, 21–4.

Soderback, I. (1988) A household based assessment of intellectual functions in patients with acquired brain damage. Developmental evaluation of an occupational therapy method. *Scandinavian Journal of Rehabilitation Medicine*, **20**, 57–69.

Stern, P.H. (1970) Effects of facilitation exercise techniques in stroke rehabilitation. *Archives of Physical Medicine Rehabilitation*, **51**, 526–31.

Stern, P.H., McDowell, F., Miller, J.M. and Robinson, M. (1971) Factors influencing, stroke rehabilitation, *Stroke*, **2**, 213–18.

Stewart, A.L., Greenfield, S., Hays, R., Rogers, W.H. and Berry S (1989) Functional status and well-being of patients with chronic conditions. Results from the Medical Outcomes Study. *Journal of the American Medical Association*, **262**, 907–13.

Strand, T., Asplund, K., Eriksson, S. *et al.* (1985) A non-intensive stroke unit reduces functional disability and the need for long-term hospitalisation. *Stroke*, **16**, 29–34.

Thompson, S.B.N. and Morgan, M. (1990) *Occupational Therapy for Stroke Rehabilitation*, Chapman and Hall, London.

Trieschmann, R.B. (1980) *Spinal Cord Injuries: psychological, social and vocational adjustment*, Pergamon, Elmsford, NY.

Trombly, C.A. (ed.) (1989) *Occupational Therapy for Physical Dysfunction*, 3rd edn., Williams and Wilkins, Baltimore.

Turner, A. (Ed.) (1987) *The Practice of Occupational Therapy*, Churchill Livingstone, Edinburgh.

Wade, D.T., Langton-Hewer, R., Skilbeck, C.E. and David, R.M. (1985) *Stroke: a critical approach to diagnosis, treatment and management*, Chapman and Hall, London.

Weber, P.L. (1989) in *Occupational Therapy for Physical Dysfunction*, (ed. C.A.,Trombly), pp. 336–47.

Whalley Hammel, K. 1994 *Spinal Cord Injury Rehabilitation, Chapman and Hall, London*.

Wilcock, A.A. (1986) *Occupational Therapy approaches to Stroke*, Churchill Livingstone, Edinburgh.

Wilson, B. (1992) Recovery and compensatory strategies in head injured memory impaired people several years after insult. *Journal of Neurology, Neurosurgery and Psychiatry*, **55**, 177–80.

Young, G.C., Collins, D. and Hren, M. (1983) Effect of pairing scanning training with block design training in the remediation of perceptual problems in left hemiplegia. *Journal of Clinical Neuropsychology*, **5**, 201–12.

42 Dental Care

P.N. Hirschmann

INTRODUCTION

The dental care of those with physical disability can suffer for reasons of access, attitude and ability (Figure 42.1). Epidemiological studies have demonstrated that almost all such patients have more periodontal disease and poorer oral hygiene than the general population. The aims of dental care for this group of individuals should be no different from those for any other members of the community:

These are:

- preventing pain and discomfort;
- improving (or maintaining) the patient's appearance;
- enhancing their ability to eat;
- assisting their speech;
- promoting a satisfactory standard (by the patient or their carers) of oral hygiene;
- in addition, and of particular relevance to physically disabled people, maintaining the dentition for use as an accessory limb (O'Donnel, Yen and Robson, 1985).

Some patients are dependent on a mouth stick to access a keyboard or environmental controls. Occasionally, the body weight is carried through the teeth during transfers.

It should not be necessary to say that such dental care should be to the best possible standard and of the same quality (as far as possible) as that offered to all other patients. It is also important to remember that dental treatment may be required early in, if not in some cases prior to, the rehabilitation process. For instance, professional oral hygiene, from a dental hygienist, should be available early in the management of patients with head injuries or receiving parenteral or enteral nutrition before gingivitis becomes established or existing dental disease is exacerbated. Patients may complain of ill-fitting dentures shortly after a stroke: often this is due to loss of muscle tone and the consequent inability to control the lower denture in particular. 'Plumping' the surface of the lower denture to eliminate the buccal sulcus may prove helpful in both eating and speech. Intra-oral palatal training appliances have been described which are helpful in the speech therapy of acquired velopharyngeal disorders (Enderby, Hathorn and Servant, 1984) and the control of drooling (Oliver, 1987). An oral assessment should be carried out by trained health professionals (usually nurses) as part of the overall process of rehabilitation (Griffiths and Boyle, 1993).

ORGANIZATION OF DENTAL SERVICES IN THE UK

Access to dental treatment

Dental treatment for disabled people is available either from a general dental practitioner

Rehabilitation of the Physically Disabled Adult. Edited by C. John Goodwill, M. Anne Chamberlain and Chris Evans.
Published in 1997 by Stanley Thornes (Publishers) Ltd, Cheltenham. ISBN 0-7487-3183-0.

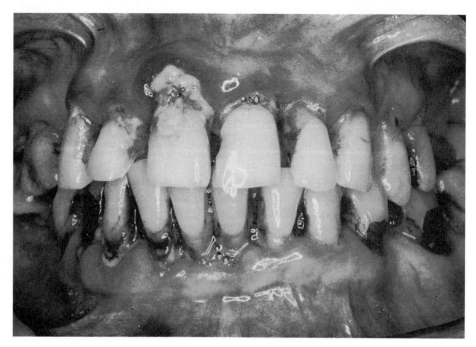

Figure 42.1 Clinical photograph showing the dental state of a 56-year-old lady with a 32-year history of rheumatoid arthritis. She last saw a dentist 2 years ago and can no longer clean her own teeth. There is widespread calculus and plaque, in particular on the upper right central incisor. Her gums are inflamed and there is much recession.

(GDP, family dentist), working either within the NHS General Dental Service (GDS) or to private contract, the Community Dental Service or the Hospital Dental Service. It is the accepted policy that treatment for such patients should be provided, as far as possible, by the first of these three. The description that follows of the UK dental services must be regarded as provisional: sweeping changes are happening.

General Dental Services

Since 1990 patients have been able to register with a dentist for continuing care, as with a family doctor. However, the availability of dental treatment on the NHS is decreasing as more dentists are only prepared to accept new patients on a private contract and an increasing amount of care is underwritten by third party insurers. The names of those dentists continuing to work within the GDS are available from the health authorities. British Telecom's Yellow Pages (or similar directories) are good source of information, **Access to dentists' surgeries** is often a problem and the dental services manager of the health authorities will have the names of those level access.

Housebound patients may request a domiciliary visit from the dentist which is still free (see below) and many practitioners advertise that they provide such a service. The extent of the treatment they provide varies: check-ups should present no problems nor should the construction of dentures. Fillings and cleaning may be more difficult to provide, although some practitioners do have their own portable dental equipment to enable them to provide such treatment. An annual inspection is recommended for edentulous patients.

The ambulance service may also impose a further limitation on their seeking treatment from a GDP; however, in some parts of the country the ambulance service appears willing to take patients to dentists' surgeries but prior negotiation may be necessary before they will agree to convey personal wheelchairs. Most social services departments will provide transport and have suitable vehicles for transporting those confined to wheelchairs, as do some of the charitable organizations, such as the Multiple Sclerosis Society.

Community dental services (CDS)

The CDS currently provides treatment not only for children but also for adults and elderly people who are unable to obtain it from a general dental practitioner under the NHS. Most Community Trusts now have a senior dental officer with specific responsibility for patients with special needs. An inquiry to the (Community) Dental Services Manager, new-style, or the District Dental Officer (DDO), old-style, will establish the nature of local provision. They can often undertake to negotiate with ambulance services.

Hospital dental services

Provision of dental care for physically handicapped persons is as uneven between hospitals as in other areas of the dental services. Most **dental teaching hospitals** have comprehensive adult handicapped services, whereas in **district general hospitals** the extent of the provision will depend on the attitudes and interests of the individual Consultant Oral Surgeon. Some limit their service to consultation and to surgical treatment of those whose handicap is primarily medical; others do have the staff and facilities to provide regular dental care. The Dental Services Manager/DDO will know the extent of the service

available. Finally, Consultant Oral Surgeons may be willing to see patients for domiciliary assessments if not actual treatment.

Cost of dental treatment

The (rising) costs of dental treatment may deter the physically disabled person from seeking a dentist. Domiciliary visits are free, as are repairs to NHS dentures. Otherwise the patient pays, at present 80% of the cost of treatment, including the examination, up to a maximum of £300.

There are certain exemptions:

- All treatment is free to those receiving Disability Working Allowance, Income Support or Family Credit, or to holders of an AG2 certificate.
- Those on low income (details on DHSS leaflet Dl 1) may get some assistance; they should obtain a form AG1 from their dentist, optician, hospital or DSS office which then has to be sent to the Health Benefits Unit in Newcastle. An AG2 certificate entitles the holder to free dental treatment, an AG3 to limited help only.

Patients should always be advised to seek clarification about charges **before** commencing treatment from their dentist, who should also provide them with a written treatment plan if they are a new patient.

ORAL HYGIENE AND THE ROLE OF THE DENTAL HYGIENIST

The maintenance of an adequate dentition depends as much on the efficacy of the patient's own toothbrushing and on their diet as on the quality of professional care provided. Rehabilitation units providing advice to newly disabled people may usefully include a talk from a dental hygienist in their educational programme for patients and carers.

In addition to those groups of hospital

inpatients mentioned above, the need to maintain an adequate level to oral hygiene should not be overlooked in the management of the terminal stages of multiple sclerosis, pseudobulbar palsy and motor neurone disease, when their expertise is particularly valuable. Many of the drugs used in the treatment of Parkinson's disease or psychiatric disorders cause a dry mouth and meticulous attention to oral hygiene is therefore important to prevent oral disease. There are increasing numbers of dental hygienists in all three branches of the dental services whose role as part of the dental team is to provide advice and active treatment in these areas. Those working in the CDS and GDS will provide home care.

Tooth brushing

A toothbrush should be of a suitable size and design to reach all tooth surfaces and gum margins with ease and comfort. For those unable to grip a normal toothbrush there are now several modifications. Details of these are available from Disabled Living Centres. If these prove unacceptable, then it is also possible for the dentist, and his/her dental technician, to construct a 'made-to-measure' handle. A range of the modifications possible is shown in Figure 42.2, and also in Griffiths and Boyle (1993). Electric toothbrushes are particularly useful when manipulating a toothbrush (whether by the patient or their carers) is difficult and, in some cases, may be obtained with financial assistance from social services departments of the local authority as an aid to daily living. The handle can be modified in the same way as conventional toothbrushes.

Dental floss, a fine nylon cord or tape, and woodsticks are used to clean between teeth. Misused they can be destructive and, as a general rule, individual instruction from a dentist or dental hygienist is preferable. Handling dental floss becomes more difficult, if not impossible, if dexterity is impaired.

Mouthwashes

Although numerous mouthwashes are available, both on prescription and over the counter, chlorohexidine gluconate (Corsodyl) is still the most efficacious in reducing plaque and maintaining oral hygiene (Seymour, 1994). It is available either as a 0.2% mouthwash or a 1% dental gel; the former can be applied with a swab, the latter a soft toothbrush.

Diet

Dietary advice for the prevention of dental disease is part of more general counselling. Wherever possible, sugar-coated foods and drinks should be confined to mealtimes to minimize the risk of dental decay and the prescription of sucrose-based medicines for chronic disease avoided. Both hospital and community pharmacists are a good source of advice. However, in some instances, the patient's medical management or dietary considerations will prove to be paramount: for example, in motor neurone disease (Chapter 25). The range of artificial sweeteners is increasing, as are alternative, non-cariogenic sugars which are added to some confectionery, medicines and diabetic foods.

Dentures

Dentures need to be cleaned as regularly as teeth, the simplest method being brushing with soap and lukewarm, not hot, water. Dentures should not be worn at night and should be soaked two or three nights a week in a proprietary denture cleanser, such as 0.1% hypochlorite (Dentural, Milton) and then washed thoroughly. Other proprietary cleansers are generally less effective (Jagger and Harrison, 1995). The presence of an angry red mucosa, sometimes flecked with white patches, beneath the denture is a sign of candidal infection and the patient should be

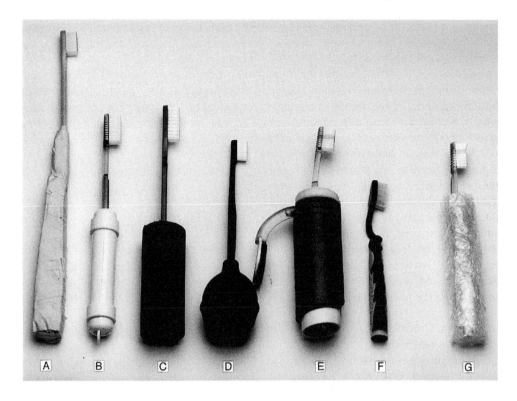

Figure 42.2 Photograph showing a range of modified toothbrushes. G is the simplest and cheapest: it consists of a sheet of 'bubble-pack' wrapped around the handle and fixed with Sellotape. It can be made in any convenient thickness for the patient and replaced whenever the bubbles have burst. F is intended for children and has a thumb-grip. E is made by Tools for Daily Living. The head of the toothbrush in C, which has been modified with a roll of foam, is too large. E and G are among the currently recommended toothbrush sizes (Oral-B 35) and designs (Oral-B Advantage).

referred for the appropriate dental advice and antifungal therapy.

WHAT DENTISTS NEED TO KNOW

If access and costs are two of the barriers facing disabled people in their search for dental treatment, then apprehension is the third: not only for the patient but also for the dentist! In dealing with people with disability there are some particularly important topics for the dentists. They include:

- suitability for local and general anaesthesia;
- anticoagulant therapy;
- when to boost steroids;
- when to use prophylactic antibiotics;
- drug interactions;

Anaesthesia

Some dentists may be able to offer the more apprehensive patients either intravenous sedation or relative analgesia, but nonetheless there will remain a small residue of patients who because of their handicap, such as spasticity or behavioural problems, cannot receive comprehensive treatment in the dental chair. An endotracheal anaesthetic is needed for these patients and this service is provided by either the Community or Hospital Dental Services. In case of difficulty, contact the Dental Services Manager/DDO.

Some GDPs are reluctant to treat patients who pose 'medical problems' due to the risk of sudden collapse in the dental surgery or potentially hazardous drug interactions, and they may telephone requesting advice as to the suitability of your patient for treatment in their dental surgery: to which your reply should be, what treatment? There are few handicapped patients who cannot receive simple dental treatment, such as fillings and cleaning, if not simple extractions, in the normal way under local anaesthetia. Patients should be advised to take their drugs in the customary fashion. Requests for advice as to the suitability of a patient for general anaesthesia in the dental chair should be referred to the appropriate Consultant Anaesthetist. Dentists should be warned of the risk of atlanto-axial dislocation when treating patients with rheumatoid arthritis; those with juvenile chronic arthritis may also have restricted neck movement.

Anticoagulant therapy

Patients on anticoagulant therapy are at risk of excessive bleeding not only after extractions but also from scaling in the presence of either severe periodontal (gum) disease or marked gingivitis. In these cases the dentist would appreciate an International Normalised Ration (INR) in the range of 2.0–2.5 where this does not otherwise constitute a hazard to the patient's primary condition, for instance a prosthetic heart valve.

Corticosteroid therapy

The relationship between the type of dental treatment and the degree of stress induced is impossible to quantify and each patient must be judged individually, but in general whereas a filling is not usually considered

stressful, a single extraction under local anaesthesia is. In the latter instance the dentist should be advised to boost the steroid cover either by an intramuscular IM injection of 100 mg hydrocortisone hemisuccinate (or the equivalent oral dose), half an hour to one hour prior to the extraction. Where more major dental procedures are involved the patient should be referred the local Consultant Oral Surgeon.

Antibiotic prophylaxis

Antibiotic prophylaxis is essential for patients at risk from endocarditis when their dental treatment (not only extractions but also fillings and gum treatment) produces a significant bacteraemia. The level of susceptibility varies: those with heart valve replacement or a history of endocarditis are considered at higher risk compared with those with rheumatic heart disease, congenital anomalies and repairs or a previous valvotomy. Those with ischaemic heart disease or coronary artery autografts are considered at negligible risk. Antibiotic prophylaxis for those with a history of rheumatic fever alone may not be necessary if there is no evidence of consequent rheumatic heart disease. The antibiotic regimen recommended by the British Society for Antimicrobial Chemotherapy is given in the British National Formulary and should be adhered to.

Antibiotic prophylaxis is not considered necessary prior to dental treatment of most patients with **prosthetic joint replacement** except those with rheumatoid arthritis, reoperated hips, diabetes mellitus and on steroid or immunosuppressive therapy who are thought to be at greater risk, (Thynne and Ferguson, 1991). A suitable antibiotic regimen for such patients is given by Field and Martin (1991). Finally, it is also indicated for patients, such as those with hydrocephalus, with **ventricular shunts**.

REFERENCES

Enderby, P., Hathorn, I.S. and Servant, S. (1984). The use of intra-oral appliances in the management of acquired velopharyngeal disorders. *British Dental Journal*, **157**, 157–9.

Field, E.A. and Martin, M.V.(1994) Prophylactic antibiotics for patients with artificial joints undergoing oral and dental surgery: necessary or not? *British Journal of Oral and Maxillofacial Surgery*, **29**, 341–346.

Griffiths, J. and Boyle, S. (1993) *Colour Guide to Holistic Dental Care. A practical approach.* Mosby-Year Book, London, 1993.

Jagger, D.C. and Harrison, A. (1995) Denture cleansing – The best approach. *British Dental Journal*, **178**, 413–417.

O'Donnel, D., Yen, P.K.Y. and Robson, W. (1985) A mouth-controlled appliance for severely physically handicapped patients. *British Dental Journal*, **159**, 186–8.

Oliver, R.G. (1987) Theoretical aspects and clinical experience with the palatal training appliance for saliva control in persons with cerebral palsy. *Speciality Care in Dentistry*, **7**, 271–274.

Seymour, R.A. (1994) Pharmacological control of periodontal disease: i Antiplaque agents. *Journal of Dentistry*, **22**, 323–35.

Thynne, G.M. and Ferguson, J.W. (1991) Antibiotic prophylaxis during dental treatment in patients with prosthetic joints. *Journal of Bone, and Joint Surgery*, **73**, 191–4.

USEFUL ADDRESS

British Society of Dentistry for the Handicapped
Secretary: Mrs. S. Greening, 62 Brandreth Road, Penylan, Cardiff, UK.

43 Art therapy[*]

Words – the images of things. Painting – silent poetry[†]

C. Wisdom

INTRODUCTION

> It has changed my body, it has changed my life.

These are the words of a patient struggling to re-adjust to the limitations caused by his stroke. At whatever age the stroke occurs, however minor or severe, a stroke is a tragedy, and life can no longer be the same. This chapter shows how art therapy can play a unique part in the re-adjustment and rehabilitation of some neurological patients.

ART THERAPY

> *Art Therapy is the use of art and other visual media in a therapeutic or treatment setting.* (Dally, 1984)

It is a relatively new profession, having only been formally recognized by the National Health Service in 1982. A detailed account of the growth of the profession is given by Waller (1991) in *Becoming A Profession: the history of art therapy in Britain 1940 – 1992*. Today art therapy is a well-established and growing profession. It is, however, under represented in neu-rological rehabilitation settings in Britain, especially compared with its use in the USA.

Art therapy uses art to help individuals communicate and express their feelings – anxiety, depression, anger, loss and trauma. The materials used include paint, clay, collage, plaster and video, allowing the client a wide range of expression. The therapist creates a safe and containing environment in which the patient can explore their feelings and acts as a witness to the therapeutic process. It is a specially accessible form of treatment for people who find it hard to put their feelings into words. It is particularly useful for those patients whose speech and language abilities are impaired through brain injury. Children, who find art media a natural vocabulary, gain a much broader range of communication; it may be either on an individual or group basis depending on personal preference, need and availability.

Art therapists (ATs) have completed a postgraduate Diploma (Dip AT) at one of the recognized establishments (Appendix). This includes training in the psychodynamic aspects of therapeutic intervention. A registered Art Therapist (RATh) has reached the academic standards approved by the British Association of Art Therapists (BAAT) (Appendix) and has agreed to work within its objectives and constitution.

---

[*]All of the names used within this chapter are pseudonyms.
[†]A quotation from an unknown source.

Rehabilitation of the Physically Disabled Adult. Edited by C. John Goodwill, M. Anne Chamberlain and Chris Evans. Published in 1997 by Stanley Thornes (Publishers) Ltd, Cheltenham. ISBN 0-7487-3183-0.

THEORETICAL STANDPOINT

ATs have considerable understanding of symbolic communication and the healing potential of art making. They are able to provide a trusting environment in which patients feel safe to express strong emotions.

Art therapists are employed with various client groups: the terminally ill; people suffering from a mental health problem; people with a learning difficulty; HIV/AIDS sufferers; the physically disabled; the homeless and emotionally, physically or sexually abused children. A number of different approaches to art therapy have developed to adapt to the very different needs of the people with whom ATs work.

In the 1940s art therapy focused on the art activity itself which was considered to be the healing or therapeutic activity (Adamson, 1984). More modern approaches take into account the relationship which develops between the therapist and the patient, as well as symbolic communication through the art materials (Schaverien, 1994, P: 41). This psychotherapeutic model currently predominates.

A search of the literature an art therapy and brain injury shows a range of other methods, including: the Cognitive Approach (Joraski, 1986) which focuses on memory and concentration; a Diagnostic Test of Emotional Status Through Drawing (Silver, 1987); a Cognitive and Psychosocial Approach (Wald, 1989); Language Orientated Art Therapy (Pachalska, 1991) where the goal is to stimulate higher cognitive functions; and a Functional Communication Approach (Pitts, 1976) for dysphasic patients. The approach taken within a rehabilitation setting needs to be very flexible if it is to meet the differing needs of the patients.

A common misconception about art therapy is that the therapist will make a diagnosis about the patient from their art work. Some early methods advocated the use of art as a diagnostic tool for psychiatrists to gain insights into the inner world of their patients, but this is not considered appropriate today. A picture may only be used to gain information about the way a patient is feeling from discussion with the patient about its meaning. Such discussions can only occur within a context of a trusting relationship with the patient. Assumptions made from art work alone lack subtlety and may lead to inappropriate generalizations.

THE ROLE OF ART THERAPY IN REHABILITATION

Within rehabilitation the primary concern of the AT is the patient's emotional well-being. After a stroke, patients frequently have symptoms of depression, reduced self-esteem, a lack of confidence and feelings of low self-worth. If a person does not receive emotional support during this period, their feelings of helplessness may lead to depression. This can have a detrimental effect on the rehabilitation process itself. In the author's own work, 8% of the patients seen had attempted suicide prior to their referral (Wisdom, 1993).

Depression following a cerebrovascular accident (CVA) or a brain injury is common. Peter Wahrborg gives a comprehensive overview of the literature on this subject. He writes that 'depression is the most frequently reported reaction . . . after stroke' (Wahrborg, 1991). Morris (1990) found that 32% of post stroke patients suffered from either a major or minor depression. 'Depression is a source of excess disability . . . and should be recognised as treatable' (Reynolds, 1992). Not only can depression reduce recovery and rehabilitation, but it can destroy a person's quality of life. Depression can also increase the length of hospital stay, pharmacological costs, post discharge attendances and re-admission rates. Practical and emotional support; the implementation of realistic goals and a safe place to express feelings can all reduce the development of mental health problems.

The structure of the sessions

Ideally the room available for art therapy is private and free from interruptions. It is preferable that the appointment time and day of the week is the same, although on a busy rehabilitation ward this may not always be possible. Confidentiality, within the context of the team, is explained. This is an important factor in therapy, essential for the development of trust within the relationship. The personal nature of the art work is also stressed and images are not shared without the prior consent of the patient.

Initially patients may feel inadequate when faced with art materials – perhaps for the first time since childhood. Great sensitivity and awareness is required to help a patient make the first mark. A range of materials are available – paper, paints, crayons, pastels, simple printing equipment, clay, glue – the patient will choose which materials to use.

It is the patient who chooses how to use the session and what to reveal during the therapy session. The rest of the chapter shows how some patients have used the time and some of the art work that they have produced. This work is described under the following seven themes:

1. exploration of feelings;
2. containment of feelings within the image;
3. art as symbolic communication and symbolic re-enactment;
4. the language of art;
5. exploring physical changes;
6. confidence;
7. 'leaving pictures'.

EXPLORATION OF FEELINGS

Patients are often admitted to the unit in a state of internal chaos and shock. When patients realize the extent of their problems an almost indescribable feeling of grief and confusion is aroused. Art therapy allows exploration of the grief and starts the process of bereavement through image-making or talking. Through this exploration, and with time, a patient may begin to come to terms with disability and the changes in their lives caused by the stroke or head injury. The process of rehabilitation often contains waiting and uncertainty as the staff can rarely give definite answers regarding a final outcome. For some patients, 'not knowing' can provoke both impatience and despair. Waiting, grieving and adjusting is a long, slow process, hence adequate out-patient support and follow-up therapy is necessary.

Personal issues, particularly of loss, may be explored through art therapy. The stroke or brain-injured patient may have lost a great deal – mobility, independence, privacy, employment, financial security, a part of the self, dignity, communication, a close relationship and much more. A process of bereavement will occur for the losses experienced by the stroke patient. Emotional support is needed as a patient begins to grieve. According to Worden (1991), there are four tasks to be addressed in the mourning process:

1. acceptance of the reality of the loss;
2. to experience the pain of grief;
3. adjustment to the loss;
4. re-investment of energy into something new.

In art therapy these losses may be explored on paper and perhaps shared with the therapist. The art work may be spoken about or it may speak for itself.

A young man used images to express his losses. He began by drawing an eye, as he had lost his vision in one eye. Within the eye, his small drawings represented everything else he had lost; his ability to fly an aeroplane, his ability to drive, his ability to learn (he now saw himself as brain damaged), his fruit bushes which he could no longer tend, his dream home which he would no longer own, the loss of half his body and the tenancy of the public house where he was the landlord. The

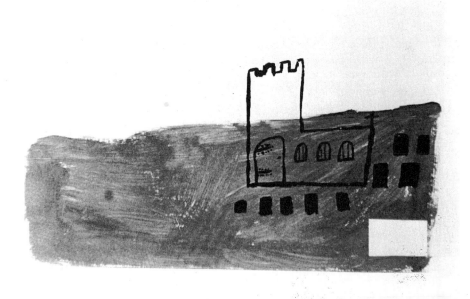

Figure 43.1 Burial.

love heart, which he drew not inside the eye, yet touching, represented his relationship, tenuous and uncertain since his stroke, which did in fact break down while he was in hospital. He drew nine losses. The patient began to explore his loss both visually and verbally, the beginning of a very long process where the loss has been so vast.

His next painting was of a graveyard with nine graves (Figure 43.1). This illustrated the close relationship between the loss this patient experienced and the death of a loved one. Each must be grieved for and buried – this man began the process through the imagery. Those parts of the self which are lost need to be identified, and let go of, before a person can make the most of what they have remaining. Feelings of frustration, grief and depression may be projected into the image, either consciously or unconsciously, and the tasks of mourning may be worked through. It may well be easier to put what are certainly

frightening and distressing issues onto paper, rather than talk about them.

This session was not directed in any way. In all sessions the patient chose the subject to discuss and the pace of the session. I provided the materials, the safe space, the time and support. In this case sadness, grief and the burial of this person's losses were shown. The first image was drawn consciously, he chose to put onto paper the turmoil of his life and to share it. The second image was produced unconsciously, the patient himself saw no connection between the two. Art, like dreams, can give a voice to our unconscious processes.

The dysphasic patient is often unable to be so verbally or visually articulate about his/her loss, but can use imagery to communicate. A retired man had dysphasia which resulted in very severely limited expression and poor functional comprehension. Paul came to the session and drew four circles. He persevered on this shape and could only name the colours he had used – 'purple' and 'green'. He repeated the word 'questions'. I tried a number of avenues to determine what these questions could be, but none seemed quite right. Paul then took off his wedding ring and put my hand on it. I asked if the picture was about his wife. This time I had guessed correctly and he wept bitterly. He had suffered a bereavement with the death of his wife, just before the onset of his stroke. Since then he had had limited means of expression to explore his feelings about his loss. Paul was communicating with every means available to him.

Other patients use the art work more symbolically to express themselves and their art work is less representational than in the first example. I worked with a woman in her sixties who had suffered a right CVA. She had very little conscious awareness of her disability. Her lack of insight into her problems resulted in her feeling that she was being persecuted by the staff. For example, she could not comprehend why she needed to have physiotherapy which she found painful. For this patient, being on the rehabilitation unit was an incomprehensible and difficult experience. Initially, Mary came to my room and sat looking out of the window. She often played an imaginary organ moving her fingers on the table. She told me that she was playing the madrigal of the Silver Swan:

> *The silver swan, who living had no note,*
> *When death approached unlocked her silent throat;*
> *Leaning her breast against the reedy shore,*
> *Thus sung her first and last, and sung no more:*
> *Farewell, all joys; Oh death, come close mine eyes;*
> *More geese than swans now live, more fools than wise.*
>
> (Orlando Gibbons, 1977)

Mary misquoted the madrigal omitting the fourth line and adding her own final line.

Thus sang the silver swan and sang no more.

She explored the song by writing out the words, reciting and singing the madrigal, drawing pictures of the swan and creating a clay model of the swan, itself (Figure 43.2).

The madrigal is the origin of the expression 'Swan Song' – one's final song. The whole piece is about death and change. Mary completed the swan, giving it some notes, the day before she left the unit (Figure 43.3). She showed, that despite being apparently lacking in perception, she was acutely aware of all that had taken place, even though she could not articulate it.

Although consciously Mary seemingly had little idea of what had happened to her, unconsciously she was grieving for the changes the stroke had brought to her life. Art become a vehicle for the unconscious expression of her grief. She could not find the words to talk about what was happening to her, but she could communicate this symbolically.

CONTAINMENT OF FEELINGS WITHIN THE IMAGE

The art work and AT sessions may be a vehicle for some of the feelings aroused by the tragic consequences of a stroke or brain injury. The intensity of such feelings can be overwhelming and frightening, but some patients find the image a means to express and contain such feelings.

Peter was a 24-year-old man who had been knocked off his bicycle. Not only did he have a brain injury and leg fractures, but he also lost his independence, his permanent relationship, home and job. These are not uncommon consequences following a brain injury. Peter was referred because of aggression and sarcasm towards his parents with whom he was living temporarily. His rage was enormous and the art therapy sessions provided both a container for, and a means

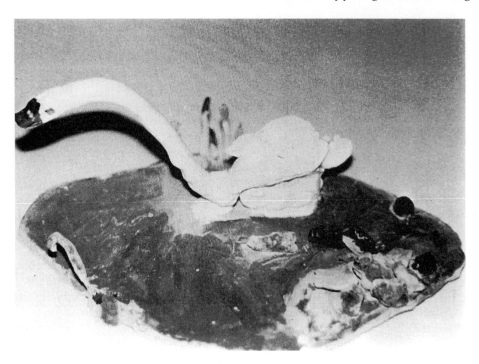

Figure 43.2 The Silver Swan.

of expression of, his anger. After a few months he created a series of images exploring his angry feelings. He painted the sun rapidly approaching the earth and a view looking into the top of a volcano. He used these symbols to express the extent of his anger as well as his fear of its destructiveness. His aggressive outbursts gradually decreased at home as his anger was contained in therapy.

Children often find art a natural vocabulary. Steven was referred because of uncharacteristic aggression at home. Once he felt secure in our relationship he began to explore the accident, spending many weeks drawing, painting and making models of cars, and he often stood at my window drawing cars in the car park opposite. Steven would become very angry if another car pulled up in front to block his view, or if the car was driven away before the painting was finished. He had good reason to be angry.

We talked very little about the accident itself or about how he felt – children of this age hardly have the vocabulary to describe the complex and painful feelings associated with such a traumatic event. He was using another means of communication to re-enact the accident and express his feelings of rage. Where words fail us, imagery may be a statement in its own right. Later his rage was discharged into increasingly large splatter paintings where the paper, he and I became more and more paint splattered.

About 8 months into therapy it was necessary for Steven to have further scans and re-examinations. He found these investigations frightening and confusing. His feelings of fear, helplessness and despair were expressed through the art media, particularly through his use of black ink. He played with the ink, watching it spread in a basin, on newspaper or in a jam jar of water making an 'ink volcano'. Once therapy became a safe

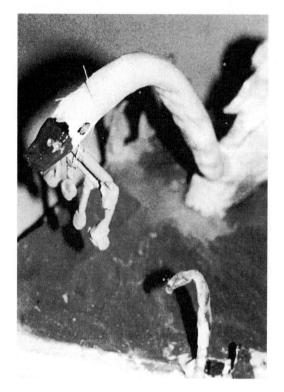

Figure 43.3 Notes.

enough place to express and contain his feelings, his aggressive outbursts stopped at home.

These statements about the art work are made with knowledge of the patient's history, as well as after months of developing a therapeutic relationship and observing their use of symbolic imagery.

ART AS SYMBOLIC COMMUNICATION AND SYMBOLIC RE-ENACTMENT

The symbolic nature of art can provide a patient with the opportunity to explore and understand their stroke and life situation in another form. The art work may be a metaphor for the self, family or feelings – form, line, colour, tone and subject can say more than words alone. Words cannot always capture the true meaning of an image or a piece of work. The images are not always talked about, but may remain as statements in their own right. Comments about such art work are cautiously offered, and not made outside the context of therapy.

Trees are powerful, archetypal images which may be seen as self-portraits. One cannot say that every tree is a self-portrait, but on these two occasions the trees appear to be symbolic of the painter. A tree was painted by a woman who had suffered a left subarachnoid haemorrhage. She was depressed, particularly about her communication disorder, and had threatened suicide. Her verbal expression was severely limited and her comprehension impaired at a higher level. She drew a tree in a very determined and attacking manner. She said that the tree was 'angry' and she had used the image to discharge and symbolize some of her sad and angry feelings.

Figure 43.4 was painted by a man post brain injury. The trees have red streams running through them and look as if they are bleeding from the top. The trees are upright, but damaged. This is a powerful and unconsciously produced image, a metaphor or silent poem, symbolizing his current situation.

Art materials may also be used to re-enact an accident or CVA in a symbolic form. Peter was very low during one session, he rolled out a circle of clay and drew in the eyes, nose and mouth. He then proceeded to slice off the top of the clay head with a knife. The head was quickly disposed of and put in the rubbish bin. Peter had re-enacted his injury in a graphic way and the disposal of the head was of important cathartic significance for him. In a very different way an elderly man knocked off his bicycle drew the accident and the sequence of events as a map. He talked through, re-lived and re-enacted the event on paper. It was painful for him to remember all of the details, but it was the beginning of letting go of the event and continuing with his life.

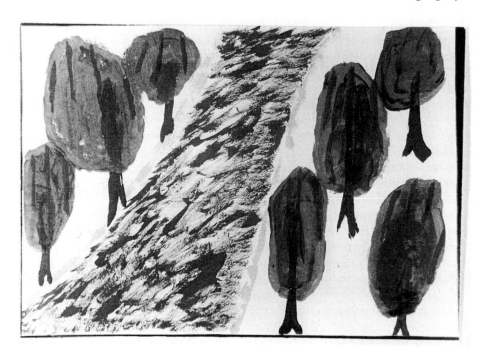

Figure 43.4 Bleeding Trees.

THE LANGUAGE OF ART

Art may be an additional means of expression to language. A sufferer of dysphasia wrote of this disorder:

> *From the beginning the loss of speech was a crushing blow – the more because I could not explain my fears and bewilderments of my situation.* (Hughes, 1992).

Art may provide relief and a keystone for the expression of individuality where language is impaired. An elderly man who acquired his severe fluent dysphasia in a road traffic accident spent many weeks drawing houses without doors. A house without a door has no entrance or exit – no way in or out. The house is isolated and unable to be reached. These houses were possibly symbols of himself and his communication disorder. The houses changed with circumstances; for example, there was a death on the unit which greatly distressed this patient, that particular week he painted the houses with black roofs and windows. He cried throughout and the houses seemed to be in mourning.

His single houses on a landscape developed when he moved from individual to group therapy. He then drew groups of houses, each having its own separate walled garden. Eventually some of the houses developed doors, but there was always at least one which had no door. He also painted a green car with a red bonnet and a red triangle in front of it. This picture was a clear depiction of his accident, an event which he could not talk about, but he found a means of expression through the art media.

At the beginning of therapy another patient with a severe non-fluent dysphasia produced many images of sea scapes with rocks and lighthouses. The pictures were deserted with no sign of life – no boats, trees, animals, sea life or people. These pictures seemed to be symbolic of the loneliness and isolation that he felt as a sufferer of dysphasia. During a year of therapy his work gradually developed and his paintings became full of life and activity. He also started joining local clubs and broadening his activities. It seemed that art therapy gave him a means of expression, the ability to reach another person and increased confidence.

The symbolic functioning of other dysphasic patients is so severely impaired that they are more limited, producing a seeming mass of scribbles or perseverative shapes with no symbolic representation. The benefits of art therapy are less clear. Many modern artists use such abstract styles to explore relationships and ideas. The therapist needs to think creatively to acknowledge the scribbles, mumblings, facial expression, grimaces, blotches of colour and movement as communication in the widest sense. The AT must sit with the patient and try to relate to their world, thus enabling the patient to share and communicate in whatever way they can.

Visual imagery is used in aphasia therapy to stimulate a return of language function by using the image to access verbal recall (Edelstein, 1977). It is, as yet, unknown how image making may assist in the re-ordering of the dysphasic patient's disordered symbolic functioning.

EXPLORING PHYSICAL CHANGES

Exploring physical changes enables a person to see an event in a visual form or re-live it on a symbolic level. The unspeakable may be expressed in art. A 60-year-old man used the image of a house to re-enact his right cerebrovascular accident (CVA). He began by drawing the house carefully with a pencil and then painted the curtains white. He proceeded to mix green paint until it was the same colour as his pyjamas. He painted over the left windows so that they were completely covered. He then painted carefully around the door and around the right

hand windows. He re-painted all of the windows pink. He had started with a complete house, wiped out the left side and then restored it, but it had changed in the process. His body underwent the same process as the house and his CVA was re-enacted through the symbol of the house. He went on to depict his physical recovery through a series of changing and developing houses. The left side of each house developed within the series, gradually becoming more complete.

A young woman, who had suffered a left CVA leaving her with a word-finding difficulty, explored her physical recovery and her relationship through abstract shapes (Figure 43.5).

She used an emerging circle to symbolize herself and a complete circle to represent her partner. A black line symbolized her stroke, red and yellow shapes became the two sides of her body. At the time she was very concerned about the slow recovery rate of her hand. She drew around this and painted the hand pink. She explored this theme in a series of three paintings using the same shapes, symbols and colours.

Visual, perceptual and spatial problems may be explored in art therapy and strategies developed to help compensate for these. Figure 43.6 was drawn by a man with a dense left hemiparesis and it illustrates some of the perceptual difficulties experienced by these patients (outline drawn by therapist). Body image changes and distortions may also be explored through image making, either directly or symbolically.

CONFIDENCE

The art therapy room provides a setting where a patient can take control and make decisions, albeit on a small scale. This is an important empowering element of art therapy. In the busy routine of a rehabilitation ward most decisions are taken for the patients and this may be experienced as de-skilling.

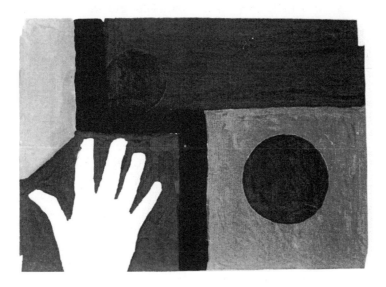

Figure 43.5 Abstract.

The opportunity to make decisions may have a ripple effect in the patient's attitude towards him/her self and an improvement in self-confidence. The first decision the patient makes is to decide whether or not to come to art therapy at all. No patient is forced to, it is entirely personal choice. A patient who decides not to come may do so because they are unwilling, or feel unable, to explore personal issues at present.

Group therapy is a valuable alternative offering patients a relaxed and informal setting to make supportive relationships with other patients. The conversation during group art therapy can cover a range of issues – coping with disability, incontinence, anxiety, feeling homesick, loneliness and many more subjects. The therapist creates an opportunity for the patients to offer each other support, encouragement and develop important friendships.

A patient may become more confident and self-esteem may improve as he/she develops and discovers artistic aptitude. John, who had farmed all his life and never painted, attended for art therapy soon after his admission. He produced many paintings in art therapy discovering a natural feel for the paint, colour and composition. Through the art work he shared his humour and life experience. John was totally absorbed by every painting and he felt enormous pride and satisfaction on completion of the work. Such feelings of achievement and accomplishment are important. So much is lost by the stroke patient, art can help to restore a sense that they can achieve a great deal – albeit in a different way.

'LEAVING PICTURES'

Leaving the unit can be a crisis time for the patient, as severe as the stroke itself, if discharge is not handled well. Many art

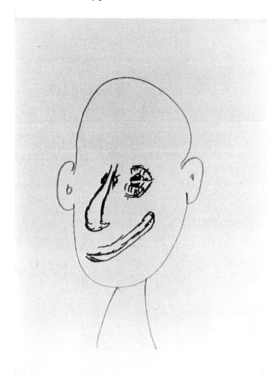

Figure 43.6 Incomplete Face.

therapy sessions are spent preparing for leaving and talking about the future. Patients may paint leaving pictures to explore their feelings. A leaving picture painted by a woman who had speech and language problems showed a gateway and very stormy landscape ahead. Her fears for the future were enormous, she was particularly concerned about managing family and business life with dysphasia. Another patient explored his feelings about leaving through an illustration of some birds flying away from a tree, leaving others behind. This may be symbolic of the patient leaving the companionship that can become important over a long period on the unit. Often patients experience a push–pull confusion of feelings as they prepare to leave. They are on the one hand longing to leave and return home to gain their independence, but on the other hand they are often afraid of the future and will miss the security, companionship and safety of the unit.

SUMMARY

These images have shown just a few of the ways patients have chosen to use the art therapy sessions. They show the wide range of feelings experienced and how such feelings can be expressed through the imagery following the devastation of a stroke or brain injury. They show how art can be a means of communication for a person who has dysphasia, providing some freedom from the isolation of this communication disorder.

Art therapy is a creative, flexible, dynamic, personal approach which has relatively unexplored potential for brain-injured and stroke patients. It can be a means of communication, personal expression and stimulation. Most of all, it can play a part in restoring a sense of well-being in a client group who have lost so much.

REFERENCES

Adamson, E. (1984) *Art as Healing*, Coventure, London.

Dally, T. (1984) *Art as Therapy*, Routledge, London.

Edelstein, D. (1977) cited in Code, C. (1987) *Language, Aphasia and the Right Hemisphere*, John Wiley, Chichester, p. 153.

Gibbons, O. (1977) The Silver Swan, in *Invitation To Madrigals*, (ed. E. Fellows), Stainer & Bell, London.

Hughes, J. (1992) Jumbley Words, and Rights Where Wrongs Should Be, in *The Experience of Aphasia from the Inside*, (ed. G. Edelman), Far Communication, Kibworth.

Joraski, M. (1990) The role of creative arts in cognitive rehabilitation, *Cognitive Rehabilitation*, April, Vol. 4, 18–23.

Morris, P.L.P. (1990) Prevalence and course of depressive disorders in hospitalised stroke patients, *International Journal of Psychiatry in Medicine*, **20**, 349–64.

Pachalska, M. (1991) *Language Orientated Art Therapy (LOAT) in Long Term Rehabilitation of Aphasics*, Fourth International Aphasia Rehabilitation Congress, September, 1992, Edinburgh, pp. 1–8.

Pitts, W.K. (1976) *I am a Man: The Creative Experience and Speech Therapy*. Proceedings of Art Therapy Association Conference, pp. 18–20.

Reynolds, C.F. (1992) Treatment of depression in special populations. *Journal of Clinical Psychiatry*, **53**, 45–53.

Schaverien, J. (1994) Analytical art psychotherapy. *Inscape*, II, 41.

Silver, R.A. (1987) A cognitive approach to art therapy, in *Approaches to Art Therapy*, (ed. J.A. Rubin), Brunner/Mazel, New York pp. 233–50.

Wahrborg, P. (1991) *Assessment and Management of Emotional and Psychosocial Reactions to Brain Damage and Aphasia*, Far Communications, Leicester.

Wald, J. (1989) Severe head injury and its stages of recovery explored through art therapy, in *Advances in Art Therapy*, (ed. H. Wadeson), John Wiley, New York, pp. 181–203.

Waller, D. (1991) *Becoming a Profession: the history of art therapy in Britain 1940–82*, Routledge, London.

Wisdom, C. (1993) Annual Report September 1992 – August 1993. Unpublished manuscript.

Worden, J.M. (1991) *Grief Counselling and Grief Therapy*, Routledge.

Appendix

Training establishments

Art Therapy Programme, University of Hertfordshire School of Art & Design Manor Road, Hatfield, Hertfordshire AL10 9TL, UK. Tel No: 01707 285308.

University of London, Goldsmith's College Art Psychotherapy Unit
23 St James, New Cross, London SE14 6 AD, UK. Tel No: 0171 919 7237.

The Postgraduate Diploma in Art Therapy Course, The University of Sheffield Department of Psychiatry, Centre for Psychotherapeutic Studies, 16 Claremont Crescent, Sheffield, S10 2TA, UK. Tel No: 01742 768555 ext. 4970/1/2.

Art Therapy Department, Wilkie House 37 Guthrie Street Edinburgh EH1 1JG, UK. Tel No: 0131 225 2079.

Association

The British Association of Art Therapists (BAAT), 11A Richmond Road Brighton. Sussex BN2 3RL, UK. General Enquiries: Tel No: 01734 265407. Honorary Secretary: Tel No: 01623 631958.

PART EIGHT
EQUIPMENT

44 Wheelchairs

L. Marks

INTRODUCTION

It is becoming increasingly common to see a person in a wheelchair, but it is only recently that wheelchairs and their users are becoming accepted in our society. However, whether the wheelchair has become a 'symbol of mobility rather than invalidity' (Nichols, 1971) is debatable. There are many reasons why people need wheelchairs. The commonest diagnoses leading to wheelchair use are shown in Table 44.1. In the UK wheelchairs are available from the National Health Service (NHS) for 'all individuals who have a permanent disability which affects their ability to walk'. Short-term needs (e.g. after a leg fracture in a person unable to use crutches) are met by loan agencies or private hire.

The number of wheelchairs on issue in the UK has been rising steadily year by year (Table 44.2) as has the cost of provision. Part of this is due to advances in medical science, whereby more people with serious injuries now survive, but with residual disabilities. By far the most wheelchairs are issued to older people, who are living longer, but develop increasing mobility problems in the later years of their lives. In some part of the UK, wheelchair services are already 'banding' the cost of the wheelchair according to usage, i.e. an occasional user will be prescribed a chair within a certain price range, but a wheelchair-dependent individual will be allocated a more expensive chair.

In February 1996 the government announced extra funding for indoor/ outdoor powered chairs. Additionally, a voucher scheme is to be introduced to allow more client choice.

ORGANIZATION OF THE WHEELCHAIR SERVICE IN THE UK

Following the McColl Report (McColl 1986), the wheelchair services were transferred from the Department of Health to the Disablement Services Authority (1987) and subsequently to the NHS (1991). There were significant changes in the structure and organization of the services. Before 1987 chairs and components were ordered on large block contracts and were distributed to the Artificial Limb and Appliance Centres (ALACS). Many chairs were issued on the basis of the referral form only, and in the few cases when the individual was assessed, it was usually by a technical officer, occasionally accompanied by a doctor. There was no direct involvement of therapists who knew the client. As stated by one of the author's colleagues, 'as the range of chairs available was very limited, it was not too difficult to identify the least inappropriate chair from that range.' (D. Thornberry, 1994, personal communication).

Rehabilitation of the Physically Disabled Adult. Edited by C. John Goodwill, M. Anne Chamberlain and Chris Evans. Published in 1997 by Stanley Thornes (Publishers) Ltd, Cheltenham. ISBN 0-7487-3183-0.

Table 44.1 Diagnoses provided on wheelchair request form. (Source: Dudley and McMahon, 1994, p. 72)

Diagnosis	No.	%[a]
Arthritis	65	(21.5)
Cerebrovascular accident	58	(19.2)
Chronic obstructive airways disease/ asthma	50	(16.5)
Ischaemic heart disease/congestive cardiac failure	41	(13.6)
Amputation	17	(5.6)
Cancer	17	(5.6)
Fracture	12	(4.0)
Dementia	11	(3.6)
Old age/frailty	9	(3.0)
Parkinson's disease	9	(3.0)
Multiple sclerosis	6	(2.0)
Reduced mobility	6	(2.0)
Peripheral vascular disease	6	(2.0)
Hip replacement	4	(1.3)
Obesity	4	(1.3)
Motor neurone disease	3	(1.0)
Others	40	(13.2)
Total	358	

[a]Note: Percentages add up to more than 100% as some forms indicated more than one diagnosis to be presented.

The major change in the wheelchair service was the creation of local district wheelchair clinics run by specially accredited therapists. Budgets were devolved and are now locally managed. There are still Regional or Supra-District centres which in the main now deal with specialized seating and more complex wheelchair prescriptions. These centres usually have a multidisciplinary team comprising a consultant in rehabilitation medicine, therapist(s), rehabilitation engineer(s), or clinical engineer, and possibly an orthotist.

The majority of individuals are now assessed for the most suitable chair and seating, either in their home environment or at the district clinic. Referral information is more comprehensively sought, so that even if the client's own therapist is unable to attend the assessment, the necessary information is available (see 'How to prescribe a chair' below). As the district centres are dealing with much smaller populations (average 250 000), the service has become more personalized. Computerization is available for processing orders/repairs of chairs but comprehensive databases are not yet universally installed. Collected clinically relevant data on wheelchair services still remains a problem in many parts of the country.

Apart from the specially accredited therapists in the district clinics, there are now courses for local therapists to become, 'approved prescribers' who are then entitled to complete wheelchair referral forms. This negates the previous need for the form to be completed by the general practitioner who, although knowing the medical diagnosis, often had little knowledge of the different

Table 44.2 Wheelchair statistics and expenditure. Extracted from: DSA reports, forms HFR 28 and KO73

	1988–89	1989–90	1990–91	1991–92	1992–93
Non-powered issues	149 096	161 097	159 045	162 661	170 504
Powered issues	7775	8463	8451	8951	8804
Total issues	156 871	169 560	167 496	171 612	179 308
Fleet size	460 000	—	530 000	—	—
Special seating items	5064	10 128	9399	11 138	13 095
Annual spend (£)	31 569 000	33 157 000	38 728 000[a]	46 931 544	39 859 679[b]

[a]Includes £1 023 000 for indoor/outdoor wheelchair pilot project.
[b]Spending appears to have dropped by £7 000 000 compared to 1991–92. This was because of an extra allocation in 1991–92 which was discontinued in 1992–93.

chairs and their suitability. Technical input to the service is now provided by rehabilitation engineers. They have all received appropriate induction training (including courses to upgrade the existing old-style technical officers), which enables them to function effectively in a clinical setting.

The service is also dependent on wheelchair manufacturers and repair services. Although the concept of 'the limited list' is now largely obsolete, the majority of chairs are still fairly 'standard' models (modified as necessary for individual needs) and contracts for these are negotiated by the NHS Supplies Authority in order to maximise the advantage of bulk purchase. Special size chairs and less commonly prescribed models may be ordered direct from the appropriate manufacturer. Repair services are provided by a large number of Approved Wheelchair Repairers. Their contracts have become much more exacting in the last few years and quality control measures are now beginning to be applied to ensure high standards of repairs and modifications.

TYPES OF WHEELCHAIR

There are numerous wheelchairs available and new designs and concepts are frequently coming on the market. Some innovations are aimed at increasing comfort (e.g. contoured upholstered seats, multi-adjustable positions), whilst others are aimed at reducing the weight of the chair (e.g. titanium frames, carbon fibre wheel struts). Wheelchairs can be classified into broad groups as shown in Table 44.3, and Figure 44.1 shows some of the common models.

The model 28B attendant controlled electric outdoor/indoor chair is not popular (Dudley and McMahon, 1993). Some district wheelchair centres will supply 'add on' power packs for standard chairs, but only during 1996 has extra funding been identified to provide outdoor/indoor electric chairs in the UK (for further information see Medical

Table 44.3 Classification of wheelchairs

Manual
(a) Pushchair (e.g. '9' series, Barrett 10)
(b) Self-propelling chairs (e.g. '8' series, Barrett 7)

Electric
(a) Indoor, occupant controlled (e.g. Apollo, Newton Badger)
(b) Indoor/outdoor, occupant +/– attendant. Only available in some regions
(c) Outdoor, attendant controlled (e.g. 28B, assistive power packs)

Special function chairs (not usually supplied by NHS)
(a) Sports chairs (e.g. RGK, Top End)
(b) Stand-up chairs (e.g. Levo, Permobile)
(c) Elevating chairs (e.g. Permobile)

Note: The models quoted are examples only and are not the only models available in that category.

Devices Directorate Report, 1993). Some wheelchair clinics have a handbook of wheelchairs, but for comprehensive coverage of the subject the reader is advised to refer to Cochrane (1993), which includes details on all chairs, whether available from the NHS or private/charity funding. Outdoor electric wheelchair users should have insurance for the chair and for third party liability in case they injure someone. There are variations by age in the percentage of people needing wheelchairs, in particular the rapidly increasing requirement for an ageing population (Table 44.4).

HOW TO PRESCRIBE A CHAIR

Accurate prescription of a wheelchair is essential to the client's comfort, function in the chair and consequent quality of life. It is critical to fit the chair to the individual and not the individual to the chair. As Goodwill (1988) wrote in the first edition of this book: 'the chair must be prescribed as accurately for the patient, as a drug for any medical

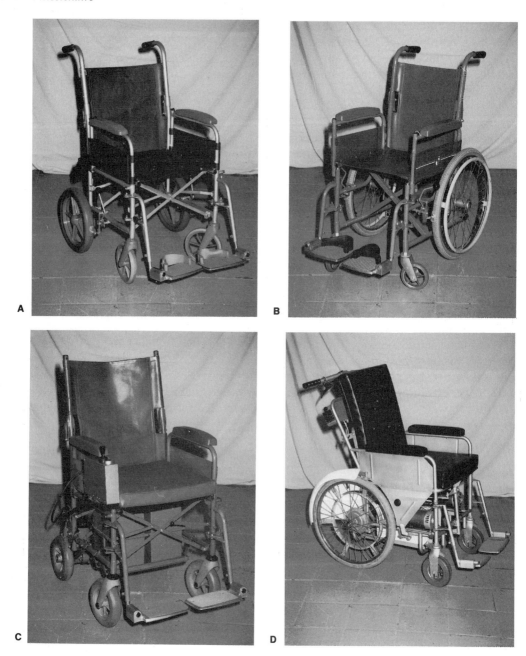

Figure 44.1 A, 9L 17 × 17 inch (44 × 44 cm) adult pushchair with folding backrest, removable armrests, and flip-up foldaway footrests. B, 8BL 16 × 16 inch (40 × 40 cm) narrow adult self-propelling chair (note large rear wheels) with folding backrest, removable armrests, slip-up foldaway footrests and 2 inch (5 cm) foam seat cushion. C, Apollo 17 × 17 inch (44 × 44 cm) indoor electric chair with right hand joystick control. Folding backrest, removable armrests, slip-up foldaway footrests and 2 inch (5 cm) foam cushion. D, 28B attendant-controlled outdoor electric chair. Upholstered seat and back cushions, flip-up foldaway footrests, rear sited controls, 'tiller' pushing handles and storage space (white area) at rear behind seat.

Table 44.4 Comparison of ages of wheelchair users. (Source: Dudley and McMahon, 1994, p. 73)

Age of user (years)	Fenwick (1973)	Kettle and Rowley (1990)	Dudley and McMahon (1994)
60	67%	74.8%	79.8%
80	17%	31.5%	33.8%

condition'. Appropriate, accurate information is therefore required to assist the prescriber. Many wheelchair centres have designed their own referral forms and the information they contain will cover the following:

1. Client's diagnosis – this will give the prescriber a good idea of the likely usage of the chair, but additionally will indicate any urgency, e.g. malignancy.
2. How often will the chair be used, e.g. twice a week, all the time?
3. Where will the chair be used – outdoors only, indoors only, or both? Environmental constraints, e.g. turning circles, doorway widths, internal hoists, will all need to be considered.
4. How does the client transfer – unaided, standing, sideways, forward or backwards or assisted (boards, carers, hoists etc.)? Requirements for footrests (e.g. flip-up and swingaway or fixed) and whether arm rests need to be removable to allow sideways transfer should be specified.
5. How is the chair to be transported – lifted into the car by occupant or carer, lifted by hoist into car or onto roof, or will the client remain in the chair (suitability of vehicle for clamping, ramps, lifts)? Electric wheelchairs do not fold unless the batteries are removed.
6. Needs of the carer, e.g. push handle heights, weight and size of chair and occupant (pushing and lifting).
7. Information should also be given on specific needs of the client, e.g. continence, present or past history of pressure sores, activities in chair.

Having obtained this information, the client should be examined. The extent of this examination will be determined by the diagnosis and usage of chair but the examination needs to identify specific deformities and ascertain whether these are correctable or fixed. If there are fixed deformities the chair may need to be modified to accommodate them.

Finally, the client should be measured, preferably sitting on a firm flat chair, bench or plinth. Details of how to do this are contained in the Disablement Services Authority Training Resource Pack (1990), but Figure 44.2 gives an indication of the type of measurements required to allow selection of a suitable chair. Next decide whether the chair needs to be modified to meet individual needs and what accessories are needed. Modifications are best discussed with the rehabilitation engineer, rather than attempt to 'salvage' a wrong prescription at a later date. Wheelchair provision should be regularly reviewed, especially for those with changing conditions such as multiple sclerosis or motor neurone disease. Table 44.5 analyses the types of chair provided.

There are numerous accessories available (see *Equipment for Disabled People – Wheelchairs* (Cochrane, 1993)), but the commonest is a wheelchair cushion (Ham, 1993). There are many different cushions on the market designed to meet differing needs – is it for comfort, pressure relief, to accommodate a deformity or any combination of these? What effect will the cushion have on other parameters of the chair (e.g. footrest and armrest height), will it raise the person too high or cause problems with wheelchair transfers? The type of cushion cover needed will be affected by incontinence problems and the cover may need to be removable for washing. Wheelchair cushions must be suited to individual needs (see Chapter 45).

For further information please refer to the *Wheelchair Cushions Summary Report*, (Tuttiett,

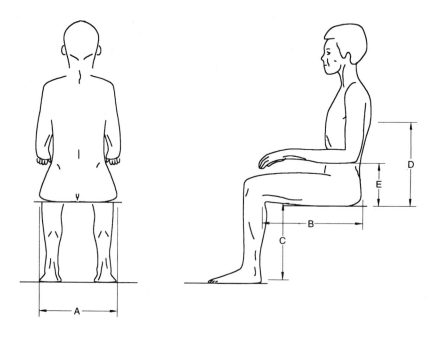

A Width across hips
B Seat length
C Seat height
D Backrest height
E Armrest height

Note; These are body measurements, not chair measurements

Figure 44.2 Measuring for a wheelchair. (Redrawn from Male and Massie, 1990.)

1989). Also, the Medical Devices Agency are currently evaluating a wide range of wheelchair cushions. Publications in their evalua-tion series include information on pressure assessments (See Further Reading).

Table 44.5 Differences in types of wheelchair prescribed.
(Source: Dudley and McMahon, 1994, p. 73)

Type of wheelchair	Kettle and Rowley (1990)	Dudley and McMahon (1994)	P value
Self-propelled	42.2%	19.5%	<0.001
Attendant-propelled	47.4%	75.2%	<0.001
Powered	3.8%	2.3%	NS
Buggy	4.5%	3.0%	NS
Commode	0.5%	—	—
Tricycle	0.3%	—	—
Unspecified	1.3%	—	—

NS = not significant.

WHEELCHAIRS FOR SPECIFIC CONDITIONS

It cannot be overemphasized that a wheelchair needs to be prescribed for the individual who is going to use the chair. The following section describes the commonest variations required to suit specific diagnoses.

Arthritis

A large number of patients with arthritis can walk indoors but not outdoors. Even then they may refuse a wheelchair for as long as possible (Brattstrom *et al.*, 1981). For these a transit or pushchair such as the 9L will be required. For independent mobility over longer distances, an outdoor powered chair, scooter, buggy or class 3 vehicle may be required (see *Which One Should They Buy? – A Powered Vehicle Prescription Guide for Therapists*) (Medical Devices Directorate Report, 1993).

For those who need a self-propelled chair for indoor use care must be taken to avoid unnecessary strain on the upper limbs and neck if involved with the arthritis; usually these patients have rheumatoid arthritis and are better with an electric wheelchair.

Attention to armrest height (posture in chair, ease of ingress and egress) as well as rear wheel position are important. For some, front-propelling wheels may be less tiring. Equally important will be the height from seat to the ground (including cushion if used), which materially affects getting out of the chair and may make it impossible if the seat is too low. A headrest extension may be required for those with neck problems and is advisable for all who are going to travel seated in the chair.

Many arthritis patients develop oedema of the ankles which may be helped by elevating legrests. Similarly these, or legrest extensions, are required by those with arthrodesed knee(s), or with a knee joint which is only comfortable in a fairly straight position. A unilateral stiff hip, which does not flex to 90°, may be accommodated by an 'arthrodesis' cushion. The cushion on the affected side is ramped below the gluteal crease to accommodate the lack of hip flexion.

When both hips are stiff, a simple option is to provide an over-sized backrest canvas (plus or minus cushion) to increase the angle between the seat and the back of the chair. If this is insufficient, then a reclining backrest will be required, but these chairs have to be longer (121 cm) and are heavy to move (30.5 kg) because the rear axle needs to be positioned further back for stability, thus making them awkward or impossible in the home environment.

Difficulty in propelling a chair, due to pain, weakness or joint limitation, should lead to early provision of an electric chair to maintain independence. Bossingham and Russell (1980), in a survey of 42 patients with advanced inflammatory polyarthritis, showed that if correctly assessed and prescribed, electric chairs are well used – 60% (25 patients) used them every day and 50% (21 patients) for more than 8 hours per day. The shape of the control may need to be modified (usually enlarged) for those with impaired grip, and if external rotation of the shoulder is limited the control can be moved to the middle in front of the occupant, being supported on a swivel arm pivoted on the side of the chair.

Stroke

Not all patients who have a stroke need a wheelchair. For those with only a mild stroke, or who make a rapid recovery, attention should be focused on normalizing balance and reflexes, aiming for walking, with or without walking aids. This does not preclude the use of a transit wheelchair for access to therapy appointments and general transport in the early phase, or use for longer distance especially to prevent poor gait due to fatigue.

For those who have a moderate to severe stroke, there appears to be considerable debate in the literature about the advantages and disadvantages of providing a wheelchair. Blower (1988) gives 10 advantages of the early use of wheelchairs, although he does give brief consideration to three 'theoretical' disadvantages. Ashburn and Lynch (1988) remind us that we are trying to achieve a balance between independence and compensatory techniques. Whilst acknowledging that delays in walking and independence are frustrating for the stroke victim, they caution that the early use of self-propelling wheelchairs not only increases spasticity but may

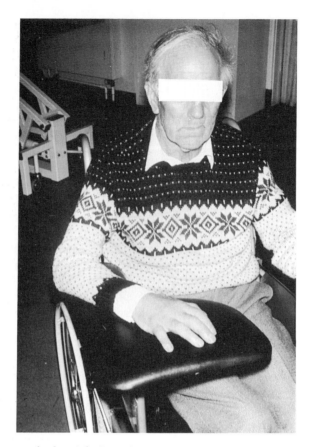

Figure 44.3 Bexhill armrest for hemiplegic patient.

also set a behavioural pattern for the future and delay the retraining of essential skills. They propose that the selective use of wheelchairs can be valuable in early stroke, but this should not extend to routine provision.

Cornall (1991) summarizes the debate well and her paper includes a small study of 10 patients (not all stroke victims) whose spasticity was assessed before and after being pushed and self-propelling over a 24-m flat course. The results of the study show that it is the action of self-propulsion that causes the increase in spasticity in many patients. She also points out that hemiparetic patients can be divided into two groups: those who demonstrate a significant increase in spasticity upon effort, and those who do not. For

the first group she suggests that provision of an electric chair (which involves no physical effort on the part of the user) would be more appropriate, whilst for the second group there are benefits in providing a self-propelling chair.

Whatever chair is prescribed for a stroke patient attention must be given to posture and function. Pushchairs or transit chairs present little problem providing the correct size is selected and consideration is given to stabilizing the pelvis and providing appropriate support for the affected arm (Figure 44.3 shows the Bexhill armrest) to maintain it in a functional position and prevent secondary shoulder problems, for example subluxation. Self-propelling in a standard manual chair obviously presents problems as usually only one arm is available for pushing, resulting in circular rather than forward movement. One option is to push with one arm and paddle as well as steer with the ipsilateral leg. For relatively tall people this may be possible in a standard 8L or 8BL chair (canvas to floor distance = 47.5 cm/19 inches). For shorter individuals a Barrett 7 (canvas to floor distance = 46.25 cm/18.5 inches) might be preferable or one of the 'hemiplegic' chairs which are specifically designed for this purpose (canvas to floor distance = 43.75 cm/17.5 inches). The height of the seat cushion adds to these measurements.

Another possibility is to have the chair modified for foot steering. This is done by linking the appropriate footplate to both front castors so that movement of the foot turns the chair. The disadvantage is that all propulsion is by the one good arm and the occupant has to steer the chair even when being pushed. There are 'one-arm drive' chairs which have a double hand rim (the outer smaller rim driving the opposite wheel) and the concept is that both hand rims are pushed together to go straight forward. However, these are heavy (24 kg) and the technique of driving them is difficult, especially if the patient has perceptual problems. All self-propelling chairs need an extended or elongated brake lever on the hemiparetic side so that it can be reached with the good arm.

For those who are unlikely to walk, and for whom self-propelling increases spasticity, an electric indoor chair should be considered. Most stroke patients can manage to operate a standard joystick with the sound hand and do not need specialized controls. To ensure safety, adequate training is required for all patients, particularly those with perceptual problems or hemianopia. If severe, these may make the use of such a chair unsafe for others.

Braus and Mainka (1993) recommend 'adaptive' wheelchairs for the most severely handicapped stroke patients. These are prescribed at the end of the rehabilitation programme for patients who are likely to be wheelchair dependent. The concept is that having tried different standard wheelchairs during their stay, a final prescription is determined which will include optimization of the rear wheel angles as well as a more vertical backrest to facilitate leg propulsion. This is achieved on a multi-adjustable wheelchair frame.

Cron and Sprigle (1993) describe a foam cushion for stroke patients using unilateral arm and leg propulsion. This has a ramped cut out on the unaffected side to permit some increase in hip extension (similar in configuration to an arthrodesis cushion which is designed to accommodate a fixed flexion deformity of one hip). Of the 11 subjects tested, only three were found to have improved propulsion, and the results also indicated that pressure distribution and pelvic obliquity were adversely affected. Nevertheless 10 of the 11 subjects preferred the 'hemi' cushion to their usual cushion!

The Brunel Institution for Bioengineering (Mandelson *et al.*, 1994) have carried out a study, 'Stroke rehabilitation at home – bridging the gap between home and hospital', which was funded by the Nuffield Foundation. Part of this study involved the design of a portable rehabilitation kit, comprising a seat cushion, back cushion and arm support. The seat and backrest cushion are contoured and made in firm foam. The armrest (and there is also a tray) is made of polypropylene, with padding for the elbow, plus contouring to prevent the arm slipping off, and is designed to fold out of the way for easy access. The whole system is designed to be movable from wheelchair to armchair and vice versa.

Lower limb amputees

The majority of leg amputations are done for vascular problems in older people. As many have vascular problems in the remaining leg, the majority are given a wheelchair in the early phase of rehabilitation as hopping with crutches is inadvisable or impossible. Although many will achieve mobility indoors on a prosthesis, most will still require a wheelchair outdoors, unless they are using a car all the time.

For those with **transtibial (below-knee) or through-knee amputations**, a stump board is required to prevent oedema and the development of a contracture at the knee. White (1992) reviewed the types of stump board available. In a group of 12 patients, all reported that using a stump board increased their comfort whilst sitting in a wheelchair and 11 also felt that the stump board offered protection to the stump, facilitated acceptance of the amputation and assisted in handling the stump.

For **bilateral through-knee and transfemoral (above-knee) amputees**, their centre of gravity will be displaced backwards if not wearing prostheses, making the chair unstable. Therefore, the rear-propelling wheels are positioned 7.5 cm (3 inches) further back. This makes the chair longer, more difficult to turn, and may cause problems reaching the rear wheels for effective propulsion. An alternative is a thick backrest cushion to move the body weight forward, or weights can be added to the front of the chair, but the latter makes it heavier to push or propel. Some of these patients find it easier to transfer in and out of the chair from the rear, requiring a zip in the backrest canvas.

Multiple sclerosis

This disease usually progresses with time and the wheelchair needs must be frequently reviewed. As walking becomes more difficult the initial need is for a chair for outdoor use. Unlike patients with arthritis it is wise to provide a self-propelling model so that this can provide independence indoors as well should the need arise. An 8L or the smaller 8BL may well be appropriate, but many patients prefer the Barrett 7, possibly because the slightly tilted back seat offers better trunk control.

Attention to an appropriate seat cushion is very important in multiple sclerosis. Correct pelvic positioning helps trunk control and for those with sensory impairment (with or without incontinence) pressure relief is important to prevent pressure sores. For those who experience extensor spasm a pelvic strap can help to keep the pelvis at the back of the seat, and flexor spasms of the legs may require a calf strap to prevent the legs moving backwards and 'fouling' the front castors. If oedema is a problem elevating leg rests should be considered. Additional trunk support, either by lateral supports or a shaped backrest cushion, may be required for truncal ataxia.

If self-propulsion is not feasible or causes excessive fatigue then an electric chair is required. Modern controls are all 'proportional', allowing smooth acceleration and deceleration, and thereby avoiding jerkiness which may precipitate spasm. The siting of the control may need to be reviewed if the original 'driving' hand becomes too weak and control needs to be moved to the other hand. If hand control is not feasible then foot, chin, head or suck-blow controls should be considered. Eyesight and perceptual problems should be assessed prior to prescribing an electric chair. Despite these options a few patients may be too weak or ataxic to drive a chair safely.

Some patients feel most comfortable in a recliner chair, but the size of the chair may cause problems. The Putney Alternate Position Chair (Figure 44.4) is often remarkably effective in reducing spasm and providing a comfortable symmetrical position for patients with multiple sclerosis, but the hips must flex to 90° in order to use this chair.

Spinal injury

Spinal patients tend to be younger and more active. Many will remain in or return to employment, drive their own cars and pursue sporting interests. Paraplegics in particular

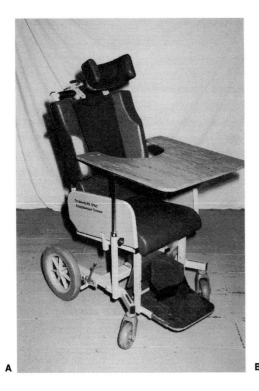
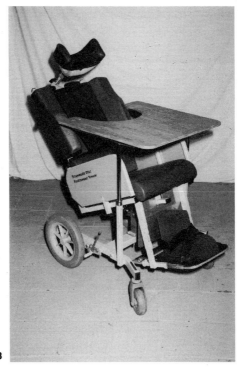

Figure 44.4 A, Putney Alternate position chair in upright position. B, Putney Alternate position chair in most reclined position. Note: upholstered seat cushion (can be used with patient's own cushion), sacral pad, soft backrest cushion with lateral supports, adjustable headrest, footboard with foot positioning block and tray.

make great demands on their wheelchairs, which need to be robust and reliable as well as light, functional and manoeuvrable. Many spinal patients would prefer more than one wheelchair; the 'everyday' model supplemented by a sports chair. Sports chairs are not often supplied by the NHS. As many spinal injuries are caused by accidents, these alternative models are often funded from compensation claims.

Low-level paraplegics may prefer lightweight chairs with adjustable rear axle position, short backrest and no armrests (Figure 44.5). However, these chairs are designed to be less stable than standard chairs, making it possible to balance on the rear wheels (wheelies) which is useful for sills and kerbs, but careful instruction is required. These

chairs are not suitable for older patients and those with high thoracic lesions whose trunk control may be precarious. If caliper walking is an option, then swing-away footplates may be preferable to a fixed footbar and the seat width must be adequate for the calipers.

For those with a lesion at C7 or below self-propelling is viable. C5/6 tetraplegics may also be able to self-propel but need careful assessment. Some manage by pushing on the tyre instead of the hand rim, in which case leather hand protectors should be worn. Alternatives are capstan hand rims which have radial projections or 'sticky' hand rims covered with special plastic. For tetraplegics above C5 an electric chair will be required. If joystick operation is not possible, then chin, hand, suck-blow, voice or infrared controls

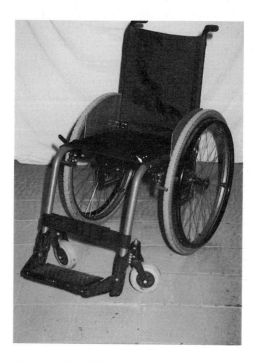

figure 44.5 Kuschall lightweight chair. Rigid frame, skirt guards, no armrests, calf strap, footplate (adjustable), adjustable height backrest, adjustable front castor and rear wheel position. Note: this is not a sports chair per se. Sports chairs feature smooth rear tyres and considerable rear wheel camber (inward tilt) for better manoeuvrability.

should be considered. C4/5 tetraplegics cannot transfer independently so need to be able to travel in their chair. Tetraplegics need an electric indoor chair, an electric outdoor chair or one that can be used indoor/outdoors, and possibly a special function chair, for example Levo 'stand-up' chair (not supplied by the NHS).

All spinal patients need a wheelchair cushion. Ideally this should be assessed objectively using some form of pressure measurement. Low-level paraplegics may find a simple foam cushion is sufficient, but foams degrade over time. Moreover, these patients develop muscle wasting around the buttocks, so reassessment is mandatory. The higher the lesion, the more critical is pressure relief as it becomes more difficult or impossible to relieve pressure. Contoured cushions

for pelvic stability with some form of pressure-relieving overlay will be required by tetraplegics.

Fyfe and Wood (1990) looked at the choice of self-propelling wheelchairs in spinal patients. In a study of 56 patients, 25 (45%) were dissatisfied with their standard (NHS) chairs. The main reason was excessive weight, with difficulty in self-propelling being the second commonest reason. Most spinal patients are issued with a Carters chair initially as these are more robust than the 8L/8BL or Barrett chairs. However, a 'standard' Carters chair weighs 21 kg as opposed to 18.1 kg for an 8L, 16.8 kg for an 8BL and 16.3 kg for a Barrett 7. Burnham *et al.* (1993) drew attention to the frequent shoulder problems in wheelchair athletes, but even for those following a less active lifestyle shoulder problems are common. It is therefore reasonable to expect a patient who is capable of self-propelling to want a lightweight chair, but as pointed out by Fyfe and Wood (1990), it is advisable to defer the choice for a few months until the individual has formulated his/her lifestyle. As a patient said 'immediately after a spinal injury we need advice as we don't know what we need, but as time goes by we are in an increasing position to determine our own needs with less dictates from the professionals!' (D. Constantine, 1992, personal communication).

Head injury

Head injuries are becoming more common and with improvements in medical care many more people survive with long life expectancy but often with some degree of intellectual and physical impairment. In a population of 250 000 the number of disabled survivors at any one time will be between 250 and 375 (The Management of Traumatic Brain Injury 1988). It is important to position a head-injured patient correctly from the start to prevent contractures and inhibit subcortical reflexes, and this should continue through progression to wheelchair or alternative mobility. Even in a persistent vegetative state sitting in a chair is beneficial in facilitating care, altering pressure areas, stimulating peripheral circulation and increasing the patient's level of awareness (Shaw, 1986). If the hips and knees can flex to 90°, then consideration should be given to a Putney Alternate Position Chair. This chair features a tilt mechanism (three positions), a supportive backrest, a very adjustable headrest, knee supports and a positioning footrest. Additionally, there is a large contoured tray which can be used for postural support, particularly in the upright position (Figure 44.4). This chair seems to be very effective at reducing hypertonicity and promoting good posture.

For those who cannot achieve 90° hip flexion (sometimes due to heterotrophic calcification), then a recliner chair will be required to accommodate the increased seat/back angle. As already noted, these chairs are often too large for a domestic environment. Some patients with brain injury can manage a powered chair, but careful assessment is necessary as perceptual problems may preclude safe usage.

Motor neurone disease

Motor neurone disease usually follows a relentless course of increasing paralysis, whilst sensation and normal intellectual function are maintained. Most patients require a wheelchair at some stage, but due to the progressive nature of the condition requirements often change rapidly and any delay in provision causes major problems. The initial prescription is likely to be for a self-propelling chair (e.g. 8L), for even if the arms are not strong enough, or weaken quite quickly, mobility may still be possible by 'foot' propulsion. When propulsion is no longer possible, an electric chair will be required controlled by hand, chin or suck-blow control. A headrest extension and head support will be required when neck muscles become weak. In the later stages of the disease, patients may be more comfortable in a recliner chair, although there are problems due to the size of this chair. It is vitally important to plan ahead.

Paediatric conditions in adulthood

Many disabled children survive into adult life. The three commonest conditions for which wheelchairs are required are cerebral palsy, muscular dystrophy and spina bifida.

Cerebral Palsy

The functional outcome will depend not only on the anatomical distribution and type of movement disorder, but whether there is additional intellectual impairment. Some will be able to walk, albeit with a very abnormal gait, but may need a pushchair (e.g. 9L) or self-propelling chair (e.g. 8L) outdoors to prevent fatigue. For those who are wheelchair dependent, but capable of self-propelling, a lightweight chair should be considered as it may make the critical difference in maintaining independence. If self-propulsion is impossible, an electric wheelchair may be needed, provided the intellectual capacity is sufficient to ensure safe control. Care is needed in siting hand controls or alternative controls should be considered (e.g. foot, chin, head). There are a significant number of adults with cerebral palsy who cannot be sat in a standard chair as their postural needs were neglected during childhood. For those specialized seating will be required.

Muscular dystrophy

Patients with Duchenne muscular dystrophy are likely to need an electric wheelchair by their teenage years. Most need accommodating in special seats. The Becker type of dystrophy progresses more slowly and with limb-girdle dystrophy walking may be possible for many years. Independence using self-propulsion should be maintained for as long as possible and front-propelling wheels may be less tiring. By the time a wheelchair is used, the need for a powered chair is not too distant.

Spina bifida

The main problems are flaccid, anaesthetic legs, anaesthetic skin over the buttocks causing increased risk of pressure sores, a short, often scoliotic spine, with a hyperlordosis and an anteriorly tilted pelvis, the ribs may actually touch the pelvic brim. Some patients will have undergone spinal surgery with the aim of preventing progression of the spinal deformity. Hydrocephalus often accompanies spina bifida and can result in

intellectual impairment. Even if a spina bifida patient can walk as a child, most lose this ability in their teens or adult life. Those who do walk have fewer pressure sores, fewer fractures and are more independent, even when they start using a wheelchair. However, the energy cost of ambulation is high and frequent hospital visits for orthopaedic and orthotic review are often required (Mazur *et al.*, 1989).

For this group of patients adequate cushioning is vital, particularly as not all can 'lift' to relieve pressure. The legs are prone to poor circulation and oedema so that elevating leg rests or a special extended footboard may be needed. These should be carefully padded to avoid pressure problems. The spine will need support, both anteroposteriorly and laterally, if there is a significant scoliotic element. Whilst this may be possible with standard backrest cushions and lateral thoracic supports, some will need more intimate contouring such as modular chair backrests or bespoke moulded cushions. Many young adults with spina bifida will be able to self-propel. A lightweight chair will make this task less fatiguing. If self-propelling is not possible an electric chair should be provided. Those with significant hydrocephalus may not even be able to manage an electric chair, in which case a pushchair (e.g. 9L) with a supportive headrest will be required.

SPECIAL SEATING

Those patients with poor postural control or fixed skeletal deformities may be unable to sit in standard wheelchairs and need 'special seating' to make them comfortable and retain or improve existing function. The function of special seats has been classified as adaptive or accommodative. An adaptive seat is designed to stabilize posture, with the intention of facilitating function and improving ability (Figure 44.6; e.g. Adapta seats, Ce-Trax, Gillingham seats). An accommodative seat is

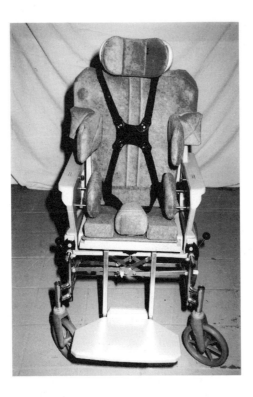

Figure 44.6 Ce-Trax seating insert on a Barrett 10 wheelchair base. This is an adaptive 'orthogonal' seat with ramped cushion, sacral pad, pelvic strap, lateral pelvic and thoracic supports, bib harness, headrest and footboard. The system also features a tray and a knee block which are not shown.

designed to accommodate existing posture in order to provide comfort and retain existing function (Figure 44.7 e.g. Matrix seats, moulded seat inserts).

For special seating to be maximally effective it needs to be prescribed early with the aims of retaining a symmetrical posture and preventing secondary deformities. The majority of seating systems have been designed for children, most notably for those with cerebral palsy. Multiple sclerosis is the commonest condition in adults that requires such seating, followed by head injury, stroke and muscular dystrophy. Learning difficulties also present quite commonly, often with fixed deformities due to lack of appropriate positioning in childhood.

Patients who need special seating require longer assessment than those using standard chairs. This is usually done by a multi-disciplinary team of doctor, therapist, rehabilitation engineer or clinical engineer and possibly an orthotist. Examination of the patient will determine what postural abnormalities are present and whether these are correctable or fixed. It is important to determine the level of sitting ability (Mulcahy *et al.*, 1988) at the first assessment, and repeat this at reviews, in order to assess whether ability is maintained, has improved or deteriorated. This group of patients need a programme of 24-hour postural management; whilst the 'special seat' may provide optimum positioning, sitting is but one activity during a 24-hour period, and in order to maximize outcome, attention should also be paid to

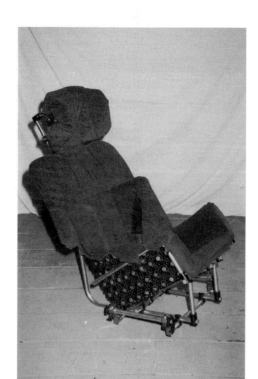

Figure 44.7 Matrix seat insert (to fit on a standard wheelchair – not shown). This is an accommodative seat which is individually designed to suit a particular client. The fabric of the seat is a sheet of interlocking modules which are shaped to suit and then 'locked' in position. The matrix is covered with a foam-backed terry cloth cover and straps added as required.

posture when lying and standing (if possible), (British Society of Rehabilitation Medicine, 1995).

REFERENCES

Ashburn, A. and Lynch, M. (1988) Disadvantages of the early use of wheelchairs in the treatment of hemiplegia. *Clinical Rehabilitation*, **2**, 327–31.

Blower, P. (1988) The advantages of the early use of wheelchairs in the treatment of hemiplegia. *Clinical Rehabilitation*, **2**, 323–5.

Bossingham, D.H. and Russell, P. (1980) The usefulness of powered wheelchairs in advanced inflammatory polyarthritis. *Rheumatology and Rehabilitation*, **19**, 131–5.

Brattstorm, M., Brattstrom, H., Eklof, M. and Fredstrom, J. (1981) The rheumatoid patient in need of a wheelchair. *Scandinavian Journal of Rehabilitation Medicine*, **13**, 39–43.

Braus, D.F. and Mainka R. (1993) Current trends of wheelchair provision after stroke. *Journal of Rehabilitation Science*, **6**, 124–7.

British Society of Rehabilitation Medicine (1995): *Special Seating Working Party Report*, The British Society of Rehabilitation Medicine, London.

Burnham, S.R., May, L., Neson, E. *et al.* (1993) Shoulder pain in wheelchair athletes. *American Journal of Sports Medicine*, **21**, 238–42.

Cochrane, G. (ed.) (1993) *Equipment for Disabled People – 'Wheelchairs'*, The Disability Information Trust (1993), Oxford.

Cornall, D. (1991) Self-propelling wheelchairs: the effects on spasticity in hemiplegic patients. *Physiotherapy Theory and Practice*, **7**, 13–21.

Cron, L. and Sprigle, S. (1993) Clinical evaluation of the hemi wheelchair cushion. *American Journal of Occupational Therapy.* **47**, 141–4.

Disablement Services Authority Training Resource Pack (1990) ''Wheelchairs'', Contact Local Wheelchair Centre for loan copy.

Dudley, N.J. and McMahon M. (1993) The Model 28B electric powered outdoor wheelchair: a users survey. *Clinical Rehabilitation*, **7**, 147–50.

Dudley, N.J. and McMahon, M. (1994) The changing pattern of wheelchair provision. *Clinical Rehabilitation*, **8**, 70–5.

Fenwick, D. (1977) *Wheelchairs and their Users*, HMSO, London.

Fyfe, N.C.M. and Wood, J. (1990) The choice of self-propelling wheelchairs for spinal patients. *Clinical Rehabilitation*, **4**, 51–6.

Goodwill, C.J. (1988) in *Rehabilitation of the Physically Disabled adult*, 1st ed. (eds. C.J. Goodwill and M.A. Chamberlain), Chapman and Hall. London, p 701.

Ham, R.O. (1993) Monitoring wheelchair and seating provision. *Clinical Rehabilitation*, **7**, 139–145.

Kettle, M. and Rowley, C. (1990) *DSA National Survey of Wheelchair Users*, Rheumatology and Rehabilitation Research Unit, University of Leeds.

Male, J. and Massie, B. (1990) *Choosing a Wheelchair*, RADAR, London.

The Management of Traumatic Brain Injury (1988) A working party report of the Medical Disability Society (British Society of Rehabilitation Medicine).

Mandelson, I., Young, V., Burkitt, J. and Torrens, G. (1994) Stroke Rehabilitation at Home – posture system. *Report by Brunel Institute of Bioengineering*.

Mazur, J.M., Shurtleff, D., Menelaus, M. *et al.* (1989) Orthopaedic management of high level spina bifida: early walking compared with early use of a wheelchair. *Journal of Bone and Joint Surgery*, **71A**, 56–61.

McColl, I. (1986) *Review of artificial Limbs and Appliance Centre Services*, HMSO, London.

Medical Devices Directorate Report (1993) *Which One Should They Buy? – a powered vehicle prescription guide for therapists*, Department of Health Store, Heywood, Lancs.

Mulcahy, C.M., Pountney, T.E., Nelham, R.L. *et al.* (1988) Adaptive seating for motor handicap: problems, a solution, assessment and pre-scription. *British Journal of Occupational Therapy*, **51**, 347–52.

Nichols, P.J.R. (1971) Some problems in rehabilitation of the severely disabled. *Proceedings of the Royal Society of Medicine*, **64**, 349–53.

Shaw, R. (1986) Persistent vegetative state: principle and techniques for seating and positioning. *Head Trauma Rehabilitation*, **1**, 31–7.

Tuttiett, S. (1989) *DH Disability Equipment Assessment Programme, Wheelchair Cushions Summary Report*, 2nd ed., Department of Health Store, Heywood, Lancs.

White, E.A. (1992) Wheelchair stump boards and their use with lower limb amputees. *British Journal of Occupational Therapy*, **5**, 174–8.

FURTHER READING

Disabled Living Foundation Fact Sheets

- Choosing an Attendant Propelled Wheelchair.
- Choosing a Standard Self-propelled Wheelchair.
- Mobility and Independence – the high performance option.
- Choosing an Electric Wheelchair.
- Choosing a Scooter or Buggy.
- Choosing a Wheelchair Cushion.
- Out and About With Your Wheelchair.
- Clothing for Women Who Use Wheelchairs.
- Clothing for Men Who Use Wheelchairs.

Available from: Disabled Living Foundation, (Cost £2.00–£2.50).

Medical Devices Agency. A wide list of publications available from their Orders Department under the headings: Autorefractors, Device Bulletins, Diagnostic Imaging, Disability Equipment Assessment, Evaluations, Mammography, Pathology, Radiology, Transport for the Disabled.

Royal College of Physicians Working Party Report (1995) *The Provision of Wheelchairs and Special Seating – Guidance for Purchasers and Providers*, Royal College of Physicians, London.

USEFUL ADDRESSES

British Society of Rehabilitation Medicine
c/o Royal College of General Physicians, 11 St. Andrews Place, Regents Park, London NW1 4LE, UK.

Department of Health Store
Health Publications Unit, No. 2 Site, Manchester Road, Heywood, Lancashire OL10 2PZ, UK.

Disability Information Trust
Mary Malborough Disability Centre, Nuffield Orthopaedic Centre, Headington, Oxford OX3 7LD, UK.

Disabled Living Foundation
380–384 Harrow Road, London, W9 2HU, UK.
Medical Devices Agency, Hannibal House, Elephant and Castle, London SEI 6TQ, UK.

45 Seating and support systems

P. Jay and S. Peters

INTRODUCTION

A suitable chair may be the most important piece of equipment used by a disabled person. It is likely to be in use for many hours a day, during which time it should provide a comfortable base for a variety of activities. A chair should not imprison the patient but be designed to facilitate rising and sitting down, so helping the patient to remain mobile. Patients with arthritis of weightbearing joints, or with paralysis, spasticity or rigidity of the lower limbs, for example due to Parkinson's disease, hemiplegia or spinal cord disease are likely to have seating problems. Weakness or pain in the upper limbs will make rising from a chair more difficult.

The patient should be consulted to ensure that the recommended seating is compatible with their needs. Too often people are trapped in chairs from which they cannot stand up, or are expected to eat while leaning backwards in easy chairs so that they spill food down their clothes. Good seating will maximize function. Good sitting posture should be combined with freedom to shift position. Similarly, armrests should not prevent arm movements. If a table is needed it must be at a suitable height. The chair needs to be well positioned within the patient's environment, whether facing the television so as to prevent neck strain, or with the best view of any stimulating action, which may be looking onto the street.

Appropriate seating should also facilitate patients to walk around. This will depend not only on the design of the chair but also, particularly for elderly patients, on relearning the techniques of getting up from a chair with least effort. When rising from a chair is easier, reaching the lavatory is less of a problem, and this may prevent or cure incontinence. Moving from an easy chair to the dining table will make eating easier. The ability to move about will encourage exercise that may help to improve circulation, prevent oedema, sustain muscle tone, prevent contractures, increase independence and go some way to overcoming social isolation. Sitting immobile in a comfortable chair all day is not good rehabilitation.

ASSESSMENT

It is very important to assess patients before advising them on the most suitable form of seating. This assessment will usually be carried out by an occupational therapist, a physiotherapist or a rehabilitation engineer. It will entail identifying both their medical condition, with the help of the referring doctor, and also what functions they want to carry out from the chair. The assessment will include body size, weight and shape, posture, balance, oedema, perceptual dysfunction,

Rehabilitation of the Physically Disabled Adult. Edited by C. John Goodwill, M. Anne Chamberlain and Chris Evans. Published in 1997 by Stanley Thornes (Publishers) Ltd, Cheltenham. ISBN 0-7487-3183-0.

confusion, continence, risk of tissue ischaemia, prognosis of deterioration, joint stiffness, muscle weakness, coordination and the ability to get out of a chair. Sitting in a better position with a more upright posture can prevent contractures, or alleviate back pain. It may also reduce the likelihood of tissue ischaemia caused either by unequal sideways pressure or shear forces generated by sliding down in the chair. However, sitting someone with a fixed deformity, such as a scoliosis, in a more upright position can result in an increase of pressure under one ischial tuberosity which may need special cushioning.

CRITERIA FOR CHAIR SELECTION
(Figures 45.1 and 45.2; Table 45.1)

Easy or fireside chairs are often used by disabled and elderly people. Many of the criteria for selecting these chairs will apply to other types of chair. Easy chairs, particularly those with high seats, can be bought as standard furniture, but are traditionally desig-

nated as 'geriatric' or 'orthopaedic' chairs. Although guidelines of choice may be given, the shape and dimensions of a comfortable chair are very individual (Harries and Mayfield, 1983).

Lumbar support in different chairs, even the best chair, will only minimize back pain discomfort. It is advisable to spend at least 15 minutes sitting in a chair before deciding it is the right one. Better still, some manufacturers will supply a chair on a trial basis. Disabled Living Centres usually have a selection of chairs which can be tried out during a visit. The following points should be considered when selecting a chair:

Seat Height

Shoes or slippers that are normally used should be worn when assessing seat height. The feet should rest flat on the floor when the knees are at right angles, allowing the legs to move easily. There should be only nominal resistance when sliding the flat hand between the thigh and seat just behind the knee. A

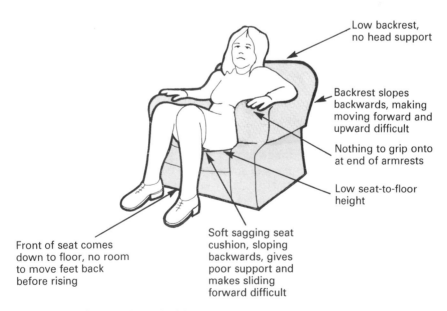

Low backrest, no head support

Backrest slopes backwards, making moving forward and upward difficult

Nothing to grip onto at end of armrests

Low seat-to-floor height

Soft sagging seat cushion, sloping backwards, gives poor support and makes sliding forward difficult

Front of seat comes down to floor, no room to move feet back before rising

Figure 45.1 An unsuitable chair for a disabled person. (Courtesy of Mr A. Chesters of Hangman Backdrops.)

Table 45.1 Checklist for selecting a chair

Getting into the chair

This sitter should not drop uncontrolled into the chair	Armrest height (from floor at front) Seat height Upholstery/suspension
The sitter should not impact with hard areas	Upholstery/suspension Width of chair
The chair should not tip	Stability Splayed/curved legs

Sitting in the chair

The sitter should be able to reach and lean against the backrest	Seat depth Seat slope Backrest slope Backrest shape
The sitter's feet should be supported	Seat height/footrest Seat depth
There should be no pressure on the calves and minimal pressure under the thighs	Seat depth Seat height Upholstery/suspension
The sitter's back should be supported in the lower and upper regions	Upholstery/suspension Backrest shape Backrest slope Backrest height
The sitter's head should be in a comfortable position when leaning on the backrest but should not be restricted when not fully reclined	Backrest slope Backrest shape Backrest height Headrest
The sitter's arms should be comfortable, supported and free for activities	Armrest height (to seat at rear) Armrest width armrest shape
The sitter should not slide forward in the chair	Upholstery/suspension Seat slope
The sitter should be able to change position as required	Upholstery/suspension Seat slope Armrest width Armrest height (to seat at rear)

Getting out of the chair

The sitter should not have to struggle forward to the edge of the chair	Upholstery/suspension Seat slope Seat height Backrest slope
The sitter should be able to place the feet beneath the front of the chair prior to rising	Stretchers/legs Seat height
The sitter should be able to give the initial push on the front of the armrest	Armrest height (from floor at front) Armrest width Grip area

Table 45.1 (continued)

The sitter should be able to rise without unnecessary exertion or struggling	Armrest height (from floor at front) Seat height Seat slope
The sitter should be able to gain support from the chair until almost standing	Armrest height (from floor at front) Grip area Extending armrests
The chair should not tip or slip	Stability Curved/splayed legs

Adapted from *Seating for elderly and disabled people*, Report No. 9, by kind permission of the Institute for Consumer Ergonomics and the DHSS.

higher seat is often easier and safer for rising and sitting down. However, when a comfortable seat height is too low for rising unaided, the compromise may be a high seat plus a footstool, but only if this can be positioned and removed safely and easily.

Seat depth

The sacrum should be touching the backrest to prevent slumping in the chair, and there should be a gap between the front of the seat and the lower leg to prevent calf pressure. A deep seat may look more comfortable but back pain is often aggravated by sitting too far forwards in the chair to get the knees comfortably over the edge which then leads to either slouching backwards or leaning forwards with a rounded back.

Seat width

This should be wider than the sitter, both to allow for changing position in the chair and

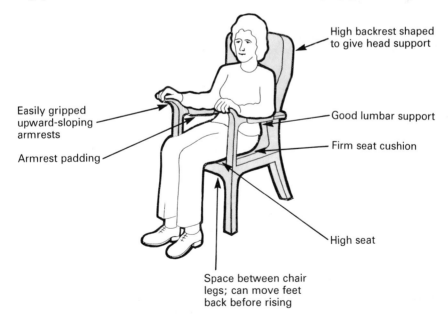

Figure 45.2 A suitable chair for a disabled person. (Courtesy of Mr A. Chesters of Hangman Backdrops.)

for sitting down clumsily (and possibly hitting an armrest). Some people like extra width to store belongings near to hand, but this may inappropriately affect armrest width. (See later).

Backrest height and width

This should be high enough to support the shoulders and for most people also the head. It should be broader than shoulder width to allow for changing position.

Backrest slope and shape

A backrest with a gentle, backwards slope from seat to shoulder height is comfortable, but if the slope is too great, leaning forwards to get up from a chair will be more difficult. The backrest should provide support in the lumbar region but if the lumbar bulge is too low it will push against the sacrum instead. People with long trunks will need higher and longer lumbar support. Above the shoulder the backrest needs to provide head support. If the backwards slope is too great the sitter will use excessive neck flexion to look straight ahead or downwards. If it is too upright it may restrict neck movement. People need to be able to turn their heads freely to look about, and also to lean back to rest with the head supported. An adjustable head or neck rest can be positioned at the correct height and will allow neck movement. It should support the base of the skull, not the back of the head. Wings on the chair are popular as headrests with people who sleep in chairs, but leaning the head so far sideways results in poor sleeping posture. Wings also restrict vision.

Armrest height

Armrests should extend beyond the front edge of the seat, be low enough to push on when getting out of the chair and high enough to provide support until nearly standing without excessive dorsiflexion of the wrists. Using armrests can reduce the forces through the knees when rising, which may be crucial in enabling the patient to get up unaided. The back of the armrest should be a comfortable height for resting the arms without elevating the shoulders, and should not get in the way when carrying out chosen activities such as dressing or knitting. Armrests that are the optimum height at both the front for getting up, and the back for comfort and convenience, are likely to be sloped or shaped upwards towards the front of the chair.

Armrest width

The distance between the armrests (as much as the height) may restrict activities. However, if armrests are too wide apart, the seating posture may be affected and pushing down to get out of the chair may be harder.

Armrest design

The top surfaces should be flat with rounded edges, and broad enough to provide comfortable support for the arms. Padding can increase comfort. The front of the armrests should be wide enough for good palmar support and of a thickness that allows the fingers to grasp the underside. Many people prefer filled-in armrests because these reduce draughts and make it easy to keep belongings within reach, but there are contraindications. Anything spilled will get trapped, a dropped lighted cigarette will be a fire hazard and unsupported vinyl sides may stretch and look unsightly. Belongings may end up beneath the seating area creating high-pressure points. Filled-in armrests, which leave a gap between sides and cushion, reduce draughts and make cleaning the chair easier.

Chair leg design

To get out of a chair easily it must be possible to position the feet almost under the front of the chair, so bringing them below the body's centre of gravity. A low front rail, boxed-in style or too deep a seat frame makes this impossible. Chairs should remain stable even when used by an unstable or atonic person, who may grab at the armrest or backrest for support. Chair legs that extend forward under the armrests, backwards under the backrest or are slightly splayed out sideways increase stability. If they project too far they could cause a fall.

Upholstery and covering

The seat and backrest should provide firm but well-padded support. Softer padding in the shoulder area may be needed to accommodate bony prominences and spinal curvature. Any armrest padding should be supportive and should not 'bottom out'. When there is insufficient support in the seat the patient may slide into a hollow. This will make getting out of the chair difficult, prevent moving in the chair and induce a dorsal kyphosis. It may mean that the thighs are resting on the front edge of the frame.

Many chairs have foam upholstery and this can burn. Flame-retardant foam burns less fiercely but may produce more smoke and toxic fumes, so foam is often covered in a flame-retardant material. Flammability is a risk for a disabled person who smokes, but for others, comfort and pressure relief are more important. After all, clothes and much else in the home will be flammable. British Standard 5852 covers upholstered furniture. (British Standards Institution, 1990). All chairs purchased for hospital or home use should conform to all relevant British Standards. Chairs are often covered with vinyl because this is hardwearing, impervious to liquids, easy to clean and flame-retardant. However, some vinyls harden after prolonged contact with urine or with body oils from scalp or hands. Many people dislike sitting on vinyl because its impermeability pools perspiration, so it feels hot and clammy. If skin and clothing stick to vinyl, movement can produce shear forces. For comfort, chair coverings should be absorbent to dissipate perspiration. Natural fabrics absorb moisture better than man-made fabrics. Vinyl can be covered by a loose cover of cotton or other natural fibre or one of the stretch fabric covers which can be bought to fit most shapes of chair.

User weight

Most chairs have a recommended user weight limit and should be checked before purchase.

SPECIALIZED CHAIRS

High-seat chairs

To get out of a chair a person will normally lean forward and move the buttocks towards the front of the seat. He/she will then bring the feet back under the front edge of the chair, grasp the armrest and push him/herself forwards and upwards. A patient with limited knee flexion will need a higher seat in order to bring the feet closer to the front of the chair and a patient with quadriceps weakness will need a higher seat to increase the mechanical advantage at the knee joint. Frail elderly patients are more likely to be able to get up from a high seat. There are many high-seat chairs on the market. Wooden frames look more aesthetic and come in a variety of seat heights, but some metal frames adjust in height, depth and backrest position. Backs may be contoured or straight and some are more upright to facilitate rising. Arms may be open, side-panelled, upholstered or removable. Upholstery may be fabric, vinyl or a combination or the two. Some manufacturers will alter chairs to suit individual needs. These options range from merely adjusting seat height to made-to-measure seating systems which can include optional lifting and reclining seats (Disabled Living Foundation, 1994).

Some patients raise the height of an existing chair by using an extra cushion, but this makes the armrests relatively lower and adversely affects the position of the curve of a shaped backrest. Chairs can be raised. Chair-raising linked systems, including ones to raise boxed-in/castor-only style chairs, or individual raising sleeves are safer than traditional blocks because they are fitted firmly to the chair frame/legs and cannot be so easily dislodged if the chair is moved or accidentally nudged.

Self-lift chairs

These actively assist patients to rise, and may be indicated for someone with painful joints or generalized weakness. They are not suitable for someone with poor balance or a limited range of hip or knee movement. Self-lift seat units and self-lift mechanical chairs are hinged at the front and have either a strong spring or a hydraulic mechanism which lifts the seat from the horizontal to an angle of about 45°. Self-lift units fit into existing chairs and are most successful on a chair with a firm base. They are portable which is useful, but the additional height gained may make the seating posture inappropriate and uncomfortable. A battery-powered inflatable seat rising cushion is an alternative. Self-lift chairs lift higher than the seat units. As the patient leans forward and takes weight over the feet, he or she will be pushed into the three-quarter standing position, and will need good quadriceps to straighten up into standing. Patients will need an assessment of lower limb function, followed by teaching and practice to use these seats safely and effectively. Some springs are noisy and safety locking mechanisms can be difficult to operate. With all systems the spring or the hydraulic system must be matched to the weight of the patient.

Electrically operated self-lift chairs are not affected by the patient's height. Some systems raise the seat, others raise the seat and arms, and others raise the whole chair and tilt it forward. There are also variations in the height of raise and angle of tilt between chairs. Those with armrests that rise and tilt far enough to provide support right up to the standing position are best. These electrical chairs are easier to use, but can be very expensive. If a person's own chair is comfortable it is now possible to purchase a lifting mechanism that is fitted to their existing furniture. This offers the same advantages as a powered self-lift chair, but at a significant saving.

Rocking chairs

These can help a patient change position, relieve pressure, encourage gentle leg exercise and relieve backache. They are unlikely to give help in rising unless the patient has very good standing balance.

Reclining chairs

These are indicated for patients who are in constant pain and unable to change their own position spontaneously. The reclining chair allows the user to rest or sleep without having to be moved to a bed by a helper. It also shifts pressure from the ischial tuberosities to the spine, and may thus be helpful in preventing pressure sores. Patients are usually more comfortable sleeping in the reclined position than in the upright one (where they very often slide down the chair). The better chairs tilt the front of the seat up and raise the leg rests as well as reclining the back. This tilting from the front effectively lowers the buttocks area and prevents sliding out of the chair. Any chair that reclines more than 20° will be uncomfortable without leg support. Mechanically operated reclining chairs can be difficult to operate. The patient must be sitting in just the right position to utilize body weight (as well as pushing hard) to recline the chair. Electrically operated chairs get over this problem, and some have a lifting seat.

Tilting chairs

These are mobile chairs which can be tilted on their back legs and locked in position. They are often used by nursing staff to prevent patients sliding down in their chairs rather than assessing the cause of slipping (such as inappropriate seat depth or pressure areas). Tilting chairs are contraindicated because they leave the patient trapped, staring up at the ceiling, out of contact with events and people around him.

Mobile chairs

These should be used only by people who are too immobile to get out of a chair, unable to propel a wheelchair or to control an electric chair. It is easier and quicker for nurses and carers to wheel a patient from one place to another, but it is much better rehabilitation to continue walking as long as possible, however slowly, using a mobile chair only when there is no alternative. Mobile chairs have fixed wheels or swivelling castors. Wheels go better in a straight line, and castors around corners. A combination of castors on the front and wheels at the back makes manoeuvring easy and also allows the chair to be tilted on its back wheels. Small wheels and castors tend to jam in every obstacle; 13 cm diameter should be sufficient to avoid this. Solid tyres are easier to maintain, but pneumatic tyres give an easier ride. Solid, spongy, semi-rigid tyres are the best compromise. Patients in mobile chairs will need help to get up, so seat height and brake position are less critical. A footrest which can only be pushed under the chair by an attendant will be quite acceptable, but a fixed footrest makes standing difficult and dangerous because the chair can tip forwards. Foot-propelled castor chairs know as 'Glide-abouts' offer very little postural support, but are extremely useful for manoeuvring within a limited environment.

Office chairs

These have advantages for more active disabled people. The height and angle of the backrest, and height and sometimes slope of the seat, are all adjustable, so these chairs encourage a more upright sitting posture. The swivelling seat increases reach. A five-pronged base provides good stability; castors are better on carpets and 'glide' on uncarpeted floors. Stability may, however, be a problem when getting up or down; backing the chair against a wall may help. Some chairs have arms; these should not prevent a chair getting close to the work top. Office chairs can be used not only when typing or working at a desk, but also when preparing food or ironing, provided the work surface or ironing board is at a suitable height.

High-seat stools

These are used by disabled people who need to conserve energy by sitting rather than standing, but who need to work at a standing rather than sitting height. Some have back-rests and some have armrests. A swivel seat can increase the flexibility of use of a high seat stool. There are also stools with angled seats sloping downwards towards the front, which are used by patients with limited or painful hip flexion or ankylosing spondylitis.

Balans seats

These seats are designed to relieve back pain. They have angled seats and kneerests, but neither backrests nor armrests. The base may be a rocker or it may be fixed. The combination of angled seat and kneerests tends to induce an increased lumbar curve and so encourage a more upright posture, although it is still possible to slump. The rocking base facilitates changing position and redistributing pressure. The seat and kneerests should be well padded but, even so, resting the shins rather than the knees on the knee pads is likely to be uncomfortable. Adjustable features are recommended to achieve the optimum position. These seats come in various sizes and dimensions from a number of manufacturers under different names. To work from such a seat, the work surface must be a convenient height and preferably sloping slightly upwards.

Moulded seats

Some patients are so severely disabled that even with the most careful assessment and prescription they cannot be adequately supported in a chair, even with extra padding and cushioning. For them, moulded seats may provide the answer. There are various systems. With vacuum-extracted systems the patient sits on an envelope filled with polystyrene granules. Air is extracted from this envelope until the seat takes up the shape of the user. This moulded seat can then be fitted into a wheelchair, or it can be used to produce a positive cast on which a moulded plastic seat is shaped. The Matrix Body Support system is a series of small plastic units attached together by ball-and-socket joints to form a sheet of material. This is so adjustable that it can take up any shape. It is then covered with foam upholstery, mounted on a tubular frame, or clamped onto a wheelchair. Funding for moulded seats to fit into wheelchairs would come from the local Wheelchair Service. Information about suppliers of moulded seats is available from the Disabled Living Foundation.

SEATING SYSTEMS

For a disabled child or young adult with complex problems, a seating system that is part of their overall postural management can be more successful than moulded support seats. These systems are carefully assessed for each individual by appropriately trained staff. The basic aim is to exert force on the pelvis via supported feet, a ramped cushion, knee

block and sacral pad to bring it into the neutral plane and thereby restoring or facilitating the lumbar lordosis of the spine. Other features fine tune the system to each person's individual needs (Green and Nelham, 1991) The seating system can be used in a wheelchair or on a mobile base suitable for the home or classroom. Further advice can be obtained from the Wheelchair Services or Disabled Living Centres.

SPECIAL CUSHIONS

Wheelchair cushions increase comfort and can also reduce the risk of tissue ischaemia (Jay, 1984). Everyone who sits in a wheelchair should have a cushion unless there are contraindications. These cushions can also be used in other chairs. Relief of pressure under the ischial tuberosities can be achieved by sitting on a more conforming cushion, so that pressure is taken over more of the seating area, or by increasing the amount of support in some parts of the sitting area to balance the decrease in support elsewhere, as with alternating pressure cushions. Humidity at the interface can also lead to tissue ischaemia. An absorbent cushion cover or a sheepskin will dissipate perspiration. Choosing an appropriate pressure-relief cushion from the vast range available can be assisted by using an indicator scale such as the Waterlow Score, which identifies an individual's level of risk (of developing a pressure area) (Waterlow 1994). A suitable cushion can then be recommended.

Cushions with carrying straps are available for arthritics, or people of short stature who need a high seat. There is also a cushion with a thigh depression to accommodate an arthrodesed hip or knee. More information about wheelchair cushions is given in Chapter 44.

Lumbar support

This must be in the right place. If it is too low in the chair it just pushes the patient forward.

Good lumbar support not only provides a more comfortable and upright posture but can also reduce pressure under the sacrum. Lumbar supports and other backrests are often sold for use in cars (Sweeney and Clarke, 1995). Sculptured foam supports come in different shapes which suit different people. Inflatable back supports will mould to fit any back, which is an advantage, but cannot be used for postural control. Lumbar supports covered in vinyl will be hot and sticky. Fabric or sheepskin covers are better.

Lateral support

Side cushions can give support and produce a more upright posture which will equalize pressures over the seating area. Corrective side cushioning, for example for scoliosis, will not be effective unless the pelvis is stabilized first and any pelvic tilt accommodated by a specially designed seat cushion. Side support cushions need to be firm to achieve correction.

Neck support

Bone-shaped neck pillows will provide support when the head is forward flexed, and they can be removed when lying back. These are small and easy to handle while sitting, but people often find it easier to use a fixing such as Velcro or a weighted flap over the back of the chair.

Legrests

These should be stable and height adjustable to hold the legs in the optimum position. They must be long enough to support the whole lower leg, from ankle to knee, and well padded to spread pressure. Taking weight solely through the calf can restrict circulation; a pillow along the length of the rest can help redistribute pressure. Many patients prefer a legrest that allows about 20° of knee flexion. If oedema is to be reduced the legrest should be horizontal so that the ankles are at hip height.

The end of the legrest adjacent to the chair should be at seat height to support the knees and prevent them hyperextending, which would lead to pain, stiffness and difficulty in rising.

Footstools

These should be high enough to support the feet at a height that prevents pressure under the thighs. Adjustable-height footstools are available or the legs of a wooden stool can be cut to give the desired height. Footstools with ferrules on the legs will give more stability, but patients need telling never to stand up on a footstool. A footstool with castors will be easier to push safely out of the way before getting up from the chair. It can be hooked back with a walking stick. Castors will also encourage leg movement during sitting.

TABLES

The height of a table or desk should relate to the height of the chair and the person in it. Elbows should be about table-top height and there should be clearance underneath so that the thighs are not compressed. A strong, solid table will provide support when rising. Someone who sits mainly in an easy chair may need a cantilevered table which adjusts in height. One with an X-shaped base will be stable, and can be drawn close to the chair. Some have a tilting surface to hold a newspaper or act as a bookrest. The best have a small permanently horizontal section big enough to hold spectacles and a cup of tea.

TRAYS

A lap desk provides an alternative to a table for someone sitting in an easy chair. It is a tray with a polystyrene bead cushion underneath which moulds itself to fit the shape of the lap. This forms a stable base for writing or taking tea. Some models of chair have a tray, which attaches to the armrests, as an optional extra.

SOURCES OF SUPPLY AND FINANCE

Social Services Departments may provide special chairs and seating equipment on a long-term loan to a disabled client. The assessment and recommendation is usually made by an occupational therapist or physiotherapist. For a private purchase chair, an assessment can be obtained at a Disabled Living Centre. Some wheelchair and pressure-relief cushions will be supplied free of charge by hospitals or social services departments. When the patient must pay, cushions, as well as other pieces of equipment, specifically designed for disabled people, including chairs, can be VAT exempt. Sometimes a standard chair ordered for a disabled person on a doctor's recommendation will be VAT exempt. Many companies, particularly specialist agents, can advise customers about this. Otherwise the relevant claim form is included in the leaflet 'VAT Relief for People with Disabilities', obtainable from local VAT Offices.

MAINTENANCE AND FOLLOW-UP

Chairs wear out, foam degrades and loses its resilience, webbing straps stretch or break. It is not sufficient just to choose a suitable chair. This should be checked at least once a year to make sure it is not worn out. Too many elderly people sit with piles of newspapers under a degraded foam cushion. Upholstery may need cleaning, repairing, or even re-covering. Mobile chairs, too, need attention. Castors may get clogged up or need lubricating. There should also be a built-in review procedure to check whether the chair is still appropriate for the patient, or whether some other type of seating would now be better.

REFERENCES

British Standards Institution (1990) (BS 5852. Methods of Test for Assessment of the Ignitability of Upholstered Seating by Smouldering and Flaming Ignition Sources, British Standards Institution London.

Disabled Living Foundation (DLF) (1994) *Hamilton Index. Part 1, section 4, Chairs and chair accessories*, Disabled Living Foundation, London (revised annually)

Green, E.M. and Nelham, R.L. (1991) Development of sitting ability, assessment of children with a motor handicap and prescription of appropriate seating systems. *Prosthetics and Orthotics International*, **15**, 203–16.

Harries, C. and Mayfield, W. (1983) Selecting easy chairs for elderly and disabled people. Institute for Consumer Ergonomics, University of Technology, Leicester.

Sweeney, G.M. and Clarke, A.K. (1995) "Backrests and Back Supports for drivers of cars, a Comparative Evaluation", Disability Equipment Assessment Report, June 1995, Department of Health Medical Devices Agency, London.

Waterlow, J.A. (1994) *Waterlow Score: Pressure sore prevention manual*, Newton Curland, Taunton, Somerset.

FURTHER READING

Atherton, J., Harrison, R.A. and Clarke, A.K. (1982) *Office Seating for the Arthritic and Low Back Pain Patients*, DHSS Aids Assessment Programme, Department of Health Publications, Heywood, Manchester.

Booklet on chairs, available from the Arthritis and Rheumatism Council.

Bridel, J. (1994) Risk assessment. *Journal of Tissue Viability* **14** (3), 84–5.

Choosing a Chair, Factsheet, Disabled Living Foundation.

Disabled Living Foundation (DLF) (1995) Hamilton Index. Part 2, section 9, Pressure relief, Disabled Living Foundation London (revised annually).

Firecode: textiles and furniture (1989) Health Technical Memorandum, 87, HMSO, London.

The Furniture and Furnishings (Fire) (Safety) (Amendment) Regulation 1989 Statutory Instruments 1989 No.2358, HMSO, London.

Harries, C. and Mayfield, W. (1983) Selecting Easy Chairs for Elderly and Disabled People, Institute for Consumer Ergonomics, University of Technology, Leicester.

Institute for Consumer Ergonomics (ICE) (1983) *Seating for Elderly and Disabled People. Report no. 9, Chair specifications and guidelines for chair selection*, University of Technology, Loughborough (May).

May, A. (1979) *Assessment of Selfrise Chairs and Cushions*, DHSS Aids Assessment Programme, Department of Health Publications, Heywood, Manchester.

Nelham, R.L. (1981) Seating of the chairbound person, a survey of seating equipment in the UK. *Journal of Biomedical Engineering*, **6**, 267–74.

Sitting and Seating: a series of articles which includes discussion of the Balans seat, personally contoured cushions and moulded seating, *Physiotherapy*, February 1984.

Wheelchair Information Pack. (1993) Disabled Living Foundation.

USEFUL ADDRESSES

Arthritis and Rheumatism Council, Copeman House, St Mary's Court, Chesterfield, Derbyshire S41 7TD, UK.

Disabled Living Centres Council, Winchester House, 11 Cranmer Road, Kennington Park, London SW9 6KJ, UK.

Disabled Living Foundation, 380–384 Harrow Road, London, W9 2HU, UK.

RADAR (Royal Association for Disability and Rehabilitation), 12 City Forum, 250 City Road London ECIV 8AF, UK.

46 Patient transfers, hoists and stairlifts

C. Tarling

INTRODUCTION

Where physically disabled patients require assistance with transfers, it has been the practice until recently for staff to lift them manually or otherwise physically assist them. However, as from 1 January 1993, the Manual Handling Operations Regulations 1992 have required a different approach to be taken when an adult dependent person is required to be moved. These regulations form part of the Management of Health and Safety at Work Regulations 1992 and are mandatory wherever an employer/employee relationship occurs. It should also be considered that what is required for employed staff may be appropriate to the tasks undertaken by family and other informal carers.

MANUAL LIFTING

There are guidelines given by the Health and Safety Executive about the factors that affect a manual handling risk assessment process. These are generally considered under four main headings:

1. **The tasks that have to be performed**. Here the question to ask is always 'Do I **have** to lift?' In many instances, a different approach will result in a safer and more comfortable position for both patient and handler. An obvious example is the traditional task of lifting the patient up the bed to sit propped up against the pillows that are stacked on the bedrest. The way to avoid this is to use either a mattress inclinator on a conventional bed or to invest in electrically controlled profile beds which will sit the patient up at the press of a button (and which the patient can operate independent of any assistance).

2. **The characteristics of the load**. The comfort of the patient, the avoidance of damage to pressure-sensitive skin and the damaging stress through joints must all be considered, as well as the much discussed weight of the patient. The Regulations are clear in their guidance and indicate that loads for women must be less than those for men. It is suggested that a fit woman may be able to lift a load of some 17 kg (2.5 stone) while in a naturally erect posture. There are few adult patients of this weight and therefore the use of hoists and manual handling equipment should always be considered for the adult dependent patient.

Rehabilitation of the Physically Disabled Adult. Edited by C. John Goodwill, M. Anne Chamberlain and Chris Evans. Published in 1997 by Stanley Thornes (Publishers) Ltd, Cheltenham. ISBN 0-7487-3183-0.

3. **The environment**. While it is to be hoped that places where patients visit and stay for treatment or care are designed for their needs and the tasks which have to be performed, those disabled people who live at home may have to consider some adjustments to their environment if handling equipment has to be introduced.

4. **The capabilities of the handlers**. Most carers are women who are not always as fit as they should be. Age, sex, stature and weight, as well as training and employment history, will all influence the ability of the carer to handle highly dependent people.

If rehabilitation is to be as complete as possible, independent forms of mobility and transfer must be discussed and tried. Elderly patients often return home to the care of an equally elderly and frail relative who may or may not receive assistance for that care through the new Community Care arrangements. While care packages for younger patients may be financially enhanced through application to the Independent Living Fund(s), the elderly patient is often left with a minimal package due to their own or the local authority's financial position. It is most important that the methods of transfers are agreed, taught and established while the patient is in the rehabilitation process and prior to hospital discharge.

One of the greatest difficulties currently being faced by patients and their families on their return home is the delay in the supply of equipment required for their care at home. While many of the smaller items discussed in this chapter may be available, the provision of a mobile or fixed hoist is often not so easily or quickly obtained. Many patients have to settle for a bed downstairs with a commode or chemical toilet while the necessary adaptations and equipment are processed. It is to be hoped that this does not retard or regress their rehabilitation programme.

SEATING

There are many small items of equipment available that will either assist with transfers or alleviate the need to move the patient. Correct seat height of furniture is important in allowing the patient to rise from the seated position without assistance. Beds, too, need to be sufficiently high to allow patients to get in and out on their own. There are a number of ways in which bed and chair legs can be extended to make sure that the seat height is right. For those patients who have difficulty in getting their legs into bed, there are now electrically operated leg-raisers which can be attached to beds, apart from the use of an adapted simple pulley system. The electrically controlled 'sit-up' beds may help some people into a seated position when they are at their most immobile in the early morning. Once seated, the independent sideways transfer becomes possible. For those patients who have very limited hip and/or knee movement, who find sitting very difficult, there are 'stand-up' beds that put the patient on his/her feet, and similarly designed chairs. Chairs with riser seats are available whether electrically or mechanically operated (Figure 46.1). Some are adjustable to the weight of the user, while others have the spring mechanism set in the factory as they are made. Choosing the right chair, particularly for its seat height, is a most important aid to independence (Chapter 45).

BATHING AND TOILET

The bathroom and toilet present problems in many disabilities. Transfers on and off the toilet seat are some of the earliest goals in rehabilitation planning. The toilet seat must not be so high that feet cannot rest firmly on the floor, nor so low that the patient requires a great effort to rise from it. Rails securely fastened on the wall or adjacent to the toilet will help the patient to pull up to transfer. Plastic rails are warmer to touch than metal, and the use of plastic also prevents additional

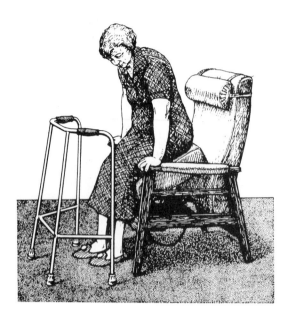

Figure 46.1 Patient using an electric tip-up chair. (Redrawn with permission from Disabled Living Foundation.)

safety wiring having to be provided. The rail should usually be fastened at a height that is just below the seated person's elbow, and should rise from a point level with the centre of the toilet pan to a point 20 cm (8 inches) in front of the pan and at an angle that rises slightly up and away from the seated person. Where the toilet seat is too low, raised seats may be provided in 5-cm (2-inch), 10-cm (4-inch) or 15-cm (6-inch) depths. There are many designs of these, some incorporating a dip in front of the seat which allows patients to clean themselves while still seated. For people who are too severely disabled to manage transfers on and off the toilet from a wheelchair, there are modified cushions that fit inside the wheelchair with a gap where a small hand-held urinal can be fitted between the legs and under the patient. Provided that the patient is wearing adapted clothing, where the crotch of the pants can be opened, then a urinal or simple funnel and tube can be

placed in position, and the patient can use the toilet without transferring.

Getting out of the bath presents problems. The simple bath board across the top of the bath, and a bath seat inside the bath, make it easier for someone to sit on the side of the bath (providing it is not too low) and then swing the legs over the edge before moving into the middle of the board and then down on to the seat. Patients need to have reasonable strength and movement in the upper limbs in order to pull themselves upwards on to the seat or board when getting out. The design of lightweight acrylic baths means that wedging bath seats cannot be used.

If it is decided that a shower is the answer to personal hygiene, then the base of the shower unit needs to take into account that wheeled shower chairs might be used, and the disabled person may not be able to step over ledges into the shower tray. There is a variety of wall-mounted shower seats available with slatted, solid or holed seats. A stool may be used, or a wheeled shower chair which will also act as a mobility aid between the bedroom and the shower, as well as being pushed over the toilet to eliminate the need for yet another transfer.

As long as the patient has good use of his/her upper limbs, small aids to transfers will be the most that are needed. Once the upper limbs as well as the lower limbs lose their power, then transfers become increasingly difficult. Many more severely disabled patients will require a hoist to enable them to transfer either independently or with the assistance of a carer. Most disabled people now have high expectations of a rewarding and full life within their own home and in the community to which they belong. The use of a hoist may be the only way in which these expectations can be fulfilled. However, the family of the disabled person has already had to accept many alterations to its way of life and many items of complex-looking equipment. Whatever is chosen to solve lifting and transfer problems must cause as little disturbance as possible to the family. Members of the rehabilitation team will know how difficult it can be to persuade patients that the use of a wheelchair, even for part of the day, can increase mobility. The same is true of using a hoist, which is seen as a symbol of dependency, but can offer the freedom to transfer when and where the patient wants without relying on community nursing staff, care attendants or frail relatives.

The majority of disabled people living in private dwellings do not live in houses that have been designed for the use of a wheelchair. For many years to come, 'normal' housing will need alterations and extension to accommodate a disabled person. The most common sites for hoists are in the bathroom and the bedroom, but there are many other areas where transfers may be difficult and a hoist helpful. Hoists may be used to pick fallen people up from the floor, get people in and out of cars, or on and off a soft, deep easy chair.

HOISTS

The following review of types of hoists will outline the choice available in order that detailed assessments and decisions can be made:

Mobile hoists

These can be divided into two main classes:

- Larger models suitable for hospitals or the heavier user. These are available in mechanical or electrical systems.
- Smaller models suitable for the domestic environment, also in mechanical or electrical models.

Larger mobile models

Hoists such as the Arjo Ambulift (Figure 46.2) are commonly used in hospitals and residential care homes. They are larger in size and incorporate either slings or a static seat (which can be detached from the hoist and placed on

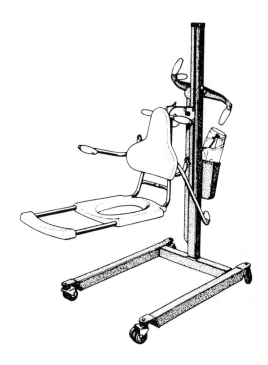

Figure 46.2 Arjo Ambulift Model D with seat and leg extension. (Reproduced with permission from Disabled Living Foundation.)

a mobile chassis). The static seat may not offer enough support to the severely disabled person. The larger models can lift a heavier load, usually up to 160 kg (25 stone), with some manufacturers offering a hoist that will lift 190 kg (30 stone). However, it is important that the equipment chosen for use on the hospital ward is the same as that the patient will use at home; it is confusing to the patient and relatives if they have to learn how to use one hoist in hospital and then quite a different model in their own home.

Smaller mobile hoists

There is a range of these small mobile hoists available both in hospitals and in the community. Most will lift a 127-kg (20-stone) person and are appropriate for the domestic environment. Most models can be easily taken apart for storage or transportation in a car although the Manual Handling Operations Regulations 1992 would deter staff from regularly carrying them from house to house to use with different patients. All models now have a wide variety of slings which may be padded to add to the comfort of the user.

Mobile hoists can be used by an individual person at any site, either inside or outside the home. If transfer problems are present at more than one site, then a hoist may provide the answer. However, none of these mobile hoists can be operated by the patient independently.

Both larger and smaller models are now available with either a mechanical or electrical method of operation. The most usual mechanical method is by a hydraulic pump which still requires effort to operate (particularly with a heavy adult user). Many of the pump handles are also sited too low, thus placing the operator in a stressful working position, unless they sit to pump the handle, thus keeping their spine in an erect position. The electrical models are now increasing in popularity because of their ease and speed of use, particularly by carers who are less than fit themselves. The batteries are easily recharged at minimal cost and are located on the chassis base or on the hoist mast. These electrically powered mobile hoists are heavier to dismantle and transport and this must be borne in mind when considering their use.

Overhead track hoists (Figure 46.3)

The majority of these overhead hoists are electric, and run on a fixed track which may be supported at each end by an A-shaped metal frame resting on the floor or fastened to the ceiling in a predetermined place. The former is used where the person is waiting to be rehoused, or is in privately rented accommodation where the landlord will not allow

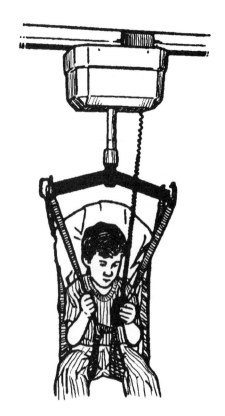

Figure 46.3 A ceiling track hoist with a traversing motor unit. (Redrawn with permission from Disabled Living Foundation.)

alternations, or in the case of terminal care where a lifting aid is needed to assist the heavy load of the carers. It can also be used as part of the assessment process where an electric hoist is to be tried out before the final order for an installation is made.

The hoist has an electric motor which raises and lowers the person in the sling(s). The hoist can be fitted with a traversing motor, or a system of pulleys may be used to move the suspended person sideways.

One of the advantages of the overhead electric hoist is that it takes up no floor space and is therefore very suitable for small bathrooms and toilets. This type of hoist offers disabled persons the option to operate the hoist themselves. In some cases the tracking can run from room to room and be taken round corners, but more frequently the track runs from wall to wall within one room. All electric hoists are now available in 24-volt models with transformers so that they may be safely used in a room with a water supply. There may be some instances where the electricity supply is unreliable and several manufacturers now provide an in-built battery which is charged between uses so that a power failure for some hours does not present a problem to the user.

Bath hoists

This is the area of most frequent hoist provision and there are many varieties. There are two basic types:

- Those that fit inside the bath, and move up and down.
- Those that fit outside the bath and swing over the bath before going up and down in the bath.

Those bath hoists that fit inside the bath require the bath base to be checked for strength. With a lightweight type of bath there may be a need to strengthen points beneath the bath to take the stresses of the weight of the hoist and user. When using the hoist the patient will usually need to be able to lift his/her legs over the side of the bath, requiring hip and sometimes knee flexion, as well as reasonable balance. Because they require little fitting, they can be used as a short-term hoist where the patient's circumstances may change. Nearly all bath hoists have an upright seat on which the patient remains seated. This type of hoist is not for those people who wish to lie back and luxuriate in a bath.

There is a range of bath hoists that take the form of a seat attached to a pillar mounted in the bathroom floor (Figure 46.4). They may be used independently by the patient. Some models are designed so that the carer can

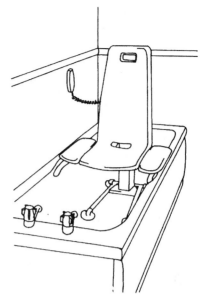

Figure 46.4 An internal bath hoist which is battery powered.

move the seat on to a chassis so that it can act as a mobility aid between the bathroom and bedroom, and may also be pushed over a toilet. Many of these types of bath hoists will have a leg bar as an extra attachment to the seat, so that the patient's legs can be raised as they are swung over the rim of the bath.

CAR ACCESS

Mobility and freedom of movement are important aims of rehabilitation. Many disabled people own and/or drive their own cars, and access to the outside world is a normal expectation. Transferring in and out of a car may be achieved by a sliding or transfer board, a car-top-mounted hoist, a mobile hoist or alterations to the design of the car.

Sliding board

Because of the awkward body positions in which the carer will have to try and assist the patient in and out of the car, the use of a small lifting aid will ensure that the transfer is achieved with little physical stress. A sliding board can be used by removing the nearside arm of the wheelchair and placing the wheelchair next to the driver or passenger seat. The patient's feet are lodged on the car sill ready to slip into the footwell as the transfer takes place (Figure 46.5). The board is slipped part way under the seated patient's hips and the lifter goes around the car and kneels on the other car seat facing the patient. Getting hold of a belt around the patient's waist, or grasping the material of his/her trousers where maximum weight is on them, the lifter then pulls the patients towards him/her and the patient will slide over the board and into the seat. In this way the lifter is not lifting in a twisting or bent position, and the patient is not subjected to the discomforts of manual handling.

Car-top hoist

A car-top hoist is fixed to the roof of the car and works with a hydraulic pump system

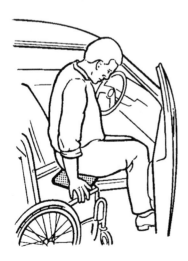

Figure 46.5 Use of a sliding board to assist a patient into a car.

operated by the carer. Table 46.1 lists the points which need to be taken into consideration when choosing between a car-top or mobile hoist for car transfers.

Alterations to the design of the car

One of the most common adaptations of the car is to alter the passenger seat so that it swivels out from the side of the car, thus creating greater space for a transfer. The person is seated as he/she is swung back into the car, thus avoiding the need to duck the head while transferring (Figure 46.6). For a totally dependent person a van's roof can be raised, and a ramp created at the back so that the person may be pushed up into the van and travel whilst remaining seated in their wheelchair. The wheelchair must be clamped to the floor of the van (Chapter 50).

This is not an exhaustive description of the hoists available. There are now models which will cope with a wide range of lifting and transfer problems, as varied as getting in and out of a swimming pool or on and off a horse and trap.

SLINGS

There are five main types of support used on hoists: the static seat; two-piece slings; divided leg sling; full-body hammock sling; one-piece sling.

The static seat

This may be used on a mobile hoist such as the Ambulift, or on a bath hoist such as the Autolift. If used on a mobile hoist then the seat may be detached from the main hoist and the patient may be rolled on the bed, the seat placed beneath him/her and then, with the patient on the set, it is reconnected to the hoist and raised off the bed. If the seat is on a fixed floor bath hoist then the patient must be able to effect the transfer with minimal assistance. Since the use of a hoist is to obviate the need to lift, unless the patient can be rolled, or can

Table 46.1 Comparison between types of hoists

Car-top hoist	Mobile hoist
Space is left free inside the car	Less space inside the car if the hoist is to be carried
The hoist can only be used for car transfers	The hoist can be used in many different situations
Quick to use as the hoist is always in position	Slower to use as the hoist has to be assembled and then stored away again
Can be used on the front or back seats of the car	Can only be used on the front seat as the back wheels of the car usually obstruct access to the back seat
Can be used on a variety of surfaces	Can only be used on relatively smooth surfaces because of the wheels of the mobile chassis

effect a transfer him/herself, then the use of a static seat on a hoist should be questioned.

Two-piece band slings

Although these have been commonly used until recent years, they are only used by those people who are experienced hoist users. The narrower band goes around the chest wall, under the axillae with the arms outside the sling, the wider band goes under the thighs as close to the hip joints as possible. In lifting with the hoist, unless the slings have been carefully positioned the chest sling will rise, and can cause uncomfortable pressure through the shoulder joints, while the thigh sling may slip towards the knees, thus causing the patient to 'jack-knife' through the slings. This design may be used by the hoist user who does not have a carer to assist in placing the slings, and who has considerable experience in hoisting himself. These two-piece band slings are not now recommended.

Divided leg sling

Most manufacturers now produce a divided leg sling to fit their own hoist. These have developed so that there are now no chains or metal parts in the sling. The sling is in one piece with a deep backpiece that supports up to the shoulder joints, and two longer sidepieces which are slid beneath the patient's legs. It is a quick and simple task for a carer to place the sling around the patient and to remove it after the transfer is completed.

A recent further development of the divided leg sling has been the 'dress' or 'toileting' sling. This has a chest band to hold the sling in place and a cut away area around the hips to allow access to clothing. While this sling is in use, the patient's trousers and underclothes can easily be pulled down just prior to being seated on the WC (Figure 46.7).

The full-body hammock sling

This is similar in shape to the divided leg sling but has the additional height at the back to offer head support to those patients with little or no head control. These slings are also useful when the patient in semiconscious or in a highly dependent state while in hospital.

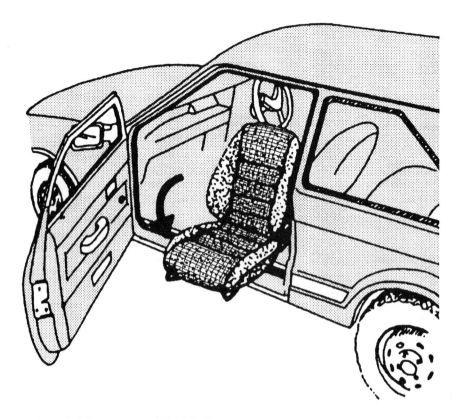

Figure 46.6 Swivel sliding car seat (ELAP Ltd).

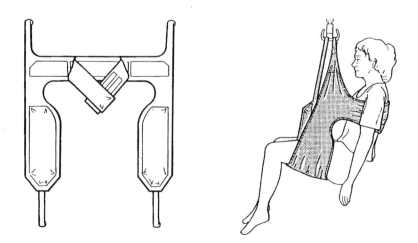

Figure 46.7 The 'dress' or 'toileting' sling that allows access to clothing.

One-piece sling

The patient is rolled on to this type of sling while in bed and then hoisted to a commode or wheelchair, but he/she must then remain sitting on the sling as it cannot be removed without lifting. This sling is often used by frail carers who need to assist with a transfer but who cannot get a divided leg sling on and off easily. If the patient is to remain seated on the sling, and particularly if the sling has a commode aperture, then a sheepskin liner to the sling might help in maintaining good skin care. The one-piece sling may also be used by an independent hoist user when a carer is not available.

Whichever sling and hoist is used, training will be needed for all those concerned with its use. Most manufacturers will provide training sessions to ensure that the users of their equipment are competent and that the hoist does all that is required. Where hoists are to be supplied through a centralized loan equipment store, then it is desirable that the hoist is not delivered to the patient's home long before the staff member is informed or available to teach its use and check its installation. These training sessions may need to be repeated from time to time, especially if there are changes in the staff members using the hoist or in the circumstances of the patient and his family. Follow-up check visits are also necessary to maintain the hoist and its slings in safe working order.

The use of a hoist or small transfer aid can open up a wide range of activities and freedom of movement to many disabled people. While some patients may have to accept the assistance of a carer to operate the hoist, it still leaves them the ability to choose the timing and method of their transfer. For those patients able to self-operate an electric overhead or bath hoist, the independence is invaluable and a most important part of the rehabilitation process.

STAIRLIFTS IN THE HOME

To the home dweller, access to all parts of the house is extremely important, especially sleeping, bathing, toileting and living areas. When a patient has problems with mobility, and lives in a house of two or more storeys, access to the higher levels is often difficult and painful, and sometimes impossible. A number of solutions are therefore available:

1. **Move the bed downstairs** – this is only practical when few people live in the house and there is more than one living room. There must also be a toilet available downstairs, as constant use of a commode is disagreeable to most people. Where there is a family, the bed downstairs causes stress, due in part to lack of privacy.

2. **Build an extension** – this necessitates enough space outside to accommodate a WC and bathing facilities, as well as a bedroom, if this cannot be provided within the existing space on the ground floor. Very often there is not the land available. It is also a costly undertaking which is usually financed through the provision of a Disabled Facilities Grant from the local authority. This Grant is subject to a financial test on the family's resources and currently has a maximum ceiling of £20 000 (1996).

3. **Move house** – this solution is often totally unacceptable to the client. Long-standing relationships have often been established with neighbours, especially where the client lives alone. Neighbours help with shopping, frequently do some cooking, and keep the client company for many a long afternoon or evening. Such relationships are almost impossible for a disabled person to initiate after a move, and consequently to move to a new environment can bring loneliness, isolation and subsequent depression.

4. **Install a stairlift or through-ceiling vertical lift** – this solution is usually the most acceptable, being the least expensive and also maintaining the use of all areas of the home. Life is therefore as normal as possible. The financing of this provision is usually through a Disabled Facilities Grant. However, some local authorities have evolved systems to use reconditioned second-hand stairlifts or vertical lifts, thus reducing the cost for themselves and offering a quick service. This also usually includes maintenance costs. It is also possible for a second-hand stairlift to be purchased privately thus reducing the costs for a family where a Grant may not be possible; servicing needs to be included in the budget.

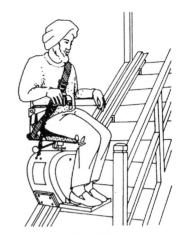

Figure 46.8 A seated stairlift in use.

Stairlifts (Figure 46.8)

A stairlift is a seat and/or platform mounted onto a drive unit, running up a track which is superficially mounted onto the staircase. These are usually made to cope with a straight staircase, with alteration often possible where there is a half-landing and two or three steps round a corner at the top. There are a few made to cater for curved staircases, but these are most costly.

Through-ceiling lift

Where the patient is confined to a wheelchair, or finds it very difficult to transfer from the wheelchair to the seat, and would therefore need another wheelchair at the top of the stairs, a through-ceiling lift is more frequently being installed. These can also be installed when the staircase configuration is costly or impossible to negotiate. It transports the client seated either in his/her wheelchair, or on a seat in the lift, or even standing, from one floor through the ceiling to the next floor. The lift runs on two tracks fitted to the wall, and when out of use is neatly stored away on the upper floor, out of sight, to be called down again when needed by the push of a button.

Method of selection

It is best practice to call in the local community occupational therapist who will, in some authorities, work together with an engineer. Between them they will assess the patient. This calls for much skill and accurate observation. The client's medical condition and prognosis need to be taken into consideration, as do mental abilities; physical ability; the needs of the rest of the family, especially children where applicable; type of house; physical characteristics of the staircase; headroom available; positioning of doors, electrical points, windows and any other relevant detail. A selection can then be made from the choices available, many of which can be seen and tried at a Disabled Living Centre.

Many months may elapse between the initial request for equipment and the final delivery and fitting, mainly because agreement of funding usually has to be sought.

In the case of the stairlift, the track must be suitable for the staircase, and must not protrude any further than necessary. Some tracks need to extend a long way past the bottom step, depending on the angle of the rise of the staircase. The height of the footplate varies considerably. A footplate which is high off the ground when the stairlift has come to rest at the top or bottom of the staircase is a disadvantage. The client usually needs to stand on the footplate in order to get onto the seat. Not all are weightbearing.

The footplate should be sufficiently deep in order to take the feet securely, without the risk of them slipping off. It should be so positioned that the knees need only be bent up to 90°.

The relationship between the seat and the footplate dictates the amount of knee flexion required, and one needs also to consider how far back on the seat the client is able to sit comfortably. Usually a gap between the backrest and seat enables the user to sit right at the back of the seat, thus putting minimal pressure on the knees as they do not have to be tucked well under.

The harness or seat belt, if required, needs to be easy to fit, fasten and release. The user must feel secure, and this applies particularly to children and all people with poor muscular control.

Stairlifts can be operated in a number of ways – the most common being by continuous pressure on a pushbutton located on or near the armrest. When this cannot be manipulated, modified controls such as a rocker switch or joystick can be used. These modifications are usually available at an extra cost, and the additional outlay required must be checked.

Stairlifts vary in levels of noise; whether this is acceptable depends on where they are situated, for example on a party wall in a pair of semi-detached houses.

Servicing arrangements need to be organized – either through the social services department or privately. Each area in the UK has its own policy on servicing, and information regarding this needs to be sought locally.

Some authorities operate a 24-hour call-out service; others rely solely on the stairlift company.

Insurance needs to be taken out, and its provisions clearly understood.

Training the clients in the use of the stairlift should be thorough, and a telephone number where the therapist, lift engineer or lift company can be reached in case of emergency needs to be available.

When selecting a stairlift a few patient-related points need to be considered. For example: Will the client sit or stand? If he/she sits, how far can the knees be bent? As most stairlift seats face sideways, those patients with limited knee flexion need to be looked at carefully, and perhaps a forward-facing stairlift installed. Can the patient operate the control buttons, which are usually constant-pressure ones? If not, do they simply need to be relocated or are other types of switch needed, such as a rocker, joystick or wobble-stick? If the patient cannot operate the controls at all, as is the case with some, especially children, a wander lead can be installed for the patient/carer to use. Call switches are usually installed at both the top and bottom of the stairs.

Access to the stairlift or into the through-ceiling lift needs to be looked at carefully. Most stairlifts have some sort of step up onto the footplate: can the patient cope with this? Sometimes the footplate does not take the weight of a person, and thus the patient has to be able to sit on the seat and bring the legs up after him/her. Access to a through-ceiling lift can be either up a small raise of 2–3 cm (1 inch), or a ramp may be lowered to ensure a smooth ride into the lift.

The provision of a stairlift or through-ceiling lift may not only be of direct benefit to a patient in terms of access, it may also be a means of keeping his or her family intact and close, giving the disabled person help and independence but also allowing the latter to contribute to the family's well-being.

FURTHER READING

Disabled Living Foundation (1994) *Handling People – Equipment advice and information*; Disabled Living Foundation, London.

Fletcher, B., Holmes, D., Lloyd, P.V. *et al.*, (1997) *The Handling of Patients*, (4th ed), National Back Pain Association, in collaboration with the Royal College of Nursing, Teddington, Middlesex.

Equipment for the Disabled (1996) *Hoists, Lifts and Transfers* (and other titles) Disability Information Trust, Oxford.

Goldsmith, S. (1976) *Designing for the Disabled*, Royal Institute of British Architects, London.

Health and Safety Executive Manual Handling (1992) *Guidance on Regulations – Manual Handling Operations Regulations 1992*; HMSO, London.

Stowe, J. (1988) *Guide to the selection of stairlifts*; Rheumatism and Rehabilitation Research Unit.

USEFUL ADDRESS

Disabled Living Foundation
380–384 Harrow Road, London W9 2HU, UK.

Disabled Information Trust
Mary Marlborough Lodge, Nuffield Orthopaedic Centre, Oxford OX3 7LD, UK.

National Back Pain Association
16 Elm Tree Road, Teddington, Middlesex, TW11 8ST, UK.

Rheumatism and Rehabilitation Research Unit
School of Medicine, University of Leeds 36 Clarendon Road, Leeds LS2 9PJ, UK.

47 Orthotics

F.T. Ponton

DEFINITIONS AND CLASSIFICATIONS

An orthosis (plural: orthoses) is defined by the International Standards Organization as: 'An externally applied device used to modify the structural or functional characteristics of the neuro-musculo-skeletal system'. Orthotics is the science of selecting, manufacturing and fitting the most appropriate device for an individual patient. An orthotist is a health care professional qualified by certification to assess, measure and fit orthoses upon completion of a 3-year degree and 1-year internship.

Orthoses are provided for a wide range of disabilities. They are normally prescribed by a doctor, with advice from an orthotist and sometimes physiotherapist or occupational therapist. The more complex devices require individual fabrication for the patient, though an increasing number are assembled from modular components or are available in ranges of sizes and fittings.

Successful orthotic prescription requires careful analysis of the patient's physical and functional status followed by the selection of realistic objectives in conjunction with the other elements of a treatment regimen. Surgery, for example, may be a prerequisite or an alternative to orthotic management. Continuous patient review, which may involve fine tuning or adjustment of a device, is essential for long-term usage.

The primary function of an orthosis is the control of rotary, translatory or axial motion of one or more body segments. The orthosis should control only undesirable motion and permit motion where normal function is possible. Hence an accurate biomechanical analysis of the patient should form the basis of orthotic prescription.

Systematic prescription is possible using the Biomechanical Analysis System devised by the American Academy of Orthopaedic Surgeons and described in *The Atlas of Orthotics* (1985). This methodology forms the basis of orthotic terminology, such that the descriptive acronym for any orthosis will be the joints across which the orthosis crosses, for example AFO for ankle/foot/orthosis or TLSO for thoracic/lumbar/sacroiliac/orthosis.

ASSESSMENT AND PRESCRIPTION CRITERIA

Assessment

Assessment for orthotic treatment commences with examination of joint ranges of movement, the condition of ligaments, muscle strength, tone and contractures. The potential patient–orthosis interface conditions are critical: vascular status, tissue viability, allergenic skin reaction, oedema, bony prominences, anaesthesia or hypersensitivity will all influence the orthotic prescription.

Rehabilitation of the Physically Disabled Adult. Edited by C. John Goodwill, M. Anne Chamberlain and Chris Evans. Published in 1997 by Stanley Thornes (Publishers) Ltd, Cheltenham. ISBN 0-7487-3183-0.

Note the location and nature of pain. Hand function problems are important since independent doff and don is preferable. For all ambulatory orthoses, visual gait assessment (Chapter 8), body segment alignment, balance and proprioception conditions are essential to assessment. Sociopsychological factors may be relevant but patient motivation is the key to acceptance and use of any orthosis.

The assessment process should summarize the functional disability and consider recommendations for complementary treatment. The adult paraplegic, for example, may require the surgical release of tendon contractures or the reduction of hypertonicity before the use of a walking orthosis is feasible. Similarly, physiotherapy is a frequent prerequisite or adjunct to successful orthotic management.

Prescription

The prescription process must determine the functional requirements, the orthosis design features and seek the patient's agreement. The functional objectives include one or more of the following:

1. to prevent, correct or compensate for a deformity;
2. to reduce the axial loading of a limb or body segment;
3. to rest or protect a joint in a given position;
4. to improve walking;
5. to control the range of motion of a joint;
6. to exercise or re-educate neuromuscular function;
7. to transmit forces in a controlled manner in order to promote one or more of the above objectives.

Orthoses function through the application of mechanical forces to the body. The success of any prescription will depend upon a clear understanding of biomechanical principles and their application in the context of an individual pathology. However, other factors also influence successful prescription and the patient's concerns over appearance may compromise the functional objectives and determine alternative design features.

DESIGN CRITERIA FOR ORTHOSES

The selection of appropriate materials requires an understanding of the elementary principles of mechanics of materials, material properties, deformation and failure of structures under load (Major and Stallard, 1985). Steel and aluminium alloys were traditionally used in the fabrication of structures, but are being increasingly replaced by plastics and composites (Bader, 1993). The thermoplastics in most common use are polypropylene, due to its long fatigue life under repeated loading, and various densities of polyethylene. Thermosetting plastics like polyester and epoxies are more brittle and less frequently used. Carbon fibre composite materials are used in conjunction with thermoforming plastics for increased rigidity at specific points and are now available in rigid strut form for structural components with enormous weight-saving benefits. Some low-temperature thermoplastics can be moulded directly to the body with obvious time-saving benefits (Malick, 1978, 1979). Cellular foamed thermoplastics are widely used as interface materials and have a broad range of accommodating and resiliance characteristics. Naturally tanned leathers continue to provide well-tolerated interface materials. Rubbers, natural and artificial elastomers, are used in a variety of applications, particularly when large elastic deformation is required with relatively low force levels.

The choice of material in orthotic design will be determined by its weight, the fabrication method, and its biocompatibility (it should not cause a toxic or allergenic reaction, nor excessive heat or moisture retention). Additional criteria are the ability of the material to withstand load (strength), to withstand shock loading without failure (toughness), to withstand cyclic loading (fatigue resistance), to deform permanently before fracture (ductility), to deform and return to normal upon the removal of loading (elasticity) and to resist chemical degradation (corrosion resistance).

The fabrication of an orthosis incorporates structural integrity, adjustability and a fail-safe design. Whilst British and European Standards provide specifications for orthotic materials and assembly methods, there is a lack of definitive data on the in-service loading of orthoses (Scothern and Johnson, 1984). Some modular designs have adjustable features to accommodate changing clinical circumstances, but the adjustability of metals and plastics by bending and heating is often limited. To avoid dangerous breakage an orthosis should fail in a ductile manner: the Parawalker, for example, designed to brace adult paraplegics, has a relatively brittle hip joint casting which is therefore backed with a ductile plate.

The user-friendliness, and hence patient acceptability, of a device will depend upon the ease of doff and don, its appearance (cosmesis), comfort, ease of toilet functions and low energy useage. The success of any prescription is always enhanced by a full explanation of the function, expected usage and care of the orthosis.

BIOMECHANICAL PRINCIPLES IN ORTHOTIC MANAGEMENT

Any force has a magnitude, a direction and a point of application. When a force causes rotation about a point, the result is a turning moment. The normal musculoskeletal system is constantly subjected to external forces and moments which are resisted or controlled by forces generated by body tissues such as ligaments and muscles. Where pathology affects one or more body segments, it may be necessary to modify external forces and moments acting across a joint or joints by the use of an orthosis. The prescription process must determine which of the following will be applied:

1. Restriction of rotational motion at a joint. The moments acting about the joint may be modified in one or more planes. For example, at the knee joint rotation is possible around three perpendicular axes in the coronal, transverse and sagittal planes. Orthotic control can eliminate motion about the coronal and/or transverse plane axes whilst allowing sagittal plane motion (Figure 47.1), or it can restrict sagittal plane motion.

2. Removal of translational motion at a joint. This is possible, for example, using a sagittal plane four-point pressure system of orthotic control at the knee following anterior cruciate ligament damage or repair (Figure 47.2).

3. Reduction of axial forces across a joint. In this case loading of body tissues is wholly or partially transferred via the orthotic structure to the ground as, for example, in the use of a patellar tendon-bearing or ischial weight-bearing orthosis, (Figure 47.3).

4. Alteration of the direction and point of application of the ground reaction force. This approach can be used to reduce high moments about a joint or to change alignment of the joint. It is particularly used for control of motion at the foot–ankle complex or at the knee, (Figure 47.4).

The patient–orthosis interface

The patient–orthosis interface is the junction between the body tissues and the orthosis and/or support surface through which forces are transmitted. Pressure is the intensity of loading applied to a particular area and should normally be minimal given the ease of tissue breakdown.

Successful orthotic design should therefore consider:

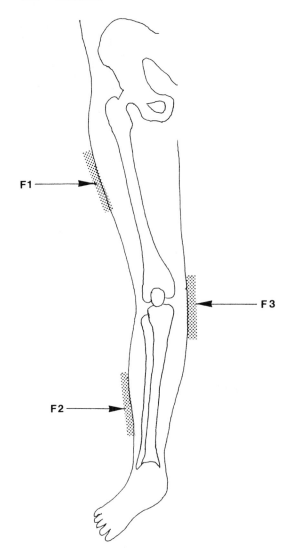

Figure 47.1 Orthotic control of rotational motion (KAFO or KO).

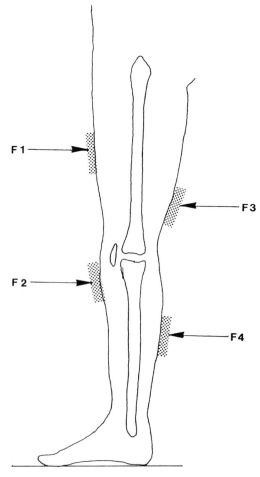

Figure 47.2 Orthotic control of translational motion (KO or KAFO).

1. maximizing the area of contact.
2. contouring the contact area to the body shape.
3. careful choice of contact material
4. positioning the contact area(s) to maximize moment arm (even more critical in the presence of fixed deformities), and so reduce force per unit area.

Measurement of body/support interface pressure has been the subject of some research, but there has been little work to determine quantitive optimization of applied forces within orthoses (Chase, 1989; Chase, Bader and Houghton, 1989).

UPPER LIMB ORTHOSES

Upper limb orthoses serve one or more basic functions:

1. Assistance for residual weakened motor power, or substitution with dynamic mechanisms for complete motor loss.

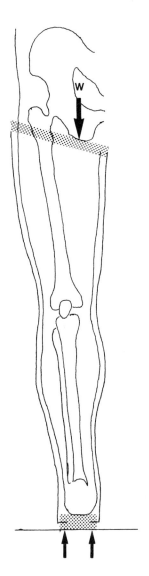

Figure 47.3 Orthotic control of axial forces (ischial weight-relieving KAFO).

2. Protection from pain or potential deformity.
3. Correction of deformity.

Since upper limb anatomy and biomechanics are complex, orthotic management, particularly following trauma, is usually highly specialized and rarely undertaken except as an integral part of a planned rehabilitation programme (Wynn Parry, 1982). Careful explanations to the patient are necessary to achieve compliance because orthoses are often complicated and bulky.

Fabrication techniques for upper limb orthoses are described by Malick (1978, 1979) and Rossi (1987).

Hand and wrist hand orthoses (WHO)

The joints of the wrist, hand and fingers are particularly prone to inflammation and/or the development of contractures. In Dundee a review of 1 year's supply of upper limb orthoses (McDougall, Carus and Jain, 1985) has shown that the indications for prescription were as follows:

Traumatic injuries	61%
Hemiplegia	17%
Wrist pain	13%
Dupuytren's contracture	9%

These figures are likely to be typical except where centres specialize in conditions such as rheumatoid arthritis.

WHOs are either static or dynamic. Static orthoses may rest and/or immobilize the joint(s) in a chosen position to alleviate pain, aid extensor weakness or prevent stiffness and deformity (Figure 47.5)

Causes of pain include arthritis, tenosynovitis or malunited fractures. Orthoses commonly offer palmar support though the dorsal option leaves the palm free for touch and function. A wide variety of pre-fabricated supports are available in fabrics, elastics, neoprene and aluminium or plastic. In rheumatoid arthritis static orthoses for night-time use may relieve morning joint stiffness. Some patients with motor neurone disorders, with poor ability to provide thumb opposition, may benefit from the use of opponens orthoses for specific activities. Their success has been reported (Pichora, McMurty and Bell, 1989) in the treatment of chronic metacarpophalangeal joint injury of the ulnar collateral ligament. Various static digital

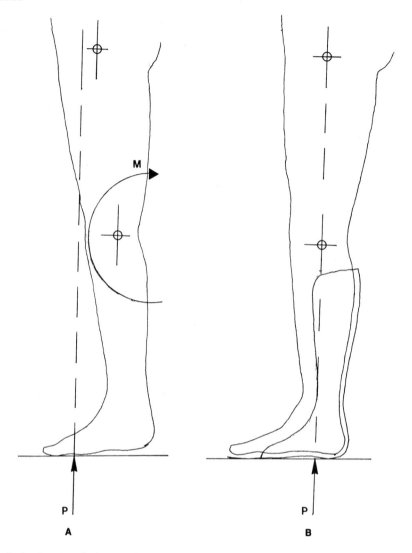

Figure 47.4 Orthotic control of ground-reaction forces. A, Knee extension moment created by GRF anterior to knee centre; B, reduced knee extension moment as a result of realignment of GRF by AFO-footwear.

orthoses, such as the mallet finger splint, are able to prevent movement in the desired plane.

Dynamic WHOs aim for active correction through the use of stored energy in the form of coiled springs or elastic. Commonly used 'outriggers' are bulky, though Moberg (1983) has addressed this problem and variations of his 'low-profile' design are in wide use today.

Dynamic wrist orthoses are often prescribed for radial nerve palsy (Figure 47.6), wrist extensor weakness, and to control ulnar drift in rheumatoid arthritis with a design which applies gentle and continuous forces acting dorsoradially on the displaced phalanges. Although in common use, there is little evidence of their efficacy. Various finger orthoses are used for flexor tendon repair,

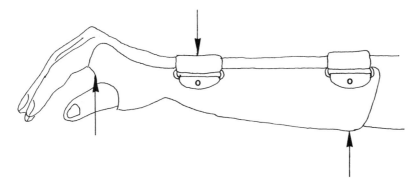

Figure 47.5 Static wrist–hand orthosis.

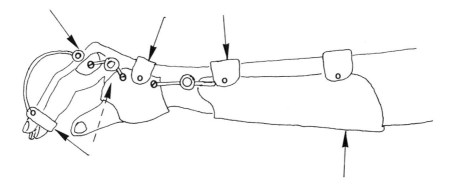

Figure 47.6 Dynamic wrist–hand orthosis.

Boutonnière deformity, swan neck deformity and Dupuytren's contracture.

Elbow orthoses (EO)

Following trauma or disease, if no recovery is expected then conforming static orthoses, fabricated in plastic or moulded leather, are used to hold the forearm in a position of optimum function or comfort. For flexion/ extension assist and/or mediolateral elbow and rotational stability, above- and below-elbow cuffs may be connected by free or positional ratchet joints. To resist elbow flexion contractures a turnbuckle may be fitted across the joint between the cuffs and

gradually extended (Green and McCoy, 1979). To promote elbow flexion strong elastic between the cuffs has been used.

Shoulder orthoses (SO)

For glenohumeral subluxation due to muscle paralysis, slings are inadequate since the objective is to provide a proximally acting axial force on the humerus to prevent inferior migration. Cool (1989) has demonstrated orthotic designs which meet this criterion, where the arm is suspended from a moulded cap which is fitted over the involved shoulder. This is attached by a variable tension band to the proximal forearm so that

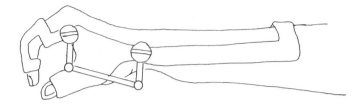

Figure 47.7 Flexor hinge wrist–hand orthosis (transfers active wrist extension to interphalangeal flexion).

the tension produces a moment sufficient to maintain it in equilibrium while supporting the humerus. Hence no axial force is directly applied to the upper arm, a chest harness ensures the shoulder cap provides a secure anchor, and excessive forearm pressure is avoided by the use of a lightweight stainless steel frame.

In brachial plexus lesions with a flail arm an orthosis can help to improve function. Such modular orthoses (e.g. the Stanmore or Roehampton models) are complicated and require skilled fitting and training, particularly if terminal devices are to be used. Their use is reviewed by McKenzie and Buck (1978).

For patients with severe upper limb paralysis, prehension orthoses can offer the potential for grasp, holding and release. The orthosis moves the stabilized index and middle fingers toward and away from the thumb by harnessing the hand or wrist (Allen, 1971) or possibly an electrical power source (Dillner and Georgiev, 1979) (Figure 47.7). As an alternative to complex prehension orthoses, some paralysed patients prefer to wear a simple utensil holder (Lehneis, 1971).

Mobile arm supports (MAS)

Where muscle weakness (grade 2) prevents useful arm movement against gravity, a balanced forearm orthosis (mobile arm support) may be prescribed (Figure 47.8). They are only helpful if there is residual hand function or if implements can be gripped by, or fixed to, the hand. This commonly occurs with motor neurone disease, progressive muscular atrophy, muscular dystrophy and sometimes in tetraplegia or multiple sclerosis. The MAS is contra-indicated if there are spastic or involuntary movements, limited upper limb joint motion due to arthritis or contracture, lack of patient comprehension or lack of staff to adjust and balance the device.

To use the MAS the patient must be firmly supported in a functional position. The supporting adjustable clamp is fixed around the metal backrest, which should not usually be angled back more than 12°. It may be angled further back to allow a headrest to support weak neck muscles, in which case a universal clamp is used to allow correct positioning of the MAS. The proximal metal arm pivots in this clamp, and extends out to provide another socket for pivoting of the distal metal arm, into the end of which the forearm trough fits with a swivel attachment. For weaker patients this swivel may be offset to allow greater adjustment.

Adjustment is provided by the following means:

1. Height of the clamp on the wheelchair is adjusted for the patient's natural forearm position.
2. Rotation of the clamp inwards or outwards will assist adduction or abduction of the shoulder.
3. Tilt of the bracket on the clamp will alter the support angle of the MAS. Tilt upwards will aid flexion and tilt downwards will aid extension of the elbow.

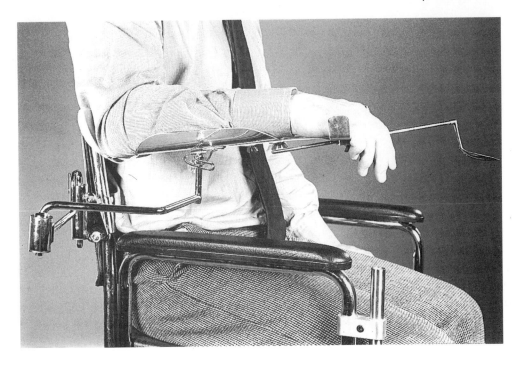

Figure 47.8 Mobile arm support.

4. The anterior-posterior position of the forearm trough on the distal arm will not only aid flexion and extension of the elbow, but also influence rotation of the shoulder.

5. The offset swivel support for the forearm allows a greater range of vertical movement of the hand, especially if the patient is very weak.

6. A T-bar extension to the forearm trough is used to support the hand if the wrist extensors are weak, and a supinator assist may be used under the trough.

The MAS is used for feeding, writing/typing, turning pages and other work and hobby activities. Once correctly adjusted, useful function depends upon acceptance of the device and the determination of the patient (Yasuda, Bowman and Hsu, 1986) and regular review is essential.

SPINAL ORTHOSES

Cervical orthoses (CO)

Cervical orthoses may be categorized as collars, braces and halo-traction devices related to the degree of immobilization which they impart.

Collars, available in foam, Plastazote, semi-rigid polythene or tubular sections, provide mimimal support and limitation of movement. They are widely prescribed for pain in cervical spondylosis (Johnson *et al.* 1981), rheumatoid arthritis (Moncur and Williams, 1988), spinal injury (Herkowitz, Kurz and Samberg, 1989), or in destructive lesions due to malignancy or in vertebrobasilar insufficiency (Nachemson, 1987). Pellicci *et al.* (1981), in a prospective study of the progression of rheumatoid arthritis in the cervical spines of 106 patients, demonstrated that diligent collar use did not prevent the natural progression of

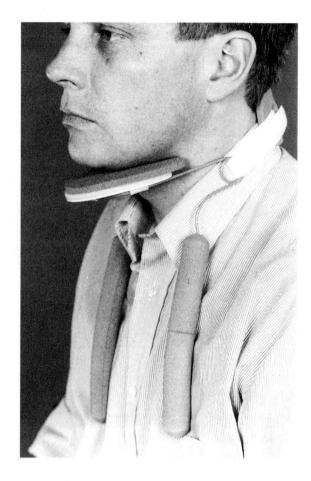

Figure 47.9 MND Association Collar.

the disease. For long-term use more extensive collars ('Doll's' or Cuirass-type) may be custom-moulded over the shoulders and fabricated in polyethylene or blocked leather. The bivalved Minerva collar extends even further over the occiput and more distally on the trunk (Pringle, 1990).

Cervical braces restrict flexion/extension, partially relieve compressive stress and provide some limitation of rotational movement. These modular devices have rigid, adjustable struts attached to sternal and/or posterior thoracic sections to apply distractive forces to the mandible and occiput. The SOMI (sterno-occipital-mandibular   immobilizer)

brace is particularly effective (Fisher *et al*, 1977).

Halo ring-vest orthoses provide maximum distraction and restriction and are commonly used postoperatively following cervical spinal fusion (Convery and Hamblen, 1991).

In the advanced stages of some neuromuscular conditions, such as motor neurone disease (MND) or multiple sclerosis, two other devices are useful. The MND Association collar provides dynamic head support with minimal weight, minimal interface contact, and no interference with swallowing or breathing (Figure 47.9). The Oxford Lees head support provides support via an elasticated head band which allows rotation and leaves the neck completely free. It can be attached to a wheelchair or a posterior spinal strut.

Thoraco-lumbo-sacral orthoses (TLSO)

As a result of force application nearly all spinal orthoses produce three effects: (1) increased intra-abdominal pressure, (2) restricted trunk motion and (3) modified skeletal alignment of spinal segments.

Orthoses for adults are used for postural and/or pain management rather than dynamic correction of deformity. For neuro-muscular conditions such as spina bifida, poliomyelitis and muscular dystrophies, cir-cumferential orthoses made of leather, poly-ethylene or polypropylene can provide stability for comfort and function (Hsu, 1988). Where there is trunkal symmetry with instability, possibly for example in high-level paraplegia, a modular shell TLSO, such as the Boston Overlap orthosis, may be indicated.

Lumbo-sacral orthoses (LSO)

These orthoses are used in medical conditions which apply to other spinal segments but are dominated statistically by low back pain and sciatica (25% of the UK orthotic budget). Predominantly made in fabric with steel reinforcements, they are also available in metal constructions (Goldthwait, Knight, Jordan orthoses) and in modular plastic.

Many authors, including Alaranta and Hurri (1988), have attempted to establish the efficacy of the LSO. Long-term use is usually only advisable where no other treatment relieves pain. Willner (1990) using a test instrument which imitates a rigid brace and has variable sagittal plane support, claims that it was possible to predict whether a rigid brace would give pain relief in patients with low back pain and that is could also indicate the manufacturing method for optimum relief.

LOWER LIMB ORTHOSES

Hip-knee-ankle-foot orthoses (HKAFO)

These devices are primarily prescribed in cases of complete and incomplete paraplegia, both traumatic and congenital, with the aim of allowing a patient to stand and/or walk. Walking with orthoses can usually only supplement, and not replace wheelchair use. It should only be recommended when there are clear therapeutic benefits or an improved level of independence, and when the patient is well motivated. Perceived therapeutic ben-efits include improved bowel function, urinary drainage and peripheral circulation, and reduced osteoporosis. Only recently (Mazur *et al.*, 1989) have some of these claims been measured and validated. Inde-pendence in this context refers to relatively low energy walking, unassisted doff and donn, and transfer from sitting to standing and vice versa when wearing the orthosis.

The HKAFO must meet three biomecha-nical requirements:

1. stabilization of a multisegmental struc-ture;
2. injection of propulsive forces;
3. control of the forces used for stabilization and propulsion.

Bilateral KAFOs with pelvic/thoracic exten-sions do not meet the above criteria and they are less commonly used. One of several devices may be used, in conjunction with a walking aid, for reciprocal, as opposed to swing-through, gait. The ORLAU Parawalker (Butler and Major, 1987) employs limited range low-friction hip joints in a rigid ad/abduction-resistant framework (Figure 47.10). The Louisiana State University Reciprocating Gait Orthosis (LSU-RGO) (Beckman, 1987) consists of bilateral plastic KAFOs with twin cables linking the hip joints to enforce relative reciprocal flexion and extension (Figure 47.11). The Advanced Reciprocating Gait Orthosis (ARGO) employs a single hip cable, has no thigh restraint and gas pistons which

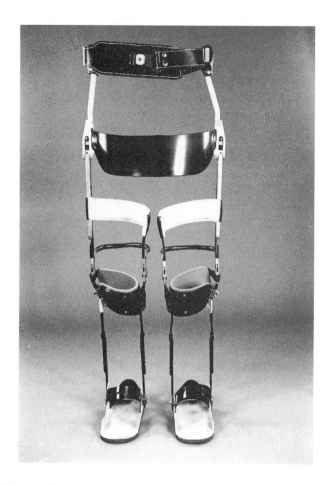

Figure 47.10 ORLAU Parawalker.

may assist standing and dampen the jolt in sitting (Figure 47.12). Devices incorporating further refinements of mechanical efficiency, such as Isocentric RGO (Motloch, 1992), are now available.

Comparative studies of reciprocating orthoses have been undertaken (HMSO, 1989, Whittle *et al.*, 1991) as well as physiological cost analyses of individual orthoses (Bowker *et al.*, 1992). The most suitable orthosis can only be selected following careful assessment of the individual patient. These orthoses, used in conjunction with functional electrical stimulation, have undergone trials (Isakov, Douglas and Berns,

1992), but this treatment is not routinely available.

For very heavily handicapped adults with upper limb involvement and inability to use walking aids, a swivel walker may be appropriate (Farmer *et al.* 1982).

Knee-ankle-foot orthoses (KAFO)

For knee disorders a KAFO may be used in preference to a knee orthosis in the following circumstances:

1.   when functional disorders of the ankle/ foot are also present;

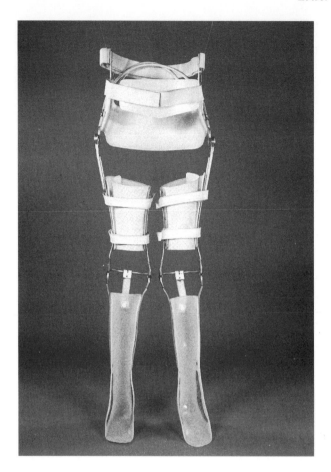

Figure 47.11 LSU Reciprocating Gait Orthosis.

2. when the severity of the knee disorder requires long lever arms and maximal interface contact (particularly for weight-bearing pain relief),
3. when only a KAFO can overcome a problem of poor orthosis suspension at the knee.

Joint replacement has reduced the need for these orthoses but they may still be indicated (Condie, 1991):

1. Loss of structural integrity of the knee joint, as in arthritic disease.
2. Muscle weakness at the knee (and possibly hip and ankle) as in lower level paraplegia or poliomyelitis.
3. Upper motor neurone lesions with hypertonicity as a result of cerebral palsy, head injury or, occasionally, adult hemiplegia.

There are three main types of KAFO fabrication. Conventional single or double-sided metal uprights with leather-covered calf and thigh bands are now less frequently used (Figure 47.13). Polypropylene or Ortholen (high-density polyethylene) thigh and AFO sections, connected by metal knee joints, are most frequently used (Yates, 1976) (Figure 47.14). A third option, with or without a plastic AFO component, is the use of carbon fibre composite uprights and transverse

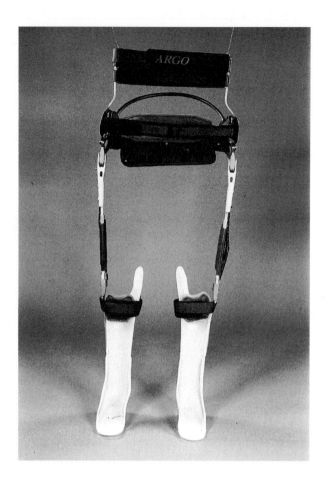

Figure 47.12 Steeper Advanced Reciprocating Gait Orthosis.

bands (Figure 47.15). This latter option is likely to be increasingly taken given the significant weight-saving benefits.

Biomechanical function in all cases centres on three-point force applications (Figure 47.16). The shoe is an essential component of the orthotic system and additional control straps, pads or extensions are used as necessary. The sites of force application are discussed by Lehmann and Warren (1976). Where there is a loss of axial load-bearing capacity, as in failed hip/knee replacements or femoral fracture non-union, then an ischial weightbearing thigh component is employed to transmit damaging ground reaction forces.

In most cases, proper function necessitates walking with the knee locked in extension, for which a range of manual or semi-automatic mechanical joints are available. Walking aids will also be necessary. Accurate mechanical-anatomical knee joint alignment is essential if unacceptable pressure and shear are to be avoided in sitting. Since the anatomical axis of rotation moves posteriorly during knee flexion, the positioning of any uni-axial mechanical joint will be a careful compromise. Controlled swing-phase flexion is not normally possible, though the use of powerful gas struts offers some potential, and at least one orthosis (the Chignon

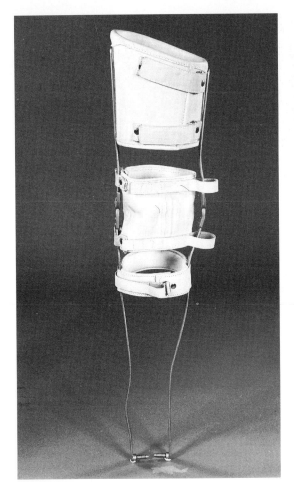

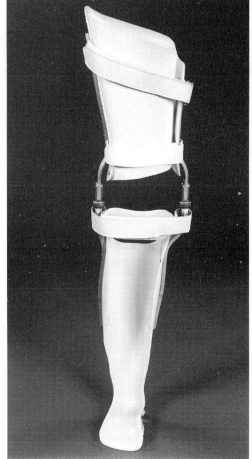

Figure 47.13 Conventional KAFO.

Figure 47.14 Cosmetic KAFO.

Dynamic Orthosis CDO) used in stroke rehabilitation) uses strong elastics for this purpose (Chignon *et al.*, 1990).

Knee orthoses (KO)

Knee orthoses may be prescribed for biomechanical deficit where there is:

1. medial or lateral collapse on weight-bearing, as commonly occurs in arthritic conditions;
2. joint hyperextension;
3. excessive anteroposterior tibial translation and/or collateral ligamentous damage, as commonly occurs in certain sports injuries;
4. weakened quadriceps function.

The majority of KOs are prescribed for arthritic patients and exceptionally poor compliance (Butler *et al.*, 1983) may be due to distinct mechanical problems. They have little leverage advantage and potentially high localized pressure applications, often over fragile soft tissues. It can be

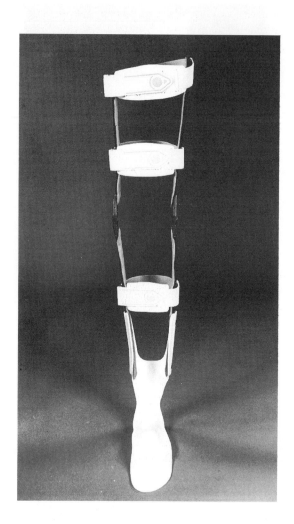

Figure 47.15 Proteor carbon fibre KAFO.

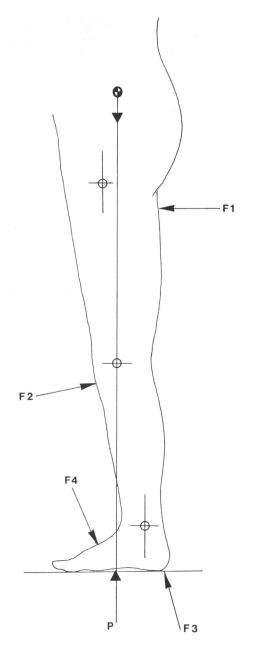

Figure 47.16 Force application for postural balance.

difficult to maintain correct positioning both vertically and rotationally, and given the difficulty of securing a fixed reaction point, it is hard to apply derotational forces. If mechanical knee joints are indicated, they should be polycentric in order to match normal sagittal motion as closely as possible.

Knee orthoses are classified as prophylactic, post-operative or rehabilitative, and functional. They are of three general types: knee sleeves, stabilized knee sleeves, and semirigid or rigid frame braces.

Prophylactic braces are designed specifically to prevent or reduce the severity of patellar tracking. Stabilized knee sleeves, with medial and/or lateral hinged bars, may also incorporate a hypertension stop. In cases of mild hyperextension deformity, the Swedish Knee Cage functions more adequately, but in severe cases longer lever arms and larger areas of interface contact will be necessary (Figure 47.17) (Chase and Whittle, 1988). For mediolateral correctable deformities of less than 20°, the TVS orthosis (telescopic valgus-varus support) (Figure 47.18) can be useful. Jawad and Goodwill (1986) obtained relief of knee pain in 14 out of 18 osteoarthritic patients, but in only five out of 13 with rheumatoid arthritis.

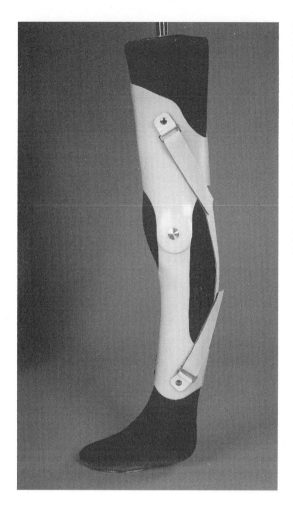

Figure 47.17 Wingfield KO.

injury resulting from an externally applied force and are used almost exclusively in American football. Their use is controversial despite considerable research (Grace *et al.*, 1988).

Postoperative knee braces are applied immediately following ligament reconstruction. They are characterized by greater length and usually incorporate a means of selective range of motion control (Cawley, 1990:).

Simple knee sleeves, now usually fabricated in stretch cotton or neoprene, apply circumferential pressure and are often used to aid

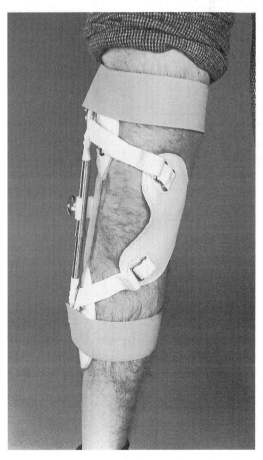

Figure 47.18 Telescopic valgus-varus KO.

Functional or dynamic knee braces are of the frame type and fabricated in materials such as aluminium alloy, composite, carbon fibre and titanium. They are used for the chronically unstable knee with all combinations of ligamentous deficiency (Halling, Howard and Cawley, 1993). Their principle application is now for reconstructed knees, often following sports injury. Cawley, France and Paulos (1991) provide a review of the current state of functional knee brace research. For anteroposterior instabilities, the Donjoy brace has had good trial results (Liggins and Bowker, 1991). Cook, Tibone and Rediern (1989) cautioned prescribers that the carbon–titanium (C.Ti) brace did not prevent abnormal anterior translation, though there have now been design improvements. For rotational instabilities, the customized Lennox Hill brace (Figure 47.19) is thought to be most effective (Hanswyck and Baker, 1982). Recent comparative studies by Pratt (1990a) and Wojtys *et al.* (1990) display a wide range of results from different braces. For both the deficient and reconstructed knee, the great majority of patients report significant functional improvement when wearing these braces. Such braces may also prove effective for patient groups other than the younger, more active and sports oriented.

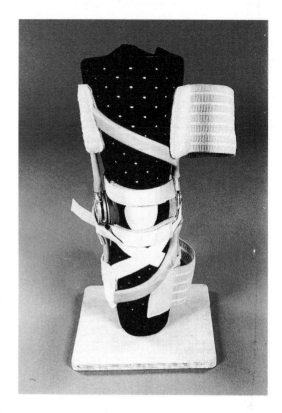

Figure 47.19 Lennox Hill KO.

Ankle-foot orthoses (AFO)

AFOs are amongst the most commonly prescribed orthoses and probably have the highest rate of successful prescription. Although there are only three basic types – metal, thermoplastic and hybrid – the variants, configurations, and additional componentry are almost limitless.

The biomechanical function of an AFO will include one or more of the following:

1. To limit normal or abnormal joint range of movement, wholly or partially.
2. To stabilize the foot/ankle segments.
3. To influence the line of action of the ground reaction force and hence alignment of knee, hip and trunk.
4. To relieve axial or transverse loading of the limb segment.

Some designs of AFO may have a neurophysiological, as well as biomechanical, function.

AFO prescription is common in three broad categories of impairment: (1) flaccid muscle weakness, (2) upper motor neurone lesions involving spasticity, (3) structural instability and/or pain. Some appropriate orthotic designs will be described for each category.

Flaccid muscle weakness

Many pathologies involve weakness or paralysis of the foot and ankle: nerve or tendon injury, lower motor neurone lesions spring-assisted ankle joint (Figure 47.20) or plantar-flexion stop in a tubed shoe heel. The three points of force application are the posterior calf band, the secure dorsal instep of the shoe, and the strong shank of the shoe under the foot. Contemporary AFOs, usually moulded in polypropylene or ortholen to a plaster cast of the patient's limb, employ a similar force system (Figure 47.21). The stiffness/flexibility of the posterior ankle section allows bending and resists plantar-flexion. They fit inside the shoe and are also routinely available in a range of prefabricated sizes (Lehmann, 1979). Because of their intimate contact odema is usually a contra-indication.

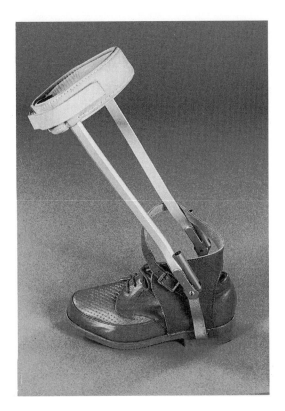

Figure 47.20 Klensac lateral bar AFO.

such as poliomyelitis, spinal lesions such as spinal bifida, and neurological disease such as multiple sclerosis can result in flaccid foot-drop. Peroneal nerve palsy due to pressure at the neck of the fibula, muscular dystrophy or Charcot–Marie–Tooth disease may also cause ankle weakness. Nerve root lesions are usually relieved by surgery, but some cause persistent foot-drop. Tendon transfer of tibialis posterior to produce active dorsi-flexion may be an option, but for many patients an orthosis is appropriate, particularly when recovery is expected.

Dorsiflexor absence or weakness, resulting in poor swing-phase clearance and causing forefoot initial contact in stance phase, can be substituted by a simple three-point force system. This is provided conventionally by a single or double metal upright orthosis with a

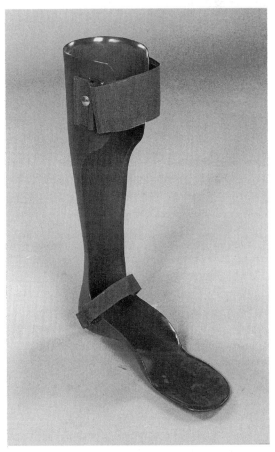

Figure 47.21 Dynamic AFO.

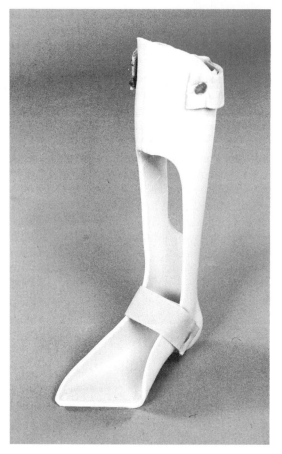

Figure 47.22 Ground reaction AFO.

Plantarflexor absence or weakness is controlled by a three-point force system which involves a posteriorly directed force on the front of the calf. The Floor Reaction AFO (Figure 47.22) with its rigid ankle trimline, achieves this function (Lindseth and Clancy, 1974). A conventional double-upright AFO with anterior stops may achieve the same results though it will be heavier. However, leg section to foot section alignment is critical and Lehmann *et al.*, (1985) conclude that this should be 5° of dorsiflexion.

General ankle weakness, together with poor control of pronators and supinators (subtalar instability), will present as valgus or varus

deformity of the hind- and/or mid-foot. It can occur in conjunction with any of the above problems and requires three-point pressure control in the mediolateral plane. This is provided conventionally by a T- or Y-strap at the malleolus fastening around a metal upright on the opposite side. Even with the use of inshoe heel wedges and strap fixation, this does not always provide effective control. A plastic AFO trimmed to give mediolateral three-point pressure control may prove more useful.

Unilateral knee extensor weakness is often overcome by a patient flexing the trunk to bring the line of action of the ground reaction force in front of the knee, so creating a knee-stablilizing moment (i.e. in maximum extension). If they are unable to support this knee extension with strong plantarflexors, then a KAFO may be indicated. With moderate weakness a Floor Reaction AFO may be sufficient to promote knee extension. Ankle joints for use with plastic AFOs can be set to resist dorsiflexion and allow plantarflexion. Care must be taken to avoid knee hyper-extension and a rocker sole has proved effective in such cases (Hullin and Robb, 1991).

Upper motor neurone lesions

The design and biomechanical function of AFOs used for this category of patient are similar to those used for muscle weakness. However, the spastic foot-drop is more difficult to treat, since a spastic equinovarus causes instability in stance phase as the calf muscles invert the subtalar joint. Spasm may be reduced by physiotherapy or medication. In some cases an AFO can reduce muscle tone by maintaining the ankle in a chosen position. Conventionally this is provided by mechanical stops rather than springs which can exacerbate spasticity. To control hind- and mid-foot inversion bilateral uprights fit into rectangular sockets in firmly constructed and fastened shoes. Persisting

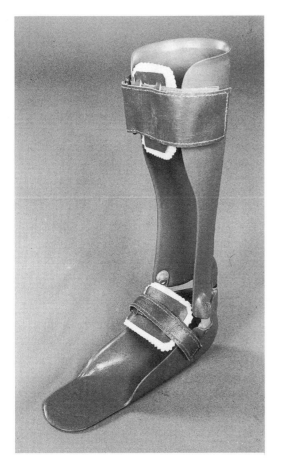

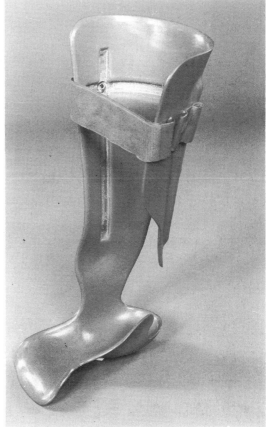

Figure 47.23 Jointed AFO.

Figure 47.24 Neurophysiological AFO.

inversion may be reduced by a lateral T- or Y-strap in conjunction with lateral heel flares and lateral sole and heel wedges. A plastic AFO with a fixed 10–20° of dorsiflexion and rigid ankle trimlines is usually prescribed if there is only moderate spasticity. Modern jointed plastic AFOs (Figure 47.23) which resist plantarflexion and allow adjustable degrees of dorsiflexion are now often preferred. Independent doff and donn is of course highly preferable for the stroke patient.

Tone facilitating or inhibiting orthoses, described as neurophysiological AFOs (Ford, Grotz and Shamp, 1986; Shamp, 1987), are being increasingly used in clinical practice (Figure 47.24). Their design is complex and not recommended unless under close supervision in a physiotherapeutic regime.

Structural instability

Arthritic conditions or trauma often result in chronic pain in the ankle–foot complex during weightbearing and/or joint motion. Most commonly a solid AFO, blocking all ankle and hind-foot movement, is used. The obvious functional deficit may be aided by a cushion heel and rocker sole, though Schuh

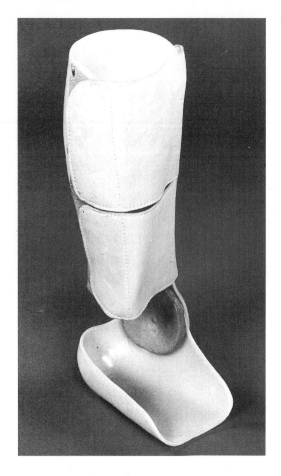

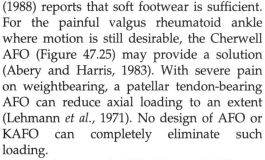

Figure 47.25 Cherwell AFO.

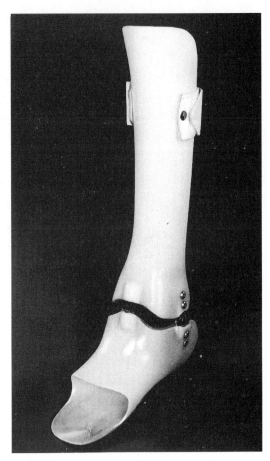

Figure 47.26 Talar control AFO.

(1988) reports that soft footwear is sufficient. For the painful valgus rheumatoid ankle where motion is still desirable, the Cherwell AFO (Figure 47.25) may provide a solution (Abery and Harris, 1983). With severe pain on weightbearing, a patellar tendon-bearing AFO can reduce axial loading to an extent (Lehmann *et al.*, 1971). No design of AFO or KAFO can completely eliminate such loading.

The talar control AFO (Figure 47.26) provides an attempt to control subtalar joint motion anterodorsally, though it may be considered too aggressive in many cases (Brown, Byers-Hinkley and Logan, 1987).

Foot orthoses

Foot orthoses usually function by realignment of ground reaction forces. The objective in mobile deformities is to place the foot in the optimum functional position, that is, subtalar (STJ) and midtarsal (MTJ) joint neutral. For fixed deformities, the objectives may include accommodation, redistribution of plantar pressure or realignment of the plantar surface of the shoe. The overriding presenting symptom in nearly all cases is chronic pain, most commonly as a result of an arthritic condition.

Foot instability or deformity may be due to

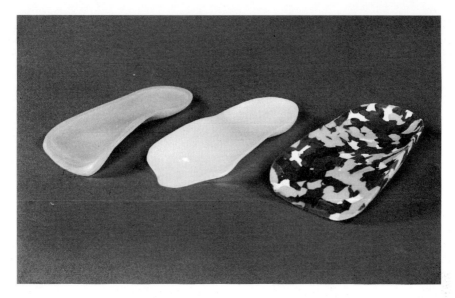

Figure 47.27 Functional foot orthoses.

muscle weakness or imbalance, structural malalignment or loss of structural integrity. Abnormal function can also be a compensatory mechanism for mediolateral or rotational problems at the knee or hip and orthotic management may be the only feasible means of treatment.

The foot, the foot orthosis and the shoe must be considered as a functional unit, and the efficacy of any orthosis or footwear adaptation depends upon the shoe's intimacy of fit. The shoe should:

1. grip the dorsal hind-foot for subtalar control;
2. have effective fastening with mechanical advantage (usually laces);
3. have a firm heel counter for calcaneal control;
4. have a semirigid sole to aid mid-foot control;
5. have a low, broad heel for stability.

Where weakened musculature results in excessive pronation or supination, the simplest way to apply a hind-foot corrective moment following heel strike is by medially or laterally wedging and flaring the shoe heel. However, more accurate control is achieved if wedging (posting) is built into an in-shoe foot orthosis. Extrinsic posting is applied as a wedge of additional material to the main shell of the device. Intrinsic posting involves rectifications of the plaster cast prior to moulding, so that corrective design features are already built into the device (Sanner, 1989). Orthosis materials are rigid (acrylics, carbon fibre, polypropylene) or semi-rigid (polyethylene, EVA foams) (Figure 47.27). Philps (1990) describes the applications and fabrication of functional foot orthoses in readable detail and there has been considerable scientific evaluation of their efficacy (Tollafield and Pratt, 1990). For greater hind-foot control a polypropylene heel cup can be used and can also include extrinsic rear-foot and/or fore-foot posting (Figure 47.28). Digital deformities, such as clawed or hammer toes, may be controlled using three-point pressure digital orthoses, described in detail by Whitney and Whitney (1990). Silicones and urethane foams are most frequently used to control or accommodate toe

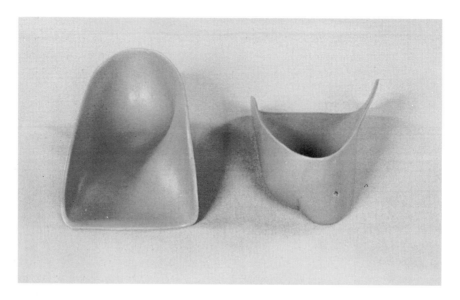

Figure 47.28 Heel cup.

deformities. For metatarsal pain and deformity a wide range of designs and materials are available to provide pressure relief and weight redistribution (Figure 47.29) (Bradley and MacDonald, 1987).

The structural integrity of the foot is commonly lost in rheumatoid arthritis where connective tissues soften, joints dislocate and digital deformity leads to metatarsal overloading. The skin becomes atrophic and

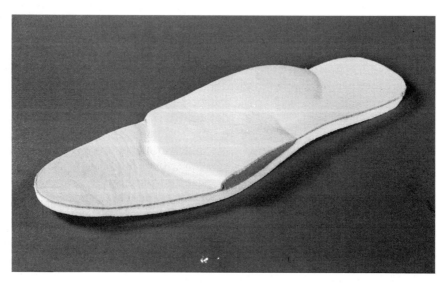

Figure 47.29 Padded shoe insert.

susceptible to ulceration, with pressures up to three times normal levels (Minns and Craxford, 1984). Orthotic treatment aims to reduce pain by controlling joint motion or to compensate for reduced motion. Plantar fascitis, heel spurs, Achilles tendonitis and metatarsalgia will also be treated with a wide range of shock-attenuating materials such as sorbothane, Viscolas, PPT, poron and other polymerics. Pratt (1990b) assesses the long-term effectiveness of some of these materials.

Rigid foot deformities, with localized pressures and gait abnormalities, require orthotic solutions which alleviate the secondary effects. Rigidity may be associated with the neuropathic foot, as in diabetes mellitus, or, more rarely, Hanson's disease. The aim is to reduce pressure and shear stresses in the abnormally high loaded areas of the foot. Suitably shaped inserts and pads need to be soft enough to cushion the foot, but firm enough to achieve load redistribution. For a stiff and painful MTP joint, a rocker sole slows down the forward progression of the centre of pressure of the ground reaction force and relieves the joint prior to toe-off. The value of such footwear adaptations for diabetic or neuropathic feet is well established (Tovey and Moss, 1987).

Footwear

Prescribed footwear comprises the largest part (up to 65%) of the UK orthotic budget and its provision to patients has been scrutinized by several studies (Bainbridge, 1979; Disabled Living Foundation, 1991). Footwear is prescribed for pain, deformity and peripheral neuropathies covering a wide range of clinical conditions. Rheumatoid arthritis and its associated pain and deformity may be particularly acute in the ankle–foot complex. Orthopaedic problems such as gross leg-length discrepancy, fixed talipes equinovarus and structural deformities commonly necessitate special footwear, as do some neuromuscular conditions such as poliomyelitis. Gross

odema and sensory neuropathies with foot involvement will similarly require special footwear and foot care programmes.

The shoe should rightly be considered as an orthosis and its successful prescription requires skilled and detailed assessment. As well as individually manufactured bespoke footwear, a huge variety of 'stock' footwear is now available, many in attractive styles but all with slightly different design features. The footwear normally incorporates an inshoe orthosis as described in the previous section. For temporary or post-operative use, ranges of neoprene, felt or plastazote bootees are available. If made-to-measure footwear is not indicated, there are many choices of semi-bespoke or stock shoes, and even a modular approach has been attempted (Ponton, Chase and Harris, 1987).

Care of the diabetic foot in particular requires the team approach by clinician, chiropodist and orthotist (Edmonds *et al.*, 1986). Foot ulceration due to ischaemia or neuropathy is common and appropriate footwear is an important part of their prevention and treatment. The causes of diabetic foot ulcers are fully reviewed by Edmonds (1986). During the ulcer-healing process ready-made, extra-depth synthetic shoes with plastozote linings and insoles may be used: less active patients may be content with these for permanent use. When the ulcers have healed, more active patients need custom-made shoes fabricated from a plaster cast which is rectified to provide appropriate pressure redistribution. A total-contact innersole supports the plantar surface with a low-density foam backed by high-density material which may be formed as a rocker sole. The shoe should be seamless, lightweight and soft with an intimate fit to prevent shear. An outsole rocker may be preferred to relieve loading of the metatarsal heads (Geary and Klenerman, 1987). Several ranges of stock footwear are offered as suitable for diabetics but some should be treated with caution.

Sound and practical advice is given by Janet Hughs in her books on this subject (Hughs, 1983). Good clinical practice demands a team approach to footcare and footwear supply, with careful monitoring and review by the orthotist and chiropodist and/or podiatrist/physician/physiotherapist. Clear explanations, realistic expectations, and choice for the patient, are the keys to successful patient compliance.

RESEARCH AND DEVELOPMENT

Design and materials

Computer-aided design and manufacture of orthoses is not widespread, though three-dimensional imaging of the foot and subsequent CAD/CAM is commercially available (Lord and Van der Zande, 1992). Some attempts to objectively optimize design have been made for example with AFOs (Leone, 1987) and spinal bracing (Chase, Bader and Houghton, 1989). The use of small, powerful gas pistons may be developed for controlled loading across joints. New composites, thermoplastics and thermoplastic elastomers are gradually being introduced, but further work is required on the optimum loading (Thornett, Langner and Billington, 1985) and strength/weight ratios of orthotic structures.

Clinical measurement

Whilst gait analysis systems are still not routinely used for clinical assessment and review, more user-friendly instrumentation like the video vector generator (Stallard 1987) may prove useful for fine tuning lower limb orthoses. Static and dynamic pressure measurement systems, particularly for the feet (Lord, Reynolds and Hughs, 1986; Hughs, Klenerman and Foulston, 1987), are increasingly being used clinically.

Modern spinal imaging systems can be of use in optimizing TLSO designs (Raschke and Saunders, 1992).

Clinical practice

Functional electrical stimulation (FES) has been in use clinically for many years. The Functional Electronic Peroneal Brace (Murdoch, Condie and Van Griethuysen, 1978), designed to control equinovarus in adult hemiplegia, is the most extensively used system. For paraplegic patients, 'hybrid' electrical-orthotic systems, such as the floor reaction AFO (Andrews *et al.*, 1988) or the hybrid KAFO (Andrews and Bajd, 1984), remain largely experimental.

REFERENCES

Abery, J.M. and Harris, J.D. (1983) The Cherwell splint: an ankle and foot arthosis for rheumatoid arthritis. *British Journal of Rheumatology*, **22**, 183–6.

Alaranta, H. and Huuri, H. (1988) Compliance and subjective relief by corset treatment in chronic low back pain. *Scandinavian Journal of Rehabilitation Medicine*, **20**, 133–6.

Allen, V.R. (1971) Follow-up study of wrist-driven flexor-hinge-splint use. *American Journal of Occupational Therapy*, **25**, 420.

Andrews, B.J. and Bajd, T. (1984) *Hybrid orthoses for paraplegics*. Proceedings of the 8th International Symposium on External Control of Human Extremities, Dubrovnik, Yugoslavia (suppl). ETAN, Belgrade, pp 55–59.

Andrews, B.A., Baxendale, R.H., Barnett, R. *et al.* (1988) Hybrid FES orthosis incorporating closed loop control and sensory feedback. *Journal of Biomedical Engineering* **10**, 189–95.

Bader, D.L. (1993) The potential of advanced composites in orthotic application. *Journal of Orthotics and Prosthetics*, **1**, 33–41.

Bainbridge, S. (1979) *National Health Surgical Footwear – a study of patient satisfaction*, HMSO, London.

Beckman, J. (1987) The Louisiana State University reciprocating gait orthosis. *Physiotherapy*, **73**, 386–92.

Bowker, P., Messenger, N., Ogilvie, C. *et al.* (1992) Energetics of paraplegic walking. *Journal of Biomedical Engineering*, **14**, 344–50.

Bradley, M.A. and MacDonald, W. (1987) The function and properties of metatarsal domes, in *The Biomechanical and Orthotic Management of the Foot*. (eds D.J. Pratt and G.R. Johnson), Orthotics and Disability Research Centre, Derby, pp. 69–78.

Brown, R.N., Byers-Hinkley, K. and Logan, L. (1987) The talus control ankle foot orthosis. *Orthotics and Prosthetics*, **41**, 22–31.

Butler, P.B. and Major, R.E. (1987) The Parawalker – a rational approach to the provision of reciprocal ambulation for paraplegic patients. *Physiotherapy*, **73**, 393–7.

Butler, P.B., Evans, G.A., Rose, G.K. and Patrick, J.H. (1983) A review of selected knee orthoses. *British Journal of Rheumatology*, **22**, 109–20.

Cawley, P.W., France, E.P. and Paulos, L.E. (1991) The current state of functional knee brace research: a review of the literature. *American Journal of Sports Medicine*, **19**, 226–33.

Chase, A.P. (1989) Biomechanical considerations and orthotic prescription for osteoarthritic knees. M.Phd. Thesis Brookes Univ., Oxford.

Chase, A.P., Bader, D.L. and Houghton, G.R. (1989) The biomechanical effectiveness of the Boston brace in the management of adolescent idiopathic scoliosis. *Spine* **14**, 636–42.

Chignon, J.C., Chignon, J.T., Bage, H. *et al.* (1990) A new dynamic walking orthosis: three dimensional evaluation of initial results. *Journal de Readaptation Medicale, Paris*, (1).

Condie, D.N. (1991) Lower limb orthotics. *Current Opinions in Orthopaedics*, **2**, 838–41.

Convery, P. and Hamblen, D.L. (1991) Halo orthoses. *International Journal of Orthopaedics in Trauma*, **1**, 220–6.

Cook, F.F., Tibone, J.E. and Rediern, F.C. (1989) A dynamic analysis of a functional brace for anterior cruciate ligament insufficiency. *American Journal of Sports Medicine*, **17**, 519–24.

Cool, J. (1989) Biomechanics of orthoses for the subluxed shoulder. *Prosthetics and Orthotics International*, **13**, 90–6.

Dillner, S. and Georgiev, G. (1979) Technical and clinical function testing of hand orthoses in Sweden. *International Journal of Rehabilitation Research*, **2**, 47.

Disabled Living Foundation (1991) *Footwear: a quality issue*, Disabled Living Foundation, London.

Edmonds, M.E. (1986) The diabetic foot: pathophysiology and treatment. *Clinical Endocrinology and Metabolism*, **15**, 889–916.

Edmonds, M., Blundell, M.P., Morris, M.E. *et al.* (1986) Improved survival of the diabetic foot: the role of a specialised foot clinic. *Quartely Journal of Medicine*, **60**, 763–771.

Farmer, I.R., Poiner, R., Rose, G.K. *et al.* (1982) The adult ORLAU swivel walker – ambulation for paraplegic and tetraplegic patients. *Paraplegia*, **20**, 248–54.

Fisher, S.V., Bowar, J.F., Award, E.A. and Gullickson, G. (1977) Cervical orthoses effect on cervical spine motion: roentgenographic and goniometric method of study. *Archives of Physical and Medicine and Rehabilitation*, **58**, 452–6.

Ford, C., Grotz, R.C. and Shamp, J.K. (1986) The Neurophysiological Ankle Foot Orthosis. *Clinical Prosthetics and Orthotics*, **10**, 15–23.

Geary, N.P.J. and Klenerman, L. (1987) The rocker sole shoe: a method to reduce peak forefoot pressure in the management of diabetic foot ulceration, *The Biomechanics and Orthotic Management of the Foot*. (eds D.J. Pratt and G.R. Johnson), Orthotics and Disability Research Centre, Derby, pp. 161–73.

Grace, T.G., Skipper, G.J., Newberry, J.C. *et al.* Prophylactic knee braces and injury to the lower extremity. *Journal of Bone and Joint Surgery*, **70A**, 422–7.

Green, D.P. and McCoy, H. (1979) Turnbuckle orthotic correction of elbow-flexion contractures after acute injuries. *Journal of Bone and Joint Surgery*, **61A**, 1092–5.

Halling, A.H., Howard, M.E. and Cawley, P.W. (1993) Rehabilitation of anterior cruciate ligament injuries. *Clinics in Sports Medicine*, **9**, 329–48.

Hanswyck, E.P. and Baker, B.E. (1982) Orthotic management of knee injuries in athletics with the Lennox–Hill orthosis. *Orthotics and Prosthetics*, **36**, 423–7.

Herkowitz, H.N., Kurz, L.T. and Samberg, L.C. (1989) Management of cervical spine injuries. *Spine State of the Art Reviews*, **3**, 231–41.

HMSO (1989) A comparative evaluation of the hip guidance orthosis and the reciprocating gait orthosis, in *Health Equipment Information*, 192, HMSO, London.

Hsu, J.D. (1988) Management of musculoskeletal complications: Spinal deformity and the role of bracing and surgery, in *Physical Medicine and Rehabilitation: State of the Art Reviews*, vol. 2, no. 4, Hanley and Beljus, Philadelphia.

Hughs, J. (1983) *Footwear and Footcare for Adults*, Disabled Living Foundation, London.

Hughs, J., Klenerman, L. and Foulston, J. (1987) The use of a pedobarograph in the assessment of the effectiveness of foot orthoses, in *The Biomechanics and Orthotic Management of the Foot*. Orthotics and Disability Research Centre, Derby, pp. 115–19.

Hullin, M.G. and Robb, J.E. (1991) Biomechanical effects of rockers on walking in a plaster cast. *Journal of Bone and Joint Surgery*, **73B**, 92–5.

Isakov, E., Douglas, R. and Berns, P. (1992) Ambulation using the reciprocating gait orthosis and functional electrical stimulation. *Paraplegia*, **30**, 239–45.

Jawad, A.S.M. and Goodwill, C.J. (1986) TVS brace in patients with rheumatoid arthritis or osteoarthritis of the knee. *British Journal of Rheumatology*, **25**, 416–17.

Johnson, R.M., Owen, J.R., Hart, D.L. *et al.* (1981) Cervical orthoses: a guide to their selection and use. *Clinical Orthopaedics*, **154**, 34–5.

Lehmann, J.F. (1979) Biomechanics of ankle foot orthoses: prescription and design. *Archives of Physical Medicine and Rehabilitation*, **60**, 200–7.

Lehmann, J.F. (1985) Ankle foot orthoses: effect on gait abnormalities in tibial nerve paralysis. *Archives of Physical Medicine and Rehabilitation*, **66**, 212–18.

Lehmann, J.F. and Warren, C.G. (1976) Restraining forces in various designs of knee-ankle orthoses: their placement and effect on the anatomical knee joint. *Archives of Physical Medicine and Rehabilitation*, **57**, 430–7.

Lehmann, J.F., Warren, C.G., Pemberton, D.R. *et al.* Load bearing functions of patellar tendon bearing braces of various designs. *Archives of Physical Medicine and Rehabilitation*, **52**, 366–70.

Lehneis, H.R. (1971) *Upper extremity orthoses*, New York University Institute of Rehabilitation Medicine, New York,

Leone, D.J. (1987) A structural model for molded thermoplastic ankle–foot orthoses. *Journal of Biomechanical Engineering*, **109**, 305–10.

Liggins, A.B. and Bowker, P. (1991) A quantitative assessment of orthoses for stabilisation of the anterior cruciate ligament deficient knee. *Engineering in Medicine (Proceedings of the Institute of Mechanical Engineers*, Part H), **205**, 81–7.

Lindseth, R.E. and Clancy, J. (1974) Polypropylene lower extremity braces for the paraplegic due to myelomeningocela. *Journal of Bone and Joint Surgery*, **56A**, 556–63.

Lord, M., Reynolds, D.P. and Hughs, J.R. (1986) Foot pressure measurements: a review of clinical findings. *Journal of Biomedical Engineering*, **8**, 282–94.

Lord, M. and Van der Zande (1992) *A comparison of two fitting procedures used for Orthopaedic Shoes*. Proceedings of the 7th World Congress, ISPO, pp. 104.

Major, R.E. and Stallard, J. (1985) *Structures and Materials – an introduction based on orthotics*, ORLAU Publishing.

Malick, M.H. (1978) *Manual on Dynamic Hand Splinting with Thermoplastic Materials*, Harmarville Rehabilitation Center, Pittsburgh.

Malick, M.H. (1979) *Manual on Static Hand Splinting – new materials and techniques*, Harmarville Rehabilitation Center, Pittsburgh.

Mazur, J.M., Shurtleff, D., Menelaus, M. *et al.* (1989) Orthopaedic management of high-level spina bifida. *Journal of Bone and Joint Surgery*, **71A**, 56–61.

McDougall, D.J., Carus, D.A. and Jain, A.S. (1985) *A Handbook of Experiences with the Application of Wrist, Hand and Finger Orthoses*, Tayside Rehabilitation Engineering Services, Dundee Limb Fitting Centre, Dundee (Mr A.S. Jain).

McKenzie, M.W. and Buck, G.L. (1978) Combined motor and peripheral sensory insufficiency. Management of spinal cord injury. *Physical Therapy*, **58**, 294–303.

Minns, R.J. and Craxford, A.D. (1984) Pressure under the foot in rheumatoid arthritis: A comparison of static and dynamic methods of assessment. *Clinical Orthopaedics*, **187**, 235–42.

Moberg, E. (1983) The outrigger problem. *Scandinavian Journal of Rehabilitation Medicine. Supplement*, **9**, 136–8.

Moncur, C. and Williams, H.J. (1988) Cervical spine management in patients with rheumatoid arthritis: a review of the literature. *Physical Therapy*, **68**, 509–15.

Motloch, W. (1992) *Principles of Orthotic Management for Child and Adult Paraplegics and Clinical Experience with the Isocentric RGO*. Proceedings of 7th World Congress ISPO, p. 28.

Murdoch, G., Condie, D.N. and Van Griethuysen, C. (1978) A Clinical Evaluation of the Ljubliana Functional Electronic Peroneal Brace. *Final Report to the Chief Scientist Office, Scottish Home and Health Department*.

Nachemson, A.L. (1987) Orthotic treatment for injuries and diseases of the spinal column. *Physical Medicine and Rehabilitation*, **1**, 11–24.

Pellicci, P.M., Ranawat, C.S., Tsairis, P. *et al.* (1981) A prospective study of the progression of rheumatoid arthritis of the cervical spine. *Journal of Bone and Joint Surgery* **63A**, 342–50.

Philps, J.W. (1990) *The Functional Foot Orthosis*, Churchill Livingstone, London.

Pichora, D.R., McMurty, R.Y. and Bell, M.J. (1989) Gamekeeper's thumb a prospective study of functional bracing. *Journal of Hand Surgery (St Louis)*, **14**, 567–73.

Ponton, F.T., Chase, A.P. and Harris, J.D. (1987) Modular orthopaedic footwear, in *The Biomechanics and Orthotic Management of the Foot* (eds D.J. Pratt and G.R. Johnson), Orthotics and Disability Research Centre, Derby, pp. 183–7.

Pratt, D.J. (1990a) A three dimensional electrogoniometric study of selected knee orthoses. *Clinical Biomechanics*, **6**, 67–72.

Pratt, D.J. (1990b) Long term comparison of some shock attenuating insoles. *Prothetics and Orthotics International*, **14**, 59–62.

Pringle, R.G. (1990) Review article: halo versus minerva – which orthosis? *Paraplegia*, **28**, 281–4.

Raschke, S.U. and Saunders, C.J. (1992) *Custom Design of Spinal Orthoses: the CANFIT PLUS (tm) CAD/CAM softwear*. Proceedings of the 7th World Congress ISPO, p. 25.

Rossi, J. (1987) Concepts and current trends in hand splinting. *Occupational Therapy in Health Care*, **4**, (3–4), 53–68.

Sanner, W.H. (1989) The functional foot orthosis prescription, *Mechanical Therapy in Podiatric Surgery*, (ed. R. Jay), Decker, Philadelphia, pp 302–7.

Schuh, C.M. (1988) Orthotic management of the arthritic foot. *Clinics in Prosthetics and Orthotics*, **12**, 51–60.

Scothern, R.P. and Johnson, G.R. (1984) A method for determining the mechanical characteristics of orthotic knee joints. *Prosthetics and Orthotics International*, **8**, 16–20.

Shamp, J.K. (1987) Neurophysiologic orthotic designs in the treatment of central nervous system disorders. *Journal of Prosthetics and Orthotics*, **2**, (10, 14–32.

Stallard, J. (1987) Assessment of the mechanical function of orthoses by force vector visualisation. *Physiotherapy* **73**, 398–402.

Thornett, C.E.E., Langner, M.C. and Billington, G.D. (1985) Portable modular transducer system for the measurement of stabilising forces in TLS-HKA orthoses. *Journal of Biomedical Engineering* **8**, 224–8.

Tollafield, D.R. and Pratt, D.J. (1990) The effects of variable rearposting of orthoses on a normal foot. *Chiropodist* **8**, 154–60.

Tovey, F.I. and Moss, M.J. (1987) Specialist shoes for the diabetic foot , *The Foot in Diabetes* (ed. H.Connor, A.J.M. Boulton and J.D. Ward), Wiley, Chilchester, pp 97–107.

Whitney, K.A. and Whitney, A.K. (1990) Orthodigita techniques, in *Principles and Practice of Podiatric Medicine*. (eds L.A. Levy and V.J. Hetherington), Churchill Livingstone, Edinburgh, pp. 697–708.

Whittle, M.W., Cochrane, G.M., Chase, A.P. *et al.* (1991) A comparative trial of two walking systems for paralysed people. *Paraplegia*, **29**, 97–102.

Willner, S.W. (1990) Test instrument for predicting the effect of rigid braces in cases with low back pain. *Prosthetics and Orthotics International*, **14**, 22–6.

Wojtys, E.M., Loubert, P.V., Sampson, S.Y. *et al.* (1990) Use of a knee brace for control of tibial translation and rotation. *Journal of Bone and Joint Surgery* **72A**, 1323–9.

Wynn Parry, C.B. (1982) *Rehabilitation of the hand*, 4th edn, Butterworths, London.

Yasuda, Y.K., Bowman, K. and Hsu, J.D. (1986) Mobile Arm Supports: criteria for successful use in muscle disease patients. *Archives of Physical, Medicine and Rehabilitation*, **67**, 253–6.

Yates, G. (1976) A modular system of exoskeletal bracing, *The Advance in Orthotics* (ed. G. Murdoch) Edward Arnold, London, pp. 211–17.

48 *Walking aids*

J. Fisher and M. Jackson

INTRODUCTION

Walking aids are used by many people, principally to provide stability in the event of muscular weakness, poor balance, or to reduce the load carried by painful and damaged joints. After trauma to the lower limbs, walking aids allow the patient to become ambulant with no weight or partial weight being taken through the injured limb.

Though the load through the lower limbs is decreased, that through the upper limb is increased. The joints of the upper limbs are not designed for this and, when inflammatory arthritis coexists, may respond with synovitis. When the upper limbs are used to propel the body the muscles of the arm and shoulder have to become stronger.

A variety of walking aids is illustrated and some discussion of their uses and limitations. The type of gait most appropriately used with the aid is suggested.

When a patient uses a walking aid automatic changes will occur in their postural mechanisms. There is a risk that changes will become established and prove resistant to returning to more normal 'non-aided' patterns. There are particular risks with patients with neurological problems, for example a stroke patient given a walking stick at an inappropriately early stage may well develop static and dynamic postures which are dependent upon the stick as part of their base of support. As well as being a great disadvantage itself, this also limits the availability of more normal posture and movement, the facilitation of which is a keystone in much current neurological rehabilitation practice.

Skilled assessment is required to decide if a patient will benefit from an aid, and ensure the patient is provided with appropriate aid for his/her needs. Instruction is necessary for the patient to receive maximum benefit from this aid, and safety has to be considered at all times. So more complex case assessment and training is most appropriately carried out by a physiotherapist.

ASSESSMENT

When selecting the most appropriate walking aid and the type of gait to be used the physiotherapist will consider the following factors: (1) physical, (2) psychosocial and (3) environmental.

Physical

1. What is the specific problem for which the aid is required, and how much does the condition limit weightbearing?
2. The age and general fitness of the patient is important, e.g. axillary crutches are rarely appropriate for elderly or frail patients.

Rehabilitation of the Physically Disabled Adult. Edited by C. John Goodwill, M. Anne Chamberlain and Chris Evans. Published in 1997 by Stanley Thornes (Publishers) Ltd, Cheltenham. ISBN 0-7487-3183-0.

3. The musculoskeletal system of the patient should be assessed, especially weightbearing joints, including upper limbs.
4. Neurological factors should be taken into account, e.g. an elderly patient with a moderately severe injury to a leg who also has poor balance may require a walking frame, whereas walking stick(s) would normally be appropriate. Perceptual or visual problems also affect choice of aid.

Psychosocial

1. Psychological: these include intelligence, anxiety and motivation, e.g. an intelligent well-motivated patient may learn to use elbow crutches where a less motivated patient would require axillary crutches or a frame.
2. Attitude to the aid: a patient's self-image may be adversely affected when using a walking aid, although this can be minimized by the careful choice (and presentation) of aid.
3. Support available, e.g. when a patient has a relative who can give assistance and supervision at home an aid can be provided that is less stable but that with practice will be more appropriate for the patient.
4. Hazard caused by aid, e.g. in some homes for the elderly use of aids may be restricted if the residents are at risk: some may fall over an aid; and others have been known to use their aids as weapons!

Environmental

1. Living accommodation: homes are frequently small and conditions cramped. The arrangement of furniture, distances to be walked, position and other features of stairs, width and position of doorways, access to the house, etc. are all factors which require consideration: a home visit may be necessary.
2. Non-domestic environments: other areas that the patient visits should be considered, including workplace. The geography of outside areas, hills, distance to shops, etc, is important.
3. Transport requirements, e.g. ordinary frames are very difficult to place in most cars, so a folding frame may be more appropriate for a patient who will be travelling in a car. Frames are rarely allowed in buses thus limiting the mobility of their users.

Sometimes the patient will be reluctant to bear weight on a weak or painful limb, and will require encouragement to progress from non-weightbearing, to partial weightbearing, and finally to full weightbearing through the limb. As a general rule, the minimum required support should be provided consistent with safety. Careful instruction in the use of the aid is also important to avoid the problem of overdependence.

EXAMPLES IN SELECTION OF AIDS

Soft tissue injury to the knee (e.g. partial tear medial ligament)

The patient may initially be non-weightbearing with axillary crutches, but when weightbearing is allowed it may well be advisable to exchange the axillary crutches for walking sticks, first two and then one, to encourage the patient to take an increasing amount of his/her weight through the affected leg.

Hemiplegic patient

The patient may benefit from a walking stick, particularly after the early stage of a stroke. However, the assessment for an aid, and its use as part of the rehabilitation process, must be very carefully considered.

The risk of using a walking aid after a stroke is that it may promote postural malalignment, and increased compensatory activity, thus inhibiting the regaining of more normal postural control. A longer than usual walking stick may be the aid of choice.

Rheumatoid arthritis

Here the patient may benefit from using an aid at a relatively early stage. Reduction of weightbearing through a damaged joint may slow the progression of the condition and reduce eventual damage. When selecting the most appropriate aid it is necessary to avoid excessive force being put through involved arm joints. If there is over 40° fixed flexion at the elbow then an elbow crutch cannot be used. A moulded hand grip is advisable with any walking aid (Chapter 14).

VARIOUS TYPES OF GAIT USING WALKING AIDS

Three-point gait

The three-point gait is used when the patient is non-weightbearing through one leg and is using crutches. The crutches are moved forward together while the body weight is borne through the good leg. Weight is then taken through the arms and crutches as the weightbearing leg is brought forward to a point either in front or behind the lines of the crutches to avoid the instability of a linear base. When ascending stairs the good leg goes up the stairs first, followed by the crutches; on descending, the crutches move down on to the lower step first. Patients are advised that this man-oeuvre is not safe without some assistance unless a good stair rail is available, in which case the crutches are used together as one crutch and the patient uses the free hands to grasp the rail.

Four-point gait

This may be used when weight can be borne through both legs. The pattern is – right crutch (or stick), left leg, left crutch, right leg.

Swing-through walking

This system is used when both legs are very weak. The patient balances on both legs whilst the crutches are moved forward together. The weight is then taken through the arms whilst the legs are swung through the crutches. The abdominal muscles may be used to tilt the pelvis to assist weak hip flexors to bring the legs forward, and must be strong.

Swing-to walking

This is an adaptation of swing-through. The legs are brought forwards towards the crutches but not through them. When one stick or elbow crutch is used it is in the hand opposite to the weak or painful leg so that the pattern of walking resembles the normal pattern where the opposite arm and leg move forward together.

Patients are always encouraged to walk with a gait which is as normal as is possible, for them to relieve strain on weightbearing joints and facilitate their full rehabilitation where this is possible.

WALKING AIDS

Axillary crutches (Figure 48.1A)

Measurement is made from the shoe heel to 5 cm below the posterior axillary fold. The position of the hand piece typically is adjusted as for a pair of sticks, i.e. allowing 15° flexion of the elbow when the crutch is held to the side and resting 15 cm out from the front of the shoe toe.

During walking the patient's weight is taken through the shoulders, arms and

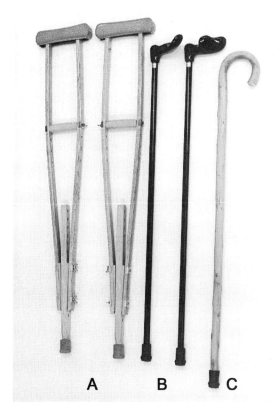

Figure 48.1 A, Axillary crutches; B, Fischer sticks; C, walking stick.

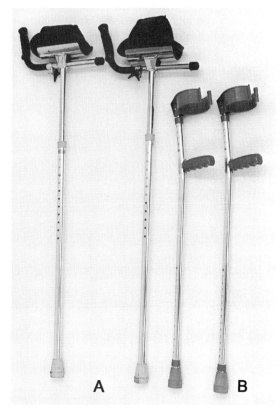

Figure 48.2 A, Forearm support (gutter) crutches; B, elbow crutches.

hands, and transferred to the floor through the lower part of the crutches. Axillary crutches are used when one leg is non-weightbearing with or without a plaster cast, in part weightbearing and in swing-through walking when the arms are weak.

Forearm support (gutter) crutches (Figure 48.2A)

These can be used as an alternative to axillary or elbow crutches, or with one elbow or axillary crutch when there is some abnormality of the patient's arm or arms; for example, the elbow is held in fixed flexion or the arm in a forearm cast. The length of the crutch is adjusted so that the forearm rests in the gutter comfortably without the patient raising the shoulder girdle. The handpiece is adjusted to the patient's grasp. These crutches are heavier and less stable to walk with than axillary and elbow crutches may be fixed on a trolley for patients with severe rheumatoid arthritis. For those with mild arthritis it may be highly desirable to take weight through the forearms rather than the extended elbow and wrist joint.

Elbow crutches (Figure 48.2B)

These can be used as an alternative to axillary crutches but are less stable and need stronger arms if the patient is non-weightbearing. They may be adjusted so that the handpiece is grasped with the elbow at 15° and cannot be used if there is more than some 40° of fixed flexion at the elbow. The length of the upper part of the crutch should be adjustable, and the arm grip should be around the upper third of the forearm.

Walking stick (Figure 48.1C)

These may be wooden, in which case they have to be cut to the length required for each patient, or metal and adjustable. When the patient stands upright and grasps the handle of the stick the elbow would usually be at 15°. However, stroke patients may benefit from a slightly longer stick or crook to aid balance while inhibiting excessive weightbearing through the walking aid.

When two sticks are used, four-point walking is preferable, otherwise the painful or weak leg is placed with the foot between the sticks, and is followed by the good leg. The patient is encouraged to take even paces.

When only one stick is required it is carried in the hand opposite the affected leg. Some weight is transferred through the stick from the hand, and by increasing the size of the patient's base it aids balance and, therefore, confidence. Some patients may not require a walking aid at home but find a stick helpful outside particularly on uneven pavements. Walking sticks are simple and extremely useful, one clear advantage being to alert other people to the fact that the person using the stick requires consideration and space.

Fischer sticks (Figure 48.1B)

Patients with rheumatoid arthritis may find a normal stick difficult or painful to grip. The hook may be padded but if this is still not satisfactory they may find a stick with a moulded handpiece, such as the Fischer stick,

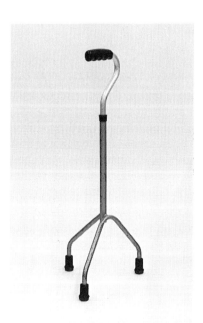

Figure 48.3 Tripod.

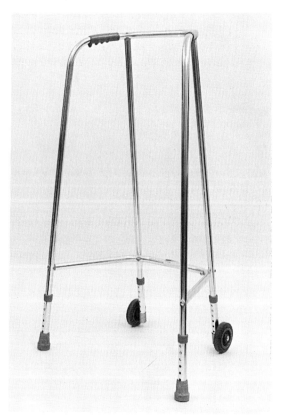

Figure 48.4 Frame with wheels (standard frame does not have wheels).

more comfortable. These provide a larger platform for the transference of weight from the hand to the stick. **Right-hand and left-hand sticks are not interchangeable.** Moulded hand-grips can be used on other walking aids for those with severely deformed hands.

Tripod (Figure 48.3)

The tripod provides more stability than a stick and in the past was used frequently for stroke patients. It is now used only rarely as a last resort following stroke as it encourages overuse of the sound side, so inhibiting more normal postural activity.

Frame (Figure 48.4)

A frame may be used in non-weightbearing walking, for example Pott's fracture, where the patient lifts the frame forwards and then hops into it. It can also be used for partial weightbearing and full weightbearing with

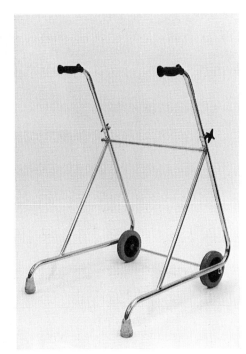

Figure 48.6 Rolator.

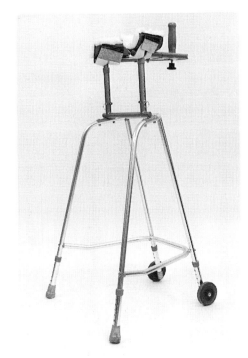

Figure 48.5 Bond frame.

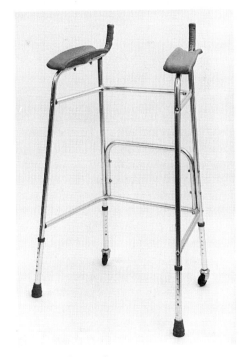

Figure 48.7 Gutter frame.

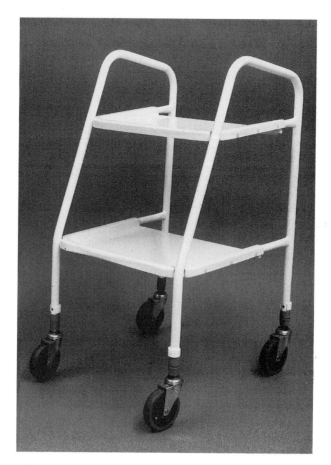

Figure 48.8 Walking trolley.

frail or unsteady elderly patients. It is much more stable than crutches. Crutches may fall on to the floor out of reach when the patient is carrying out functions in the home, and the elderly may have difficulty in recovering them. The frame remains where it is put, and within reach. However, walking with a frame is slow and it cannot be used on stairs or transported unless it will fold. Frames may be set on wheels; they may be reciprocating or they may be triangular (Figures 48.5 and 48.6).

Gutter frame (Figure 48.7)

This gives more support than the ordinary frame because patients take weight through both forearms. It is particularly useful on orthopaedic wards for early ambulation after fractures of the lower limbs, and for patients with rheumatoid arthritis, where it is desirable to protect the joints. It is rarely suitable for use in the home, because of its size and poor manoeuvrability.

Walking trolley (Figure 48.8)

Many types of walking trolleys are available to assist people who have difficulties with their mobility and/or their ability to safely carry objects around the home, they are especially helpful in the kitchen. Forearm supports can be fitted to some types of trolley.

CARE OF AIDS AND GENERAL ADVICE

Patients should be advised to inspect walking aids regularly, looking for signs of wear and tear including splintering of wood and wear of any mechanical parts. Ferrules should be replaced when they become worn (they should always have a metal washer inside to prevent the tip from piercing the ferrule). Bolts on axillary crutches require tightening if they work loose. When using walking aids patients should be advised to avoid slippery and irregular surfaces, for example uneven paving stones and slopes. The floor should be kept clear in the patient's home, loose rugs should be removed, holes in carpets should be repaired. Shoes should be well fitting, have low heels and non-slip soles.

FURTHER READING

Hollis, M. (1981) *Practical Exercise Therapy*, Blackwell Scientific Publications, Oxford.

Walking Aid (1985) booklet in series on *Equipment for the disabled*, Mary Marlborough Centre, Nuffield Orthopaedic Centre, Oxford, OX3 7LD, UK.

49 Environmental controls

R. Potter and E. McClemont

INTRODUCTION

Life is full of routine activities: opening the front door to a caller; locking up safely before going to bed at night; answering the telephone; pulling the curtains when it gets dark so that the people across the street cannot see in. A boring documentary can be switched off if a preferred TV chat show is on another channel, or a track selected on the compact disc player. All this can be accomplished by an able-bodied person in a few minutes without thought or effort.

Consider the same tasks for someone with a severe physical disability. The caller has gone by the time the front door is reached. Lack of grip and fine coordination makes control of a Yale lock impossible. If the telephone handset can be picked up, tremor may make accurate dialling difficult and poor or indistinct speech further handicaps the user. He/she is forced to sit in the dark because no one has turned the lights on or may worry about sitting in full view of passers-by in a brightly lit room with open curtains. The television programme of no interest remains unchanged and someone else must work the music centre. Life is a series of impossible tasks and endless frustrations.

When disability is severe, there is high dependence on others for all activities of daily living – getting up, washing, dressing, toileting and being fed. The telephone always seems to ring when a carer is out. Tradesmen continue to ring at the doorbell because they hear a radio playing. A key left under a doormat or an open front door poses major security worries to carers and the person with disability.

It also challenges the disabled person who wishes to live independently, whether for short periods or permanently. Awareness of the heavy burden of care on others may lead to reluctance to ask for help in changing the television programme or making a telephone call to a friend. Further social isolation and loss of independence is the inevitable result.

Advances in modern medicine have led to an increased number of survivors of severe physical disability. Though there are fewer school leavers disabled with spina bifida, there are more surviving with disability from conditions such as myopathy and cerebral palsy. (Thomas, Bax and Smyth, 1989). Survivors of spinal injuries may have tetraplegia or paraplegia and will come home with severe disability (Kirby, 1989). Those who have had traumatic brain injury may have active brains in a severely disabled body. Better management of urinary tract and pressure sores mean that patients with multiple sclerosis survive with severe neurological problems for much longer than they did 20 years ago (British Society of Rehabilitation Medicine, 1993a).

Outcome measures and rehabilitation

Rehabilitation of the Physically Disabled Adult. Edited by C. John Goodwill, M. Anne Chamberlain and Chris Evans. Published in 1997 by Stanley Thornes (Publishers) Ltd, Cheltenham. ISBN 0-7487-3183-0.

assessment generally focus on major problems such as mobility, washing, dressing and toiletting. There is therefore little documented data on the numbers with these additional daily living problems. They are some of the most disabled people in the community, and are particularly disadvantaged when it comes to expressing their opinions and needs. Neither Barthel, Nottingham ADL or other commonly used assessment scales address these difficulties. About 2% of the adult population in Britain is estimated to have a disability leading to some problems of daily living (OPCS, 1988). However, the survey, for example, does not distinguish between those who can control security of their own home and those who cannot.

ACCESSING TECHNOLOGY

The field of environmental controls is one example of many areas in which modern technology has a tremendous potential to benefit disabled people. The greater the degree of physical impairment, the greater is the need for assistance from technology. However, increased physical impairment also leads to difficulties in operating the controls of whatever assistive equipment is required.

The simple task of switching a light presents difficulty to a severely disabled user. Lack of mobility makes it impossible to get up and walk over to a conventional light switch. A powered wheelchair can allow access to the switch but there may still be insufficient function to reach it, or loss of grip and fine movements may make it impossible to work it. In severe disability only a single movement, possibly as small as an eye blink, may be all that is available to control an extensive range of equipment.

A two-way interaction between the user and the environmental control system is required. A person with visual impairment may be unable to distinguish the display panel unless there is additional sound feed-

back. To make environmental control systems practical they must be capable of being configured for an individual user.

ASSESSMENT OF NEED

General

For the past 30 years, people with severe physical disabilities in the UK have been provided with environmental control equipment, funded centrally by the Department of Health (Department of Health, 1993). Responsibility has recently been devolved to regions. The increased independence which these systems provide allows the user to stay at home, confident in the knowledge that the home is secure and that help can be obtained if required. Consequently, carers are freer to go out and the burden of providing continuous care is much relieved. Effective environmental control systems improve the lives of many severely disabled people, by restoring independence and dignity. They may also improve life for the rest of the family, and reduce dependence on care services and institutional care.

The criteria for eligibility restrict prescription to the most severely impaired in the population, but even so the numbers of users in England and Wales is a fraction of the incidence of severe disability. Take up is also very patchy. It is recognized that many others would benefit from this equipment and, in particular, there has been scant provision amongst disabled teenagers and the elderly.

Referrals

Referrals for assessment of need or eligibility are generally from other professionals in either health or social services, but the process can be initiated by the person with disability. Lack of knowledge both of the benefits of equipment and how the system of provision works or can be accessed, is often a problem (Disabled Living Foundation, 1992). The referral should be made to the nearest environmental control assessor (ECA). The ECA will be a specialist in rehabilitation, neurology or a related discipline, and will have been recognized by the district who should know their name and place for contact. The Department of Health (1993) has published a booklet aimed at all those with an interest or involvement in the provision of equipment for people with a disability. Copies have been sent to health authorities, NHS Trusts, family health service authorities, social services departments and voluntary organizations.

To ensure effective provision of environmental control systems (ECS), it is essential to have knowledge of benefit and use widely disseminated. Members of hospital and community based multidisciplinary rehabilitation teams should receive training in selection, use and provision. Clinicians with responsibility for people with severe disability, including neurologists, rheumatologists, paediatricians, geriatricians and general practitioners, should be aware of the local referral system.

Individual

Assessment of the appropriate system for the individual is a process of careful evaluation of all physical, cognitive, functional and social problems. Selection of a system should reflect the comprehensive coordination of the thoughts and reports of all members of the multidisciplinary team.

The greater choice and flexibility of new equipment means that medical assessors should work closely with a specialist team of clinical engineers, occupational and speech and language therapists, when deciding on the choice of equipment and actuation for the user. In practice such teams are scarce.

Both user and carer choice at the time of assessment can influence the outcome. Poor timing of assessment, lack of familiarity with or hostility to 'modern technology' and the wish to be cared for by a person rather than a machine can all lead to a negative outcome.

A request to perform an environmental control assessment **provides the opportunity to undertake a full assessment of rehabilitation need**, and to explore the possibility of providing integrated mobility aids, communication devices and environmental controls. A holistic approach is therefore required. A wide training in all aspects of rehabilitation medicine, in the management of disabling neurological disorders and specific training in ECS should be mandatory for those who prescribe such specialist equipment (British Society of Rehabilitation Medicine, 1994).

THE ENVIRONMENTAL CONTROL SYSTEM

System design

Environmental control systems usually comprise three distinct components. The **selection unit** operates as the 'nerve centre' of the system, receiving **input from the user** to control the selection of new settings for the various appliances and transmitting appropriate commands to the **controlled appliances** to effect these changes. The selection unit may also receive information from the appliances so as to be able to indicate back to the user which appliances are switched on or the fact that the door bell has been rung, as well as providing feedback on the selection process itself.

Where the user's requirements are limited, alternative approaches, such as the provision of a combined infrared handset for home entertainment equipment, may lead to a more simple and cost-effective solution than provision of a full ECS. Social services departments already have an obligation (under the terms of the Chronically Sick and Disabled Persons Act 1970) to provide individual pieces of equipment to enable disabled people to control aspects of their environment, such as door entryphone, alarm or intercom systems. Local authorities are also responsible for any additional organization and funding of modifications necessary for ECS provision such as door closers or additional power outlets.

Types of switches

The user input commonly takes the form of a simple electrical switch which is mounted appropriately for effective user control. Some of the types of switches in common use are listed in Table 49.1. In choosing a switch it is important to ensure that the user can both actuate and release the switch and that inadvertent operation does not occur during the normal activities of the user. Some users will be capable of reaching out to a lever

Table 49.1 Switches and their applications

Type of switch	Typical application
Lever switch	Operation by hand or foot where there is sufficient fine motor control
Joystick	Combined use for powered mobility and environmental control
Chin bead switch/ headrest switch	In high tetraplegia to harness head movement when seated
Suck/puff	Where head movement is restricted but lip sealing is possible. This method may also be effective when the user is lying down
Pressure pad	An alternative switch method for use in bed
Specialized inputs, e.g. eye movement switch	Devices such as eye-movement switches and sound-operated switches can be used in cases of very severe disability where other inputs cannot be operated

switch on their wheelchair tray as illustrated in Figure 49.1 and no special mounting of the switch will be required. In other cases there may be a tendency for the user to slip away from the switch and lose the ability to operate it. Figure 49.2 illustrates the use of a 'necklace' mounting which ensures that the bead switch remains accessible for operation by the user's chin.

The mounting of the switch should provide easy operation at all times without causing irritation to the user's skin. Care should be taken to ensure that neither the switch nor its mounting present a mechanical hazard to the user, both in normal use or if the user spasms or slips from his or her normal posture. Some systems provide wireless connections between the switch and the selection unit. These avoid the hazards of trailing leads and can also allow the user freedom of movement around the room.

Some environmental control units have the option of using built-in switches or alternatively an array of buttons which may, for the less severely disabled, facilitate more rapid direct selection of functions.

Selection system

The selection unit generally comprises a scanning indicator system in which an array of lights is used to indicate each function in turn, as illustrated in Figure 49.3. The switch is operated at the appropriate time to select the desired function. Some locations on the selection unit may be programmed so that holding the switch down causes a continuous action such as stepping through each channel of the television in turn, the elevation of the bed head or the steady dimming of the room lights. Release of the switch at the appropriate time gives the user precise control of the particular function. The scanning speed can be varied, slow while the person is learning to use it and faster when used to it. The use

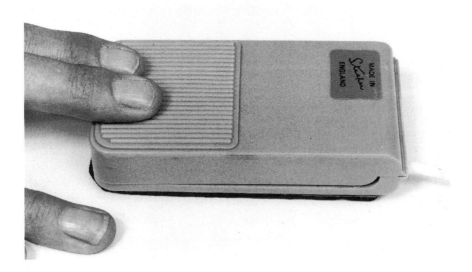

Figure 49.1 Some users will be capable of reaching out to a lever switch on the wheelchair tray. (Reproduced from Department of Health, 1995.)

of an electronic display screen extends the number of possible selections by allowing the user to step through multiple pages on the display. Thus several pages may be allocated to the storage of a personalized telephone directory. The link between the scanning indicator and the equipment is either by infrared (e.g. Possum) or FM radio (e.g. Steeper).

The selection system shown in Figure 49.4 combines the use of illuminated symbol panels with synthetic speech annunciation of the scan position. This can be of great assistance at night and also extends access to environmental control to those with intellectual or visual impairments. Particular difficulties may be experienced **when the user has a requirement to access the system while lying down in bed** or where one switch is required to have several functions, such as wheelchair control and communication aid as well as the environmental control system. In these cases

specialist assessment by an experienced clinical engineer is required.

FEATURES OF ENVIRONMENTAL CONTROL SYSTEMS

Home security

Home security needs vary widely according to the user's home circumstances. In a society where it is generally no longer acceptable to leave a disabled person at home with the front door unlocked, the provision of a door entryphone or security camera together with electronic remote control of the front door lock relieves the requirement on carers to be in continual attendance. For those who use powered wheelchairs, the addition of a door opener/closer provides the means for them to enter and leave the home independently.

Another critical feature of home security is the ability to obtain help quickly in case of

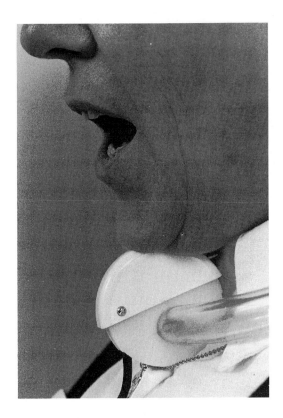

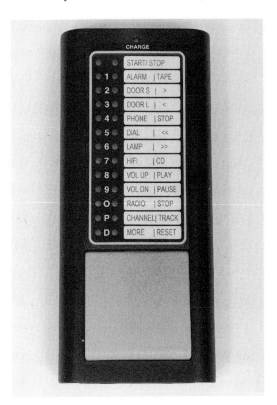

Figure 49.2 The use of a 'necklace' mounting ensures that the bead switch remains accessible for operation by the user's chin. (Reproduced from Department of Health, 1995.)

Figure 49.3 An array of lights is used to indicate each function in turn and the switch is operated at the appropriate time to select the desired function. (Reproduced from Department of Health, 1995.)

difficulty. Table 49.2 shows some of the types of alarm which may be operated via an ECS and the situations in which they are likely to be useful. A particular installation may require one or more of these alarms dependent on local circumstances. For the wheelchair-mobile user **it is important that the alarm works throughout the home and garden** and for this reason FM radio signalling is commonly used.

Communication

Attention to communication needs is another vital requirement in avoiding isolation of the physically disabled individual. The provision of a remote control loudspeaking telephone linked to a directory of prestored numbers puts the person on an equal footing with other telephone users. In a family or group care setting, consideration should be given to the siting of the unit to avoid loss of privacy.

Should there also be a serious impairment of speech the environmental controls will have to act as, or be used with, a synthetic speech communication aid or a speech amplifier if the voice is very soft.

Appliance control

Many appliances in the home can now be operated from an environmental control

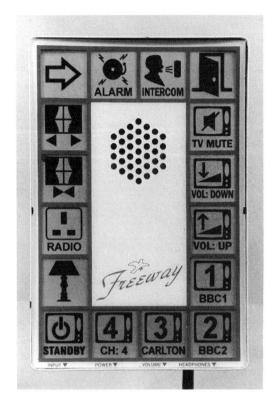

Figure 49.4 A selection system combining illuminated symbol panels with synthetic speech annunciation of the scan position extends access to those with intellectual or visual impairments. (Reproduced from Department of Health, 1995.)

Table 49.2 Calling for help

Type of alarm	Typical application
External sounder/ beacon	Allows carer to enjoy the garden knowing that he/she can be contacted
Internal sounder	Allows ECS use to summon the carer to another room or to the garden
Telephone autodialler	To obtain emergency help via 24-hour manned switchboard.
Nurse/warden call system	To call help in residential or respite care setting.

system. Home entertainment equipment, including televisions, videos, audio tape, CD, satellite and cable systems, have infrared remote control as standard and therefore requires no modification. Replacement wall light switches and curtain openers/closers are now available with infrared control, as are customized loudspeaking telephones. Specialist equipment is still required for mains power switching, motorized bed and chair control and for internal and external intercoms and these items are consequently expensive.

An important feature of the use of appliances is that operation by the environmental control system should be **transparent** and not interfere with other members of the family using the equipment. While this requirement is readily met for standard consumer equipment such as videos, specialist equipment generally requires a separate handset or **family override** to be provided for use by other members of the family.

PROVIDING ENVIRONMENTAL CONTROLS

Choosing a system

An environmental control system is a permanent installation involving the installation of additional wiring, modifications to door locks and often the fixing of equipment by means of wall brackets. It is vital, therefore, that in choosing a system an informed choice is made so that the subsequent installation is reliably operable by the user, provides the required range of functions and does not disrupt the life of other family members or ruin the appearance of a previously well furnished home.

User involvement in this process is vital and is facilitated by the availability of demonstration equipment in a Disabled Living Centre or other suitable location such as a Rehabilitation unit or Younger Disabled Unit (YDU), where it can be used by potential recipients before the prescription is confirmed. A comparison of systems available in the UK, following a thorough programme of technical and user evaluation, has recently been published (Department of Health, 1995).

Newly developed equipment which does not have the relevant test house approvals should be treated with caution. Medical electronics departments in most major hospitals are able to undertake safety testing and give advice on the standards appropriate for particular situations.

Designing and installing the equipment

Initial assessment undertaken by medical and other professionals should be sufficient to allow identification of a type of system appropriate for the user's needs and abilities. However, much detailed work remains to be done to achieve the final design of the system. This work can only be undertaken in the user's home and requires the presence of a technician from the environmental controls contractor with the support of other relevant members of the multidisciplinary team. The final prescription should address the user's needs for security, communication and appliance control throughout the day, identifying appropriate means of user input when seated and also for use in bed.

CONTINUING CARE AND AUDIT OF PROVISION

When independence and security are literally dependent on the flick of a switch, the operational ability of the user can be affected by very minor fluctuations in the level of disability. Intercurrent infection, varying spasticity or a minor relapse in multiple sclerosis may all render the equipment inaccessible. The relentless progress of motor neurone disease can mean that a switch which functioned one day is useless the next.

Users of ECS must, therefore, be supported by a team of professionals sensitive to these changes and aware of how to procure technical assistance. This has traditionally been provided on service contract by the manufacturers of ECS, in direct communication with the user. Now that independence also increasingly depends on control of wheelchair, computer and communication aid, there is a growing need for integrated technical support to sustain these functions. This can best be addressed by ensuring that there are robust interdisciplinary working arrangements within local rehabilitation services (British Society of Rehabilitation Medicine, 1993b). Speech therapists, wheelchair service staff, district nurses, social workers, and most of all ECS users and their carers, need to have access to technical support and advice at all times.

Some environmental control installations are more successful than others. For many users the benefits are undoubted and the system provides a vital lifeline. In a small minority of cases the system does not stay in long-term use and the family request its withdrawal. Systems cost typically between £3000 and £6000, depending on complexity and it is therefore vital to develop a system of audit to ensure that limited funds are utilized so as to maximize the number of successful outcomes.

There are no widely accepted outcome measures in this field and development of these tools requires an elaboration of the philosophy and values of ECS provision. Table 49.3 indicates some service standards which may be appropriate and indicates the way in which audit criteria could be developed from these.

Table 49.3 Developing outcome measures

Service standards	Specimen audit criteria
The user will be secure within his/her home	The user will be able to identify callers and control who is admitted to the home
The user will be able to make use of postal and telecommunications services	The user will be able to obtain a new telephone number from the directory enquiry service
The user will have a comfortable home environment	The user expresses satisfaction with control of posture, heating, lighting and ventilation
The installation of the system will be undertaken so as to minimize intrusion in the home	The principal carer will find the system aesthetically acceptable and will not impede others from using equipment such as telephone, TV, etc.
The system will be available to the user on a continuous basis	The user will be able to operate the system when in bed

UK SERVICE PROVISION AND DEVOLUTION

In common with other centrally provided services, the Department of Health in the UK took the decision to devolve the environmental controls budget, and hence the services in 1993. Prior to devolution in 1995 a specialist working party had already voiced its concerns over certain aspects of the service, including the lack of specialist training for assessors, the lack of awareness and hence uptake amongst both potential clients and professionals, and the need for an integrated 'holistic' approach to equipment (British Society for Rehabilitation Medicine, 1994).

A small budget, thinly spread, has meant inadequate resources to meet individual needs. Uptake of ECS has not been subject to national, or even local, audit in the past, but there is awareness of an uneven distribution of systems throughout the UK, and even within regions, tending perhaps to reflect the activity, awareness and interest of local professionals rather than actual need.

Over the past decade both the Wheelchair Services and the Artificial Limb Services have been subject to major re-organization and been integrated into health services either at regional or district level. There have been undoubted benefits to the users in terms of improved access to services, greater local awareness of need amongst providers and purchasers alike, and demands for both improvements in quality of service and increased resources. Devolution of environmental controls and absorption into local health services must bring similar opportunities, mostly in the form of integrated service provision and improved holistic assessment of individual need. The need for local measures for audit and quality control must also mean improved value for money.

Loss of a national centrally controlled source of funding is always a concern, particularly when the recipient has traditionally been amongst the most disadvantaged and most in need. Increased awareness, effective monitoring and efficient service provision will be essential. Changes in service provision, the impact of 'Care in the Community' and the development of new technology may all influence current services. Access to technology as an everyday tool may no longer be confined to a few, but recognized as a necessity for many who experience everyday living difficulties.

With increased use and acceptance of

technology by many, the question of whether such equipment should be a 'health' or 'social services' provision needs to be considered. Where health and social services work as one board, as in Northern Ireland, a centralized budget and strong interagency collaboration means such questions need not arise. A joint purchasing approach to the needs of any one individual would certainly simplify life for the user who is often very bewildered by 'who provides what?'

With the advent of modular equipment, similar to the many sets of remote controls now found in any home, individuals may wish to purchase their own equipment, as they currently often purchase powered wheelchairs or electric beds outwith health resources. This may leave the user vulnerable in the face of changing disability or subject to commercial pressure at times of need. Access to informed professional advice for those wishing to exercise individual choice should be built into local service developments.

The next few years will probably see major developments continue to encourage such innovation. Technology that can improve the quality of survival must be made available to all who would benefit from it (Platts and Andrews, 1995).

FUTURE TECHNOLOGY

The future prospects for the development of environmental control systems are inextricably bound up with advances in consumer products for home security, communications, entertainment and appliance control. While there has been extensive European Union investment in the development of a home systems specification, manufacturers have not yet adopted a common standard and very few 'Smart House' products are reaching the domestic marketplace. Delays in commercial exploitation of new technology will inevitably have a consequence for the development of environmental control systems.

The new types of environmental control equipment recently introduced into the marketplace have gone a long way towards meeting the obvious deficiencies in traditional prescription equipment, catering for some of the needs of the mobile user and facilitating sharing of equipment in a family setting. However, intercom and telephone facilities are still available only at fixed locations in the home and require special wiring to be installed. Specific developments are therefore needed to bring to physically disabled people the benefits of new wireless telephone technologies.

Although it is now possible to operate environmental control functions from certain communication aids and some environmental controls provide synthetic speech output, further development is needed to achieve effective integration at the wheelchair level, especially for the more severely disabled user.

More sophisticated control systems will be needed to provide effective access to the multitude of services now becoming available from developments such as cable television and interactive CD-ROM. The Internet has an enormous potential for the disabled as well as for the rest of the population and is growing exponentially. There is information about disability and resources on the World Wide Web. The bulletin boards and newsgroups allow international and local communication, and many systems have been developed which may be used by people with disability (Figure 49.5).

Significant developments have also taken place in the field of robotics. The use of such devices as food preparation and feeding aids, to apply make-up, to undertake domestic cleaning etc. will need to be addressed in the near future. Clearly safety of the user is a paramount consideration with such equipment and full evaluation of new systems must be a prerequisite of clinical introduction.

It is by no means certain that future developments in consumer electronics will automatically lead to widespread benefits for

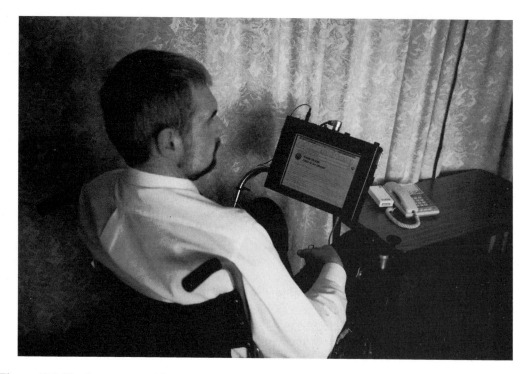

Figure 49.5 The Internet provides communication between disabled and non-disabled users without discrimination.

physically disabled members of society. The commercial pressures to which specialist manufacturers are now subject may encourage development but could prove restrictive unless a sufficiently large market is perceived to guarantee returns on investment. A wider European market for specialist products combined with maximum use of standard consumer products is required if people with physical disabilities are to benefit fully from technological advances.

REFERENCES

Barnes, M.P. (1994) Switching devices and independence of disabled people. *British Medical Journal*, **309**, 1181–2.

British Society of Rehabilitation Medicine (1993a) *Multiple Sclerosis: a working party report of the BRSM*, British Society of Rehabilitation Medicine, London.

British Society of Rehabilitation Medicine (1993b) *Advice to purchasers: setting NHS contracts for rehabilitation medicine*, British Society of Rehabilitation Medicine, London.

British Society of Rehabilitation Medicine (1994) *'Prescription for independence': A Working Party Report of the BSRM Environmental Control Special Interest Group*, British Society of Rehabilitation Medicine, London.

Department of Health (1993) *Environmental Control Systems Funded by the Department of Health*, Department of Health, London.

Department of Health (1995) *Environmental Control Systems: an evaluation. Disability Equipment Assessment*, HMSO, London.

Disabled Living Foundation (1992) *Environmental Controls Systems – investigating provision*, Disabled Living Foundation, London.

Kirby, N. (1989) The individual with high quadriplegia. *Nursing Clinics of North America*, **24**, 179–91.

OPCS (1988) *Surveys of Prevalence of Disability in Great Britain*. Report 1, Office of Population Census and Surveys, London, Table 3.14.

Platts, R.G.S. and Andrews, K. (1994) How technology can help rehabilitation. *British Medical Journal*, **309**, 1182.

Thomas, A., Bax, M. and Smyth, D. (1989) The health and social needs of young adults with physical disabilities, in *Clinics in Developmental Medicine*, no. 106, Mackeith Press, London, pp. 36–46.

VIDEOS

Steeper Fox Environmental Control: Hugh Steeper Ltd, Roehampton Disability Centre, Queen Mary's University Hospital, Roehampton Lane, London SW15 5PL, UK.

Possum 2000: Possum Controls Ltd, 8 Farmborough Close, Aylesbury Vale Industrial Park, Stocklake, Aylesbury, Buckinghamshire HP20 IDQ, UK.

Operating the Director using Liberator and *Operating the Director using Touch/Light Talker.* Liberator Ltd, Whitegates, Swinstead, Lincs NG33 4PA, UK.

Electronic Voices for Emergency Calls: Templar Film and Video Production, Templar Vision, 159 Whiteladies Road, Clifton, Bristol BS8 2RF, UK.

PART NINE

LIVING AT HOME IN THE COMMUNITY

50 Driving independently

C. Murray-Leslie

INTRODUCTION

Independent mobility through driving a car can be of crucial importance in enabling a disabled person to work, maintain social contact and function independently in the community. Quite apart from the more obvious advantages, people often comment that motoring does much to raise their self-esteem and reduce their sense of frustration at being disabled.

The numbers of disabled people wishing to drive are likely to continue to increase, not only because of increasing expectations for greater independence, but also because of the changing age structure of the population. The greater availability of affordable smaller cars with both automatic transmission and power-assisted steering, and expensive technical aids is making motoring possible for many older and disabled people. (Oxley, 1989).

INFORMATION AND ADVICE FOR DISABLED MOTORISTS AND DISABLED CAR PASSENGERS

Disabled people have frequently stated that one of their key needs is for good and easily accessible information, (Living Options, 1985). They are likely to need information and advice on one or more of the following:

1. Whether they will be or are safe to drive.
2. The most suitable type of car or vehicle to purchase.
3. The aids and adaptations needed to enable them to get in and out and use the vehicle controls.
4. Whether they can stow a wheelchair if they use one, and if not how this might be accomplished.
5. How other family members, disabled or not, might be accommodated in the vehicle.
6. Sources of finance and grants.
7. Insurance to drive and information on how to obtain tax exemption.
8. The whereabouts of a driving instructor with an appropriately adapted vehicle and experience of teaching disabled people to drive.
9. Advice on alternative means of transport if driving does not seem feasible.

It is important that disabled people are supported in making decisions for themselves, and they are given balanced independent advice on the choice of cars and equipment available, and are not subjected to undue commercial sales pressure from dealerships with a limited range of products, knowledge and experience. A comprehensive approach to a person's overall mobility needs is desirable so that an individual's lifestyle and the needs of the family and carers, along with any likely future change in or progres-

Rehabilitation of the Physically Disabled Adult. Edited by C. John Goodwill, M. Anne Chamberlain and Chris Evans. Published in 1997 by Stanley Thornes (Publishers) Ltd, Cheltenham. ISBN 0-7487-3183-0.

sion of disability, is taken into account. Any advice should be based on individual preference but also most importantly on the practical assessment of abilities and requirements for technical assistance. This usually means test driving vehicles and trying out controls in a safe environment.

THE FORUM OF UK MOBILITY CENTRES

Within the UK a regional network of mobility centres has been developed and accredited in collaboration with Motability so that each offers a defined range of facilities and services. These include the ability to give disabled people an off-road test in a vehicle with a variety of driving controls, together with an assessment of their equipment needs for vehicle access and wheelchair storage. (See 'Information' section UK Forum of Mobility Centres).

In addition to these regionally based Mobility Centres, a number of other centres, individuals and small organizations, and some driving instructors may offer very good advice to disabled people, although sometimes on a rather limited basis. A number of car adaptations firms offer a variety of specialist services to disabled people. An inventory of organizations offering advice, information and assessment to disabled and elderly motorists was updated in 1993 by the Department of Transport (See 'Information' section). It is axiomatic that occupational therapists, both in hospitals and in the community, should be able to give simple and competent advice regarding driving mobility and be aware of sources of further help and advice for disabled drivers.

Mobility Road-Show

The Department of Transport holds its Mobility Road-Show every 2 years at the Transport Research Laboratory at Crowthorne, Berkshire and has done so since 1983. This event lasts for 3 days and provides an unrivalled display of mobility equipment, both cars and wheelchairs, along with extensive facilities to test drive a variety of vehicles and try specialized controls.

The role of the driving instructor

Driving instructors clearly have a central role to play in helping disabled people to learn to drive and in assisting the assessment process of mobility centres, both for novice drivers and for experienced drivers who have developed disabilities. The National Disability Tuition Register is maintained at Banstead Mobility Centre and lists driving instructors' experience, training and interest in teaching disabled people to drive, together with the vehicles and adaptations they possess.

The Association of Driver Educators of People with Disabilities (ADEDP)

This influential UK organization concerns itself with the education of those who teach and those who assess disabled drivers and with information exchange between each. It is currently implementing an accreditation scheme for both these groups. This is designed to ensure minimum levels of experience and a minimum number of attendances at educational and instructional meetings and seminars. The bulk of the current membership of around 300 is made up of driving instructors and therapists, but doctors, psychologists, engineers and disabled motorists also belong.

Disability Allowance, Financial Grants and Concessions for Disabled Motorists

Financial grants may be critically important to disabled motorists, both drivers and passengers, since they are frequently financially disadvantaged and motoring is an expensive business.

The mobility component of the Disability Living Allowance

This benefit is of great importance to disabled motorists and is described in Chapter 53 on Social Services and Benefits. When awarded at the higher level it entitles the holder to several important concessions including the holding of a driving licence from the age of 16, exemption from vehicle excise licence duty (Road Tax) and if the benefit is awarded for 3 years or more the facility to use one of the Motability schemes (Disability Alliance ERA, 1995)

Motability

Motability is a voluntary organization set up by Government initiative to help disabled people use the mobility component of the Disability Living Allowance towards obtaining a car or wheelchair. Hire purchasing and leasing arrangements are made with Motability Finance Limited. It is interesting to note that in 1993 more than 50% of the 14,000 vehicles in circulation were issued in respect of disabled passengers rather than drivers.

Mobility Equipment Fund

The fund set up by the Central Government is administered by Motability and is now in its third year. Initially running at the rate of £1 million per annum, 1993/4 saw increased funding to £2 million and an increase in the upper limits of grants to £30,000, thereby enabling the mobility needs of the most severely disabled individuals to be met.

Orange Badge Scheme

This scheme offers national parking concessions for disabled and blind people with the exception of certain inner London Boroughs. Important changes have been introduced since 1992 and the old windscreen badge has been replaced by a personalized passport-type document with the holder's photograph affixed. This document is kept by the holder, who may be a non-driver, and has to be displayed on the top of the dashboard when a parking concession is being used. The documents are being renewed every 3 years and are being issued to those who have the higher rate of the mobility component of the Disability Living Allowance, those who are registered blind, those using a vehicle supplied by a Government Department, and those in receipt of the War Pensioners Mobility Supplement or who have a grant towards their vehicle. Additionally those who have a severe disability in their upper limbs and who regularly drive but cannot turn a steering wheel, even with a steering knob, are eligible and others with a permanent disability causing inability or very considerable difficulty in walking may apply.

CAR INSURANCE

The Research Institute for Consumer Affairs (RICA) has demonstrated that there is considerable variation between insurance companies both in the cover provided and the cost of the premiums to disabled motorists. Fortunately in future under the Disabilities Discrimination Act, which was phased in during the second half of 1996, it will become illegal to load a motor insurance premium on the grounds of disablement unless there is actuarial evidence of increased risk.

THE DRIVER: FITNESS TO DRIVE AND THE ISSUE OF LICENCES

The following discussion only applies to the drivers of private cars (Group 1 licence) and not to those requiring vocational licences, i.e. for large good vehicles (LGV) and passenger carry vehicles (PCV) for which more stringent conditions apply (Group 2 licence). It should be noted that some of the advice from the Drivers and Vehicle Licensing Agency

(DVLA) and some of the regulations have changed over the last few years. The regulations and the current advice of the Medical Advisory Group of the DVLA are set out concisely in the publication 'At a Glance'. A more detailed discussion is contained in 'Medical Aspects of Fitness to Drive' (Taylor 1995).

LICENSING AND THE NOTIFICATION OF DISABILITY

The licencing of drivers in the UK depends on their honesty in declaring disabilities and relevant conditions to the DVLA in Swansea. Any individual applying for a licence for the first time (a provisional licence) must declare on the application form whether or not he/ she has any of a number of specified conditions, for example epilepsy, liability to sudden attacks of disabling giddiness or dizziness, mental handicap or inability to meet the visual requirements, or if he/she have any other condition which could make driving a source of danger to others if the individual was to drive. Similarly an existing licence holder also has a duty (stated on the licence itself) to immediately inform the DVLA of any mental or physical disability or condition which at the time affects fitness to drive or might do so in the future (provided the condition is expected to last for more than 3 months). It should be noted that in some conditions a decision to notify the licensing agency does require a certain amount of judgement on the part of the individual and doctors and other professionals may well be asked for their advice. Any person who requires control adaptations in order to drive is advised to notifying the DVLA. It is also important for drivers to notify their insurance company if they have a disability and if they are driving with special controls.

It is well known that many drivers appear to be ignorant of their duty to inform the DVLA of a relevant condition, or choose not to do so (Legh-Smith, Wade and Langton-Hewer, 1986, Eadington and Frier, 1988; Frier, 1992; and Mars, 1993). It is therefore incumbent upon doctors and other professionals to remind people of their duty to inform the DVLA when this is indicated. This situation should be discussed with the spouse or adult children if possible. In the event of an individual refusing to do so despite advice and encouragement, the doctor has to consider his duty towards the safety of the public at large in deciding whether or not to inform the DVLA. However, clearly this should be a last resort. It is important for specialist medical practitioners and other professionals to liaise with the patient's general practitioner in these matters. In difficult cases the doctors from the Medical Advisory Group at the DVLA will give helpful advice over the telephone.

When a person has notified a disabling condition which might affect driving safety he/she may well be asked further questions or enquiries made of the general practitioner. Sometimes a specialist medical examination or opinion is sought or a driving assessment at a Mobility Centre requested. Exceptionally a driver may be required to take another driving test.

Advising the DVLA or the patient themselves over fitness to drive may sometimes be difficult for a doctor unless the situation is clear cut; for example, when a disability bar exists, such as an inability to meet the eye sight requirements. In some circumstances the overall picture has to be taken into account, with an assessment of a person's general competence and mental faculties being made along with any history of problems with driving. There are unfortunately at present no off-road tests which are wholly reliable in predicting driving competence and safety, although clearly a substantial degree of dementia, severe spatial/ perceptual difficulties or visual inattention are incompatible with driving safety. Frequently the best solution is to assess an individual's driving ability and safety in a suitably adapted vehicle. If serious doubt exists about a person's competence or safety, initial assessment is probably best carried out on a private test circuit where there is no other traffic, before proceeding to the public road. In these situations the comprehensive approach of a fully Forum-accredited mobility centre is recommended.

When physical disability alone is present without there being any cognitive, perceptual or behavioural impairment, for example when a person has arthritis or an amputation or a weakness of the limb(s), it is usually possible to find a technical solution to the driving control needs.

Full driving licences are usually issued to both able-bodied and disabled people to the age of 70 and thereafter for periods of 3 years with no upper age limit. In the event of an individual having a prospective disability, i.e. a disability which may be intermittent or progressive so that in time it may cause a driver to be a source of danger to others, a short duration licence of 1, 2 or 3 years may be issued with renewal subject to satisfactory review. If an individual requires to drive an adapted vehicle or use special controls, the licence is endorsed to indicate that person may drive a vehicle suitably adapted for their disability.

Regulations for eye sight

The minimum standard for visual acuity with or without spectacles is the ability to read a car number plate 3.5 inches (79.4 mm) high at 25 yards (20.5 m). The minimum visual field allowed is an arc of 120° horizontal to the eye, with the same arc 20° into the superior and 20° into the inferior visual field. Monocular vision is allowable provided that, as it usually the case, the field is greater than 120°. Visual inattention is a bar to driving. Double vision is also allowable, provided this is corrected by appropriate spectacles or an eye patch when the person drives. It is permissible for a person

to drive with defective colour vision. (Chapter 20).

Epilepsy regulations

Epilepsy is a prescribed condition for driving; however, since 1970 a series of concessions have been granted that allow people with epilepsy to hold driving licences. The most recent concession came into force in August 1994 and this allows a person with epilepsy to drive provided that no seizure (of any kind) has occurred whilst awake during the preceding 12 months. (This applies to a single fit and post-traumatic epilepsy as well.) The regulations regarding seizures occurring during sleep have not been altered and the seizures must have occurred exclusively during sleep for at least 3 years for a person to be able to drive. In the event of a seizure occurring whilst awake the 12 month regulation would then apply. It goes without saying that any diagnosis of epilepsy should be made as accurately as possible and certainly when there is doubt the patient should have the benefit of an expert neurological consultation. (Chapter 24).

EQUIPMENT FOR DISABLED DRIVERS AND PASSENGERS

The choice of a car

When a car is chosen consideration needs to be given as to how the driver and their passengers, who may also be disabled, will get in and out. Thought also needs to be given on how a wheelchair, if used, will be stowed and even whether the driver or a passenger needs to travel in a wheelchair. Vehicles with one door on each side will have the widest door aperture and easiest access for both the individual and the wheelchair, even though the door may not open quite so wide as on some four-door models. Getting into a car can be further helped by extending the seat runners to allow greater retraction of the

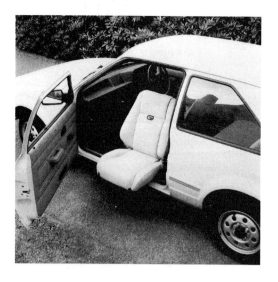

Figure 50.1 A car with one door on each side and fitted with a 90° swivel seat. (Reproduced by kind permission of ELAP Engineering Ltd.)

seat and sometimes by fitting one of the several types of swivel seats (Figure 50.1). An estate car enables a wheelchair to be stowed much more easily, particularly if it is a heavier electrically powered one or one with a non-folding frame (TRRL Research Report No. 2, 1985; Murray-Leslie, 1990; Haslegrave, 1991).

Automatic transmission

An automatic gearbox is necessary for a substantial proportion of more severely disabled people to drive. It is probably true that the majority of disabled people would be wise to choose a vehicle with automatic transmission, even if this was only to anticipate further deterioration in a progressive disorder, such as multiple sclerosis.

Power-assisted steering

This may be desirable or essential for people with upper limb weakness, but also a great help to others with painful joints in the arm or spine. If a person is required to steer one

handed, as in hemiplegia, it is advisable to have power-assisted steering. Power-assisted steering and automatic transmission in addition to electrically operated car windows and heated rear windscreens are now standard features on many smaller cars. Power-assisted steering is particularly helpful to people when reversing and manoeuvring at low speed. It is also possible for power-assisted steering to be customized and the steering resistance reduced to extremely low levels, but this may be expensive.

Specialized vehicles

Drivers who need to enter vehicles and drive from their wheelchairs (usually electric) require a van conversion with an appropriate remote control system to operate the vehicle doors and a platform hoist. At the time of writing there are only three vehicle conversions available to allow a wheelchair driver to be fully independent in most electric chairs (Ford Transit, Chrysler Voyager and Mercedes Sprinter). **Passengers** who wish to travel in their wheelchairs have a wider range of vehicle from which to choose, which allow wheelchair access from the side or rear, along with good all-round visibility when the passenger is inside.

Seat belts

Some people may have difficulty and discomfort in using conventional seat belts, however there are a number of ways of overcoming these difficulties without interfering with the effectiveness of the restraint. A clip-on extension handle may help those with impaired upper limb function reach the stowed belt (Figure 50.2). 'Even in countries like the United Kingdom where permanent exemption from wearing a seat belt may be granted there is very seldom any justification for this' (TRRL Contractors Report 158, 1990; Taylor, 1995)

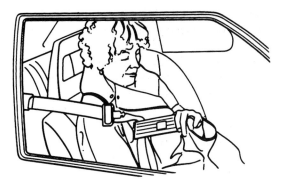

Figure 50.2 A clip-on extension handle to assist reaching for a stowed inertia reel seat belt. (Reproduced by kind permission of the Department of Transport.)

It should be noted that the wearing of seat belts increases the frequency with which neck strains occurs in motor accidents (Porter, 1989). The use of a head restraint is recommended for all drivers, especially for those with arthritis in the neck or any cervical instability or inability to control the neck through muscle weakness (Kahane, 1982). There may sometimes be a considerable gap between a head restraint and the back of the head of a person who has a kyphosis, such as sometimes occurs in ankylosing spondylitis. In this situation it would be important for the head restraint to be adjustable. It also follows that those travelling in wheelchairs should have an adequate headrest. Collars if substantial may give a little added protection to patients with rheumatoid neck instability.

Seat cushions

Disabled drivers may wish to sit on a cushion for comfort, for pressure relief or because their car seat is too low for them. It is recommended that if a cushion is used it should, wherever possible, be firm and positively anchored in place. If a soft cushion has to be used this should be enclosed in a firm cover

which should be anchored to the car seat. (TRRL Leaflet LF1020, 1986).

Modifications to car foot pedals

Foot pedals can be extended or widened to suit different disabilities. A common conversion to an automatic vehicle is the provision of a left accelerator for a patient with a right hemiplegia (Figure 50.3). This device can be folded down to allow an able-bodied person to drive with the right foot in the usual way. Where individuals drive with their arms only and have a tendency to spasms or involuntary movement of their legs, it may be advisable to fit pedal guards over the foot pedals.

Steering aids

If the driver only has one arm available for steering, as for example in hemiplegia or paraplegia, a rotating steering knob (spinner) is mounted on the steering-wheel rim (Figure 50.4). A variety of shapes and configurations to enable effective gripping are available (Bulstrode, Harrison and Clarke, 1987). An attachment for an upper limb prosthesis to a steering knob is also available. It is most important to make sure that any aid fitted to the steering wheel does not get in the way of the airbag systems, which are now fitted to many newer cars. RICA has looked at the effects of car adaptations on secondary safety or the car's ability to protect its occupants from injury and crash (Turner-Stokes *et al.*, 1996).

Hand-operated brakes and accelerators systems

Disabled people unable to use their legs for driving, as for example those with paraplegia, tetraplegia or bilateral amputation, will need to use a one-hand operated brake and accelerator system. There are a number of different types of systems available and a

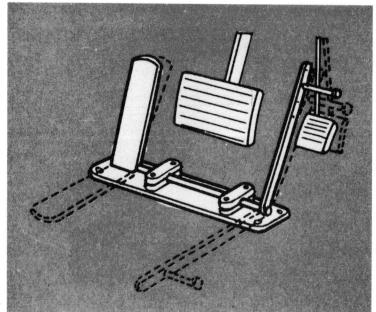

A

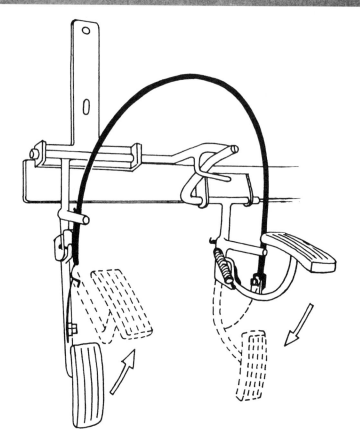

B

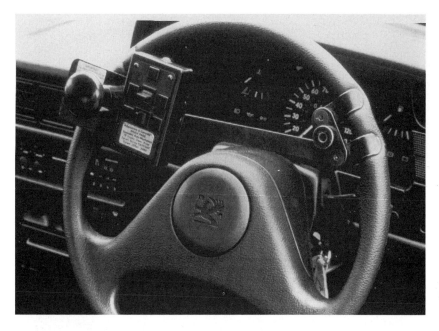

Figure 50.4 A steering knob (spinner) combined with an infra-red switching unit (transmitter unit) for car secondary control operation.

commonly used one employs a push and pull mechanism, which operates a lever system linked into the conventional foot pedals (Figure 50.5). Such systems may leave little room for the knees of taller people and then may present an additional hazard in a frontal impact accident. Indicator switches and horn controls are often mounted on this system as a simpler alternative to using an infrared switching control system.

Parking brake/gear shift adaptations

Easy release devices are available to facilitate the release of the inhibitor buttons on parking brakes and also on the gear shift lever of an automatic gear box. These controls are cheap and simple and frequently very helpful to people with arthritis in their hands.

Vehicle secondary controls

The operation of conventional control systems for the car indicators, horn, lights, etc., may present difficulties to disabled people. Several adaptations are available, including infrared switching systems incorporated into steering ball mechanism (Figure 50.4).

Car telephones

Although expensive, a car telephone can be a great reassurance to a disabled driver as it can be used to alert people to the expected time of

Figure 50.3 A,B A left accelerator conversion for use in an automatic vehicle, note the device can easily be folded back to enable an able-bodied driver to drive with the right foot. (Reproduced by kind permission of Alfred Bekkers Controls.)

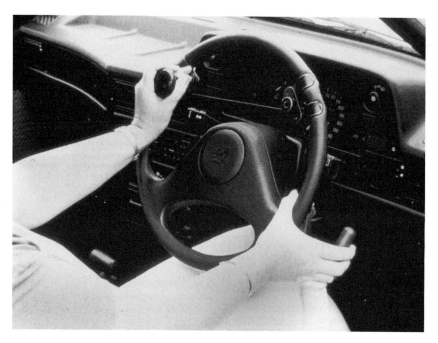

Figure 50.5 Driving with the hands only (right-handed operation of brake and accelerator and left-handed steering).

arrival and also can be used in the case of a breakdown or emergency.

Transfer aids

Different methods of getting in and out of the car are well described in the Department of Transport's guide 'The Ins and Outs of Car Choice'. Simple aids familiar to therapists include transfer boards, either straight or boomerang shaped, and also a swivel disc to assist standing transfers. People often devise their own solution to problems and the legs may be transferred in over the vehicle's sill by means of a simple loop of cord or a carrier bag. A smooth car seat with relatively low friction will aid transfers and occasionally people sit on plastic bags to enable them to swivel round on a car seat. However sitting on a plastic bag could potentially lead to a seat belt injury in the event of a rapid deceleration. Seats which swivel out through the car door are helpful to some (Figure 50.1).

Equipment to stow wheelchairs

Whilst some disabled people are able to stow their own wheelchairs, especially if these are of a light, high-performance type, which are easy to dismantle, this will not be possible for many who will require the assistance of another person or a mechanical aid (TRRL Research Report no. 2, 1985). A variety of electrically powered hoists exist for the transfer of a folded wheelchair into the car's interior, boot or roof. The stowage of electrically powered wheelchairs can pose considerable problems because of their weight and their inability to fold unless the batteries are removed. Advice on the stowage of such chairs can be obtained from a mobility centre.

Technically advanced aids

The great majority of aids and adaptations required by disabled people are relatively

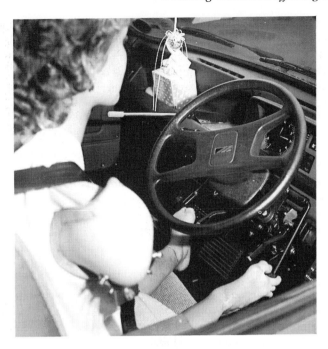

Figure 50.6 Steering from the right shoulder (using joystick mechanism), and operating the brake/accelerator with the right foot and the secondary controls with the left foot in a person with a limb deficiency syndrome. (Reproduced by kind permission of Steering Developments.)

simple in design and inexpensive, costing in the order of a few hundred pounds, with many under £100. However a small proportion of disabled people are so severely disabled from severe limb weakness due to conditions such as muscular dystrophy, polyneuropathy, or from arthrogryphosis or limb deficiency syndromes that they may require very specialized and expensive control systems which are tailormade for them. (Figure 50.6). Examples are the combined joystick control for steering and operating the brake and accelerator, and a mechanism to allow steering with the feet. The same individuals frequently need to drive from a wheelchair and will often require a van conversion for full independence in mobility. Whilst some may be able to fund such equipment from personal accident compensation, state funding which is means tested has become available over the last few years (see 'Mobility Equipment Fund' on page 711).

DISABLING CONDITIONS AFFECTING DRIVING ABILITY

The following discussion is not intended to be fully comprehensive and the conditions covered have been chosen either because of the frequency with which they occur or the frequency with which people suffering from them present for advice on driving or because of the degree of difficulty they present in relation to the assessment of driving safety.

Old age/dementia

In western countries the proportion of drivers who are elderly is increasing rapidly. In 1990 in the UK there were 3 million licence holders over 60 years of age and 680 000 were over 70 years of age. Driving skills in both sexes diminish with increasing age beyond the sixth decade, after which there is a considerably increased frequency of fatal and non-fatal accidents (Simms, 1991; O'Neill *et al.*, 1992; Brouver and Ponds, 1994).

All aspects of vision deteriorate with ageing (visual acuity, visual fields and night vision) and these may be compounded by perceptual failures leading to errors at junctions and when pulling out. Additionally there is a general reduction in overall cognitive capacity leading especially to difficulty in performing time-pressured tasks such as lane merging, difficulty in dividing the attention between two tasks and also forgetting to check mirrors and to make signals. Elderly people drive less miles and may avoid driving at night or in busy or inclement conditions. Some may decide to give up, but others are very reluctant to do so even in the face of advice. Dementia poses a particular problem, both because it is common in the elderly, but also because of the **impairment of insight which occurs and the difficulty of making an early diagnosis**. Many early cases are unknown to their general practitioners. The 3 year licence review of drivers over 70 years provides an opportunity for a person's driving ability to be checked and for enquiry to be made, but even in the face of the anxiety of relatives some drivers with dementia may well not admit to any difficulty. There is currently no official system for checking elderly peoples' actual driving ability, unlike the safety of elderly vehicles! (O'Neill *et al.*, 1992; Freidland, Koss and Kumar, 1988).

Stroke

Hemiplegic stroke is the commonest condition seen at most mobility centres and at the Derby centre it makes up 25% of its referrals. Hemiplegia of itself seldom prevents a person from driving unless there is also hemianopia, visual inattention or other perceptual or cognitive problems. It is important to note that in the context of driving not all spatial problems following stroke can be picked up on 'pencil and paper tests' and that some form of practical driving assessment is advisable, especially if the patient has had **a right hemisphere stroke**. The stroke driver screening assessment developed by Nouri and Lincoln (1993) only accurately predicted road performance in 81% of patients. Aphasia per se does not seem to impair driving ability unless accompanied by cognitive deficits. The DVLA currently recommends that driving is delayed for at least 1 month after a stroke.

Drivers with hemiplegia usually require automatic transmission using the unaffected hand to steer by means of a knob (spinner) fitted to the steering wheel rim. In the case of left hemiplegia the accelerator and brake are operated in the usual manner with the right foot; with right hemiplegia the left foot has to be used and a left accelerator conversion is required. A leaflet on driving after stroke has been published by the Stroke Association (Chapter 32).

Head injury

Traumatic brain damage may be both focal and diffuse and a wide array of possible deficits occur which might affect driving competence. (MacFlynn *et al.*, 1984; Van Zomeren, Brouver and Minderhoud, 1987; Simms, O'Toole and Clayton, 1992). In addition to the more obvious motor impairment of limb paresis, spasticity, dystonia, incoordination and tremor, there may be disorders of hearing, vision, balance, arousal, psychomotor slowing, cognitive deficits and disorders of mood and behaviour. Whilst high-level cognitive difficulties may not pose a problem for driving, poor concentration, distractibility and marked psychomotor slowing and visual/perceptual difficulties certainly will. Additionally a history of recent behavioural aberration especially poor control of anger and aggression or apathy and lack of concern will have to be taken into account. Assessment is difficult and it should be remembered that functionally significant improvement may continue for a number of years. The DVLA guidance on the return to driving after head injury is set out in the publication *At a glance*. A good history, particularly with input from relatives and professional attendants, together with expert psychometric testing, may be very helpful. Following a careful 'in car assessment', a period of accompanied driving without problems or incidents is very reassuring. Moreover, the issue of a short duration licence offers the opportunity for a early formal review of driving safety. Further information for people with head injury is contained in the Headway publication 'Driving after Head Injury' (Chapter 29).

Multiple sclerosis

It is evident that many people with multiple sclerosis with slow progression may drive safely either with or without adaptations for many years. Driving may however become very difficult or impossible if there are frequent relapses and rapid progression and when there is major impairment of function in three or four limbs, either in terms of weakness, spasticity, sensory loss, incoordination or tremor. Visual acuity may be inadequate for driving and sometimes there are cognitive impairments in combination with physical difficulties which may make driving inadvisable. People with multiple sclerosis may find that their spasticity and clonus is worse when they are cold or fatigued and their visual acuity seems also to be affected by fatigue.

It is important that people do not drive during relapses and that there is some forward planning so that people do not struggle on driving with their feet when hand controls would make driving both easier and safer. Patients with tremor may sometimes be helped with a tiller type of steering control (Figure 50.7). It is recom-

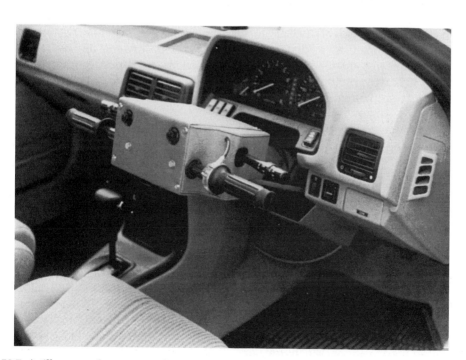

Figure 50.7 A tiller control system, with twist grip throttle. (Reproduced by kind permission of Jim Doran Hand Controls Ltd.)

mended that people with multiple sclerosis have at least one assessment at a mobility centre with the chance of a further review if they wish, as it is important that all aspects of mobility are talked through with them and their family and sensible proactive plans are made (British Society of Rehabilitation Report on Multiple Sclerosis, 1993). The DVLA will issue an "until 70" years old driving licence if medical assessment (preferably practically based) is satisfactory, but a shorter duration licence if disease progression is rapid (Chapter 26).

Parkinson's disease/Parkinsonism

Many people with Parkinson's disease drive perfectly safely provided there is reasonable disease control and no dementia. There seems to be no evidence that the Parkinson's disease is an important cause of accidents and Police notifications to the DVLA are rare (Editorial, 1990). It has even been asserted that patients with Parkinson's disease may have fewer rather than more road accidents (Ritter and Steinberg, 1979) and there is evidence that people with Parkinson's disease adopt sensible strategies by driving within their medication period, avoiding night driving and certain road and weather conditions (Hoyle, 1990). The licensing agency will issue an until 70 years old driving licence if a satisfactory medical report is received, or a limited duration licence if disease progression appears rapid (Chapter 33).

Cerebral palsy

The expectations for driving of this the largest group of physically disabled young adults are now high and many have learnt to drive successfully. Usually young people with hemiplegic, diplegic and milder quadriplegic forms can be helped relatively easily with conventional car modifications. When three or more limbs are affected and choreoathetosis is severe, finding a suitable control system can be a considerable technical challenge. Movement disorders and tremors in cerebral palsy, as in some acquired neurological conditions, can sometimes be overcome by using a tiller type control (Figure 50.7). The presence of learning difficulties may make learning to drive impossible or a protracted and expensive business. It is therefore important that such people are expertly assessed in the first place and are given sensible and balanced advice before being put in the hands of a driving instructor who has the necessary patience and experience in teaching slow learners (Chapter 23).

Spina bifida and hydrocephalus

Spina bifida, which is frequently associated with hydrocephalus is now much less common due to prenatal screening. The varying degrees of flaccid weakness from the spinal lesion may be complicated by a degree of spastic weakness of one or more limbs due to hydrocephalus. Many young people in this category have substantial difficulties in learning to drive due to cognitive deficits, most noticebly visual perceptual difficulties, but also poor memory, attention and judgement (Simms 1989)

Arthritis

Car driving is possible for most people with arthritis. The difficulty that people experience is due to various combinations of pain, joint and muscle dysfunction and deformity, (Cornwell, 1987; Jones, McCann and Lassere, 1991; Murray-Leslie, 1991). Patients may choose not to drive during periods of exacerbation of their arthritis or following joint surgery (Murray-Leslie, Brain and Stephan, 1994, unpublished). The wisdom of this approach is supported by the literature (Macdonald and Owen, 1988; Spalding *et al*, 1994). It is also apparent that people with arthritis often do not get adequate help and advice on driving and that much of this help is of a simple nature which could easily be provided in a local occupational therapy department, (Jones, McCann and Lassere, 1991; Murray-Leslie, Brain and Stephan, 1996, unpublished).

It is important that patients choose a suitable car with good access and many would benefit from power-assisted steering or automatic transmission, even if this is not essential. Advice is necessary on measures to protect the neck, ways of getting in and out more easily, the use of mirrors, easier techniques for steering, adapted ignition keys and easy release mechanisms for the parking brake and gear shift levers and aids for grasping seating belts. Young drivers who are of short stature due to chronic arthritis may need foot pedal extensions and vertically adjustable car seats. Additionally adjustable steering columns (height and rake) can be fitted to some car models.

If neck rotation is restricted, particularly in ankylosing spondylitis, adequate rear-view mirrors are especially important. Negotiating junctions, especially if the roads meet at less than 90°, can be assisted by convex interior and wing mirrors supplemented sometimes by extra adjustable mirrors. Difficulty with seat belts can almost always be overcome (Figure 50.2) The Arthritis and Rheumatism Council have published a booklet on car driving and the Forum of UK Mobility Centres is currently producing a more comprehensive booklet (Chapters 13 and 14).

Spinal cord injury

People with paraplegia with the use of their arms usually have no problem driving with hand controls. Those with tetraplegia and paralysed hands can generally hook their hands around a modified steering control (usually a three-pegged version of the steering spinner) and use a hand-operated braking/accelerator control system, provided there is shoulder and some elbow movement. For complete independence in driving many patients with tetraplegia and a few with high paraplegia will require to drive from a wheelchair in a van conversion (Chapter 28).

Limb amputation

Loss of one or two limbs can be relatively easily compensated for by the use of technical aids. Loss of the clutch foot may be compensated for by the use of an automatic gear box, or if preferred a hand-operated clutch or electrical clutch. The loss of the right leg necessitates an automatic vehicle and a left accelerator conversion. In the case of bilateral above-knee amputation the car will have to be driven with hand controls. Some people with below-knee amputations drive using foot pedals and sometimes use manual gear box vehicles, but the conventional advice is to use hand controls if the amputation is above ankle level because of the attendant loss of proprioceptive function. The Forum of UK Mobility Centres has produced booklets for both amputees and their professional advisers. (Chapter 15).

Planning journeys and summoning assistance

Route planning is important for disabled people, who may wish to take frequent breaks or who may require assistance at petrol filling stations and level access with adapted WC facilities. There are a number of books which help in this respect (*AA Guide for the Disabled Traveller/Motoring for Disabled People*) and "Tripscope" provides a telephone advice service.

Obtaining help at petrol filling stations can be a particular problem and both Shell and Esso provide help at some of their filling stations. This can be summoned using a hand-held infra red 'service call' device, obtainable from Autochair Limited. Filling stations displaying the official disabled persons logo, provide assistance, which meets the standards of the Disabled Persons Transport committee. Many disabled motorists take a mobile (cordless) phone with them in their car in order to use in the event of an emergency or breakdown.

Alternatives to driving a car

Sometimes it is necessary to advise a person not to drive as when assessment has shown it is unsafe to do so or when very expensive adaptations will be required for a person with a rapidly deteriorating neurological condition. Sometimes the situation is eased by a relative being able to drive, but it is useful to remember that if a person drives less than 4000 miles a year, which many elderly or disabled people do, it is cheaper to travel by taxi rather than to attempt to run a car. 'Metro' Black Cabs are designed to take a wheelchair passenger, but also have features to help other ambulant disabled people such as a fold-down step and swivel seat, and convenient grab handles. Some people who are elderly or who have severe arthritis seem to prefer the saloon car type of taxi.

Banstead Mobility Centre runs a scheme for the short-term loaning of rear-entry passenger vehicles for people with motor neurone disease who are deteriorating rapidly and who need to travel in their wheelchairs.

Outdoor electric wheelchairs may be used on the pavement provided the maximum speed does not exceed 4 mph. Class 3 vehicles (which includes some four-wheel and three-wheel electric chairs) have a top speed of 8 mph and may be used on the road as an alternative to driving a car, but users are strongly advised to take out an adequate insurance policy. (Department of Transport publication on the code of practice for 8 mph vehicles is in the 'Information' section.)

REFERENCES

British Society of Rehabilitation Medicine Report Multiple Sclerosis (1993) Royal College of Physicians, London.

Brouver, W.H. and Ponds, R.W.H.M. (1994) Driving competence in older persons. *Disability and Rehabilitation*, **16**, 149–61.

Bulstrode, S.J., Harrison, R.A. and Clarke, A.K. (1987) *An Assessment of Car Steering Wheel Knobs*. DHSS Disability Equipment Assessment Programme.

Cornwell, M. (1987) The assessment of people with arthritis who wish to drive a car. *International Disability Studies*, **9**, 194–7.

Disability Alliance ERA (1995) *Disability Rights Handbook*, Disability Alliance, London.

Eadington, D.W. and Frier, B.M. (1988) Type I diabetes and driving experience: An eight year Cohort study. *Diabetic Medicine*, **6**, 137–41.

Federal Motor Vehicle Safety Administration, Federal Motor Vehicle Safety Standard 202 (DOTHS 806–108), Washington DC.

Friedland, R.P. Koss, E. and Kumar, A. (1988) Motor vehicle crashes in dementia of Alzheimer type. *Annals of Neurology*, **24**, 782–6.

Frier, B.M. (1992) Driving and diabetes. *British Medical Journal* **305**, 1238–39.

Haslegrave, C.M. (1991) Driving for handicapped people. *International Disability Studies*, **13**, 111–20.

Hoyle, E. (1990) *Driving and Parkinson's disease*. Proceedings of ADEPD Summer Conference, 1990.

Jones, J.G., McCann, J. and Lassere, M.N. (1991) Driving and arthritis. *British Journal of Rheumatology*, **30**, 361–4.

Kahane, C.J. (1982) *An evaluation of head restraints*. United States Department of Transportation, National Highway and Traffic Safety Administration.

Editorial (1990) Driving and Parkinson's disease. *Lancet*, **336**, 781.

Legh-Smith, J., Wade, D.T. and Langton-Hewer, R. (1986) Driving after stroke. *Journal of the Royal Society of Medicine*, **79**, 200–3.

Living Options (1985) Prince of Wales Advisory Group on Disability 1985, London.

Macdonald, W. and Owen, J.W. (1988) The effect of total hip replacement on driving reactions. *Journal of Bone and Joint Surgery*, **70B**, 202–5.

MacFlynn, G., Montgomery, E.A., Fenton, G.W. and Rutherford, W. (1984) Measurement of reaction time following minor head injury. *Journal of Neurology, Neurosurgery and Psychiatry*, **47**, 1326–31.

Mars, J.S. (1993) Drivers who defy the law. *British Medical Journal*, **307**, 844–45.

Murray-Leslie, C.F. (1990) Aids for disabled drivers. *British Medical Journal*, **301**, 1206–9.

Murray-Leslie, C.F. (1991) Driving for the person disabled by arthritis. *British Journal of Rheumatology*, **30**, 54–5.

Nouri, F.M. and Lincoln, N.B. (1993) Predicting driving performance after stroke. *British Medical Journal* **307**, 482.

O'Neill, D., Neubauer, K., Boyle, M. *et al.* (1992) Dementia and driving. *Journal of the Royal Society of Medicine*, **85**, 199–202.

Oxley, P.R. (1989) Disabled people and cars: An overview, in *Transport for disabled people*. Proceedings of a Conference organized by the European Ministers of Transport.

Porter, K.F. (1989) Neck sprains after car accidents. *British Medical Journal*, **28**, 973–74.

Ritter, J., and Steinberg, H.J. (1979) Parkinsonism and driving fitness. *Munch Med Wochenschr*, **121**, 1329–30.

Simms, B. (1989) Driver Education: The needs of the learner driver with spina bifida and hydrocephalus. *Zeitschrift fur Kindorchirurgic*, **44**, 35–7.

Simms, B. (1991) *Driving after a Stroke in Private Transport for Elderly and Disabled People*. Proceedings of an International Seminar, Transport and Road Research Laboratory, Department of Transport, Contractors report 308.

Simms, B., O'Toole, L. and Clayton, S. (1992) *Cognitive deficit after head injury: implication for driving*. Research Report funded by TVS Trust, available from Banstead Mobility Centre.

Spalding, T.J.W., Kiss, J., Kyberd, P. *et al.* (1994) Driver reactions after total knee replacements. *Journal of Bone and Joint Surgery*, **76B**, 754–6.

Taylor, J.F. (ed) (1995) *Medical Aspects of Fitness to Drive, a guide for Medical Practitioners*, 5th edn, Medical Commission on Accident Prevention, London.

TRRL Contractors Report 158 (1990) Seat belts and disabled people. (eds J, Issacs, and B. Massie), Department of Transport, London.

TRRL Research Report no. 2 (1985) *Problems Experienced by Disabled Elderly People Entering and Leaving Cars* Department of Transport, London.

TRRL Leaflet LF 1020 (1986) *Tests on Cushions Used by Seat Belted Car Occupants* Turner-Stokes, L. *et al.* (1996) Secondary safety of car adaptations for disabled motorists. *Disability and Rehabilitation* (in press).

Van Zomeren, A.H., Brouver, W.H. and Minderhoud, J.M. (1987) Acquired brain damage and driving – a review. *Archives of Physical Medicine and Rehabilitation*. **68**, 697–705.

INFORMATION

A guide to services in the UK offering advice, information and assessment to disabled and elderly motorists (Information correct in second quarter of 1993) TRRL, Department of Transport

AA Guide for the Disabled Traveller 1995, AA, Fanum House, Basingstoke, Hants RG21 2EA, UK.

Ability Car Guide, Castlemead, Gascoyne Way, Hertford SG14 ILH, UK (also car fact sheets available). Tel : 01992 822820.

Access to taxis transport for people with Mobility handicaps (1992) European Conference of Ministers of Transport 1992 (ISBN 9282111660).

ADEPD (The Association of Driver Educators for People with Disabilities), c/o Banstead Mobility Centre.

DIAL UK (The National Association of Disablement Information and Advice Services), 117 High Street, Clay Cross, Chesterfield, Derbyshire S45 9DZ, UK Tel : 01246 864498.

Disability Unit, Room S10/21, Department of Transport, 2 Marsham Street, London SW1P 3EB, UK.

Disabled Drivers Association, Askwellthorpe Hall, Askwellthorpe, Norwich, Norfolk NR16 1EX, UK.

Disabled Drivers Motor Club, 1a Dudley Gardens, Ealing London W13 9LU, UK.

The Disabled Living Foundation, 380–384 Harrow Road, London W9 2HU (and see list of Disabled Living Centres (DLC), Chapter 55).

Disability Rights Handbook (1995) Produced by the Disability Alliance, 25 Denmark Street London WC2H 8NJ, UK.

Door to door. A guide to transport for people with disabilities (updated 1995) Obtainable from HMSO (ISBN 0 1155 0884 8).

Driving after amputation – information for professionals. Compiled by the UK Forum of Mobility Centres, c/o Banstead Mobility Centre.

Driving after head injury, Headway National Head Injuries Association, King Edward Court, King Edward Street, Nottingham NG1 1EW, UK. Tel: 01602 240800.

Driving after a Stroke, The Stroke Association, CHSA, Whitecross Street, London EC1Y 8JJ, UK.

Esso Service Station Address List. Copies available from Esso Merchandising Service, PO Box 2, Feltham, Middlesex, UK.

How to Get Back Behind the Wheel – information for amputees wishing to drive a car. Compiled by the UK Forum of Mobility Centres, c/o Banstead Mobility Centre.

How to Get Equipment for Disabilities. Compiled by Michael Mandelstam. Jessica Kingsley publishers and Kogan Page for the Disabled Living Foundation.

The Ins and Outs of Car Choice. A guide for elderly and disabled people (1985) Department of Transport at TRRL.

The Medical Advisor, Drivers Medical Unit, Drivers and Vehicle Licensing Agency (DVLA), Longview Road, Morriston, Swansea SA99 ITU, UK.

Medical Aspects of Fitness to Drive: a guide for medical practitioners, 5th edn (1995) (ed J.F. Taylor). Published by Medical Commission on Accident Prevention, 35–43 Lincoln Inns Field, London WC2A 3PN, UK.

Motability, Goodman House Station Approach, Harlow, Essex CM20 2ET, UK. Tel: 01279 635666.

Motoring for Disabled People 1994, An Independent guide for disabled people - published by Countryside Publications, Unit 26, Orton Enterprise Centre, Bakewell Road, Orton Southgate, Peterborough, Cambridgeshire PE2 0XU, UK.

Motoring and Mobility for Disabled People. Compiled by Ann Darnbrough and Derek Kinrade RADAR, 25 Mortimer Street, London W1N 8AB, UK.

The National Disability Tuition Register, c/o Banstead Mobility Centre.

Outdoor transport: Equipment for the Disabled, 6th edn (1987) Mary Marlborough Lodge, Nuffield Orthopaedic Centre, Oxford OX3 7LD, UK.

Secondary safety for vehicle adaptations for disabled motorists, Research Institute for Consumer Affairs, 2 Marylebone Road, London NW1 4DF, UK.

Service Call Systems Limited, Details from Autochair Ltd., Milford Lane, Bakewell, Derbyshire DE45 IXA, UK. Tel: 01629 812422.

Triscope (for solving mobility problems), The Courtyard, Evelyn Road, London W4 5JL. Tel: 0181 994 3618.

The UK Forum of Mobility Centres, c/o Banstead Mobility Centre.

8 mph Vehicle – your rights and responsibilities. A code of practice for users issued by the Department of Transport.

Forum of UK Mobility Centres

Bansted Mobility Centre, Damson Way, Fountain Drive, Queen Mary's Avenue, Carshalton, Surrey, SM5 4NR, UK. Tel: (0181) 7701151

Cornwall Friends' Mobility Centre, Tehidy House, Treliske Hospital, Truro, Cornwall, TRI 3LJ, UK. Tel: 01872 260060.

Derby Regional Mobility Centre, Kingsway Hospital, Derby, DE3 3LZ, UK, Tel:01332 371929.

Disability Action, 2, Annadale Avenue, Belfast, BT7 3JR UK. Tel: 01232 491011.

Edinburgh Driving Assessment Service, Mobility Centre, Astley Ainslie Hospital, 133 Grange Loan, Edinburgh, EH9 2HL, UK. Tel: 01315 379192.

The Mobility Centre, Regional Rehabilitation Centre, Hunters Road, Newcastle Upon Tyne, NE2 4NR., Tel: 01912 210454.

Kilverstone Mobility Centre, Kilverstone Country Park, Kilverstone, Thetford, Norfolk, IP24 2RL, UK. Tel: 01842 753029.

Mobility Advice and Vehicle, Information Service (MAVIS), Macadam Avenue, Old Wokingham Road, Crowthorne, Berks, RG45 6XO, UK. Tel: 01344 661000.

Mobility Information Service, Unit 2A, Atcham Estate, Shrewsbury, SY4 4UG, UK. Tel: 01734 761889.

Wrightington Mobility Centre, Wrightington Hospital, Hall Lane, Wrightington, Wigan, Lancashire, WD6 9EP, UK. Tel: 01257 256280.

51 Enabling the young disabled adult

A.E. Ward and M.A. Chamberlain

INTRODUCTION

Of all the challenges in life, one of the greatest is that of the transition from childhood to adulthood. In this period from puberty through to the middle of the third decade, adolescents have four major developmental tasks (Hardoff and Chigier, 1991). These are:

- to consolidate their identity;
- to achieve independence from parents;
- to establish adult relations outside the family;
- to find a vocation.

To achieve these aims young people need many skills. Young people with physical and cognitive disabilities are at a considerable disadvantage. They many not have acquired certain skills; they may not have a clear sense of identity; they may have missed out on a variety of basic experiences, perhaps because of lack of independent mobility. Finally, those with neurological problems may continue to experience difficulties in learning and in their acquisition of knowledge about the world.

The Warnock Report (Warnock, 1978) recognized the size of the task required of the adolescent during the transition from childhood to adulthood. It went on to say, 'For those with special educational needs it is likely to be a period of particular stress. Unless skilled support is available to them and their parents at this stage all the efforts made to meet their special needs during their school career may come to nothing. . .'

In childhood, for both able-bodied young people and those with physical disabilities, school provides the framework for much of their existence. For those with special needs, paediatric services in many industrial countries are well developed and well integrated, both internally and with schooling, so that the health, social and educational needs of teenagers are cohesively provided for until they leave school. Then they 'hurtle into a void', services are fragmented and there is no obvious route to acquiring consistent health service care and advice.

Thomas, Bax and Smyth (1989) found that contact with the health services by these young adults was often very poor, with the most handicapped having least contact. Provision by social services, education, employment and health often appeared unrelated, with those in one service knowing little about the provisions or aims of those in another. This was compounded by the low expectations and demands of disabled young people, especially those with congenital disabilities, and their parents. The survey also found a considerable number of young people without access to physiotherapy and therefore developing new contractures. The OPCS survey (Martin, White and Meltzer, 1989) found they had poor dental health; they had problems with their feet through lack of

Rehabilitation of the Physically Disabled Adult. Edited by C. John Goodwill, M. Anne Chamberlain and Chris Evans. Published in 1997 by Stanley Thornes (Publishers) Ltd, Cheltenham. ISBN 0-7487-3183-0.

chiropodist care, and they had occular and orthopaedic problems. It is now widely recognized that such a dismal state of affairs does not help prepare the young person for responsible adult life.

Much of the research concerned with the social needs of children with disabilities lies in an array of literature related to their specific diseases. Eiser (1990) makes the point that these children, although having different diagnoses, have many needs in common which should help the planning of services. Yet many families are confused by the multiplicity of services which fail to work in harmony. The situation is similar in adolescence. At this age, there are too few services and too little information which is available on them.

DEFINING THE PROBLEMS

Which diseases?

Needs are related to diagnosis, so this is a useful starting point. The prevalence of diseases in childhood is a good indicator of their prevalence in young adulthood if survival rates are known. These are given in Table 51.1.

Recent requests to the Rowntree Family Fund to help with funding expensive equipment for children with severe disabilities suggests that, whilst there is now a declining incidence of spina bifida, no drug-induced phocomelia and no disability due to intrauterine rubella, there are now children, born very small, with severe multiple disabilities. A recent report from the Royal College of Physicians (1990) suggests there is also a need to plan for increasing survival into adult life of those born with cystic fibrosis.

Some conditions appear during adolescence, for example traumatic head injury and spinal injury which occur more often in young men. Adult-type rheumatoid arthritis and multiple sclerosis occur more frequently in young women.

It is useful to categorize these diseases to extract common features that may help in management; conditions may be static, fluctuant or progressive, either rapidly or slowly. Some have serious complications which mean the young person needs to know what to do in an emergency (such as hydrocephalus in spina bifida); some conditions need regular medical review (e.g. where silent renal damage may be occurring, as in spina bifida). Many inherited neurological diseases are individually rare but together form a large group in which there are common features. For most of these young people there is a common core of needs and tasks to be addressed which transcends diagnostic labels. These matters can be approached not only at the level of disease but also at the levels of impairment, disability and handicap.

What impairments?

These include:

1. Pressure sores in those with paraplegia, perhaps deriving from spina bifida.
2. Contractures, where there is spasticity or loss of muscle power over a joint.
3. Incontinence of bowel and bladder.
4. Scoliosis from weakness of truncal muscles potentially leading to respiratory failure.
5. Limb growth problems.
6. Failure to thrive is commonly seen and, like cognitive and behavioural impairments, is of major significance in the drive to maturation.

Many of these are dealt with elsewhere in this book. The incidence in the USA is given as 90.8/1000 persons (White, 1996), with deformities or orthopaedic impairments being most frequent.

What disabilities?

The nature and severity of the young person's functional limitations and whether the young person has to contend with more than one

Table 51.1 Incidence and prevalence of certain diseases of young adults

Disease	Incidence per 10^6	Prevalence per 10^6	Prevalence trend	Problems seen
Congenital				
Cerebral palsy	200	200	Static	Mobility, dexterity, communication, learning, epilepsy
Spina bifida	Variable	2	Down	Mobility, dexterity, continent, renal failure, hydrocephalus
Muscular dystrophy (all types)	1–3/8000 live births	90	Down	Mobility, posture, resp. problems. Coping with death and disease progression
Neurological rarities	Make large group together		Down	Mobility, dexterity, learning, epilepsy, ataxia
Cystic fibrosis	40/2500 live births		Increasing in over 15 year-olds	Failure to thrive, respiratory problems, mortality issues
Acquired				
Head injury	300	150	Up	Cognition/behaviour problems, communication, mobility. Peak age 18–22 years
Spinal injury	10–15		Up	Mobility, dexterity, bowel/bladder problems, presure sores
Juvenile chronic arthritis	16	up to 113	Static	Mobility, dexterity, pain, ill health, effects of drugs, time off school
Multiple sclerosis	4–8	99–178	Static	Progressive, mobility, ataxia, bowel/bladder problems, visual loss

disability needs to be known. Many young people have multiple disabilities; 82% of those with cerebral palsy (Lagergren, 1981) have more than one disability. Whilst all disabilities have an additive effect, some combinations make learning new tasks particularly difficult. Table 51.2 identifies some multiple disabilities which occur in different diagnoses. These disabilities (together with handicaps) are as important in determining service needs at various stages in life as diagnoses.

What handicaps?

A study of 19–25 year olds and their carers revealed that their aspirations were very different from their expectations. The young persons' self-image was often poor. Often a

Table 51.2 Examples of the potential effect of certain diseases in terms of disability and handicap

	Juvenile chronic arthritis	Cystic fibrosis	Cerebral palsy	Spina bifida	Head injury	Spinal injury
Disabilities						
1. Behaviour			+	+	+	+
2. Communication			+		+	−
3. Personal care	+		+	+	+	+
4. Locomotor	+	+	+	+	+	+
5. Body disposition	+	+	+	+	+	+
6. Dexterity	+		+	+	+	+
7. Situational	+	+	+	+	+	+
8. Vocation	+		+	+	+	+
Handicaps						
1. Orientation		+	+	+	+	−
2. Physical independence	+	+	+	+	+	+
3. Mobility	+	+	+	+	+	+
4. Occupation	+		+	+	+	+
5. Social integration	+		+	+	+	+
6. Economic self-sufficiency	+	+	+	+	+	+

+ - abnormality may be present.

client's needs were not matched with an appropriate response and with available support (Table 51.3). Knowing this, parents were often unwilling to let the young person try to be independent. A review of services in Gloucestershire (Beardshaw, 1989) revealed numerous services shortcomings for disabled adults (Table 51.4).

In developing areas of the world attitudes to disability may often preclude disabled individuals from being part of society (Helander, 1992). Whilst children often participate in integrated education, as young adults they often find the greatest difficulty in obtaining training or employment. There may be an abundance of people available to do the less skilled work they might do. Resources are limited so that acute issues of funding are raised. It is essential that disability awareness is increased and the community's and family's abilities harnessed to aid young people. Experience elsewhere suggests that equal opportunities legislation will probably be needed.

Table 51.3 Constraints on disabled young people

Constraint	Examples
Resources	Lack of appropriate facilities
Personal ability	Low self-esteem and self-image
Family concern	Letting go of adulthood
Service mismatching	Failure to match client with facility

Table 51.4 Shortcomings of services to disabled people: Gloucestershire Survey (Beardshaw, 1989)

A lack of a coordinated rehabilitation service
A shortage of skilled specialists in all social service and health professions
Poor liaison between services leading to fragmented services to clients
Lack of a readily available information resource for service users and providers
Inadequate provision of certain services
Inadequate provision and lack of choice of residential accommodation
Inadequate day care provision outside city centres

What numbers?

The UK OPCS Survey (Martin, White and Meltzer, 1989) was notable for the extent and thoroughness of its findings. These have been secondarily analysed by Hirst (1990) as they apply to young people. The results indicate that although disability is strongly associated with age, nonetheless there are some 340 000 young people between the ages of 16 and 29 years with a disability. They constitute about 5% of all disabled people and 2.5% of young people in the total UK population of 57 million. Only about 20 000 of these young people were living in residential care or communal establishments. Males outnumbered females slightly. More than half had a very severe disability (category 7 or above).

These findings are likely to be similar in countries with similar wealth, development and socioeconomic structure. Trends alter constantly and, over the past two decades, treatments aimed at secondary prevention have altered the disabilities seen.

What skills are required?

A range of skills is required of adults (Table 51.5). They are usually acquired at different times by young people, dependent on their home, educational, work and sexual situations. It is worth considering the hierarchy of skills needed by the individual. For instance, most young people wishing to live alone will first need to be able to make themselves a snack, and budget, and later begin to organize their shopping, cleaning and other tasks. Even those who are grossly dependent will need to be aware of the necessity of these things being done if they are to organize and direct a paid helper to do these tasks for them.

RESPONDING TO THE NEED

What services need to be provided?

Some idea of the demands which will be made of a young adult service can be seen in Table 51.6, and also from considering the service/requirements in tabulated form for two diseases, juvenile chronic arthritis and cerebral palsy, (Tables 51.7 and 51.8). These case studies given in the Appendix indicate how various needs came to light as they progressed towards independent living. They indicate what professional resources were used to solve the problems raised, but it is possible that solutions could have been provided via other routes.

What sort of problems do the young people present?

From the surveys undertaken it seems that many young people have little idea of how to keep themselves fit and well. In the survey carried out by Thomas, Bax and Smyth (1989), many were obese, some ill-nourished, they were rarely fit or playing games or occupying their time pleasurably. Many had problems with inadequate or inappropriate medication; some were incontinent, some were kept in nappies, many were inadequately informed about sexual matters in general or the genetics of their condition in particular and few had knowledge of contraception. They might be unable to look after their personal or domestic activities of daily living; they might not hold down a job and not be undertaking training. Their parents were ageing and worried. The young persons themselves were frustrated by their lack of autonomy. The Prince of Wales Advisory Group on Disability has produced 'Living Options' as a response to the problem (Fiedler, 1990). A summary of their principles is given in Table 51.9.

The skills young physically handicapped adults require to enter adulthood can be organized under several headings: health and health maintenance; personal and domestic activities of daily living; social; education and vocational (Table 51.6); leisure; housing; transportation. Consideration of the case histories in the Appendix

Table 51.5 Skills required of young adult

Maintenance skills				Life skills			
Health	Self-care	Domestic skills	Mobility	Relationships	Leisure	Work	Self-development
Nutrition	Feeding	Food collection,	Indoors	Sexual	Hobbies	Direct work skills +	Assertiveness
Exercise	Dressing	preparation, storage	Threshold	Family	Sports	Movement to work	Negotiation
Disease management	Hygiene	Maintenance of clothes	Outdoors	Social		and within workplace,	Time management
(e.g. joint movement)	i.e. PADL	Home cleaning and	On foot/in wheelchair	Work		posture and seating	Money management, etc.
Disability management		maintenance	Using transport,	Community			Information gaining
Use of health service		Home safety	public or private	Other			(including
resources (e.g. GP, GDP)		Money management,					experimental)
		i.e. DADL					Career development

DADL = domestic activities of daily living; PADL = personal activities of daily living.

Table 51.6 Main needs of young people

Independent living

Information

Health care and personal issues

Social needs – personal care, finance, occupational activity

Aids and equipment for daily living, education and employment

Transport/mobility/access

Further education and training

Employment

Housing

Leisure and recreation facilities

indicate several common needs (see also Figure 51.1), and it is these skills requirements which largely determine service models. Many of the handicaps experienced by the young person can be overcome by effective interagency working. Unless there are professionals with a specific brief for young persons' services, this is unlikely to occur regularly.

SERVICE MODELS

There are many potential models of service (Chamberlain *et al.*, 1993). In the UK there has been an adolescent's clinic (mainly for those with spina bifida) for many years in Newcastle (Castree and Walker, 1981). Two Young Adult Teams are now well established in the UK in Stoke and Leeds, and these will be described. Others are being set up. In Exeter, an education-based training unit exists. At Queen Elizabeth Foundation, Banstead Place, residential training is provided and there are many local colleges of further education and higher education which provide specific training and tutors for handicapped young people. However, there has been a dearth of coordinated health services able to address the majority of the needs of this group of young people. An evaluation of the Stoke service indicated that

clients also wanted an input from the voluntary sectors (Aung, Boughey and Ward, 1994) and the two clearly need to work in partnership.

In Hereford a voluntary organization provides training and advice for disabled people, voluntary organizations, social services, education and health have been involved in its development. Some voluntary organizations which have significant numbers of young people may put on short (weekend usually) courses on such topics as self-management, assertiveness or social skills. In the USA, the National Centre for Youth with Disabilities publishes regular newsletters and updates of new developments in legislation and education programmes.

It seems that the most successful models are based on a philosophy which responds to the needs of the client and enables them to achieve their aims and acquire abilities which gradually build up towards independence. Freedom of informed choice is the key to a successful life, and the framework which is widely accepted in the UK is that enunciated in the Living Options Principles (Fiedler, 1990), with the disabled person at the centre of the service and aiming for choice, consultation, participation, recognition, and information and autonomy.

The range of health, therapy-based and social abilities to be acquired suggests that a multidisciplinary team is required and should contain the skills necessary to respond to the young person (Baines and Chamberlain, 1994).

A case manager might be able to seek out professionals, but it is the interaction between these staff with a great range of expertise in a coordinated, focused way, often over a long period, which produces good results. Experience has shown that when the young person attends a rehabilitation clinic in a hospital, transitional needs do not get properly addressed and the visit to hospital may be associated with painful memories, particularly of surgery.

Table 51.7 Cerebral palsy: possible service requirements (service implications depend upon a great range of variables; e.g. epilepsy, spasticity)

| | Disease | | | Disability | | | | | | | | | |
| | | | | Health service provision | | | Other service provision | | | | | | |
	Prevention	Investigation	Treatment	Surgery	Rehabilitation	Support[a]	Housing/ adaptations	Education	Vocational assessment	Transport and access	Leisure	Social services/ carer support	Benefits
Birth	0	+	0	0	+	0	0	0	0	0	0	0	0
Child	0	+	+	+	++	+	±	+	0	±	0	±	0
Teens	0	0	0	+	+	+	+	+	++	++	+	+	+
Adult	0	0	0	−	±	+	+	±	+	+	+	+	+

[a] e.g. continence service, wheelchair provision, nursing input.
0 = No input/not relevant or appropriate; ± = possible minor input; + = service requirement; ++ = major service requirement.

Table 51.8 Juvenile chronic arthritis: possible service requirements (this is based on the assumption that if much treatment, rehabilitation and surgery are given in teens and early adult life, the situation will be relatively stable thereafter)

| | Disease | | | Disability | | | | | | | | | |
| | | | | Health service provision | | | Other service provision | | | | | | |
	Prevention	Investigation	Treatment	Surgery	Rehabilitation	Support	Housing/ adaptations	Education	Vocational assessment	Transport and access	Leisure	Social services/ carer support	Benefits
Birth	0	0	0	0	0	0	0	0	0	0	0	0	0
Child	0	+	++	+	±	+	+	+	0	±	0	±	+
Teens	0	+	++	++	++	±	+	++	++	++	±	±	+
Adult	0	±	+	+	+	±	+	0	++	++	0	±	+

0 = No input/not relevant or appropriate; ± = possible minor input; + = service requirement; ++ = major service requirement.

Table 51.9 Living options principles

Choice as to where to live and how to maintain independence

Consultation with disabled people and their families on planning services

Information, clearly presented and readily available to the most severe disabled users

Participation in the life of local and national communities in respect of both responsibilities and benefits

Recognition that long-term disability is not synonymous with illness

Autonomy: the Freedom to make decisions regarding the way of life best suited to an individual's circumstances

A YOUNG ADULT TEAM

The multidisciplinary teams established in Leeds and Stoke are community based, working out of small hospitals and health centres, often with related services on site. The team at Stoke meets regularly with locality and rehabilitation teams. Young Adult Teams need a base, and secretarial support, even though individual members spend much of their time at clients' homes. The team should include not only health service staff but also those in other agencies such as social services, education and employment. Managerial support and a budget are also necessary. A clear operational policy, agreed routes of referral, into the team and from it, and processes (such as the formats for assessment and review) have to be worked out. The client should be involved in setting goals and priorities and should have a copy of any reports generated. Follow-up is important: change of skills, of priorities and of needs will occur over, perhaps, a decade, as it does in the able-bodied young person (though the process may be more protracted). The membership of a multidisciplinary team is suggested in Table 51.10.

The process of the team's working is illustrated by John's case in the Appendix. It

Table 51.10 Multidisciplinary teams for young adults

Professionals workers involved (variable amounts of time required)
   Doctor with rehabilitation expertise
   Physiotherapist
   Occupational therapist
   Speech and language therapist

Core workers
   Social worker (facilitates interagency working)
   Psychologist
   Secretary
   Nurse
   Careers officer/disability advisor
   Further education (tutor)

Others
   Link person in housing

Include
   Link person with voluntary, disability organization and others
   Counselling

will be seen that he was helped over several years by the team. Medical assessment, speech therapy, occupational therapy and physiotherapy interventions were in place early (staff agreeing with John and between themselves that the first aims were to improve communication and socialisation). Later John learnt the domestic abilities necessary to survive alone so that he is still independent in his own home and prefers this to his previous institutional living.

Clients are referred in from many sources and will require a great range of services. The links of a service are shown in Figure 51.1. Some needs recur so frequently that the team may devise their own in-house responses. One team runs social skills training sessions and draws in isolated individuals to its discussion groups, which have helped the young people organize activities to increase their fitness and their enjoyment. They have run family planning advice sessions and given much education on the nature of the person's disease and disability. Also, they

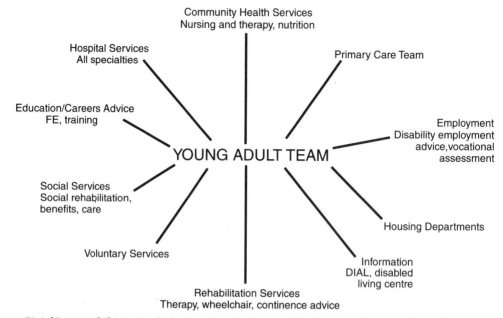

Figure 51.1 Young adult service links for investigation and/or treatment or provision of services.

have established a 'hot-line' via the sister on the local neurosurgical ward for those with spina bifida who are anxious that they should be able to obtain knowledgeable neurosurgical help for possible hydrocephalus.

NEED FOR SERVICES PROVIDED OUTWITH THE TEAM

Figure 51.1 indicates the diversity of services needed by the young people. Many of these are frequent, such as wheelchairs and seating, and a well-established, comprehensive rehabilitation service will deliver them. Well-developed community services will supply nursing and homecare support, making possible the move to independent living. The local hospital and the teaching hospital will have consultant-led services dealing with the services, renal function, management of epilepsy, movement disorders, and spasticity. Genetic counselling, pain clinics and psychosexual counselling may be sought.

An aware local authority providing good access to public buildings, good transportation and sufficient purpose-built housing arguably does as much as health services for these young citizens. Enlightened, accessible higher and further education and equal access to job opportunities will ensure that what has been achieved with the help of the Young Adult Team will be on-going.

Young Adult Services frequently end at the age of 25 or 30 years. Gains hard won can be easily lost with preventable complications ensuing. Arrangements for linking these young people to generic rehabilitation services and to general practice are required. A good relationship with general practitioners (GPs) is valuable and disabled young people are twice as likely to have had face-to-face contact with their GP (Martin, White and Meltzer, 1989; Hirst and Baldwin, 1994). However, they were less likely to attend a GP appointment on their own. GPs are in a good position to be the point of contact and coordination, but clear management guidelines are required for accessing specialist services for those that need them. Where a community has no framework of general practice, other responses to the young person's need have to be put in place.

TRANSPORT, MOBILITY ACCESS

Help is often required for personal mobility and the health service has a clear commitment to the assessment for and provision of walking aids, wheelchairs and appropriate seating. Transport, both personal and public, is an essential part of life today and, without adequate arrangements, employment, education and leisure activities are virtually impossible. However, this has often been overlooked, as has the fact that disabled young people may need to learn how to use transport, including driving (Chapter 50). The Department of Transport (Disability Unit) noted that many disabled children relied heavily on private transport and had little understanding of public transport and of making decisions on how to obtain it (McBride and Ward, 1991).

Much public transport is inaccessible to disabled people and, in particular, to wheelchair users. Disabled people are often not sufficiently involved in the planning of transport facilities; accessible transport is helpful not only to disabled people, but also to the community at large, including people who push prams or wheelchairs.

FURTHER EDUCATION, TRAINING AND EMPLOYMENT

The majority of young people with physical disabilities do nothing during the day and are unable to develop a role in the community (Tripp, 1985). When the individual leaves school not only is there an increased burden on parents but lack of a daytime occupation also has major consequences (Chapter 52).

In most parts of Europe there has been a great expansion of tertiary education and disabled people have benefitted from this. In the UK those in special schools may stay on until they are 19, after which courses in further education are available to take them up to 23 years. However, for many people major difficulties remain in finding gainful employment or even an acceptable way of spending their time. Disabled people find it more difficult (Walker, 1982) to find and keep paid employment (Martin, White and Meltzer, 1989). Disabled young people are less able than others to take on part-time jobs as children, they therefore lack this learning experience and introduction to employment. Less than full-time employment may lead to a net loss of income. In a few countries the situation is better than in the UK and lessons could usefully be learnt from them. The difficulties appear to include poor access to information about work, inadequate vocational evaluation and training, and high levels of unemployment amongst able-bodied peers. Potential employers may be poorly supported when they take on disabled young people, whose abilities may not be recognized. There are frequently misconceptions about disability amongst employers and workpeople alike and restrictive practices may have to be addressed. Finally, structural boundaries between health and employment are often too great to be bridged easily by professionals or their patients.

LEGISLATION: WHAT SOCIETAL RESPONSES ARE HELPFUL?

In the last two decades in the UK much potentially helpful legislation has been enacted (Table 51.11).

In the USA, the Americans with Disabilities Act 1990 is beginning to exert profound beneficial effects. Civil liberties have been strengthened and access to jobs is opening up. Consequently, there has been the development of much new assistive technology by industry. Further benefits will ensue.

Table 51.11 Helpful legislation in the UK

Report/act	Principal effect
Chronically Sick & Disabled Persons Act 1970	Provision by statutory services of information and a range of services and equipment for disabled persons
Disabled Persons (Services, Consultation & Representation) Act 1986	States need for collaboration of agencies in service planning and provision. Sections V & VI state the requirement for Social Services and Education Departments to assess needs of disabled school leavers, which includes adequate participation by disabled person and representative
Warnock Report 1978	Recommends the integration of children with special needs into mainstream education and gives point of contact to specialist careers service
Education Act 1981	Provision is made for statementing of children with special educational needs due to a disability
Children Act 1989	Provision is made for safeguarding children in need, including disabled children up to the age of 19 years
NHS & Community Care Act 1990	Provision of Care in the Community with lead role given to social services for assessment of needs of disabled people. Concept of purchasers and providers of health and social care introduced and development of philosophy of community rather than institutional care
Education Act 1993	
Disability Discrimination Act 1995	Employment and public transport

STANDARDS OF A GOOD SERVICE

Little research has been done to address this issue. However, we do know that a Young Adult Team increases the access of its clients to needed services, both inside and outside the health service. The number of assistive devices prescribed increases, the young people become more able to manage their own health; they feel more in control of their own lives and they go into further and higher education in increasing numbers. Significant numbers leave home to live independently and a few get jobs. These are obvious markers of the team's success but cannot be the only ones. Even for very disabled young people, autonomy and enjoyment of life can be enhanced and these are legitimate measures of a team's success.

These findings fit well with the definition of transition to adulthood given at the beginning of the chapter, and it is suggested that quality standards for a service should relate closely to this process. Whatever model of service is adopted this goal remains. To achieve this, it is essential to understand that transition is viewed not as an event but as a gradual process. Its timescale varies greatly from person to person and family to family and services need to be flexible to accommodate this diversity.

A recent Scandinavian study (Lindstrom, 1991) showed that it is possible to achieve a good quality of life, independent living and social integration for many young people. We believe that Young Adult Services can help bring about this happy state of affairs. In so doing they will open up opportunities which may last over 50 years for the individual and their family.

REFERENCES

Aung, T.S., Boughey, A.M. and Ward, A.B. (1994) A study of the North Staffordshire Young Adult Service for Physically Disabled School Leavers and Young Adults. *Clinical Rehabilitation*, **8**, 147–53.

Baines, P. and Chamberlain, M.A. (1994) The physically disabled adolescent – service provision in the community. *Maternal and Child Health*, January 10–19.

Beardshaw, V. (1989) *Last on the List: community services for people with physical disabilities*, Kings Fund Institute, London.

Castree, B.J. and Walker, J.H. (1981) The young adult with Spina Bifida. *British Medical Journal* **283**, 1040–2.

Chamberlain, M.A., Guthrie, S., Kettle, M. and Stowe, J. (1993) *An Assessment of the Health and Related Needs of Physically Handicapped Young Adults*, Department of Health, London.

Eiser, C. (1990) *Chronic Childhood Disease: an introduction to psychological theory and research*, Cambridge University Press, Cambridge.

Fiedler, B. (1990) *A Framework for Action: developing services for people with severe physical and sensory disabilities*, Living Options in Practice Project, Kings Fund Centre, London.

Hardoff, D. and Chigier, E. (1991) Developing community based services for youth with disabilities. *Paediatrician*, **18**, 157–62.

Helander, E. (1992) *Prejudice and Dignity: an introduction to community-based rehabilitation* (United Nations), HMSO, London.

Hirst, M.A. (1990) *National Survey of Young People with Disabilities: matching and weighting samples*, DHSS 531, Social Policy Research Unit Working Paper, University of York.

Hirst, M. and Baldwin, S. (1994) *Unequal Opportunities: growing up disabled*, Social Policy Research Unit, HMSO, London.

Lagergren, J. (1981) Children with motor handicaps: epidemiological, medical and socio-paediatrics of motor handicapped children in a Swedish County. *Acta Paediatrica Scandinavica*, **70**, (suppl. 289), 1–69.

Lindstrom, B. and Kohler, L. (1991) Youth, Disability and Quality of Life. *Pediatrician*, **18**, 121–8.

Martin, J., White, A. and Meltzer, H. (1989) *Disabled Adults: services, transport and employment*, Report 4, OPCS Survey of Disability in Great Britain, HMSO, London.

McBride, A. and Ward, A.B. (1991) *Developing Services for Physically Disabled School Leavers and Young Adults*. Report of a Conference at Keele University, April 1991, Stafford. (Copies from Dr A Ward, North Staffs Rehab Centre, Heywood Hospital, Stoke).

Royal College of Physicians, (1990) *Cystic Fibrosis in Adults: recommendations for care of patients in the UK*, Royal College of Physicians, London.

Thomas, A.P., Bax, M.C.O. and Smyth, D.L. (1989) *The Health and Social Needs of Young Adults with Physical Disabilities*, McKeith Press, Oxford.

Tripp, J.H. (1985) *The Needs of Handicapped Young Adults*, Paediatric Research Unit, Royal Devon and Exeter Hospital and Medical School.

Walker, A. (1982) *Unqualified and Underemployed: handicapped young people and the labour market*, Methuen, London.

Warnock, H.M. (1978) *Report of the Committee of Enquiry into the Education of Handicapped Young People*, HMSO, London.

White, P. (1996) Future expectations: adolescents with rheumatic diseases and their transition into adulthood. *British Journal of Rheumatology*, **35**, 80–3.

FURTHER READING

Beardshaw, V. (1988) *The Hidden 3000: joint study of services for physically handicapped people in Gloucestershire (1988)*, vol 1–3, Social Services Department, Gloucestershire County Council, Shire Hall, Gloucester.

Bone, M. and Meltzer, H. (1989) *The Prevalence of Disability among Children*, OPCS Survey of Disability in Great Britain, Report No. 3, HMSO, London.

Chamberlain, M.A., Guthrie, S., Kettle, M. and Stowe, J. (1993) *An Assessment of Health and Related Needs of Physically Handicapped Young Adults,* Department of Health Publication Unit, London.

Connections: The Newsletter of the National Center for Youth with Disabilities. University of Minnesota, Box 721, 420, Delaware, St SE. Minneapolis, MN 55455, USA.

Eiser, C. (1990) *Chronic Childhood Disease: an introduction to psychological theory and research,* Cambridge University Press, Cambridge.

Helander, E. (1992) *Prejudice and Dignity: an introduction to community-based rehabilitation* (United Nations), HMSO, London.

Hirst, M. and Baldwin, S. (1994) *Unequal Opportunities: growing up disabled,* Social Policies Research Unit, London.

Martin, J. Meltzer, N. and Elliott, D. (1988) *The Prevalence of Disability among Adults,* Report 1, OPCS Survey of Disability in Great Britain, HMSO, London.

Martin, J. and White, A. (1988) *The Financial Circumstances of Disabled Adults Living in Private Households,* Report 2, OPCS Survey of Disability in Great Britain, HMSO, London.

Prouse, P., Ross-Smith, K., Brill, M. *et al.* (1991) Community support for young physically handicapped people. *Health Trends* **23**, 105–9.

Appendix: *case reports*

JOHN aged 23: cerebral palsy with gross athetosis

JOHN: 1

Referral by himself
Assessment
Totally dependent
Speech unintelligible
Highly intelligent
Obligatory wheelchair user
Lives in institution, few social contacts
Attends resource centre only
Interest: computers, photography, cinema

Wanted	more socialization
	development of interests
	ability to go out alone
Had	manual and electric wheelchairs (poor)
	borrowed communication aid (useless)

JOHN: 2 – Interaction with young adult team	Professionals involved
Year 1: Agreed *requires* improved communication and confidence	Speech and language therapist
Action: communication aid bought	
Use practised in shops, pubs, etc.	
Confidence in these situations built up	
Met more people	
- -	
Seating and wheelchair provision need improvement	
Years 1–2 Action: needs assessed, wheelchair bought and used (in conjunction with speech and language therapist). Outdoor mobility enhanced	Occupational therapist physiotherapist
Year 2: Application for residential training made.	Social worker Doctor (referral)
Could involuntary movements be better controlled?	
(referral not helpful)	Occupational therapist
Wants to live independently	
Years 2–3: Component skills	
for independent living analysed. Work on these begins	
Year 3: Continued work on activities of daily living skills	Social worker Occupational therapist
Planning for independent living continues	
Unsuccessful re residential college	
Year 4: Moved successfully to (supported) independent living	

JAN: juvenile chronic arthritis since age 1

JAN: 1 *Referral* from rheumatologist

Assessment

Disease still slightly active

Small. Deformities mainly at weightbearing joints.

Mobile short distances

Independent in feeding, toilet but needs help with dressing; needs help or equipment for washing

Living at home, unadapted

Contributes to family finances

Trained in office skills. Doing full-time job

JAN: 2	Professionals involved
Desires more independence and possibly own home	Occupational therapist, physiotherapist
Outdoor electric wheelchair funded and bought	
Environment assessment: ramp into family home	
Offer of housing from housing association	Social worker
Specific fitting and structures to be agreed.	
Care package to be defined/negotiated	Occupational therapist, social worker
Benefits to be sorted	
Taught to manage own health, own home.	
Fear of hospitals, of men, of anxiety, isolated	Psychologist
Assertiveness training	Doctor
Evening meetings with young people at Young Adult Team	Doctor – others of team
Urological problems	
Result: lives happily, independently, managing full-time work and some social activities. Drives own car	Doctor – urology clinic

52 *Providing training for employment*

J. McCarthy

INTRODUCTION

Unemployment is a national issue, and never far from the political agenda and close media attention. Finding a job is difficult for many people and for those with disabilities even more so. There is now a growing realization that employment opportunities should be available for people with disabilities who are well motivated and trained in today's skills. The disabled adult needs proper assessment and training, and subsequent integration in work. This chapter describes the improvements and the limitations of the new provisions, it also gives advice and information on how to access and use the new range of specialist services in the UK.

The Disabled Persons (Employment) Act 1944 and 1958 Amendment laid the foundations of the services that have developed since. The 1980s were a decade of progress, and in 1984 a *Code of Good Practice on the Employment of Disabled People* was published. The creation of a Disablement Advisory Service to facilitate good practice encouraged employers to give disabled people more opportunities for employment. There was the growth of assessment and rehabilitation services, ASSET Centres, with a more professional and client-centred approach to rehabilitation processes, and also the introduction of a sheltered placement scheme supporting people with severe disabilities within many firms. There has been a substantial expansion in services such as those providing technical aids to overcome barriers to work, and a welcome increase in the number of schemes to train people for employment. More recently Placing Assessment and Counselling Teams (PACTs) have been set up to provide local integrated services and an Agency Rehabilitation Network has been introduced. The Constitution of the Committees for the Employment of People with Disabilities (CEPDs) has been strengthened and the new Jobseeker's Charter to raise standards of service of jobcentres was introduced in 1994. The Government's Consultation Document (Employment and Training for People with Disabilities, 1990) was an important innovation in providing a comprehensive review of assessment, rehabilitation, training and employment. The Document addressed many of the employment issues affecting the daily lives of disabled people and has led to many improvements. However, largely through ignorance, discrimination still prevails.

Society is becoming increasingly aware of the role that Government must play in recognizing the value of the individual. The Citizen's Charter, the attempted Civil Rights (Disabled Persons) Bill 1994 and the subsequent Consultation Document (1994) have

Rehabilitation of the Physically Disabled Adult. Edited by C. John Goodwill, M. Anne Chamberlain and Chris Evans. Published in 1997 by Stanley Thornes (Publishers) Ltd, Cheltenham. ISBN 0-7487-3183-0.

brought into sharp focus our responsibility to see that every individual must have the opportunity to become as effective a contributing member of society as is possible. At the time of writing, the UK Government favours voluntary self-regulation backed by a statutory right to protect disabled people against unjustified discrimination in employment with respect to recruitment, transfer, dismissal, training, career progression and general treatment at work. The Government considers that a workable and beneficial employment right should be based on a definition that:

1. It is confined to people who have a substantial and long-term disability, or a disability which has substantial or long-term effects.
2. In principle it covers physical, sensory and mental impairment.

3. It is straightforward and easy to interpret.

Progress by some member states within the European Union towards the equalization of opportunities and independent living for disabled people, strengthened by legislation and practice, has already led to greater self-empowerment. More details of the European dimension are contained in the first issue of HELIOS magazine (Helioscope, Summer 1994), the text of which is also available on audio cassettes and diskette.

EMPLOYMENT ISSUES

As shown in Figure 52.1, the population of working age is growing quite slowly whilst the population aged 16–19 has decreased sharply from the high levels of the early 1980s to reach its lowest point of 2.6 million in

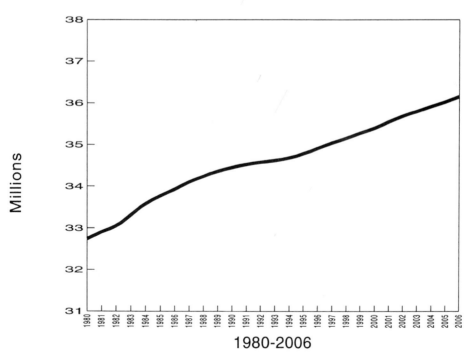

Figure 52.1 Working population – all ages, Great Britain. (Figures supplied by the Employment Service, Sheffield: men aged 16–64 and women aged 16–59 years. Source: Employment Gazette, April 1994.)

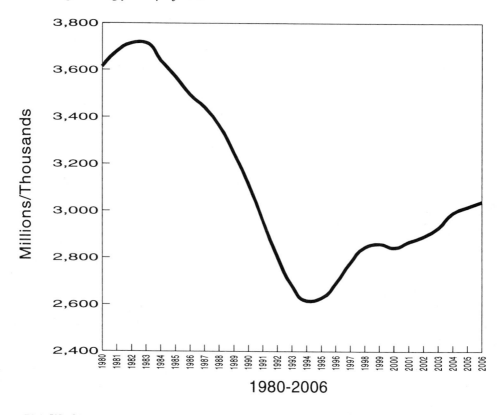

Figure 52.2 Working population aged 16–19 years, Great Britain. (Figures supplied by the Employment Service, Sheffield. Source: Employment Gazette, April 1994.)

1994 (Figure 52.2). At the same time it is evident that more students of the post-16 age group are staying on longer in full-time education; currently this has been put as high as 70%.

Already many employers are reporting shortages of certain skilled people. It is predicted this will get worse in years to come. There is a need for better training of people, including those with disabilities; underlying demographic pressures render this group, if well trained, a valuable economic resource. Surveys by the Office of Population Censuses and Surveys (OPCS) published during 1988 and 1989 have found that there are over six million disabled people in the UK, about two million of whom are under pensionable age. These figures com-

prise people with a wide range and degree of disability. Unfortunately, the general perception of disability as a single entity has given rise to many misconceptions where a disabled person is synonymous with a wheelchair, whereas the majority would not even be recognized as disabled. The Social and Community Planning and Research (SCPR) study *Employment and Handicap* (Prescott-Clarke, 1990) greatly increased our understanding of the types of disability people have in the key areas outlined in Table 52.1.

The SCPR Study considered those who were economically active and having a health problem or disability that affected the work that they could do. The Study put the number of self-declared people with disabilities at 1 272 000, of whom 845 000 were

Table 52.1 All people with disabilities[a]

Key areas[b]	%
Limbs, back or head	52
Respiration	18
Circulation	13
Skin condition	12
Digestion	10
Depression/anxiety	10
Hearing	9
Sight	7
Mental handicap	3
Mental illness	3

[a]Some people have more than one disability.
[b]Source: Social and Community Planning and Research Study, 1990.

employees and 142 000 self-employed; this left 285 000 not in employment, but who wanted to work – that is 22% of the total. The chances of someone with a disability being unemployed are significantly higher than somebody without one, and the ratio has been put as high as 4:1. Consequently, it is essential that disabled people are trained in a range of high-technology skills, where appropriate, to improve their chances of employment.

A University of North London survey cited in *Disability Now* (the national disability newspaper published by Scope, formerly the Spastics Society, London) in August, 1993 highlighted the perceptions of people with disabilities and found that they placed 'fear of discrimination' as the main reason preventing them from looking for or obtaining employment. Lack of support and inadequate training also featured strongly (Figures 52.3 and 52.4). 'But some "barriers", such as lack of suitable jobs, are myths' (Figure 52.5).

Fear of discrimination and lack of confidence continue to thwart the desire of disabled people to find and keep jobs (Friend, 1993) and inhibits many people with disabilities from taking full advantage of training and employment opportunities. Lack of self-confidence and low self-esteem can often be more of an obstacle to an individual than a disability. Furthermore, the poverty trap is also a recognized barrier to employment, with potential employees

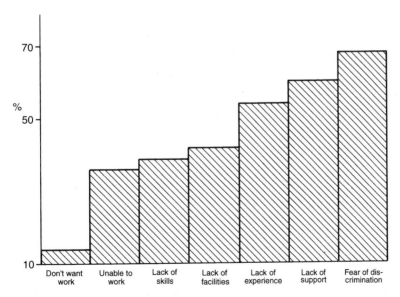

Figure 52.3 Reasons for disabled people not seeking employment. Reproduced with permission from *Disability Now*, August 1993.)

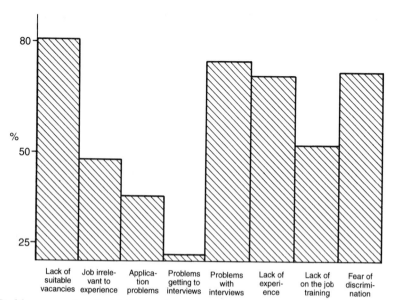

Figure 52.4 Problems seen by disabled people as barriers to employment. (Reproduced with permission from *Disability Now*, August 1993.)

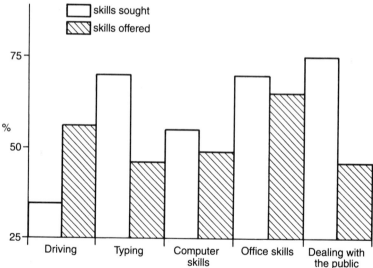

Figure 52.5 Skills sought by employers/skills offered by disabled job seekers. (Reproduced with permission from *Disability Now*, August 1993.)

being better off living on benefits than in low-paid employment. However, this is likely to be less so in the future as steps have already been taken by the UK Government, particu-larly with relation to payment of unemploy-ment benefit, income support and invalidity benefit. A Jobseeker's Allowance published in a Government White Paper in 1994, will make payment of benefits dependent upon claimants making determined efforts to find work. Additionally, claimants of invalidity benefit will be required to complete a questionnaire about their ability to carry out work-related activities and, where appropriate, will be referred to the Benefits Agency Medical Services for further assessment. Thus for some there is likely to be a greater requirement for training.

The SCPR Study *Employment and Handicap* reports that 42% of people with disabilities have no qualifications compared with 32% for non-disabled people. Thus vocational training as a preliminary to employment is essential for many people with disabilities and an advantage to most. The idea that disabled people are capable of only designated unskilled work is entirely mistaken and must be abandoned for all time. On the contrary, they reach a standard of skill which compares favourably with, if it does not surpass, that of the able bodied. Too often trainers and employers are prone to assess the capacity of disabled people by considering what they cannot do rather than concentrating on abilities.

There is now an opportunity and a real potential for people with disabilities and learning difficulties to achieve successful outcomes because:

1. Demographic trends have highlighted the advantages of employing well-trained disabled people: an important economic resource. Skills shortages can be adequately filled by people with disabilities.
2. New technology has changed traditional roles in work and altered patterns of employment. Technology is readily accessible as an aid to learning and employment for disabled people.
3. The new system of competence-led National Vocational Qualifications makes opportunities for successful outcomes accessible to all.
4. Changing attitudes and perceptions held by employers, society in general and approved trainers of what people with disabilities and learning difficulties can achieve, are becoming more evident in mainstream provision.
5. Growing problems of skills shortages in the manufacturing and service sectors in the UK could prove a serious impediment to economic recovery.

REFERRAL

The best advice one can offer to a person with a disability who has been out of a job for some time, or who is seeking training or employment, is to make contact with the Disability Employment Adviser (DEA) at a local jobcentre. There is no formal process or form to fill in; anybody can refer a client to a DEA – a telephone call or letter will suffice. The only requirement is that the client has a physical or mental health problem or learning difficulty which affects his or her ability to find or retain employment. It also helps if the referrer can advise why the referral is being made, and how the DEA might assist successful rehabilitation.

The DEA provides occupational help and advice and can either assess ability directly or arrange for a more detailed assessment by the local Placing Assessment and Counselling Team (PACT). For example, some clients need a gradual reintroduction to the world of work, perhaps vocational training for an occupation, help in finding employment or the provision of special equipment to help them into a job. For those who, because of the severity of a disability, cannot be as productive as other workers, supported employment is available. Moreover, the Supported Placement Scheme also offers integrated opportunities to disabled people to work in a normal open employment environment. If necessary, a DEA can register a client as a disabled person, and it is worth stressing here that registration now affects only those quota obligations and supported employment rules where participants have to be registered; other than these requirements and obligations a disabled person need not register. DEAs can help anybody, whether employed or unemployed, providing the person has a physical or mental health problem or learning difficulty which affects their capacity to find or retain employment. Consultants and general practitioners seeing employed people in this latter category, where health is a factor in continuing in a particular job, should make referral to the DEA before rather than after the job has been lost (R. Frost, 1994, personal communication).

ASSESSMENT AND EMPLOYMENT REHABILITATION

Based on a client's wishes and ideas, assessment leads to an agreed Action Plan for training or work drawn up by the DEA. This might well include skills and aptitude tests conducted by the PACT and a one-day verification of skills and potential with the emphasis on ability not disability. Proper assessment is the key to successful rehabilitation and vocational progress; it is essential to identify and overcome barriers to vocational progress which may result from poor literacy and numeracy, the absence of work experience or the inability to maintain the structured routine of a normal working day. There may be other factors in addition to these which cause lack of confidence and create emotional barriers to training or work. However, many of the identified barriers can be overcome.

Employment rehabilitation for up to 5 weeks is now available through a network of providers. For example, at St Loye's in Exeter, the rehabilitation programme will be undertaken by vocational trainers and occupational therapists through an evaluation of vocational preferences and interests, followed by interview with the programme manager to confirm needs, discuss options,

negotiate and agree a programme based on the client's Action Plan. Individual programmes are devised as required from the following elements of the overall rehabilitation process:

1. Evaluation of existing work skills, work habits, interpersonal and social skills and potential for employment.
2. Evaluation of work-related capabilities, including personal mobility, self-care skills, adult learning, literacy and numeracy.
3. Independent living and community skills, including self-awareness, managing disability, personal activities, daily living and team working.
4. Work simulation incorporating work tolerance, work hardening, stamina, work adjustment, work habit and opportunities to experience the wide variety of vocational options available through appropriate specialist or mainstream provision.

Alternatively, programmes can be organized on a one-to-one basis with an employer or through group-based sessions to confirm that stamina, physical and mental capacity are sufficient to sustain a working routine. Voluntary work can provide a structured activity for some clients as an opportunity to refresh skills used in the past and to learn new ones.

A programme 'Access to Work' offers practical help for disabled people and their employers. The programme is administered by the PACTs; it offers financial help in a variety of ways to suit individual needs and circumstances. Examples of arrangements that can be made are as follows:

1. Providing communicators for the deaf or partially deaf people at work as well as for job interviews.
2. Paying for blind or partially sighted people to have a part-time reader or assistant at work.

3. Providing a support worker to give practical help either at work or getting to and from work.
4. Buying or adapting equipment to suit a disabled employee.
5. Providing alterations to premises or to a working environment and help towards taxi or other costs if employees cannot use public transport to get to work.

Under the new arrangements there is more flexibility in the ways in which help can be used for people with disabilities. Access to Work is for unemployed, employed and self-employed people who need to get a job, keep a job or make progress in their career – whether they are registered disabled or not. Access to Work is an innovative form of practical help of great potential value to enable more disabled people to access employment.

THE PRINCIPLES OF VOCATIONAL REHABILITATION

In planning for the successful life of a disabled person, it is not enough to consider the disability alone. Full consideration must be given to the psychological aspects that accompany disability. Experience over 50 years at St Loye's has shown that those who have faced a long period in hospital, a sudden traumatic injury or debilitating illness may develop personality traits that do not clear up easily and can be a barrier to work. Lack of self-esteem and loss of confidence are common, and in some instances there may be bitterness at having become disabled. These traits often override more obvious physical limitations and must be overcome if the goal of employment is to be achieved. In some cases the capabilities of the individual may be so physically limited that it is impossible for the person to leave home or other residential accommodation. Fortunately, with the advent of new tech-

nology and Government help, this does not preclude the opportunity of gainful employment, consequent satisfaction and dignity. Although one cannot underestimate the problems created by such circumstances, experience has shown that disabled people can be prepared for competitive employment through assessment, appropriate training, selective placement and, if necessary, with appropriate aids to employment to match their capacity.

Setting an achievable vocational goal as early as possible after disablement is most important. This should consider physical, mental, social and vocational expectations; all the factors must be addressed simultaneously. To be successful, a rehabilitation programme must aim to enable the person with disability to live and work within the limits of that disability and to use all their abilities.

Dame Georgiana Buller was a visionary; her principles of work rehabilitation, articulated over 50 years ago were:

1. Prolonged hospital treatment must be followed when required by short-term vocational training geared to today's employment needs.
2. A wide variety of trades and occupations must be provided to satisfy the varying needs of disabled people with differing educational standards.
3. Emphasis must be placed on ability – not on disability – to work at the highest possible level.
4. Disabled people must be allowed to compete on equal economic terms with the able bodied and paid the rate for the job.

The development of her two Colleges, Queen Elizabeth's Leatherhead and St Loye's, Exeter, where over 400 men and women are currently in training, bears adequate testimony to the soundness of the principles she expounded and championed.

VOCATIONAL TRAINING AND OUTCOMES

On the continent of Europe, further education and training opportunities for people with disabilities or learning difficulties are usually provided in specialized centres. This contrasts markedly with the pattern in the UK, which is primarily through mainstream, integrated provision. Provision for handicapped young people expanded rapidly following the publication of the Warnock Report in 1978 (Warnock, 1978). It emphasized a client-centred approach in preference to the more rigid statutory categories defined in the 1944 Education Act. The provision has been further improved with the publication of the 1993 Education Act and positive steps have been taken through the Further Education Funding Council and Higher Education Funding Council to ease entry to further and higher education and training for students with learning difficulties. It is also estimated in the Starts Database (DFEE-Moorfoot) that in 1993/94 there were 37 000 adults with disabilities in other mainly integrated training programmes. Provision by voluntary organizations and independent colleges has existed much longer and the needs, where appropriate, of disability groups are met through residential provision to satisfy educational, vocational and social requirements. The Association of National Specialist College (NATSPEC) was formed to promote such opportunities for students post-16 with disabilities or learning difficulties, within a residential setting where needed.

Most adults qualifying for the Government programme 'Training for Work', and who need residential provision, are identified by DEAs and all correspondence and applications for funding through the Residential Training Colleges' Unit budgets are sent through a client's DEA. Residential training is intended for adults with disabilities who, because of the nature or severity of their disabilities, would have difficulty in training locally; there is provision to suit all needs, as support and medical care are constantly available. This environment enables clients to concentrate on gaining occupational skills and vocational qualifications without worrying about the everyday needs arising from their disabilities. In addition to training, job search and placement services are also available to clients to ensure that they have a smooth transition from training into work in either open or supported employment.

In recent years the annual number of places available in vocational training for adults aged 19–63 has remained fairly constant: today the four Residential Training Colleges (RTCs) and 11 Private Training Colleges (PTCs) have some 1250 clients in training, the latter dealing in the main with sensory disabilities (visual or aural). The majority of these clients, (76%) are undertaking a programme of training for work in the four RTCs; the geographical spread of Finchale in the North East, Portland Training College in the Midlands, Queen Elizabeth's Training College in the South East and St Loye's in the South West ensures a good distribution of provision. The Colleges are well resourced and maintained; each has specialized by means of short vocational courses in training disabled people for today's jobs: and details of training programmes are set out in the *Directory of Residential Training for People with Disabilities* (Residential Training Colleges Unit, Newcastle, 1996). In the last five decades over 30 000 people with a range of disabilities – orthopaedic, sensory, neurological, medical, mental health problems and specific learning difficulties – have gone into employment in direct competition with the able bodied. Doors to opportunities have been opened to many who thought they had been closed for ever.

In the four Residential Training Colleges (RTCs) in the financial year 1995–96; 839 clients started a programme of training, 652 completed, 528 (81%) obtained approved vocational qualifications and NVQs and 253

(39%) achieved satisfactory outcomes – jobs, further education, supported employment or self-employment – within 3 months of completion. In the last 5 years three of the Colleges have each won a corporate National Training Award and four individual awards, reflecting commitment and excellence in quality training for today's skills.

The majority of severely disabled adults, particularly those who have been handicapped from childhood, can be helped to face life, often for the first time. A specialist residential training centre is often successful because not only can it give vocational training, but also it allows mental and social rehabilitation. Activities such as sport, recreation, discussion groups and other social activities all help to build confidence and prepare people to be independent. Residential provision is not always popular, and not always needed, often local arrangements are enough. Some do not wish to be separated from families, and for others there are financial penalties. For the residential training providers it is, of course, manpower and space intensive. However, residential provision is suitable for a significant minority of people, particularly for those who have an attendant psychological problem.

Trainees must have the potential to be self-supporting and be able to make a positive contribution to their local economy, but they need specialist help and support for a brief period whilst acquiring the skills to hold their own in employment. Residential provision, rehabilitation and vocational training remove most of the external pressures, encourage mutual self-help, engender camaraderie, boost confidence, self-esteem and sustain a high morale. The integration of training, medical, social, therapies, leisure and recreational provision on the one residential site is difficult, if not impossible, to achieve in a mainstream college or provider. The end result must be the creation of an environment supported by specialist expertise to deal properly and effectively with people with a wide range of disabilities, learning difficulties and their attendant psychological problems.

In addition to the work of the RTC Unit, improved facilities for people with disabilities are increasingly available through the 82 Training and Enterprise Councils (TECs) in England and Wales and 22 Local Enterprise Companies (LECs) in Scotland; regrettably, their disparate nature does not lead to any uniformity of provision for people with disabilities. Nevertheless, one is encouraged to note that nine TECs were recently presented with awards for improving the quality of provision for people with special needs in training at the NCVO Seminar in 1994. 'Releasing Potential Awards' were given to Birmingham, Bradford and district, Devon and Cornwall, Dorset, Hampshire, Milton Keynes, North Buckinghamshire, South East Cheshire, Suffolk and Wearside. Additionally, Manchester TEC has launched a new initiative to help find work for people with disabilities called 'Skill Shadow'. The TEC is particularly keen to pair trainees with people coming up to retirement. The initiative has the potential of providing another realistic opportunity to enhance the chances of employment and hopefully could be used to advantage elsewhere. Significant improvements in the performance of the TECs and LECs are now evident since taking over the provision of training programmes from the Training Agency in 1990, and disabled people have priority on all the Government's employment and training programmes.

EMPLOYER AND EMPLOYEE ATTITUDES

Some employers resist employing disabled people and some employees are similarly reluctant to work with them. These attitudes can be major hurdles to successful vocational rehabilitation. This emphasizes again the difficulties in legislating for equal opportunities. Studies have been conducted in many parts of the world on the effectiveness of disabled workers compared with the able bodied. The findings can be summarized as follows:

1. Disabled workers, selectively placed, are as productive as non-disabled workers.
2. They are no more prone to absences from work than their able-bodied colleagues.
3. They are not particularly prone to suffer minor work injuries.
4. Injuries at work are no more serious for disabled workers.
5. They do not constitute a hazard to their fellow workers.
6. They do not lose more time than able-bodied workers when injured.

Training, experience, personality, temperament and motivation are the factors that count most for success in a job.

The Disabled Persons (Employment) Act is the only Parliamentary legislation that has tried to tackle the issue of discrimination in employment. It was 50 years old on 15 August 1994. The Act set out a quota system whereby 3% of employees in firms with 20 or more employees should be registered disabled. For several reasons, and not only those laid at the door of employers, the Act has been unworkable. The Civil Rights (Disabled Persons) Bill (1994) proposed measures to protect disabled people against discrimination. The Government rejected it on the grounds compliance would cost 17 billion. RADAR's document ('What Price Civil Rights?', as cited by Finn (1994)) states the true cost would be nearer 5 billion.

In the Consultation Document, reported at the beginning of this Chapter, the Government has proposed measures to replace the quota system through more enlightened recruitment policies. Many organizations are reporting progress, for example the Employers Forum on Disability, the BBC, the Disability Information Trust, Disability Matters, the Coverdale Organisation and the Head Work Centre. There is now every hope that 'Those who failed to take up the

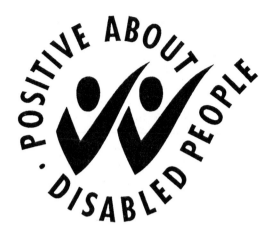

Figure 52.6 The disabled symbol.

challenge of employing disabled people will, like the Dinosaur, and the quota system introduced by the 1944 Act, eventually become extinct' (Duckworth, as cited by Finn (1994).

There is some evidence that awareness is being raised because there is a growing number of employers using the symbol 'Positive about Disabled People': the National List of Disability Symbol Users was 950 as at July 1994 (Figure 52.6).

Employers wishing and qualifying to use the symbol make five commitments to action.

1. To interview applicants with a disability who meet the minimum criteria, for example, qualifications and experience.
2. To ask every disabled employee, at least once a year, what can be done to ensure that they can develop and use their abilities at work. This can be done, for example, through staff appraisal and development programmes and through full consultation with disabled employees.
3. To make every effort, if employees become disabled, to ensure they stay in employment. This might include amending job content, altering hours or devising different ways of carrying out the work.

4. To take action to ensure that key employees develop the awareness of disability issues needed to make the five commitments work. Key employees include people such as line managers and personnel officers who would benefit from a greater awareness of disability issues.

5. Each year, to review these commitments and what has been achieved, plan ways to improve on them and let all employees know about progress and future plans.

The first four commitments are a starting point. The final one is the key to finding out what progress is being made towards implementing them, identifying opportunities and problem areas and planning further progress. The overall aim of the commitments is to eliminate discrimination on a voluntary basis and enhance the chances for people with disabilities at work and in career development (Frost, 1993).

The Disability Rights legislation (The Disability Discrimination Bill (1995)) received Royal Assent in November 1995. The Act introduces new rights to end discrimination in employment, education, public transport and access to public goods, facilities and services. It will also consider access to buildings and ease of travel. The employment code of practice of this Act was implemented in 1996.

The Cabinet Office published *Focus on Ability: A Practical Guide to Good Practice In the employment of disabled people* in 1994. The Guide is intended to complement the 'Programme for Action To Achieve Equality and Opportunity in the Civil Service for Disabled People'. It is of value as a code of good practice and also as an information resource. The Employers Forum on Disability has published *The Action File* (1993), a comprehensive guide to help employers recruit, train and develop disabled people.

CONCLUSION

For over 50 years the voluntary sector in the UK has been influential in the provision of proper assessment and training for work of a significant minority of disabled adults. In the main, such training, where numbers have remained fairly static, has been of a specialist nature and residential, in contrast to the substantial growth of integrated mainstream provision during the last decade.

Attitudes to disability have moved a long way. Disability issues are more clearly understood and the Government's recent Consultative Document and legislation suggest a more serious intent to tackle discrimination in employment and elsewhere.

Experience has shown that the capacity of an individual often exceeds expectations, and the growth of advanced technology training can keep clients' objectives and aspirations high so they can access national vocational qualifications in today's skills. By concentrating on ability, drawing out talent, building confidence and creating the atmosphere to develop self-esteem trainers can open doors to opportunities which many disabled people believed were closed for ever.

REFERENCES

Cabinet Office (1994) *Focus on Ability: a practical guide to good practice in the employment of disabled people*, Cabinet Office, OPSS, London.

Code of Good Practice on the Employment of Disabled People (1984) Employment Service Sheffield (revised and reprinted February 1990).

Consultation Document on Government Measures to Tackle Discrimination against Disabled People (1994). The Disability Unit, The Adelphi, 1–11 John Adam Street, London, WC2N 6HT.

Employment and Training for People with Disabilities (1990) Department of Employment, London.

Finn, W. (1994) Not in our organisation. *The Times*, 11 August.

Friend, P. (1993) "What the job barriers are and how they can be overcome". *Disability Now*, August 1993.

Frost, R. (1993) Fit for work. *Devon Link*, Winter.

Helioscope, Summer (1994) HELIOS Information Service, 79 Avenue de Cortenberg, B-1040 Brussels, Belgium.

Prescott-Clarke, P. (1990) *Social and Community Planning and Research (SCPR) Study – Employment and Handicap*, SCPR, London.

Residential Training Colleges Unit, Newcastle: *Directory of Residential Training for People with Disabilities*, Government Office for the North East Newcastle.

Starts Database (1993/94) (A. Blacklock, Special Needs Branch, October 1994) Department for Education and Employment, Moorfoot, Sheffield S1 4PQ.

Employers Forum on Disability (1993) *The Action File: barriers to employment of disabled people*, University of North London.

Warnock, H.M. (1978) *Report of the Committee of Enquiry into the Education of Handicapped Young People*, HMSO, London.

INFORMATION

Association of National Specialist Colleges (NATSPEC)
Secretary, Welsby Hall FE College, Grimsby, DN32 9RU, UK.

BBC Disability Programmes Unit
Room 1507, Television Centre, Wood Lane, London W12 7RJ, UK.

Coverdale Organisation plc (Management training and leadership development)
St James Court, Wilderspool Causeway, Warrington WA4 6PS, UK.

Disability Advertising Campaign 1994
For details of materials and videos available contact: Disability Services Branch (DS1), Level, 1, Courtwood House, Silver Street Head, Sheffield, S1 2DD, UK.

Disability Information Trust
Mary Marlborough Centre, Nuffield Orthopaedic Centre, Windmill Road, Headington, Oxford, OX3 7LD, UK.

Disability Matters
Berkeley House, West Tytherley, Nr Salisbury, Wiltshire SP5 1NF, UK.

Employability Awards
Opportunities for People with Disabilities, 1 Bank Buildings, Princess Street, London EC2E 8EU, UK.

Employers' Forum on Disability
Nutmeg House, 60 Gainsford Street, London SE1 2NY, UK.

Focus on Ability Appendices I–VIII
Details of organizations, videos, bibliography and literature on disability issues. Cabinet Office (OPSS).

Head Work Centre
Alexandra Warehouse, The Docks, Gloucester GL1 2LG, UK.

Information of Disability and Employment: Available from local Placing Assessment and Counselling Teams (PACT) at local Job Centres.

1. Guide to Employment Department Group
2. The Employment Service: an introduction to its services
3. Access to Work – practical help for disabled people and their employers
4. Role of Committees for the Employment of People with Disabilities
5. The Role of The Ability Development Centres

Jobcentre leaflets (current):

1. Make It Work - Employment Advice for People with Disabilities (PCL 2 Rev 1) 1993.
2. Jobseeker's Charter (JCC 100) 1994.
3. Employing People with Disabilities (PGP 2 Rev 1) 1993.
4. Registering as Disabled (PCL 4) 1993.
5. Just the Job (EMPL – 48 (F)) 1993.

Management Development Scheme for those with disabilities
Fast-Track SCOPE, 16 Fitzroy Square, London, W1P 6LP, UK.

National Council for Voluntary Organisations (NCVO)
Regent's Wharf, 8 All Saints Street, London, N1 9RL, UK.

New Start (Working for People with Disabilities)
Disability Working Allowance, FREEPOST 1399, Slough S11 4LN, UK.

Royal Association for Disability and Rehabilitation (RADAR)
12 City Forum, 250 City Road, London EC1V 8AF, UK.

SKILL National Bureau for Students with Disabilities
336 Brixton Road, London SW9 7AA, UK.

Supported Employment Programme
Disability Services Branch, Skills House, 3–7 Holy Green, Off The Moor, Sheffield S1 4JA, UK.

53 The role of the social services and an overview of benefit entitlements

E. Evans

The chapter looks at the legislation controlling the provision of services and resources to disabled people and their carers by Social Services Departments in the UK. It considers the process of assessment that is the cornerstone for obtaining services and resources. Case examples are used to illustrate the assessment and range of resources available. The Appendix at the end of the chapter outlines the financial benefits obtainable through the Department of Social Security (DSS).

LEGISLATION

Legislation provides the framework for the provision of services, resources and for service delivery. It is helpful to have an understanding of what services are covered and when local authorities have a statutory duty to arrange or provide a service or resource.

The National Assistance Act 1948 made it a duty of every local authority to provide residential care for certain categories of people, including those who are disabled. It gave local authorities the power to promote services for disabled people. This included informing people about available services, teaching people how to overcome some effects of their disabilities, providing work-shops and hostels, and providing recreational facilities.

The Chronically Sick and Disabled Persons Act (CSDP) 1970 placed a duty on all local authorities to keep a record of disabled people in their area and their needs. Under Section 2 of this Act the local authority, when satisfied that it is necessary to meet the needs of a disabled person, has a duty to arrange for the following: practical assistance in the home: help to obtain a radio, television, library or similar recreational facilities: transport to enable people to benefit from welfare services: adaptations to the home or additional facilities to 'secure greater safety, comfort or convenience', holidays, meals and telephones.

The Disabled Persons (Services, Consultation and Representation) Act 1986 was never fully implemented and only certain sections of the Act are in operation. Section 4 states that a local authority must assess the needs of a disabled person for any of the services listed above (under Section 2 of the CSDP Act 1970) if asked to do so by a disabled person, a carer or an authorized representative. Under Section 8 the local authority has a duty to assess the needs of carers when assessing the needs of the disabled person. A carer is defined as someone who is giving a substantial amount of care regularly to a disabled

Rehabilitation of the Physically Disabled Adult. Edited by C. John Goodwill, M. Anne Chamberlain and Chris Evans. Published in 1997 by Stanley Thornes (Publishers) Ltd, Cheltenham. ISBN 0-7487-3183-0.

person who is living at home. Section 9 extends the duty of the local authority to provide information about services, whether provided by the authority or by others. Section 10 of this Act states there is a duty to have consultation with organizations of (not for) disabled people and to co-opt people with special knowledge about the needs of disabled people on to committees.

Section 5 of the Act covers services requirements for people leaving special education and this will be covered elsewhere in this book.

The National Health Service and Community Care Act 1990 has had the most far reaching effects on the structure and service delivery of social service departments in local authorities. The Act aims 'to enable people to live as normal a life as possible in their own homes or in a homely environment in their local community, with the right amount of care and with a greater say in the decisions which affects their lives'. Local authorities have become the main agency responsible for assessing and designing appropriate care arrangements and securing their delivery.

The local authorities have the following duties to perform:- To consult with District Health Authorities, Family Health Service Authorities, other local authority departments, Voluntary Organizations and other interested parties; to prepare and publish a Plan of Community Care Services in their area, to take on responsibility for financial support of residential and nursing home care, to create units which have the power to inspect private, voluntary and local authority homes 'at arms length', to assess the need for Community Care Services, to assess for a financial change for the services as appropriate and to promote and use private and voluntary sector services as appropriate and to establish a formal complaints procedure.

The success of all these Acts has been limited. Legislation that gives power but not the obligation to promote services for disabled people has no real impact. Local budgetary issues may decide what services are developed and what are cut. Consequently, there is great variation between departments in provision of services and resources. In times of financial cutbacks, local authorities may choose not to afford non-mandatory services.

A social services department may meet its obligations in many ways. It may perform its duty by assessing need and recommending a service by another department. For example, a disabled person may be assessed as requiring a stair lift. Application may be made for a grant to the District Council. If the latter has no money available, a Social Service department may state it has no obligation to finance and provide the stairlift. They may opt to make arrangements for voluntary organizations, or indeed commercial ones, to provide services, such as meals or home care.

Voluntary organizations such as RADAR (Royal Association for Disability and Rehabilitation) provide information about entitlement to services and resources under the various pieces of legislation and will help people to pursue their rights.

CARE MANAGEMENT STRUCTURE OF SOCIAL SERVICES

Local authorities have responded by opting for different care management systems under the NHSCC Act and consequently there is a variation in the structure of departments. Some authorities employ social workers to be both assessors and purchasers of care packages. Other authorities require social workers to undertake only complex assessments of care. All have **care managers**, who have budgetary management, and decide which recommendations are to be carried out, with consultation where necessary from higher management. **Case coordinators** may be employed to arrange the details of the care package. They undertake simple assessments where the presenting need is not part of a complex situation. **Social workers** and **occupational therapists** form part of the teams providing the assessments, working with 'clients', families and other professionals to meet identified needs. Some departments have specialized teams and workers working with people with physical disability, others provide a generic service that encompasses people with disability. Similarly social workers may be located in a hospital or rehabilitation setting, or they may be placed in an area office from where they provide a service to people in the community and in a health setting.

Assessment of need for people with disabilities and their carers

Assessments can vary between the most simple and the most comprehensive, with a variable numbers of grades in between these. The National Health Service and Community Care Act 1990 states that the type of assessment response will normally be related as closely as possible to presenting need. There is one legally prescribed exception. Where a person is disabled under the terms of the Disabled Persons (Services Consultation and Representation Act) 1986, the local authority is required to offer a **comprehensive assessment**, irrespective of the scale of need that is initially presented. The term 'disabled' includes 'persons aged 18 over who are blind, deaf, or dumb or who suffer from mental disorder of any description and other persons aged 18 or over who are substantially and permanently handicapped by illness, injury or congenital disorder'.

The needs of unpaid carers are currently assessed as part of the assessment. This involves any personal or health worries, the contribution they are planning to make and what help they need to fulfil their role as a carer. The needs of carers are to be seen as distinct from clients. Their participation may be central to maintaining a care package and

in providing long-term continuity of care. Carers should be aware of what the disabled person is able to do unaided, supervised or aided. Clients will be able to participate in their assessments to a varying degree, and where necessary they and their carers should be given the help they require to understand and articulate their care needs.

The purpose of assessment

In the past assessment of need has been made in relation to existing services and resources, and consequently have been resource led. The National Health Service and Community Care Act (1990) states that assessments are now to identify an individual's need, and should not reflect available resources and services. In theory, therefore, services are to be developed to meet individual needs. It was hoped that a wider choice of options would be developed to enable more people to stay living in the community, and it was believed that to do so would be cost effective. Sadly, the reality is that current financial restriction results in identified needs not being wholly met by service provision. Distinction may have to be made between what is a need that **must** be met to enable a person to cope and what is a need that someone could manage without. For example, a priority need might be assistance with washing and dressing, whereas a need for extra domestic help might have lower priority.

Comprehensive assessments must remain needs related and be independent of any cost implications. Funding and provision of services and resources is constantly reviewed and frequently challenged. Legal battles are in process to decide whether local authorities can reduce existing services to disabled people where the need has been previously identified and has not changed. The outcome of such legal battles will clearly have major implications for future services and funding. Given this situation, clients need clear information about legislation. An advocate may be necessary to help them obtain their right to a service or resource. It is vital for future planning that statutory authorities record unmet as well as met need.

Who carries out the assessment?

Where the NHSCC Acts states a **comprehensive** assessment should be offered, this should be undertaken by a professionally qualified worker (Welch, 1991). This may be a generic social worker, or a specialist social worker who works with people with disabilities. Occupational therapists will also provide assessments, usually when the primary needs are for equipment and adaptations. Assessments will invariably involve liaison with other professionals, with the individual's consent, to facilitate a full understanding of the needs of the person in his or her environment. If a disabled person wishes to accept a **simple** assessment, usually for a practical input of service, this can be undertaken without a social worker.

What is included in an assessment?

An assessment should never be reduced to the completion of a checklist. It should start from the client's own perception of their needs, recognizing help may be required to identify needs. It presents the opportunity for the disabled person, with carer or advocate, to discuss the implications of disability, which may include the loss of independence, the fear of losing control, discussing future plans and looking at the options available to deal with these issues. An assessment not only results in the identification and consideration of ways of meeting them, but can in itself, have a therapeutic effect. The assessment will include biographical details. Racial and cultural differences should be acknowledged and provided for via access to a specialist advice if appropriate.

A **comprehensive assessment** should consider:

- personal and domestic skills;
- mobility;
- accommodation;
- legal matters;
- employment;
- finance;
- social and leisure activities;
- relationships;
- risk factors.

Existing or potential supporting networks will be explored. Good practice would involve sharing the written record of the assessment of need with the disabled person or advocate. The physical and mental health needs of the client will be taken into account. Often requests for assistance arise out of such problems and a referral to a health professional might be an integral part of the need of the client. Some understanding of people's own personal resources and how they have coped with previous difficulties may help in understanding the need in the current situation.

CASE HISTORIES ILLUSTRATING THE ASSESSMENT PROCESS IN MAJOR AREAS OF NEED.

Personal and domestic tasks

The dependency needs of the disabled person have to be identified in terms of washing, dressing, hair care, nail care, bathing, coping with menstruation, elimination, administering medications, as well as domestic tasks such as shopping, laundry, cooking, cleaning, collecting benefits and so on. Information about the type of help required for transfers, equipment used, the risks of falling, problems of access both internally and external is required. Information may come from professionals such as physiotherapists, nurses, and occupational therapists. This is important where memory or insight deficits are suspected, and the responses need to be verified.

The range of services provided by statutory services, private agencies or voluntary organizations can include home care, bathing, sitter (day and/or night). shopping, domestic help, meal provision, transport facilities, laundry services, alarm systems, telephone installation, respite care, day care, programmed care, holidays, befriending services and so forth. The health services will have responsibility for servicing some of the medical related needs, such as care of catheters, oversight of pressure care. Entitlement to financial benefits would also be discussed.

Local authorities vary in charging policies but there is usually an expectation that clients are assessed to contribute towards the cost, dependent on their finances.

Case history

Mr A was to be discharged to live alone following a stroke. He also received ongoing outpatient treatment for leukaemia. Although requiring assistance to put on his pyjama jacket, Mr A was able to cope with all other garments, but he needed assistance to get in and out of the bath and with washing his hair. He could make a hot drink and a cold snack but was unable to safely make a hot meal or cope with domestic tasks.

Mr A was understandably anxious about being left alone for long period. Informal help would be available from his married daughter who lived locally with her own family and who worked part time. She agreed to provide assistance with cleaning, shopping and some meals. Arrangements were made for a morning home care visit to check Mr A had washed, dressed and breakfasted. This was set up for a limited period to establish his confidence in coping alone and assistance to put on his pyjama jacket each evening was arranged. A local meals service was used to complement the provision of meals from the daughter. Assistance with a weekly bath was also arranged. The district nurse called weekly for medical reasons.

At the review meeting a month after discharge, Mr A opted to use his recently awarded Attendance Allowance payment to pay a neighbour to provide the evening assistance instead of receiving help from social services. The neighbour also agreed to continue the morning visit as Mr A found it very reassuring.

Mobility

It is necessary to know how a person gets around in their own home, in their locality and when travelling further afield, to establish what the person requires in the home for personal care tasks and what their transport needs are for participating in work and leisure activities. Benefit entitlement should be checked and sources of information about related subjects, such as driving assessments, the Orange Badge parking scheme, public travel and fare concessions provided. Other matters may have to be considered, such as person's safety moving around, and any problems of wandering, or other unusual behaviour which potentially poses risks.

Case history

Mr B suffered with cerebral ataxia and was wheelchair dependent and very heavy. He was unable to propel himself very far. His wife who was not strong, could not push him far because of his weight. Both wished to go in the car and for him to accompany her shopping. The assessment clarified the mobility and financial factors. Mr B was referred to a mobility centre and assessed as needing an outdoor powered chair and with equipment to enable his wife to get the chair in and out of the car. Funds had to be raised to help pay for the chair, the car hoist and shed to house the wheelchair.

Employment

Training, employment or reintroduction to former employment should be considered in a comprehensive assessment. Referral can be made with appropriate persons such as the disability employment adviser, employers, sheltered workshops, training centres and other local initiatives.

Loss of employment may affect the disabled person or the carer or both. The former may be unable to cope with returning to work and a carer may wish to cease work to fulfil their caring role. Implications are major in terms of the person's finance, role within the family, loss of work status, a sense of fulfilment and a way of life. Dependency on state benefits with a corresponding reduction in income can add to the sense of loss. The assessment process should provide the opportunity to discuss the implications for the person and the family and to identify what future support may be required. This may take the form of counselling, providing information about social security benefits and referral to appropriate organizations such as mentioned above.

Young disabled adults leaving school will have their training and employment needs assessed through the formal structure established by the Disabled Persons Act 1986 (Chapter 52).

Case history

Mrs C had short-term memory deficits following a subarachnoid haemorrhage. She was a trained nurse but had recently obtained a new job as a college lecturer. She was now unable to work at that level. She attended a local day centre, twice a week, where she did pottery and other craft activities. This helped with her concentration, confidence, and re-establishing social contacts. Working in conjunction with the community occupational therapist, arrangements were made for her to attend an open learning computer course and a memory group. A paid carer was also provided initially to supervise Mrs C with cooking at home. The long-term goal was to reintroduce Mrs C into her lecturer's job. In the event Mrs C found work as a nurse at a level determined by the local hospital.

For carers employment issues may have to be considered. For instance, what facilities and support are available to provide the necessary care for their partner to enable the carer to continue working? Those who feel they should stop working may wish to talk through the implications of becoming a full-time carer, which will almost certainly affect the financial status and the quality of future life.

Case history

Mrs D, a 60-year-old woman, had a severe memory problem following a subarachnoid haemorrhage. She could not be left safely at home without supervision. Her husband had 3 years to work before retirement. He queried the option of ceasing work and wished to talk through the anticipated problems of his wife's behaviour and his role if he opted to be a full-time carer. He also wanted to discuss financial issues – benefit entitlement and future pension entitlements. Channels for obtaining further information were set up to enable him to clarify these issues. In the event, Mr D decided to continue working and a care package was set up to cover his working hours which included day sitters, supervisions for Mrs D to undertake some simple domestic tasks and her attendance at a local day centre.

Financial factors

Disability has financial implications which have to be addressed. Financial problems which may have predated injury or illness, such as outstanding loans or arrears, may be worsened if the job is lost. For most people disability adds to their cost of living. Not all needs, for example, an outdoor powered chair, are met by State provision and to buy equipment or extra services can prove costly. Factual information and assistance to obtain benefits may be required.. Referral to other appropriate agencies, such as the Citizens Advice Bureau, for assistance with debt repayment may be made. Needs may be identified that can be funded through relevant statutory bodies such as an installation of a telephone or a help towards a holiday through social services. Where there is limited or no statutory responsibility, the need might be met by fund raising through charities.

The assessment ensures that people are informed of entitlement to State benefits and that relevant claims are made. The DSS is a separate organization from social services, although people often confuse them. Social services staff will try to guide people through the maze of benefits, and assist with problems relating to benefit entitlement. They may also refer to voluntary organizations established to undertake benefit advice. Social Security Benefits relating to disability are briefly described in the appendix to this chapter.

Sometimes an assessment identifies issues about a person's competence to manage their financial affairs. The disabled person may need a relative or carer to become either an agent or an appointee (depending on circumstances) to act on their behalf for their Social Security Benefits. This is set up with the DSS with clearly established guidelines. At other times a person has the mental capacity but lacks the physical means to manage their affairs. Information about Power of Attorney can be provided. The person nominates someone of their choosing, to deal with all or specified parts of their financial affairs.

In other circumstances the assessment may identify problems that need to be resolved through the Court of Protection. For example, when a person has money but does not have the mental capacity to manage their own financial affairs. Information about the Court of Protection can be provided to relatives. The inclusion of these aspects in a comprehensive assessment ensures that the needs of vulnerable people are protected, (Chapter 10).

Accommodation

Assessment here may consider needs for residential or nursing home placements, rehousing needs, alterations to existing housing, and claiming appropriate housing benefits.

With increased range of provision through community services more people can remain in their own home. This should hopefully be reflected in a reduction in the number of disabled people entering residential care. When such placements are required the assessment process enables the person and carer to identify care options. Each local authority will have its own procedures for determining the type of placement, residential or nursing, and procedures for arranging the placement. A contract of care is drawn up and signed by the disabled person, the provider of care and by Social Services. The funding of placements involves each future resident being assessed as to their contribution to the fees. Entitlement to State benefits is checked, with Social Services paying the balance which the client cannot meet. A ceiling is set as to the charges that Social Services will contribute and people with capital over a certain limit will pay the total cost of the fees.

If a nursing home placement is required to provide continuing medical care the payment of fees becomes the responsibility of the health services. This is an area that is currently being addressed by the health authorities and social services departments.

Other housing needs may be identified. A person living in an upstairs flat who becomes wheelchair dependent will have access problems, which may be resolved by referral to an occupational therapist, so a social worker will refer to and liaise with them. Liaison with other agencies such as housing associations may be required for rehousing, and letters of support confirming the needs are required from relevant sources. Entitlement for housing benefit should be checked.

Case history

Mr E was a tenant publican before he suffered a stroke. He was now unable to resume his employment and consequently lost his tied accommodation. While he was in hospital, liaison was made with the housing department. He became classified as homeless and was subsequently offered suitable accommodation. The assessment also included considering Mr E's needs for help to establish himself in the bungalow. It was necessary to apply for financial assistance through the Social Fund from the Department of Social Security and to arrange for Mr E to buy items of bedding and furnishings. The practicalities of the accommodation were addressed with the Occupational Therapists. One year on, as part of the reassessment process, a referral was made to the National Mobility Housing Scheme to enable Mr E to move and live near his married children.

Social and leisure activities

To neglect leisure times means that some disabled people are without any means of filling their day, increasing the sense of loss, grief and social isolation that may result from disability. Assessment has to address social and leisure activities and will need to encompass mobility and transport requirements to enable a person to resume former activities and club memberships. Volunteers may be required to accompany the disabled person, to help where there are communication difficulties, or indeed to assist with activities previously done independently. Information about specific resources available, such as organizations for fishermen, golfers and other sporting activities should be obtained.

The aim must be to promote integration within the community but sometimes a person may need assistance with using the toilet, or require more supervision than can be offered within a local club. In these situations day centres or specific clubs, with staffing to meet the needs of disabled people, may be more appropriate. The social needs of the carer must also be considered: carers need opportunities to retain former interests or develop independent ones.

Case history

Mrs F was severely brain damaged following a head injury but lived at home with her husband and three children. Her husband had given up his self-employed business to become her main carer. Mrs F required one-to-one attention because of her multiple problems and tendency to wander. She attended a local young disabled unit one day a week, but because the unit was unable to provide the necessary level of supervision, social services funded a carer to be with her there. The department also funded two afternoon sessions with a carer in her own home encouraging her to undertake some cooking activities. At a later stage when Mrs F no longer wished to attend the young disabled unit, the same carer was retained to undertake other activities locally, including swimming at a local hotel's leisure centre. Funding through social services and charitable organizations enabled Mrs F to attend a week's activity holiday, thus giving a longer period of respite to the family.

Relationships

Strengths and weaknesses of the patient's relationship, and attitudes about disability may be discussed if relevant or volunteered by either the disabled person or carer. For example, a carer who can encourage independence, or resume a collaborative relationship, or be flexible in their relationship, will have different needs from the carer who finds it difficult to come to terms with a partner's disability. Understanding previous personality traits and coping strategies is part of the assessment required to build up a picture about how people are likely to cope and where help may be required.

Potential areas of difficulties may need to be identified. Unresolved marital issues may precede the disability and re-emerge during the rehabilitation period or when planning discharge. Some people may be unable to provide certain areas of help, such as intimate care tasks, and it should be accepted that it is difficult to hold together marital and caring roles when such demands are made on the carer.

The following case examples of assessments of marital, sexual, parental and personal issues in relationships demonstrate some of the problems raised and support sought.

Marital issues

Occasionally couples may use the new situation to draw upon the supporting services to achieve separation. Sensitive discussions and assessments can enable both partners to be supported through separations.

Case history

Mr G explained his history of marital problems at the time of his wife's admission. Although he was prepared to help her return home he intended to use the opportunity as the time to separate. His stated intentions crystallized the future practical and emotional needs for his wife. A baseline for independent living was set with Mrs G and eventually achieved with the care package not requiring Mr G's participation. It included many leisure activities and the opportunity for on-going counselling.

Others couples may feel unable to separate and remain trapped in the situation. This is true for able-bodies people but the issues of dependency and of providing care because of disability adds to the difficulties. It is importance that both partners have the opportunity to discuss the problems and receive support, which may include counsel-ling as well as practical support, such as respite care.

Case history

Mr and Mrs I had a history of marital problems. He had had various affairs and they had been separated once. She had taken him back when he had to have treatment for cancer of the bowel. Mrs I had also had treatment for cancer of the uterus and suffered with angina. Following a stroke, Mr I needed total assistance with all his personal care, was wheelchair dependent and used a hoist for transfers. He had very little insight into his problems and con-stantly demanded attention. At the time of discharge various options were discussed with Mr and Mrs I but Mr I demanded to return home and his wife complied. A substantial care package was set up. Mr I spent 4 days at home with home care mornings and evenings, and 3 days and nights at a hostel for people with physical disabilities. Every 6 weeks he spent 10 nights at the hostel to give his wife a longer break. A ground floor bedroom bathroom extension was built for Mr I. Car hoists and wheel-chairs were sorted out. Whilst at home Mr I continually asked his wife to transfer him on and off the toilet and at night he would call for her continually from 5.00 am onwards. Not surprisingly, Mrs I felt trapped in her role and expressed a continual smouldering resentment towards her husband. She pro-vided intimate care for someone she not longer liked, although in some sense this gave her a feeling of power and control over him. Mr I also resented his position. He frequently told her he was having relation-ships (untrue) at the hostel and that he wished to leave her. Regular support and reviews have been maintained with Mr and Mrs I at home and at the hostel because of the intractability of these problems, the level of aggression displayed and the need to modify the care package at times of illness or extra stress.

Sexual issues

Assessments may also identify sexual issues. Some resist resuming a sexual relationship for fear that it may cause or exacerbate medical problems. This can often be resolved by discussion with medical staff. Other problems, such as inability to perform sexually, or coping with incontinence, may be discussed. It is important that people are given information and advice as to where to seek appropriate help.

Younger disabled people may face a different set of problems. Negative attitudes still prevail about their sexual relationships, with concerns expressed about risks of pregnancy and emotional repercussions of failed relationships.

Case history

Mr J, a 45-year-old man suffering with multiple sclerosis, was obsessed by his wife's refusal to have a sexual relationship. Mr J recorded any television programmes about sex and read all available information. Mrs J was contemplating separation because of her husband's changed personality and severely impaired memory. His lack of insight into the issues and his memory impairment made discussions difficult. Referral was made to the clinical psychologist who saw Mr and Mrs J jointly and separately over a period of time. Practical support was provided to enable Mr and Mrs J to spend time constructively apart from each other.

Parenting issues

Children may have difficulties coping with the fact that a parent has become disabled. Some disabilities involving communication and memory create particular difficulties in parenting. The Motor Neurone Disease (MND) Association have recognized this, and publish special booklets to explain MND to children of different ages.

Case history

Mr K, a father to two sons aged 11 and 13 years, had previously enjoyed many activities with them, he had enjoyed water sports with them and had participated weekly with their Cubs and Scouts groups and led many of the activities. Following his stroke, Mr K had no verbal communication and was unable to write or produce understandable gestures. For a long time he was emotionally labile and his tolerance was low because of the huge frustrations he experienced. Mr K felt a great need to prove himself capable and was often tempted to take unnecessary risks. As a result, Mrs K had many reservations about encouraging him to involve the sons in his activities. She felt she had become virtually a single parent, making decisions by herself. The communication problems made it extremely difficult for her to share decisions with her husband. She felt it would have been easier to have excluded him, but knew this was unacceptable because his comprehension was good.

She also expressed great sadness that her sons would probably in time have their memories of a good loving and active father replaced by memories of someone who had become unreliable, quick to express frustration and anger. She felt that from her sons' point of view, death may have been a kinder outcome. They could have grieved for their father and had memories left intact.

Further she recognized that their sons needed time and understandable information about what had occurred and why. They needed to know that they had not caused their father's stroke and be given the opportunities to be able to grieve for the losses they were experiencing.

Personal issues

An understanding of how people have coped with issues in the past, and the problems they have experienced enables the assessor to have a deeper understanding of how they may tackle current issues and what form of support they would like.

Case history

Mr L had been abandoned by his mother at birth. He had been raised in a Children's Home but also had spent long periods in hospital for treatment of tuberculosis of the hips. Although his mobility was restricted because of this, he could walk independently and drive a car. At the age of 50 Mr L married a young woman and had a daughter. Two years later Mr L suffered a stroke and with fixed hips he needed hoisting for all transfers. Mr L was an extremely anxious and demanding patient. He minimized the amount of care required and initially was reluctant to involve his wife in discussions about future plans. Appreciation of his childhood problems and the effects of institutional life enabled his behaviour to be understood. After discussion of his fears that his wife would not be able to cope, and that he would need institutional care, he was able to develop a more realistic and constructive approach and returned home with support.

Risk factors

It is important to identify risk factors. Some are aggravated by environmental hazards, as when using gas appliances if the individual has memory problems, or others are heightened by other health factors, such as epilepsy, balance problems, unsteady gait or because of behaviour which may result in aggressive tendencies or lack of cooperation. Where there is a loss of insight problems may be more apparent to others than to the client. Balanced judgements about the client's rights to make informed decisions, the risks to carers and the wider community and the possible overprotectiveness of others have to be made and decisions need to be based on the criteria laid down by social services and should be specifically recorded as part of the assessment.

Disabled people should make the decision about how they wish to live, providing they are aware of the risks that their actions might involve and have been informed the options of support available. The assessment will include the participation of other involved professionals such as nursing staff, therapists and medical staff, and take the form of a case conference. A written record of discussions and decisions should be made.

Case history

Mrs M suffered with rheumatoid arthritis and osteoporosis. Transfers were painful and difficult for her and she became extremely breathless after minimal exertion. She had a small pressure sore, her skin tissue was thin and fragile and a recent fall had caused several lacerations to her arms and legs. Mrs M was in hospital but wished to return to her home, although she realized that going to the toilet both during the day and in the night was going to be very difficult, that assistance to help her to the toilet could not be provided on demand and that there were increased risks to her pressure sore should she become wet. Mrs M did not want anyone to stay with her even if 24-hour care had been available to her in her own home. Mrs M's decision to live in her home was made in full awareness of her risks and various options for assistance. In the event Mrs M only spent a few days at home with the agreed care package before the situation broke down and she was readmitted to hospital. A residential placement was later sought.

Case history

Miss N had a brain haemorrhage following surgery to clip seven aneurysms, with resulting balance problems. She was advised to wear a helmet to protect her head (she had a piece of her skull missing from the surgery) as she had frequent falls. Miss N also had blackouts of short duration of which she was not aware and she experienced bouts of vomiting which were often prolonged and left her exhausted.

Miss N had little insight into any of her problems. She saw no reason why she should not drive, was determined to use an electric lawnmower and saw no difficulties in carrying hot pans or bending to use the oven (despite having to be saved from falling during cooking sessions). She saw no problems in her intention to use an electric mower to cut her lawn.

Miss N's previous personality and lifestyle did not help her to adjust to a very disabling state but her statements and behaviour suggested that most of her risks were due to poor insight. However, she was fully orientated and able to hold coherent discussions. To help resolve the issue she was seen by a psychiatrist for an assessment under the Mental Health Act. He stated there were not legal grounds to prevent Miss N from returning home.

Risk management of Miss N's discharge required full discussions and planning with the multidisciplinary team at a case conference. Risks and actions proposed were recorded in medical notes and on the social work assessment. The General Practitioner was forewarned of the problems.

A great deal of time and effort was spent with Miss N talking through the issues and encouraging her to accept a care package which she finally agreed to. This included regular input during the day and evening, and practical assistance for tasks with which she was at greatest risk. She also accepted a Lifeline alarm system. Extra input was available for times when she was unwell.

CARE PLANNING, IMPLEMENTING, MONITORING AND REVIEWING

Once the process of assessment has been carried out, the care plan can be designed and implemented. Clients should be given a written care plan defining the needs and objectives to be met by any service provider. Care plans should be regularly monitored to ensure the objectives are being met. This involves overseeing the quality of the services being provided, managing budgets and supporting clients, carers and service providers. Monitoring should be undertaken systematically and be recorded. At specific intervals the needs should be reassessed and changes in the care plan implemented as appropriate. This is especially relevant if the disabled person has undergone a stay in hospital. A reassessment of need rather than a resumption of former services should take place. Further review dates should be set and the findings of each review recorded.

SUMMARY

An assessment provides the means to identify needs which can then be met in a variety of ways. It is more than a matter of checklists, involving the active participation of the disabled person and carer. A relationship of trust and empathy has to be established: good counselling skills help with the assessment of the more sensitive emotional needs. Account must be taken of the attitudes and aspirations of the individual and the abilities of the person and carer (where appropriate) to cope. The outcome will be a series of recommendations for future actions to meet identified needs. Recommendations may include service delivery or mobilization of resources, and may include referrals to and liaison with other professions and organizations. Usually financial restrictions limit provisions and some prioritization of needs has to occur. Once the care plan has been implemented, it is monitored and reviewed. The process of care management and assessment, well done, is a most helpful tool, helping people who are disabled to pursue their lives more effectively, safely and congenially.

REFERENCES

Welch, R. (1991) *Care Management and Assessment, Department of Health and Social Services Inspectorate*, HMSO, London, p. 43.

Copies of the Government Acts quoted in this chapter can be obtained from HMSO Publications, PO Box 276, London SW8 5DT, UK.

USEFUL ADDRESS

The Royal Association for Disability and Rehabilitation
12 City Forum, 250 City Road, London ECIV 8AF, UK.

Appendix

Social Security Benefits

Attendance Allowance (Form DS 702)

This is a tax-free benefit for people **aged 65 and over** who need assistance and/or supervision with personal care because of disability or illness. To get this benefit people must normally have needed help for 6 months before claiming. It can be claimed regardless of savings or income. There are two rates of benefit, a lower rate is paid if assistance is needed during the day **or** night. A higher rate is paid if assistance is needed for day **and** night.

Disability Living Allowance (DLA) (Form DS 704)

This is a tax-free benefit paid to people **aged under 65** (a claim can be made for a person aged between 65 and 66 years if help was needed before the 65th birthday). To get this benefit people must normally have needed help for 3 months and be likely to need it for a further 6 months. It is not dependent on National Insurance contributions and can be claimed regardless of savings or income.

There are two components of the DLA.

- **Care component** is awarded if help is needed because of disability or sickness. This may be help with personal care, or with supervision because of things such as communication difficulties, memory impairment, or confusion. For people over 16 it can include preparing a main meal. The care component is paid at three levels depending on whether assistance is needed day and night, during the day or night, or for limited periods only.

- **Mobility component** is awarded if help is needed with getting around. The age range starts at five and the upper limit is as above. It is awarded if people cannot walk at all, or have difficulties in walking. It can also be paid if people can walk but need someone with them for safety reasons or to help them find their way. This can include people with learning disabilities, or with visual impairments. The two rates of the benefit reflect the assistance required.

Disability Working Allowance (Form DS 703)

This is a tax-free income-related benefit for people **aged 16 and over** who work for at least 16 hours a week and have a disability or illness that limits their earning capacity. It is not dependent on National Insurance contributions. The person claiming must be in receipt of one of the following: Disability Living Allowance, Attendance Allowance, War Disablement Pension with constant attendance allowance or mobility supplement, Industrial Injuries Benefit with constant attendance allowance, or have an invalid three wheeler from the Department of Social Security, or have been in receipt of Invalidity Benefit, Severe Disablement Allowance or a disability premium being paid as part of Income Support. The amount paid is affected by the amount of savings and is not payable if the person (and partner) has more than the allowed limit.

Invalid Care Allowance (Form DS 700)

This is a taxable benefit for people of working age but who are providing substantial care to a disabled person. It does not depend on National Insurance contributions. To get it the disabled person needs to be in receipt of a Disability Living Allowance at the middle or higher rate, or a Constant Attendance Allowance under the Industrial Injuries or War Pensions schemes or the Attendance Allowance at either of the two rates. The carer must be aged between 16 and 65, spending at least 35 hours a week as a carer, earning no more than 50 pounds a week and not be in full-time education.
See also FB 31: Caring for Someone?

Severe Disablement Allowance (SDA 1)

This is a tax-free benefit, normally for people of working age who have been unable to work for at least 28 weeks but cannot get sickness benefit because they have insufficient National Insurance contributions. It is paid to women under the age of 60 and men under the age of 65.
For further information see leaflet NI 152.

Statutory Sick Pay (SSP) (Leaflet NI 244)

If you work for an employer and pay Class 1 National Insurance contributions, SSP is usually paid after 4 consecutive days of sickness. It can be paid for up to 28 weeks although sometimes the employer's obligation to pay this can cease earlier. SSP is paid by the employer.

Incapacity Benefit (Form SC 1)

This is for people under pension age who cannot work because of sickness or disability. It can be claimed if a person works but cannot get Statutory Sick Pay from the employer or if they are self employed or unemployed. It

replaces Statutory Sick Pay after 28 weeks. There are different rates of payments relating to length of sick period and whether the highest rate of the care component of Disability Allowance is paid. Extra money may be paid for dependants and for age factors. Medical certificates are required and a medical assessment may be arranged by the Department of Social Security to assess a person's fitness to work.

There are various other benefits; information about these, and the benefits above, can be found in the following leaflets. All leaflets are obtainable from the Department of Social Security, listed in the telephone directory under Benefits Agency. Benefits entitlements change and the reader is urged to seek up-to-date information.

Other Useful Leaflets

Family Credit FC 1

Going into Hospital NI 9

Guide for the Blind and Partially Sighted FB 19

Guide to Income Support IS 20

Guide to Housing Benefit and Council Tax RR 2

Guide to the Social Fund SB 16

Housing Benefit RR 1

Incapacity Benefit SC 1 (replaced sickness and invalidity benefit)

Sick or Disabled? FB 28 (a guide to benefits if you are sick or disabled for a few days or more)

What to do after a death D 49

Help with NHS costs:
P11   NHS prescriptions
G11   NHS sight tests and vouchers for glasses
D11   NHS dental treatment
WF11 NHS wigs and fabric support
H11   NHS hospital travel costs

54 Housing

C. Turton

INTRODUCTION

Housing has been described as the key to community care. Successful rehabilitation for most people will involve a return to the community and for the majority of these independent self-contained accommodation is the cornerstone of this return.

Inadequate or poorly designed housing is taken for granted by most people. Whilst it may cause occasional inconvenience, it is generally accepted without question. Particular elements of housing design – for example, door widths or threshold details – have, until quite recently, been repeated across all house types without consideration for the need of those with physical or mobility problems.

Community care, improvements in medical treatment, longer lifespans and increasing personal expectations have combined to bring into question some of the basic design details in housing. A sustained but as yet unsuccessful campaign by a wide range of disability organizations has been mounted to amend the current Building Regulations. These regulations set certain basic minimum standards for new and rehabilitated housing in England and Wales. At the present time only new public buildings are required in the first instance to be accessible to wheelchair users. The object of the campaign has been to extend this requirement to housing generally.

PROVISION

No one should be under any illusions as to the scope of the problems that people with physical disabilities face in terms of housing. It has been estimated that at current rates of replacement it will be 2000 years before all of the existing housing in England and Wales is replaced. It is clear, then, that adaptation or refurbishment of existing stock for people with physical disabilities will remain a major factor in the provision of appropriate accessible housing.

There are, however, a number of housing providers which do specialize in purpose-built accessible or wheelchair-standard housing. These are mainly housing associations. The majority of housing associations only manage existing housing stock, just over 600 associations actively develop new housing. They range in size from small locally based organizations managing a handful of properties to large national groups with thousands of properties. The majority of the housing provided is intended for low income groups to rent. A significant minority of this housing is intended for special needs groups. Among these are wheelchair users. The National Association of Wheelchair Housing Associations Group (NATWAG) represents these providers.

Most wheelchair-standard accommodation is still located in the local authority sector. A

Rehabilitation of the Physically Disabled Adult. Edited by C. John Goodwill, M. Anne Chamberlain and Chris Evans. Published in 1997 by Stanley Thornes (Publishers) Ltd, Cheltenham. ISBN 0-7487-3183-0.

substantial proportion of this, though, is located amongst elderly persons, housing. Research carried out by Raglan Housing Association (1990) and Morris (1988) found that much wheelchair-standard stock owned by housing associations was one-bedroom accommodation. In addition, it was also found there was considerable under-occupation in that many of these properties were not occupied by a wheelchair user.

The private (owner occupied) sector provides a further housing option for disabled people. With the exception of one or two areas of good practice involving estate agents and voluntary groups, it is almost impossible to locate accessible housing. Finding appropriate housing becomes a lottery.

To begin with housing applicants who are wheelchair users should start at their local authority. Under the Housing Act 1996 a person who has a physical disability is likely to qualify as vulnerable. They should, therefore, receive advice and/or housing suitable to their needs. The ability of local authorities to respond to this demand is of course restricted by what is available to them. Many local authorities do not keep registers of accessible accommodation in their area. Whilst an application to the local authority should be pursued, the potential difficulties need to be recognized.

Local authorities, in providing advice or assistance, may use other agencies. Local authorities have on average nomination rights to 50% of housing association stock, often more on brand new developments. In addition applicants for housing should request from the local authority a list of housing associations operating in their area. They should find out what application systems are operated by these organizations as these tend to vary.

In all cases contact should be made with the many voluntary organizations which exist to support disabled people like SCOPE, RADAR, etc. who may be able to offer housing advice. Local housing advice centres should hold detailed lists of these agencies, or they may be contacted through their head offices (Chapter 55). In some areas disabled persons housing services (D.P.H.S.) have been established which aim to bring together a range of services for people with disabilities. Local authority housing or social services departments will be able to direct applicants to these if they exist.

The specialist providers have developed wide experience in both the design and management of wheelchair-standard housing. Successful integration or re-integration of people into society will depend not only on the type of housing available but also the support available to people to enable them to lead as full a life as possible.

DESIGN

Careful attention to design is vital in the construction of new-build housing and in the rehabilitation or adaptation of existing property. Adaptation of property will almost invariably have a particular person or client in mind. With new-build accommodation flexibility is the key to successful provision. Too often in the past strict attention to the established needs of one particular client has meant that the resulting new property is useful for only one person. In the event of the identified occupant moving on or dying the property is difficult to re-let or sell without substantial re-alteration.

What is necessary is careful attention to core design features which benefit all households irrespective of their ability or disability. Central to design is adequate space. Around these key features must be walls which can take fixed adaptations. The value of this approach to design is the flexibility it brings to the property. Subsequent adaptation or fine-tuning for successive occupants can then be achieved quickly and relatively cheaply.

The purpose of this chapter is not to provide a detailed design brief for wheelchair-standard housing, as this has already been done by a number of respected organizations, although some indicators are provided at the end of this chapter. Habinteg's Design Guide has been sold around the world and represents the sum of 25 years of design experience. A key to the success of the publication is its loose-leaf format. Habinteg recognized that product development and standards are constantly being revised. It is with this in mind that purchasers receive updated sections or even pages as the contents of these are revised.

A design guide should never be used to restrict an architect or building consultant. Instead, it should represent a set of standards or criteria which the building should reach as a minimum. Imaginative and innovative ideas which build upon these standards are how improvements can be made which can subsequently become the new standard.

For the majority of the population the use of a wheelchair will never be necessary. However, most people will, at some time in their lives, experience a mobility problem. This may be temporary or permanent. As people grow older the probabilities increase. Lifetime Homes are a form of housing design which addresses issues of accessibility and adaptability in ordinary or traditional housing. (The criteria for Lifetime Homes are available from Habinteg: see 'Useful Addresses' at end of Chapter.)

LIFETIME HOMES

The key design criteria for Lifetime Homes differ only marginally from those of a wheelchair-standard bungalow or flat. This serves to underline the point that the important design issues in housing are universal.

Key design criteria for Lifetime Homes (summary)

- Accessible external environment.
- Parking close to the property and capable of enlargement to 3.6 m width.

- Width of doors and hallways to meet Access Committee for England Requirements (Figures 54.1 and 54.2).
- Turning circles in rooms and circulation areas for wheelchairs (1.5 m).
- Walls capable of taking adaptations.
- Bathroom/bedroom ceilings strong enough to take a hoist.
- Stairs wide enough to take a stair lift.
- Bathroom designed to enable wheelchair user to use the toilet (Figure 54.3).
- Window sills no higher than 750 cm and windows easily operated.
- Electrical switches, sockets, etc. located between 600 and 1200 mm from the floor.

Like wheelchair-standard housing, Lifetime Homes are not built with one person in mind. Properly constructed, a modern house has a lifespan of up to 100 years. Within this time a wide range of occupants may be expected to live in the property. Nothing built today should compromise the basic Lifetime Homes criteria. To do so is to build in barriers to a significant element of the population.

There should be no illusions about the scale of the problem which faces physically disabled people who are trying to return to the community. New design which further restricts choice and access, often for the sake of small cost savings in construction, cannot be condoned.

DESIGN GENERALLY

In considering design the usefulness of a property for all occupants can encompass some of the following points:

- Incorporation of other key design elements for specific special needs groups can be readily assimilated into standard design for mobility or wheelchair-standard housing, without creating an institutional environment. This approach may include, for example, consideration over colour schemes for both decoration and fixtures/fittings which address the needs of partially sighted people.

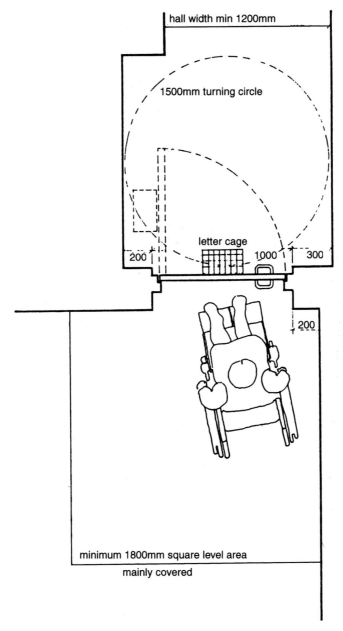

hall width min 1200mm

1500mm turning circle

letter cage

200   1000   300

200

minimum 1800mm square level area

mainly covered

Figure 54.1 Habinteg Design Guide for an entrance in a wheelchair user's dwelling. (Reproduced courtesy of Habinteg Housing Association Ltd.)

- Avoidance of sharp edges in fittings would bring benefits for those liable to falls as well as creating a safer environment for everyone.

- Consideration over types of fittings like taps or door handles and locks will improve ease of use for some and disadvantage none.

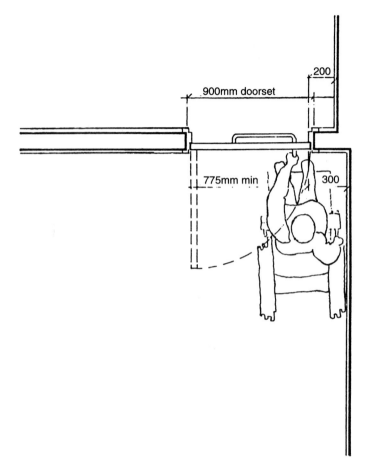

Figure 54.2 Habinteg Design Guide for an internal doorway in a wheelchair user's dwelling. (Reproduced courtesy of Habinteg Housing Association Ltd.)

- Fuseboards should always be provided not only in an accessible position but also with spare 'ways' to enable additional electronic environmental aids to be added later without major upheaval.

Adaptations

Much can be done with existing housing in terms of adaptations. However, this is always likely to be a relatively expensive option in which standards inevitably have to be compromised. Since most existing houses are different in some way it is not possible to generalize about what is and is not achievable. Variations in construction types and structural design mean that even in properties which appear similar, radically different solutions may be required to achieve comparable results.

Some public sector landlords have taken the opportunity presented by urban regeneration projects to rehabilitate numbers of old properties to Lifetime Homes standards. For the most part, though, adaptation will take place within individual properties. Some public funding is available to fund physical alterations to properties.

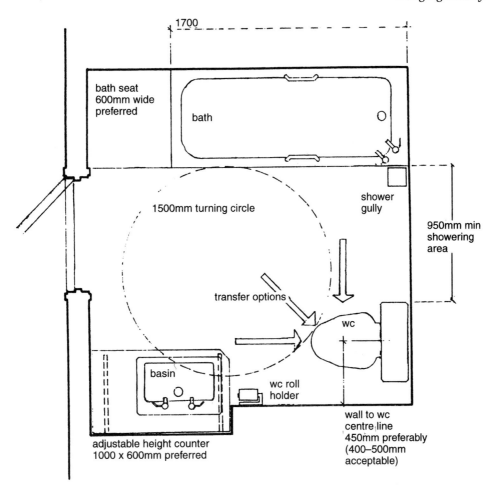

Figure 54.3 Habinteg Design Guide for a bathroom in a wheelchair user's dwelling. (Reproduced courtesy of Habinteg Housing Association Ltd.)

For local authority rented and privately owned stock, the Disabled Facilities Grant exists. The grant is means tested and most local authorities cannot allocate sufficient funds each year to keep pace with demand. Further rationing must then take place within the department administering the grant, usually the housing or environmental health sections.

For housing associations the Housing Corporation provides a non-means-tested grant for qualifying adaptations. Specialist associations which may make a number of applica-

tions in any given year bid for, and usually receive, a capital allocation to cover their projected need. Like many other forms of public spending this process is coming under review. It appears increasingly likely that this source of funding will be restricted to major adaptation works only. Funds for minor but equally important items, such as grab rails, will have to be found elsewhere – via the Disabled Facilities Grant process, other grants or from housing association's reserves.

Naturally, not all adaptations are structural or even fixed. Portable aids can be supplied by hospitals or social services departments. These items provided in conjunction with fixed items or adaptations to the building can add greatly to a person's independence and self-esteem. What is vital in this process is that the person requiring the adaptations is fully consulted at all stages and by all the professionals and advisers involved. The term client, whilst occasionally derided as impersonal, is certainly an improvement on 'patient'. It also serves to remind providers that even if the recipient is not paying or perhaps not able to express clearly their needs, every effort should be made to offer choice and to genuinely consult.

None of the above should preclude consideration of property adaptation as an option. Rehabilitation should, wherever possible, enable people to return to their existing homes. The case for more adaptable and flexible accommodation in all sectors is only strengthened by this maxim.

Consulting the community occupational therapist, general practitioner and housing or environmental health departments, is the first step in this process. Support from neighbours and family, location of the property in terms of shops and services and the accessibility of the local environment are all factors to be considered before decisions regarding adaptation of existing property or seeking alternative accommodation are made.

CHOICE IN HOUSING

For most people housing which offers the greatest independence is their objective. Unfettered consumer choice is perhaps an unrealistic target for practitioners and providers. However, within the constraints that all sectors must operate is an awareness of what might be available, and communication of these options and their consequences to consumers is vital if aspirations are to be met to any degree.

These options will include self-contained housing, self-contained clustered housing, shared supported housing, residential homes or adult placement.

For some people, training can make independent living a reality. A number of examples of good practice exist which set out, within a defined time frame, to offer support, training and advocacy to residents. In this way they can define for themselves what their housing needs and aspirations are. For such projects to succeed often requires joint working and support from a range of agencies committed to quality service delivery. In these cases the quality comes as much from the sum of the individual inputs, which is inevitably greater than could be achieved if providers had acted alone.

When the independent housing is chosen the availability of informal support and sensitive advice on housing and other issues such as care can mean the difference between genuine independence and empowerment, and enforced dependence. Specialist landlords can offer such advice. An awareness of what might be possible and where to look for the solutions means that effective management of wheelchair and mobility standard housing is much more than just being an ordinary landlord.

OBSTACLES TO A MOVE

Recent research (Hudson, 1996) highlighted **five key obstacles** which need to be addressed or overcome in disabled people achieving appropriate accommodation:

- fear of a major change of environment and living circumstances;
- poor planning and communication;
- lack of suitable housing;
- inadequate support to make the move;
- financial constraints.

Positive influences which the same research highlighted were:

- a committed professional;

- personal initiatives by the individual;
- established organizational pathways into housing.

HEALTH AND SOCIAL SERVICES PROVISION

Adaptations in detail

In general medical and nursing loans are obtained from the Health Service and aids to daily living from social services. Arrangements may differ from place to place and local provision should be ascertained. Some health authorities and social services departments operate a joint loans system with a common store accessible to professionals from both sources, for example Leeds supplies home nursing aids on loan through their Equipment Service. Common items include incontinence products, commodes and hospital beds. Contract should be made with the local health centre, the health visitor, the district nurse or general practitioner.

Equipment can be supplied direct by an occupational therapist or physiotherapist following a home assessment visit. The occupational therapist can provide aids to daily living and advice on home adaptations, the physiotherapist advising on appropriate walking aids and appliances. Communication aids are usually supplied through the speech therapist (Chapter 22). Environmental controls are supplied after assessment by a consultant medical assessor (Chapter 49).

HOUSING ADAPTATIONS

With any adaptation the client's prognosis and long-term needs have to be clearly established from the outset. With more severely handicapped persons the needs of the carer(s) take equal priority when determining appropriate adaptations. Usually a decision has to be made whether to adapt the existing house or to move to more suitable accommodation. In either case it is imperative that the household consult the community occupational therapist who will liaise with the consultant, General Practitioner, housing manager and possibly environmental health officer when making the decision to adapt or rehouse. Consideration should be given to the considerable support often given by neighbours and family, vicinity of shops and local resources and the amount of space inside the house.

Simple aids can be provided to allow a person to get up and down from the lavatory: these include raised toilet seats, toilet frames and rails secured to the adjacent wall at the height to meet the needs of the individual. When adapting for wheelchair use there should be sufficient space to allow wheelchair access, usually assuming a sideways transfer. It is important to note the method of transfer, and whether the person requires the assistance of a carer, to provide adequate space when planning for future needs. If an over-toilet chair is to be used then there should be no obstruction. Hardware can include a toilet-paper holder for one-handed operation, low mirror, lever taps on shallow hand basin, etc, to suit the individual needs.

Bathing

This is the most common area of concern since most elderly and physically handicapped people seek help when they are unable to bathe independently. The occupational therapist can assess needs. Most people are helped by simple aids, a non-slip mat, a bath board and seat and a grab-rail secured to the wall are provided, and the person is instructed in their use, the aim being to enable the person to enter and leave the bath safely, preferably from a seated position. When conventional aids are unsuitable then consideration should be given to bath hoists (Chapter 46).

Shower

In some instances where a disabled person cannot get up from the bath or bath seat an overbath shower may be suitable, provided the user can transfer onto a bath board to shower or stand in the bath with the use of grab-rails. When the use of mechanical hoists to get into and out of the bath has been discounted, then thought can be given to the removal of the bath and installation of a shower. The decision between a bath or shower is usually a matter of personal preference. However, with the more disabled person a toilet/shower chair can be used, eliminating a second transfer when using the toilet and giving good support. Where space is limited a complete shower unit can be provided, and is easily removed when no longer required. There are also a variety of shower bases available which allow access for mobile shower seats.

Folding shower seats secured to the wall allow the user to walk into the shower and take a seated shower when balance is poor. A shower bench will allow the user to transfer from his/her wheelchair into the shower.

Shower floors which have a slight incline to drain water away allow the use of over-toilet/ shower chairs which give easy access to the toilet and shower. The floor should slope approximately 76 mm to the drain outlet, and the surface should be non-slip. The shower must be thermostatically controlled and non-conductive grab-rails should be used.

Plumbed-in units are usually more suitable than the instant-heat types, provided the cold water tank is in the correct position to given a adequate water pressure. Appropriate controls to allow, for example, a rheumatoid sufferer to operate the shower independently, or the carer to remain outside the shower, should be provided. Shower chairs can be easily operated by the carer, or can be self-propelled by the user, giving greater independence and privacy.

Kitchen

Design should be carefully chosen in order to cut down the number of journeys and amount of energy expenditure each task entails. There are various texts covering this subject: *Designing for the Disabled* (Goldsmith, 1976), *An Introduction to Domestic Design for the Disabled* (Walter, 1970), and *Kitchen Sense for Disabled or Elderly People* (Conacher, 1986). Many books give recommended heights for kitchen design, but ideally the kitchen should be tailored to the individual's needs where possible. BSI standards for height apply only to people of average height. Several kitchen units are manufactured specifically for disabled people: contact the local Disabled Living Centre or local Disabled Persons Housing Service for information.

In summary, consumers should be offered as much choice as possible and given control over the processes of adaptation and housing generally. It is the environment which often compounds disability and enforces dependence. It is with this in mind that practitioners should operate.

REFERENCES

Conacher, G. (ed.) (1986) *Kitchen Sense for Disabled People*, Croom Helm, London for the Disabled Living Foundation.

Goldsmith, S. (1976) *Designing for the Disabled*, 3rd edn, fully revised, RIBA Publications, London [the standard book on the subject].

Habinteg, H.A. (1992) *Design Guide*, London.

Hudson, W.A. (1996) *Moving Obstacles*, Joseph Rowntree Foundation, York.

Morris, J. (1988), *'Freedom to Lose'*, Shelter, London.

Raglan Housing Association Ltd. (1990) *Survey of Wheelchair Housing*, NATWAG, London.

Walter, F. (1970) *An Introduction to Domestic Design for the Disabled*, Disabled Living Foundation, London.

FURTHER READING

Access Data Sheets: (1) Approach to buildings; (2) Doors; (3) Internal circulation areas; (4) Lifts; (5) Internal staircases; (6) Lavatories; (7) Auditoria; (8) Induction loop systems; RADAR, London.

CEH (1995) *Access for Disabled People: design guidance notes for developers*, Centre for the Accessible Environment, London.

Chartered Institute of Housing/RIBA (1988) *Housing Design Brief: Housing for Disabled People*. 8th Revision.

Department of Environment (1974) *Mobility Housing*, DOE/HDD Occasional Paper 2/74, HMSO, London.

Designing for Disability: (1) *Entrances;* (2) *Windows;* (3) *Bathrooms* (4) *Kitchens;* (5) *Floor finishes;* (6) *Bedrooms;* (7) *Lifts;* (8) *Controls;* (9) *Safety*, Centre for the Accessible Environment, London.

Hunt, J. (1980) *Housing the Disabled*, Torfaen Book Co., Cwmbran, Wales.

Penton, J. and Barlow, A (1980) *A Handbook of Housing for Disabled People,* 2nd edn, Housing Consortium West Group, London.

Tarling, C. (1980) *Hoists and their Users*, Disabled Living Foundation, London.

Thorpe, S. (1981) *Access in the High Street: advice on how to make shopping more manageable for disabled people*, Centre for the Accessible Environment, London.

Selected legislation: housing and environment

Practitioners in this field should be aware of the following:

Childrens Act 1989.

Chronically Sick and Disabled Persons Act 1970 – Sections 1, 2, 3–8.

Disability Discrimination Act 1995 [Relates to access to goods, facilities and services. Copies of a brief guide to the act (Disability on the Agenda) Obtainable from FREEPOST Bristol BS38 7DE, UK.]

Disabled Persons Act 1981 – Sections 1, 2, 3, 4, 5, 6, 7.

Disabled Persons (Employment) Act 1944 – Section 1.

DOE Circular 10/90 (1990) House adaptations for people with disability.

Local Authority Social Services Act 1970.

Local Government and Housing Act 1989.

National Assistance Act 1948 – Section 29.

NHS and Community Care Act 1990.

Housing Act 1996

Housing Act 1957.

Note: All except the Disability Discrimination Act are available from HMSO Publications, PO Box 276, London SW8 5PT.

USEFUL ADDRESSES

Centre for the Accessible Environment, Nutmeg House, 60 Gainford Street, London SE1 2NY, UK.

Department of the Environment, 2 Mashan Street, London, SWID 3EB, UK.

Design Centre Design Council, Haymarket House, 1 Oxenden Street, London SW1Y 4EE, UK.

Disabled Living Foundation (DLF), 380–384 Harrow Road, London W9 2HU, UK.

Habinteg Housing Association, 10 Nottingham Place, London W1M 3FL, UK.

Hull City Council, Urban Regeneration Programme, Anchor House, The Maltings, Sylvester Street, Hull HU1 3HA, UK.

The National Association of Wheelchair Housing Associations Group (NATWAG), 10 Gloucester Drive, London N4 2LP, UK.

Royal Association for Disability and Rehabilitation (RADAR), 12 City Forum, 250 City Road, London EC1V 8AS, UK.

SCOPE 12 Park Crescent, London W1N 4EQ, UK.

Transhouse, c/o Robert Jones and Agnes Hunt Hospital, Oswestry, Shropshire SY10 7AG, UK.

55 *Resources and support information*

M. Winchcombe and C. Evans

INTRODUCTION

'Knowledge itself is power' (Francis Bacon 1561–1626). It is widely perceived that there is lack of knowledge about disability. In fact, there is plenty of information available about conditions, treatments and help, but the route to it is confused and duplicated. A Department of Health initiative (National Disability Information Project 1991–1994) was set up to encourage the development of interagency approaches in providing disability information. In Scotland, Wales and Northern Ireland disability information is provided nationally and locally by Disability Scotland, Disability Wales, and Disability Action (NI). No such unified service exists in England.

This chapter provides a starting point where someone who works in rehabilitation, or is disabled, or a carer, can begin the search for information, a service, a piece of equipment or contact with other groups. It provides a list of names, addresses and telephone numbers for many national organizations. They will usually be able to give the addresses of local branches where they exist. Most national organizations produce information packs; so do most of the Disabled/Independent/Integrated Living Centres. Some of the best known starting points are:

The Disability Alliance ERA 1st Floor East, Universal House, 88–94 Wentworth Street, London E1 7SA. They publish the Disability Rights handbook annually, which is a most comprehensive guide to benefits and services. (Tel: 0171 247 8776).

The Disability Information Trust (Mary Marlborough Centre), Nuffield Orthopaedic Centre, Headington, Oxford OX3 7LD publish 'Equipment for Disabled People'. (Tel: 01865 227592; Fax: 01865 227596).

The Disabled Living Foundation (DLF), 380–384 Harrow Road, London W9 2HU publish: 'The Hamilton Index', and many other publications. (Tel: 0171 289 6111; Fax: 0171 266 2922).

RADAR, Royal Association for Disability and Rehabilitation, 12 City Forum, 250 City Road, London EC1 V 8AF (Tel: 0171 250 3222) provides literature, bulletins and political presence.

Other references have been listed alphabetically under the following headings:

Statutory organizations

National organizations

Centres for information and equipment

Organizations for specific diagnostic conditions

Organizations for holidays, leisure and sport

The Internet

Rehabilitation of the Physically Disabled Adult. Edited by C. John Goodwill, M. Anne Chamberlain and Chris Evans. Published in 1997 by Stanley Thornes (Publishers) Ltd, Cheltenham. ISBN 0-7487-3183-0.

STATUTORY ORGANIZATIONS

Legislation places a duty and responsibility upon local authorities and government bodies to provide services and information for people with disabilities and their carers. There is a legal obligation to provide information about their services, giving clear details about eligibility and criteria for service, standards of service and complaints procedures.

The telephone numbers of local authority services are listed under the name of the county council or borough.

Government bodies such as the Department of Health, Education and Employment, Transport, Social Security, the Scottish Home and Health Department produce leaflets.

The Disability Discrimination Act became law in November 1995 and from December 1996 started to phase in rights for disabled people in the areas of employment, buying and selling services, buying or renting accommodation, education and public transport.

Headquarter addresses

Benefits Agency, Chief Executive's Office, Room 4C06, Quarry House, Leeds LS2 7UA (Tel: 0113 232 4000).

Department of **Education**, Sanctuary Buildings, Great Smith Street, London SW1P 3BT (Tel: 0171 925 5000).

Department of **Social Security**, The Adelphi, 1–11 John Adam Street, London, WC2N 6HT (Tel: 0171 962 8000).

Other useful contacts

Disability Benefit and Disabled Living Allowance Unit, Warbreck House, Warbreck Hill, Blackpool FY2 0YJ. (Helpline: 0345 123456).

Independent Living 93 Fund, PO Box 183, Nottingham, Nottinghamshire, NG8 3RD.

General queries about return to work, disabled or not. Tel: 0800 884411.

National Debtline. Tel: 0121 359 8501.

For local contact addresses look under subject name in the telephone directory, i.e. Transport, Ministry of.

NATIONAL VOLUNTARY ORGANIZATIONS

Listed alphabetically by main topic, e.g. British Council of **Disabled** People is listed under Disabled. Where the acronym is well known, that is used e.g. **ASBAH**.

Access Committee for England, 12 City Forum, 250 City Road, London EC1V 8AF (Voice 0171 250 0008; Minicom 0171 250 4119).

Disabled **Access to Technology Association**, Broomfield House, Bolling Road, Bradford BD4 7BG (Tel: 01274 370019).

Age Concern Cymru, 1 Cathedral Road, Cardiff CF1 9SD (Tel: 01222 371566).

Age Concern England, Astral House, 1268 London Road London SW16 4ER (Tel: 0181 679 8000).

Age Concern Northern Ireland, 3 Lower Crescent, Belfast BT7 1NR (Tel: 01232 245729).

Age Concern Scotland, 113 Rose Street, Edinburgh EH2 3DT (Tel: 0131 220 3345).

Automobile Association, Fanum House, Basingstoke, RG21 2FA (publish the Guide for the Disabled Traveller).

Association for Victims of Medical Accidents (**AVMA**) Bank Chambers, 1 London Road, Forest Hill, London SE23 3TP (Tel: 0181 291 2793).

British Red Cross 9 Grosvenor Crescent, London SW1X 7EJ (Tel: 0171 235 5454).

British Railways Board, 222 Marylebone Road, London NW1 6JJ.

Care and Repair Cymru, Norbury House, Norbury Road, Cardiff CF5 3AS (Tel: 01222 576286)

Care and Repair England, Castle House, Kirtley Drive, Nottingham NG7 1LD (Tel: 0115 979 9091 Fax: 0115 9859457).

Glasgow **Care and Repair** South Side Housing Association, 553 Shields Road Glasgow G41 2RW. (Tel: 0141 422 1112). This project is also the forum for the other Care and Repair schemes in Scotland.

Carers National Association. 20–25 Glasshouse Yard, London EC1A 4JS (Tel: 0171 490 8818; Advice 0171 490 8898)

Charity Search, 25 Portview Road, Avonmouth, Bristol BS11 9LD (Tel: 0117 982 4060) Free advice for elderly in need and the mature disabled. They use the Victorian definition of elderly, which was 'Those surviving to the age of 40'.

National Association of **Citizens' Advice Bureaux**, (NACAB), Myddelton House, 115–123 Pentonville Road, London N1 9LZ (Tel: 0171 833 2181)

Foundation for **Communication for the Disabled**, Beacon House, Pyrford Rd, West Byfleet, Surrey KT14 6LD (Tel: 01932 336512)

Community Health Councils for England and Wales, Association of, 30 Drayton Park, London N5 1PB (Tel: 0171 609 8405).

Community Service Volunteers, 237 Pentonville Road, London N1 9NJ (Tel: 0171 278 6601)

Association for **Continence Advice**, Winchester House, Kennington Park, Cranmer Road, The Oval, London, SW9 6EJ (Tel: 0171 820 8113; Fax: 0171 820 0442; Helpline: 0191 213 0050). These numbers will get you to all other continence services.

British Association for **Counselling**, 1 Regent Place, Rugby, Warwickshire CV21 2PJ (Tel: 01788 578328).

Crossroads Care Attendant Schemes Ltd/ Caring for Carers, 10 Regent Place, Rugby, Warwickshire CV21 2PN (Tel: 01788 573653).

Cruse Bereavement Care, 126 Sheen Road, Richmond, Surrey TW9 1UR (Tel: 0181 940 4818; Bereavement Care Line 0181 332 7227).

DIAL UK, Park Lodge, St Catherine's Hospital, Tickhill Road, Doncaster DN4 8QN (Tel: 01302 310123 Fax; 01302 310404). **Disability Information and Advice Line**. They can advise if there is a local DIAL centre.

DIAL Scotland, Briad House, Labrador Avenue, Howden, Livingston, West Lothian, EH54 6BU (Tel: 01506 433 468).

DIEL The advisory committee on Telecommunications for the **Disabled** and **Elderly**. This is an independent body which advises OFTEL. 50 Ludgate Hill London EC4M 7JJ (Speech: 0171 634 8770, Text, minicom: 0171 634 8769, Text 300 baud: 0171 634 8771, Fax: 0171 634 8845). They produce an information pack. Enquiries: 0171 634 8773.

Disabled Christians' Fellowship, 211 Wick Road, Brislington, Bristol BS4 4HP.

Disabled Drivers Association, Ashwellthorpe, Norwich NR16 1EX (Tel: 01508 489449 Fax: 01508 488173).

Disabled Drivers' Motor Club, Cottingham Way, Thrapston, Northampton NN14 4PL. (Tel: 01832 734724 Fax: 01832 733816). Founded in 1922. Publish *The Disabled Driver*.

Disabled Living Centres Council, 1st Floor Winchester House, 11 Cranmer Road, Kennington Park, London SW9 6EJ (Tel: 0171 820 0567). For full list see next section.

DLF Disabled Living Foundation, 380–384 Harrow Road, London W9 2HU, (Tel: 0171 289 6111). Wide range of activities and publications.

British Council of **Disabled People**, (BCODP) Litchurch Plaza, Litchurch Lane, Derby DE24 8AA (Tel: 01332 295551 Fax: 01332 295580) Umbrella for organizations which are managed by disabled people.

Association of **Disabled Professionals**, 170 Benton Hill, Wakefield Road, Horbury, West Yorkshire WF4 5HW (Speech and minicom: 01924 270335).

Disablement Income Group and DIG Charitable Trust (DIG), Unit 5, Archway Business Centre, 19–23 Wedmore Street, London N19 4RZ (Tel: 0171 263 3981).

Disability Action, 2 Annadale Avenue, Belfast BT7 3JH (Tel: 01232 491011; Fax: 01232 491627; Text: 01232 645779).

Disability Alliance, 1st Floor East, Universal House, 88–94 Wentworth Street, London E1 7SA (Tel: 0171 247 8776).

Disability Information Trust, Mary Marlborough Centre, Nuffield Orthopaedic Centre, Headington, Oxford OX3 7LD (Tel: 01865 227592; Fax: 01865 227596).

Disability Scotland, Princes House, 5 Shandwick Place, Edinburgh EH2 4RG (Tel and Minicom: 0131 229 8632; Fax: 0131 229 5168)

Disability Wales Llys Ifor, Crescent Road, Caerphilly, CF83 1XL (Tel: 01222 887325)

Centre for Accessible **Environments**, Nutmeg House, 60 Gainsford Street, London. SE1 2NY (Tel: 0171 357 8182)

Disability **Equipment** Register, 4 Chatterton Road Yate, Bristol BS17 4BJ (Tel: 01454 318818; Fax: 01454 883870). To help match needs for equipment with sources.

Help for Health Trust, Highcroft Cottage, Romsey Road, Winchester, Hants SO22 5DH (Tel: 0115 9121000).

Kings Fund Centre, 11–13 Cavendish Square London W1M 0AN (Tel: 0171 307 2400). Information and research.

Disability **Law Service**, 49–51 Bedford Row, London WC1R 4LR (Tel: 0171 831 8031). Free legal advice for people with disabilities.

Law Centre Federations, Duchess House 18–19 Warren Street, London, W1P 5DB (Tel: 0171 387 8570). Provide legal advice on all aspects of disability. Contact the nearest Law Centre first, address via telephone directory).

The **Law Society**, 114 Chancery Lane, London WC2A 1PL (Direct line: 0171 320 5793). A group of solicitors who will advise solicitors and entrants to the profession.

Leonard Cheshire Foundation 26–29 Maunsel Street London SW1P 2QN.

MIND (National Association for Mental Health), Granta House, 15–19 Broadway, London E15 4BQ (Tel: 0181 519 2122).

Disabled Motorists Federation, National Mobility Centre, Unit 2a, Atcham Estate, Shrewsbury SY4 4UG (Tel: 01743 761181, Fax: 01743 761149). Produce RAMP (Route-finding & Access Map Project).

Banstead **Mobility Centre**, Damson Way, Fountain Drive, Queen Marys Avenue, Carshalton, Surrey, SM5 4NR (Tel: 0181 770 1151, Fax: 0181 770 1211).

Motability, Goodman House, Station Approach, Harlow, Essex CM20 2ET (Tel: 01279 635666).

Open University, Adviser on the Education of Disabled Students, Walton Hall, Milton Keynes MK7 6AR (Voice 01908 653442; Minicom: 01908 655978).

Open College, 101 Wigmore Street, London W1H 9AA.

Opportunities for People with Disabilities, 1 Bank Buildings, Prince's Street, London EC2R 8EU (Voice: 0171 726 4961; Minicom: 0171 726 4963).

PHAB, Physically Handicapped and Able Bodied. Summit House, Wandle Road, Croydon CR0 1DF (Tel: 0181 667 9443)

POWAG (Prince of Wales Advisory Group on Disability), Nutmeg House, 60 Gainsford Street, London SE1 2NY (Tel: 0171 403 9433). A catalyst and ideas organization started in the Year of the Disabled (1981).

RADAR, Royal Association for Disability and Rehabilitation, 12 City Forum, 250 City Road, London EC1V 8AF (Tel: 0171 250 3222). Provides literature, bulletins and political presence.

REMAP, Hazeldene, Ightham, Sevenoaks, Kent TN15 9AD (Tel: 01732 883818). One-off technical equipment for disabled people. There is usually a local panel.

Remploy Ltd, 415 Edgware Road, Cricklewood, London NW2 6LR (Tel: 0181 235 0500).

Research Institute for Consumer Affairs (RICA), 2 Marylebone Road, London NW1 4DF (Tel: 0171 935 2460). Recent publications include booklets on wheelchairs, a car guide, vehicle adaptations and ADL. Set up in 1961 as an offshoot of the Consumers Association.

Riding for the disabled, Avenue R, National Agriculture Centre, Kenilworth, Warwickshire, CV8, 2LY. (Tel: 01203 696510; Fax: 01203 696532).

Scope, 12 Park Crescent, London W1N 4EQ (Tel: 0171 636 5020; Helpline: 0800 626216). Formerly the Spastics Society.

The Shaw Trust, Shaw House, Epsom Square, White Horse Business Park Trowbridge BA14 0XJ (Tel: 01225 716300) 'Releasing work potential of disabled people'

Skill: National Bureau for Students with Disabilities. Information Office open 1.30–4.30, Monday–Friday. 336 Brixton Road, London SW9 7AA (Tel: 0171 978 9890; Minicom 0171 738 7722).

Snowdon Award Scheme, 22 City Business Centre, 6 Brighton Road, Horsham, West Sussex RH13 5BA (Tel: 01403 211252). Grants for further or higher education for students with physical disabilities.

SPOD (Sexual and Personal Relationships of the Disabled), 286 Camden Road, London N7 0BJ (Tel: 0171 607 8851).

Sue Ryder Foundation, Cavendish, Sudbury, Suffolk CO10 8AY (Tel: 01787 280252).

Tripscope, The Courtyard, Evelyn Road, London W4 5JL (Tel: and Minicom: 0181 994 9294; Fax: 0181 994 3618) There is also a Bristol number for the South West of England (Tel: 0117 941 4094; Fax: 0117 941 4024). Travel information helpline. Any enquiry about travel looked into.

National Council of Voluntary Organisations, (NCVO), Regent's Wharf, 8 All Saints' Street, London N1 9RL (Tel: 0171 713 6161).

LOCAL CENTRES FOR INFORMATION AND EQUIPMENT

Disabled Living Centres (DLCs) and Integrated Living Centres (ILCs)

There are several independent networks throughout the UK which provide local information and advice services relating to disability. Disabled Living Centres (DLCs) or Independent Living Centres provide people with the opportunity to see and try equipment. They also give impartial advice about a wide range of topics. The Disabled Living Centres Council, (First Floor, Winchester House, 11 Cranmer Road, London SW9 6EJ (Fax: 0171 735 0278) represent DLCs nationally and support and promote their activities.

There is a growing network of Integrated/ Independent Living Centre (ILCs) which enable people with disabilities to set up their own services. The British Council of Disabled People, Litchurch Plaza, Litchurch Lane, Derby DE24 8AA (Tel: 01332 295551; Fax: 295580) is the umbrella organization for

Integrated Living Centres. To be eligible for this Council their management committees must have more than 51% people with disabilities.

Both groups are included in the following list. Visitors are advised to arrange an appointment prior to visiting any centre.

Disability Information Centres or Disability Resource Centres provide general information relating to benefits, local housing and services, leisure, holiday and travel. Most have a telephone helpline. DIAL UK represents most of the centres. They will know if a local centre exists.

Aberdeen
Hillylands Disabled Living Centre, Croft Road, Mastrick, Aberdeen AB2 6RB (Tel: 01224 685247, Fax: 01224 663144).

Aylesbury
Stoke Mandeville Independent Living Exhibition, Stoke Mandeville Hospital, Mandeville Road, Aylesbury, Bucks HP21 8AL (Tel: 01296 315066).

Belfast
Disabled Living Centre, Regional Disablement Services, Musgrave Park Hospital, Stockmans Lane, Belfast BT9 7JB (Tel: 01232 669501 ext 2608, or 01232 669501 ext 2740 (Senior OT). Fax: 01232 683662)

Birmingham
Disabled Living Centre, 260 Broad Street, Birmingham B1 2HF (Tel: 0121 643 0980)

Bodelwyddan
North Wales Resource Centre for Disabled People, Ysbyty Glan Clwyd, Bodelwyddan, Denbighshire LL18 5UJ (Tel: 01745 583910 ext 4525 or 4706, Fax: 01745 582762).

Borden
Hampshire Centre for Integrated Living (CIL). 4 Plantation Way, Whitehall, Borden, Hampshire GU35 9HD (Tel: 01420 474261).

Bristol
Avon Disabled Living Centre, The Vassall Centre, Gill Avenue, Fishponds, Bristol BS16 2QQ, (Tel: 0117 965 3651: Fax: 0117 965 3652).

Bristol
West of England Centre for Integrated Living, Leinster Avenue, Knowle, Bristol, (Tel: 0117 983 9839; Fax: 0117 983 6765).

Bromley
Bromley Association for people with handicaps (BATH) Lewis House, 30 Beckenham Road, Beckenham BR3 4LS (Tel: 0181 663 3345; Fax: 0181 633 1442).

Cardiff
Disabled Living Centre, Rookwood Lodge, Rookwood Hospital, Fairwater Road, Llandaff, Cardiff, South Glamorgan CF5 2YN (Tel: 01222 566281 ext 3751; Fax: 01222 578509).

Carmarthen
Cwm Disability Centre for Independent Living, Coomb Cheshire Home, Llangynog, Carmarthen, Dyfed SA33 5HP (Tel: 01267 83743; Fax: 01267 241743).

Edinburgh
Lothian Disabled Living Centre, Astley Ainslie Hospital, Grange Loan, Edinburgh EH9 2HL (Tel: 0131 5379190).

Exeter
Independent Living Centre, St Loye's School of Occupational Therapy, Millbrook Lane, Topsham Road, Exeter EX2 6ES (Tel: 01392 59260).

Flintshire
Disability Action Centre, 6 Mill Lane, Flintshire, N. Wales (Tel: 01244 545759; Fax: 01244 548188; Minicom 01244 545151).

Glasgow – The Information Project
Fernen Street Complex, 30 Fernen Street, Glasgow G32 7HF (Tel: 0141 778 5147; Fax: 0141 778 5369).

Grangemouth
Dundas Resource Centre, Oxgang Road, Grangemouth, Fife, FK3 9EF (Tel: 01324 504311).

Hillingdon
Hillingdon Independent Living Centre, Colham Road, Uxbridge, Middlesex, UB8 3UR (Tel: 01895 233691; Fax: 01895 813843).

Huddersfield
Level Best, Zetland Street, Huddersfield, West Yorks HD1 2RA (Tel: 01484 223000; Fax: 01484 223049).

Hull
National Demonstration Centre, St. Hilda House, Kingston General Hospital, Beverley Road, Hull HU3 1UR (Tel: 01482 225034).

Inverness
Disabled Living Centre, Occupational Therapy Department, Raigmore Hospital, Old Perth Road, Inverness IV2 3UJ (Tel: 01463 704000 ext 5477).

Leeds
The William Merritt Disabled Living Centre, St. Mary's Hospital, Greenhill Road, Leeds LS12 3QE (Tel: 0113 279 3140; Fax: 0113 231 9291).

Leicester
The Disabled Living Centre, British Red Cross Medical Aid Department, 76 Clarendon Park Road, Leicester LE2 3AD (Tel: 0116 270 0515, Fax: 0116 244 8625).

Lewes
East Sussex Disabled Association, 47 Western Road, Lewes, East Sussex, BN7 1RL (Tel: 01273 472860; Fax: 01273 487422).

Liverpool
Liverpool Disabled Living Centre, 101–103 Kempston Street, Liverpool L3 1HE (Tel: 0151 298 2055; Fax: 0151 298 2952).

London
The Disabled Living Foundation, 380–384 Harrow Road, London W9 2HU (Tel: 0171 289 6111, Fax: 0171 266 2922).

Greenwich Association of Disabled People (CIL) Christchurch Forum, Trafalgar Road, Greenwich, London SE10 9EQ (Tel: 0181 305 2221, Fax: 0181 293 3455; Minicom: 0181 858 9307).

Lambeth Centre for Integrated Living (CIL), Barstow Crescent, Hellis Road, London SW2 3NS (Tel: 0181 671 8892).

Lowestoft
Waveney Centre for Independent Living, 161 Rotterdam Road, Lowestoft, Suffolk NR32 2EZ (Tel: 01502 404454 (minicom); Fax: 01502 405452).

Macclesfield
Disabled Living Centre, Macclesfield District General Hospital, Victoria Road, Macclesfield, Cheshire SK10 3BL (Tel: 01625 661740).

Manchester
Regional Disabled Living Centre, Disabled Living, Redbank House, 4 St. Chads Street, Cheetham, Manchester M8 8QA (Tel: 0161 832 3678, Fax: 0161 835 3591).

Middlesborough
Department of Rehabilitation, Middlesborough General Hospital, Ayresome Green Lane, Middlesborough, Cleveland TS5 5AZ (Tel: 01642 850850 (direct line)).

Milton Keynes
Milton Keynes Centre for Integrated Living.

Newcastle upon Tyne
Disability North, The Dene Centre, Castle Fam Road, Newcastle Upon Tyne NE3 1PH (Tel: 0191 284 0480; Fax: 0191 213 0910).

Nottingham
Disabilities Living Centre, Lenton Business Centre, Lenton Boulevard, Nottingham NG7 2BY (Tel: 0115 942 0391).

Paisley
Disability Centre for Independent Living, Community Services Building, Queen Street, Paisley, Strathclyde, PA1 2TU (Tel: 0141 887 0597; Fax: 0141 887 7267).

Papworth
Papworth Disability Living Centre, Ermine Street North, Papworth Everard, Cambridgeshire CB3 8RH (Tel: 01480 830495).

Portsmouth
The Frank Sorrell Centre, Prince Albert Road, Southsea, Portsmouth PO4 9HR (Tel: 01705 824853; Fax: 01705 821770).

St Andrews
St Davids Disabled Living Centre, Albany Park, St Andrews, Fife KY16 8BP (Tel: 01334 412606).

Shrewsbury
Shropshire Disability Resource Centre, Lancaster Road, Harlescott, Shrewsbury, Shropshire, SY1 3NJ (Tel: 01743 444599; Fax: 01743 461349).

Southampton
Southampton Aid and Equipment Centre, Southampton General Hospital, Tremona Road, Southampton SO16 6YD (Tel: 01703 796631; Fax: 01703 794756).

Stockport
Independent Living Centre, St. Thomas Hospital, Shawheath, Stockport, Cheshire SK3 8BL (Tel: 0161 419 4476).

Swansea
Swansea Disabled Living Centre, St. John's Road, Manselton, Swansea SA5 8PR (Tel: 01792 580161; Fax: 01792 585682).

Swindon
Options Plus Independent Living Centre, Marshgate , Stratton Road, Swindon, Wiltshire SN1 2PN (Tel: 01793 643966).

Welwyn Garden City
Herts. Association for the Disabled, The Woodside Centre, The Commons, Welwyn Garden City, Herts AL7 4DD (Tel: 01707 324581; Fax: 01707 371297).

West Wiltshire
Independent Living Centre, St George's Hospital, Semington, Wiltshire BA14 6JQ (Tel: 01380 871007; Fax: 01380 871113).

ORGANIZATIONS FOR SPECIFIC DIAGNOSTIC CONDITIONS

Some chapters have additional information. Indexed by first key word i.e. National Ankylosing Spondylitis Society is listed under A. Where the acronym is well known eg AFASIC or ASBAH it is under first letter of the acronym.

ACE Aids to Communication in Education Centres, Ormerod School, Waynfleet Road, Headington, Oxford OX3 8DD.

AFASIC, Overcoming Speech Impairments, 347 Central Markets, Smithfield, London EC1A 9NH (Tel: 0171 236 3632).

National **Ankylosing Spondylitis Society**, 3 Grosvenor Crescent, London SW1X 7ER (Tel: 0171 235 9585).

Arthritis Association, 1st Floor Suite, 2 Hyde Gardens, Eastbourne BN21 4PN.

Arthritis and Rheumatism Council, Copeman House, St Mary's Court, St Mary's Gate, Chesterfield, Derbyshire S41 7TD (Tel: 01246 558033).

Arthritis Care, 18 Stephenson Way, London NW1 2HD (Tel: 0171 916 1500; Freephone Helpline 0800 289170).

Young **Arthritis Care**, 18 Stephenson Way, London NW1 2HD (Tel: 0171 916 1500).

ASBAH (Association for Spina Bifida and Hydrocephalus), Asbah House, 42 Park Road, Peterborough PE1 2UQ (Tel. 01733 555988).

National **Asthma** Campaign, Providence House, Providence Place, London N1 0NT (Tel: 0171 226 2260: Helpline 0345 010203).

Ataxia (formerly Friedreich's Ataxia Group), The Stable, Wiggins Yard, Bridge Street, Godalming, Surrey GL17 1HW.

National **Back Pain** Association, 16 Elmtree Road, Teddington, Middlesex TW11 8ST.

RNIB Royal National Institute for the **Blind**, 224 Great Porland Street, London W1N 6AA.

RNIB Northern Ireland, 40 Linenhall Street, Belfast BT2 8GB.

RNIB Scotland, 9 Viewfield Place, Stirling FK8 1NL.

Cerebral Palsy, see **Scope**.

Chest, Heart and Stroke Association, see **The Stroke Association** and **British Heart Foundation**.

Chest Heart and Stroke Scotland, 65 North Castle Street, Edinburgh EH2 3LT.

RNID, Royal National Institute for **Deaf** People, 105 Gower Street, London WC1E 6AH.

RNID Northern Ireland, Wilton House, 5 College Square North, Belfast BT1 6AR.

RNID Scotland, 9 Clairmont Gardens, Glasgow G3 7LW.

Wales Council for the **Deaf**, Maritime Offices, Woodland Terrace, Maesycoed, Pontypridd, Mid-Glamorgan CF37 1DZ.

British **Diabetic** Association, 10 Queen Anne Street, London W1M 0BD (Tel: 0171 323 1531).

Down's Syndrome Association, 155 Mitcham Road, London SW17 9PG (Tel: 0181 682 4001).

Action for **Dysphasic** Adults, (ADA) 1 Royal Street, London SE1 7LL (Tel: 0171 261 9572).

Dystonia Society, Weddel House, 13–14 West Smithfield, London EC1A 9JJ (Tel: 0171 329 0797).

British **Epilepsy** Association, Anstey House, 40 Hanover Square, Leeds LS3 1BE (Tel: 0113 243 9393; Freephone Helpline 0800 309030). Also at Graham House, Knockbracken Healthcare Park, Saintfield Road, Belfast, BT8 8BH (Tel: 01232 248414; Fax: 01232 799076).

The **Epilepsy** Association of Scotland, 48 Govan Road, Glasgow, G51 1JL (Tel: 0141 427 4911).

The Irish **Epilepsy** Association, Brain Wave, 249 Crumlin Road, Crumlin, Dublin 12 Ireland. (Tel: (00) 3531 557500).

The National Society for **Epilepsy**, Chalfont Centre, Chalfont St. Peter, Gerrards Cross, Bucks. SL9 0RJ (Tel: 01494 873991).

Friedreich's Ataxia - see **Ataxia**

Guillain–Barre Syndrome Support Group, Foxley, Holdingham, Sleaford, Lincolnshire NG34 8NR (Tel: 01529 304615).

Haemophilia Society, 123 Westminster Bridge Road, London SE1 7HR (Tel: 0171 928 2020).

Headway, National Head Injuries Association Ltd. 7 King Edward Court, King Edward Street, Nottingham NG1 1EW (Tel: 0115 924 0800).

British **Heart** Foundation, 14 Fitzhardinge Street, London W1H 4DH (Tel: 0171 935 0185).

Huntington's Disease Association, 108 Battersea High Street, London SW11 3HP (Tel: 0171 223 7000).

National Association of **Laryngectomy** Clubs, Ground Floor, 6 Rickett Street, Fulham, London SW6 1RU (Tel: 0171 381 9993).

British **Limbless** Ex-Service Men's Association, (BLESMA) Frankland Moore House, 185–187 High Road, Chadwell Heath, Romford, Essex RM6 6NA (Tel: 0181 590 1124).

Lupus UK, 1 Eastern Road, Romford, Essex RM1 3NH (Tel: 01708 731251).

The National **Meningitis** Trust, Fern House, Bath Road, Stroud, Gloucestershire GL5 3TJ (Tel: 01453 751738; Helpline 01453 755049).

Motor Neurone Disease Association, PO Box 246, Northampton NNI 2PR (Tel: 01604 250505; Helpline 0345 626262).

Multiple Sclerosis Resource Centre, 4a Chapel Hill, Stansted, Essex CM24 8AG (Tel: 01279 817101).

Multiple Sclerosis Society of Great Britain and Northern Ireland, 25 Effie Road, Fulham, London SW6 1EE (Tel: 0171 736 6267; Helpline London 0171 371 8000; Helpline Midlands 0121 476 4229).

Muscular Dystrophy Group, 7–11 Prescott Place, London SW4 6BS (Tel: 0171 720 8055).

Myalgic Encephalomyelitis Association, Stanhope House, High Street, Stanford-le-Hope, Essex SS17 0HA (Tel: 01375 642466; Helpline 01375 636013).

Myasthenia Gravis Association, Central Office, Keynes House, Chester Park, Alfreton Road, Derby DE21 4AS (Tel: 01332 290219).

Narcolepsy Association UK, P. Saunders, South Hall, High Street, Farningham, Kent DA4 0DE (Tel: 01322 863056).

The **Neurofibromatosis** Association, (formerly Link), 82 London Road, Kingston-upon-Thames KT2 6PX (Tel: 0181 547 1636).

National Association for the Relief of **Paget's** Disease, 1 Church Road, Eccles, Manchester M30 0DL (Tel: 0161 707 9225).

Pain Concern (formerly Self Help in Pain – SHIP), PO Box 318, Canterbury, Kent CT2 0GD (01227 712183).

Young Alert **Parkinsonian** Partners and Relatives, (YAPP&RS), 38 Wessex Drive, Harp Hill, Cheltenham, Gloucestershire GL52 5AU (Tel: 01242 236729).

Parkinson's Disease Society of the UK, 22 Upper Woburn Place, London WC1H 0RA (Tel: 0171 383 3513).

British **Polio** Fellowship, Bell Close, West End Road, Ruislip, Middlesex HA4 6LP (Tel: 01895 639453).

British League Against **Rheumatism**, (BLAR), 41 Eagle Street, London WC1R 4AR (Tel: 0171 242 3313).

SCOPE, 12 Park Crescent, London W1N 4EQ (Tel: 0171 636 5020 Helpline: 0800 626216).

The **Sequal** Trust (formerly the Possum Users' Association), Ddol Hir, Glyn Ceiriog, Llangollen, Clwyd, Wales LL20 7NP (Tel: 01691 718331).

Spinal Injuries Association, 76 St James' Lane, London N10 3DF (Tel: 0181 444 2121; Counselling Line: 0181 883 4296).

The **Stroke** Association, CHSA House, 123–127 Whitecross Street, London EC1Y 8JJ (Tel: 0171 490 7999).

HOLIDAYS, SPORT AND LEISURE

'**Access to the skies committee**' RADAR, Royal Association for Disability and Rehabilitation, 12 City Forum, 250 City Road, London EC1 V 8AF (Tel: 0171 250 3222).

Across Trust, Bridge House, 70–72 Bridge Road, East Molesey, Surrey KT8 9HF (Tel: 0181 783 1355).

Camping for the Disabled, 20 Burton Close, Dawley, Telford, Shropshire (Tel. day: 01743 761889; Evenings: 01952 507653).

Gardening for the Disabled Trust, Hayes Farmhouse, Hayes Lane, Peasmarsh, East Sussex TN1 6XR.

Handihols, 12 Ormonde Avenue, Rochford, Essex SS4 1QW (Tel: 01702 548257). House Exchange or Hospitality for the disabled.

Help the Handicapped **Holidays,** 147a Camden Road, Tunbridge Wells, Kent TN1 2RA (Tel: 01892 547474).

Holiday Care Service, 2nd floor, Imperial Bldgs, Victoria Road, Horley, Surrey RH6 7PZ (Tel: 01293 774535).

Scouts **Holiday Homes Trusts,** Baden Powell House, Queen's Gate, London SW7 5JS (Tel: 0171 584 7030).

Horticultural Therapy, Goulds Ground, Vallis Way, Frome, Somerset BA11 3DW (Tel: 01373 464782).

John Grooms Association for Disabled People, 50 Scrutton Street, London EC2A 4PH (Tel: 0171 452 2000).

Jubilee Sailing Trust, Jubilee Yard, Merlin Quay, Hazel Road, Wooton, Southampton, SO19 7GB (Tel: 01703 449108).

The DLF Hamilton Index has a section on Leisure, The Disabled Living Foundation (DLF), 380–384 Harrow Road, London W9 2HU (Tel: 0171 289 61111, Fax: 0171 266 2922).

Riding for the Disabled, Avenue R, National Agriculture Centre, Kenilworth, Warwickshire, CV8, 2LY. (Tel: 01203 696510; Fax: 01203 696532).

British **Sports Association** for the Disabled, Mary Glen Haig Suite, Solecast House, 13–27 Brunswick Place, London N1 6DX (Tel: 0171 490 4919).

National Association of **Swimming Clubs** for the Handicapped, The Willows, Mayles Lane, Wickham, Hampshire. PO17 5ND (Tel: 01329 833689).

Tripscope, The Courtyard, Evelyn Road. London W4 5JL (Tel: and Minicom: 0181 994 9294; Fax: 0181 994 3618). There is also a Bristol number for the South West of England (Tel: 0117 941 4094; Fax: 0117 941 4024). Travel information helpline. Any enquiry about holiday travel looked into.

British Disabled **Water-Ski** Association, The Tony Edge National Centre, Heron Lake, Hythe End, Wraysbury, Middlesex, TW19 6HW (Tel: 01784 483664).

British **Wireless for the Blind** Fund, 34 New Road, Chatham, Kent ME4 4QR (Tel: 01634 832501).

THE INTERNET

As an information service the Internet is developing very rapidly, but is so vast and novel it can be daunting and it is difficult to know where to start. Factual information can be found on a huge range of disabilities. There are also user groups and news groups which anyone can join. These groups allow people with common interests to share their experiences and knowledge. Indeed, one of the major, if less obvious, benefits of communicating via the Internet is that it allows equal communication between people whether physically disabled or not.

This chapter can only give a few pointers to the Internet in general, and disability in particular. A computer, modem, software and an information provider are needed, or access to a 'cyber cafe'. Given these, the Internet will open up new horizons for many.

This is a very small selection of sites which give information. They will show the way to others.

Department of Health. http://www.open.-gov.uk./doh/dhhome.htm

Disability Net. http://www.globalnet.co.uk/~pmatthews/DisabilityNet/index.html
This is another UK site, with a comprehensive listing of organizations and other services.

Disability Information. http://www.eski-mo.com/~jlubin/disabled.html
General information about disability. US based but very interesting.

DO-IT (Disabilities, Opportunities, Internetworking and Technology). http://weber.u.-washington.edu/~doit/

This is from the University of Washington. It aims to give opportunities for those with disabilities to participate in projects in science and engineering.

Stephen Hawking. http:/www.amtp.cam.ac.uk/DAMTP/user/hawking/
He is the Cambridge professor of mathematics who wrote 'A Brief History of Time'. He has MND, and gives a personal insight into his ideas and disability.

This short list can only introduce a vast subject. It is growing very quickly and will become increasingly important. If used wisely can only enrich the lives and expand the horizons of all, with or without disability.

Index